Pulmonary Arterial Hypertension

Editor

TERENCE K. TROW

CLINICS IN CHEST MEDICINE

www.chestmed.theclinics.com

December 2013 • Volume 34 • Number 4

ELSEVIER

1600 John F. Kennedy Boulevard • Suite 1800 • Philadelphia, Pennsylvania, 19103-2899

http://www.theclinics.com

CLINICS IN CHEST MEDICINE Volume 34, Number 4
December 2013 ISSN 0272-5231, ISBN-13: 978-0-323-27792-1

Editor: Patrick Manley

Clinics in Chest Medicine (ISSN 0272-5231) is published quarterly by Elsevier Inc., 360 Park Avenue South, New York, NY 10010-1710. Months of issue are March, June, September, and December. Periodicals postage paid at New York, NY and additional mailing offices. Subscription prices are $345.00 per year (domestic individuals), $556.00 per year (domestic institutions), $165.00 per year (domestic students/residents), $380.00 per year (Canadian individuals), $690.00 per year (Canadian institutions), $470.00 per year (international individuals), $690.00 per year (international institutions), and $230.00 per year (international and Canadian students/residents). International air speed delivery is included in all Clinics subscription prices. All prices are subject to change without notice. **POSTMASTER:** Send address changes to Clinics in Chest Medicine, Elsevier Health Sciences Division, Subscription Customer Service, 3251 Riverport Lane, Maryland Heights, MO 63043. **Customer Service: Telephone: 1-800-654-2452** (U.S. and Canada); **1-314-447-8871** (outside U.S. and Canada). **Fax: 1-314-447-8029. E-mail: journalscustomerservice-usa@elsevier.com** (for print support); **journalsonlinesupport-usa@elsevier.com** (for online support).

Reprints. For copies of 100 or more of articles in this publication, please contact the Commercial Reprints Department, Elsevier Inc., 360 Park Avenue South, New York, NY 10010-1710. Tel.: 212-633-3874; Fax: 212-633-3820; E-mail: reprints@elsevier.com.

Clinics in Chest Medicine is covered in *MEDLINE/PubMed (Index Medicus), Current Contents/Clinical Medicine, EMBASE/Excerpta Medica, Science Citation Index,* and *ISI/BIOMED.*

Printed and bound by CPI Group (UK) Ltd, Croydon, CR0 4YY

Transferred to digital print 2013

Contributors

EDITOR

TERENCE K. TROW, MD
Director, Yale Pulmonary Vascular Disease
Program; Associate Professor of Medicine,
Section of Pulmonary, Critical Care and Sleep
Medicine, Department of Internal Medicine,
Yale University School of Medicine,
New Haven, Connecticut

AUTHORS

NADINE AL-NAAMANI, MD
Clinical Research Fellow, Division of
Pulmonary, Critical Care and Sleep Medicine,
Tufts Medical Center, Boston, Massachusetts

WILLIAM R. AUGER, MD
Professor of Clinical Medicine, Division of
Pulmonary and Critical Care Medicine,
University of California, San Diego Health Care
System, La Jolla, California

MURALI M. CHAKINALA, MD, FCCP
Associate Professor of Medicine, Division of
Pulmonary and Critical Care Medicine,
Department of Medicine, Washington
University School of Medicine, St Louis,
Missouri

RICHARD CHANNICK, MD
Division of Pulmonary and Critical Care
Medicine, Massachusetts General Hospital,
Harvard Medical School, Boston,
Massachusetts

C. GREGORY ELLIOTT, MD
Chairman, Department of Medicine,
Intermountain Medical Center, Murray;
Professor of Medicine, Department of Internal
Medicine, University of Utah School of
Medicine, Salt Lake City, Utah

HARRISON W. FARBER, MD
Pulmonary Center, Boston University School of
Medicine, Boston, Massachusetts

WASSIM H. FARES, MD, MSc
Assistant Professor of Medicine, Yale
Pulmonary Vascular Disease Program, Section
of Pulmonary, Critical Care and Sleep
Medicine, Department of Internal Medicine,
Yale University School of Medicine, New
Haven, Connecticut

PAUL R. FORFIA, MD
Director of Pulmonary Hypertension and Right
Heart Failure Program, Associate Professor of
Medicine, Section of Cardiovascular Medicine,
Temple University Hospital, Philadelphia,
Pennsylvania

BRIAN B. GRAHAM, MD
Program in Translational Lung Research,
Division of Pulmonary Sciences and Critical
Care Medicine, Department of Medicine,
University of Colorado School of Medicine,
Aurora, Colorado

PAUL M. HASSOUN, MD
Division of Pulmonary and Critical Care
Medicine, Johns Hopkins University,
Baltimore, Maryland

ANNA R. HEMNES, MD
Assistant Professor of Medicine, Division of
Allergy, Pulmonary and Critical Care Medicine,
Department of Medicine, Vanderbilt University,
Nashville, Tennessee

MARC HUMBERT, MD, PhD
Professor, Faculté de Médecine, Université Paris-Sud; AP-HP, DHU Thorax Innovation, Service de Pneumologie, Hôpital Bicêtre, Le Kremlin-Bicêtre; INSERM U999, LabEx LERMIT, Le Plessis-Robinson, France

KIM M. KERR, MD
Professor of Clinical Medicine, Division of Pulmonary and Critical Care Medicine, University of California, San Diego Health Care System, La Jolla, California

JAMES R. KLINGER, MD
Division of Pulmonary, Sleep and Critical Care Medicine, Rhode Island Hospital, Alpert Medical School of Brown University, Providence, Rhode Island

USHA KRISHNAN, MD
Associate Professor of Pediatrics, Columbia University Medical Center; Associate Director, Pulmonary Hypertension Center, Division of Pediatric Cardiology, New York, New York

RAHUL KUMAR, PhD
Program in Translational Lung Research, Division of Pulmonary Sciences and Critical Care Medicine, Department of Medicine, University of Colorado School of Medicine, Aurora, Colorado

TIM LAHM, MD, FCCP
Assistant Professor of Medicine, Division of Pulmonary, Allergy, Critical Care, Occupational and Sleep Medicine, Department of Medicine, Richard L. Roudebush VA Medical Center, Center for Immunobiology, Indiana University School of Medicine, Indianapolis, Indiana

DAVID J. LEDERER, MD, MS
Assistant Professor of Medicine and Epidemiology, Departments of Medicine and Epidemiology, Columbia University Medical Center, New York, New York

ROBERTO F. MACHADO, MD
Section of Pulmonary, Critical Care Medicine, Sleep and Allergy, Department of Medicine, Institute for Personalized Respiratory Medicine, University of Illinois at Chicago, Chicago, Illinois

JESS MANDEL, MD
Professor of Medicine, Associate Dean, University of California, San Diego School of Medicine, La Jolla, California

PETER S. MARSHALL, MD, MPH
Assistant Professor of Medicine, Section of Pulmonary, Critical Care and Sleep Medicine, Yale University School of Medicine, New Haven, Connecticut

MICHAEL A. MATHIER, MD, FACC
Associate Professor of Medicine, Pulmonary Hypertension Program, University of Pittsburgh Medical Center, University of Pittsburgh School of Medicine, Pittsburgh, Pennsylvania

VALLERIE V. MCLAUGHLIN, MD
Professor of Medicine, Director, Pulmonary Hypertension Program, Cardiovascular Center, University of Michigan Hospital and Health Systems, Ann Arbor, Michigan

STEVEN D. NATHAN, MD
Medical Director, Advanced Lung Disease and Transplant Program, Department of Medicine, Inova Fairfax Hospital, Falls Church, Virginia

STEPHANIE G. NORFOLK, MD
Instructor of Medicine, Division of Pulmonary and Critical Care, Duke University Medical Center, Durham, North Carolina

DERMOT S. O'CALLAGHAN, MB, MD
Department of Respiratory Medicine, Mater Misericordiae University Hospital, Dublin, Ireland

CAROLINE O'CONNELL, MB
Department of Respiratory Medicine, Mater Misericordiae University Hospital, Dublin, Ireland

HAROLD I. PALEVSKY, MD
Professor of Medicine, Director, Pulmonary Vascular Disease Program, Chief, Pulmonary, Allergy and Critical Care Medicine, Penn Presbyterian Medical Center, Perelman School of Medicine, University of Pennsylvania, Philadelphia, Pennsylvania

IONA PRESTON, MD
Division of Pulmonary and Critical Care Medicine, New England Medical Center, Tufts University, Boston, Massachusetts

MEREDITH E. PUGH, MD, MSCI
Assistant Professor of Medicine, Division of Allergy, Pulmonary and Critical Care Medicine, Department of Medicine, Vanderbilt University, Nashville, Tennessee

IVAN M. ROBBINS, MD
Professor of Medicine, Division of Allergy, Pulmonary and Critical Care Medicine, Department of Medicine, Vanderbilt University, Nashville, Tennessee

KARI E. ROBERTS, MD
Associate Professor of Medicine, Division of Pulmonary, Critical Care and Sleep Medicine, Tufts Medical Center, Boston, Massachusetts

JEFFREY ROBINSON, MD
Program in Translational Lung Research, Division of Pulmonary Sciences and Critical Care Medicine, Department of Medicine, University of Colorado School of Medicine, Aurora, Colorado

ERIKA B. ROSENZWEIG, MD
Associate Professor of Pediatrics, Columbia University Medical Center; Director, Pulmonary Hypertension Center, Division of Pediatric Cardiology, New York, New York

MAOR SAULER, MD
Senior Post-Doctoral Fellow, Section of Pulmonary, Critical Care and Sleep Medicine, Department of Internal Medicine,

Yale University School of Medicine, New Haven, Connecticut

ELVIRA STACHER, MD
Institute of Pathology, Medical University of Graz; Ludwig Boltzmann Institute for Lung Vascular Research, Graz, Austria

DARREN B. TAICHMAN, MD, PhD
Executive Deputy Editor, *Annals of Internal Medicine*, American College of Physicians; Adjunct Associate Professor of Medicine, Penn Presbyterian Medical Center, University of Pennsylvania Perelman School of Medicine, Philadelphia, Pennsylvania

VICTOR F. TAPSON, MD
Professor of Medicine, Division of Pulmonary and Critical Care, Duke University Medical Center, Durham, North Carolina

TERENCE K. TROW, MD
Director, Yale Pulmonary Vascular Disease Program; Associate Professor of Medicine, Section of Pulmonary, Critical Care and Sleep Medicine, Department of Internal Medicine, Yale University School of Medicine, New Haven, Connecticut

RUBIN M. TUDER, MD
Program in Translational Lung Research, Division of Pulmonary Sciences and Critical Care Medicine, Department of Medicine, University of Colorado School of Medicine, Aurora, Colorado

MEREDITH E. PUGH, MD, MSCI
Assistant Professor of Medicine, Division of Allergy, Pulmonary and Critical Care Medicine, Department of Medicine, Vanderbilt University, Nashville, Tennessee

IVAN M. ROBBINS, MD
Professor of Medicine, Division of Allergy Pulmonary and Critical Care Medicine, Department of Medicine, Vanderbilt University, Nashville, Tennessee

KARI E. ROBERTS, MD
Associate Professor of Medicine, Division of Pulmonary, Critical Care and Sleep Medicine, Tufts Medical Center, Boston, Massachusetts

JEFFREY ROBINSON, MD
Program in Translational Lung Research, Division of Pulmonary Sciences and Critical Care Medicine, Department of Medicine, University of Colorado School of Medicine, Aurora, Colorado

ERIKA B. ROSENZWEIG, MD
Associate Professor of Pediatrics, Columbia University Medical Center; Director, Pulmonary Hypertension Center, Division of Pediatric Cardiology, New York, New York

NAOR SAGLER, MD
Senior Post-Doctoral Fellow, Section of Pulmonary, Critical Care and Sleep Medicine, Department of Internal Medicine,

Yale University School of Medicine, New Haven, Connecticut

ELVIRA STACHER, MD
Institute of Pathology, Medical University of Graz, Ludwig Boltzmann Institute for Lung Vascular Research, Graz, Austria

DARREN B. TAICHMAN, MD, PhD
Executive Deputy Editor, Annals of Internal Medicine, American College of Physicians; Adjunct Associate Professor of Medicine, Penn Presbyterian Medical Center, University of Pennsylvania Perelman School of Medicine, Philadelphia, Pennsylvania

VICTOR F. TAPSON, MD
Professor of Medicine, Division of Pulmonary and Critical Care, Duke University, Medical Center, Durham, North Carolina

TERENCE K. TROW, MD
Director, Yale Pulmonary Vascular Disease Program, Associate Professor of Medicine, Section of Pulmonary, Critical Care and Sleep Medicine, Department of Internal Medicine, Yale University School of Medicine, New Haven, Connecticut

RUBIN M. TUDER, MD
Program in Translational Lung Research, Division of Pulmonary Sciences and Critical Care Medicine, Department of Medicine, University of Colorado School of Medicine, Aurora, Colorado

Contents

> Changes in the epidemiology of pulmonary arterial hypertension (PAH) have resulted from changes in classification schemes and an increased emphasis on diagnosis because of the availability of effective therapies. The terms primary pulmonary hypertension and secondary pulmonary hypertension are considered inappropriate, confusing, and should not be used. Recent registries of patients with PAH have provided improved data regarding prognosis in the era of advanced therapies.

> The pathology of pulmonary hypertension includes numerous abnormalities of the intima, media, and adventitia of the pulmonary vascular tree. A recently completed systematic analysis revealed high variability of morphologic measurements within a given pulmonary arterial hypertension (PAH) lung and among all PAH lungs, as well as distinct pathologic subphenotypes, and included a subset of lungs lacking intimal and medial remodeling. There was correlation between perivascular inflammation, remodeling, and hemodynamics. This article summarizes the pathologic features of the normal and abnormal pulmonary circulation, and correlations with animal models.

> Painstaking research led to the discovery of gene mutations responsible for heritable forms of pulmonary arterial hypertension (PAH). Mutations in the gene *BMPR2*, which codes for a cell surface receptor (BMPRII), cause the approximately 80% of heritable cases of PAH. Less commonly mutations in *ALK1*, *CAV1*, *ENG*, and *SMAD9*, and newly discovered mutations in *KCNK3*, may cause heritable PAH. Other family members of many patients diagnosed with idiopathic PAH may be diagnosed with PAH. Genetic counseling and testing should be offered to patients diagnosed with heritable or idiopathic PAH.

> Accurate diagnosis of pulmonary arterial hypertension can be challenging and often requires a high index of clinical suspicion. Use of a variety of noninvasive tests can help define the population of patients in whom invasive cardiac catheterization should be pursued. An understanding of the historical, physical exam, electrocardiographic, radiographic, and echocardiographic clues in the diagnosis is important. A ventilation-perfusion scan and careful assessment for left-to-right shunting are mandatory to avoid missing reasons for pulmonary hypertension that may require

nonpharmacologic management. Right heart, and sometimes concomitant left heart, catheterization is required to establish the diagnosis and distinguish pulmonary arterial from pulmonary venous hypertension.

The relationship between pulmonary hypertension and left heart disease is complex. When initial assessment suggests the presence of pulmonary hypertension, it is critical to determine its precise nature: pulmonary arterial hypertension versus pulmonary hypertension owing to left heart disease. Clues to diagnosis can be found in the history, physical examination, initial laboratory testing, and imaging studies. Treatment requires optimal therapy of the underlying left heart disease. It is uncertain whether therapies for pulmonary arterial hypertension have any role in treating pulmonary hypertension owing to left heart disease, and there are safety concerns with these agents in this population.

Pulmonary hypertension may complicate the course of patients with many forms of advanced lung disease. The cause is likely multifactorial with pathogenic pathways both common and unique to the specific disease entities. The occurrence of pulmonary hypertension is associated with worse outcomes, but whether this is an adaptive or maladaptive phenomenon remains unknown. The treatment of pulmonary hypertension with vasoactive medications in lung disease remains unproved. Specific disease phenotypes that might benefit, and those in which such therapies might be deleterious, remain to be determined.

In the past decade, there have been more patients with congenital heart disease (CHD) surviving to adulthood; whether due to late repair, or complex underlying CHD, many of these patients will be faced with pulmonary arterial hypertension (PAH) associated with CHD (APAH-CHD). In this review, the authors discuss the most commonly encountered forms of APAH-CHD, how to interpret the hemodynamic data, and how to classify the patients into meaningful subgroups that have similar management strategies. The current state of targeted medical treatments available to patients with APAH-CHD is also discussed.

Diagnosis of portopulmonary hypertension (PoPH), is challenging because of the multitude of cardiac and pulmonary diseases that cosegregate with advanced liver disease. PoPH is unique in that its natural history is not wholly dependent on portal hypertension. Despite a dearth of randomized, prospective data, an ever-expanding clinical experience shows that patients with PoPH benefit from therapy with PAH-specific medications. Because of high perioperative mortality, transplantation should be avoided in those patients who have severe PoPH that is refractory to medical therapy. This article reviews the pathophysiology and pathogenesis of PoPH and discusses approaches to diagnosis and management.

Pulmonary hypertension (PH) has emerged as a major complication of several hematologic disorders, including hemoglobinopathies, red cell membrane disorders, chronic myeloproliferative disorders, and splenectomy. With the exception of sickle cell disease, there are a limited number of studies systematically evaluating the prevalence of PH using the gold standard right heart catheterization in these disorders. The cause of the PH in patients with hematologic disorders is multifactorial, and a thorough diagnostic evaluation is essential. More importantly, there are virtually no high-quality data on the safety and efficacy of PH-targeted therapy in this patient population.

World Health Organization (WHO) group 5 pulmonary hypertension (PH) entails a heterogeneous group of disorders that may cause PH by unclear and/or multiple mechanisms. In particular, group 5 includes PH caused by hematologic disorders, systemic diseases, metabolic disorders, chronic renal failure, and disorders leading to pulmonary vascular occlusion or compression. This article discusses common pathogenic mechanisms leading to group 5 PH, followed by a detailed overview of epidemiology, pathogenesis, and disease-specific management of the individual group 5 conditions. Off-label use of vasomodulatory therapies, typically indicated for pulmonary arterial hypertension (WHO group 1 PH), in group 5 conditions is also discussed.

Chronic thromboembolic pulmonary hypertension (CTEPH) is a disease with high mortality and few treatment options. This article reviews the epidemiology of CTEPH and identifies risk factors for its development. The pathobiology and the progression from thromboembolic events to chronically increased right-sided pressures are discussed. The diagnosis and assessment of CTEPH requires several modalities and the role of these is detailed. The pre-operative evaluation assesses peri-operative risk and determines the likelihood of benefit from PTE. Pulmonary thromboendarterectomy (PTE) remains the treatment of choice in appropriate patients. Nonsurgical therapies for CTEPH may provide benefit in patients who cannot be offered surgery.

Recent advances in pulmonary arterial hypertension (PAH) research have created a new era of PAH-specific therapies. Although these therapeutics have revolutionized PAH therapy, their innovation was predated by supportive but nonspecific medical therapies adapted from their use in more common cardiopulmonary diseases. These therapies include oxygen therapy, diuretics, digoxin, anticoagulation, and high-dose calcium channel blockers. Expert opinion continues to support the use of adjunct therapies based on current pathologic understandings of PAH combined with some evidence extrapolated from small studies. This article discusses why these therapies continue to play an important role in the treatment of patients with PAH.

The development of orally active pulmonary vasodilators has been a major breakthrough in the treatment of pulmonary arterial hypertension (PAH). Orally active medications greatly enhanced patient access to PAH treatment and increased an interest in the diagnosis and treatment of this disease that still continues. Four different orally active drugs are currently available for the treatment of PAH and several more are undergoing evaluation. This article discusses the mechanisms by which endothelin receptor antagonists and phosphodiesterase-5 inhibitors mitigate pulmonary hypertensive responses, and reviews the most recent data concerning their efficacy and limitations in the treatment of PAH.

Since continuous IV epoprostenol was approved in the U.S., parenteral prostanoid therapy has remained the gold standard for the treatment of patients with advanced pulmonary arterial hypertension (PAH). Prostanoid agents can be administered as continuous intravenous infusions, as continuous subcutaneous infusions and by intermittent nebulization therapy. This article presents data from clinical trials of available prostanoid agents, and their varied routes of administration. The varied routes of administration allow for the incremental use of this class of agents in advanced PAH, and if PAH progresses. Prostanoids will remain a major component of PAH therapy for the foreseeable future.

Despite major advances in understanding the mechanisms of disease and development of specific drug therapy, pulmonary arterial hypertension (PAH) remains a progressive, fatal disease. At present there are 3 classes of drug therapy for PAH: prostaglandins, endothelin receptor antagonists, and phosphodiesterase-5 inhibitors. To maximize therapeutic benefit, and according to national and international guidelines, many patients are treated with combinations of these medications. This review presents a detailed account of the published data on the use of combination therapy in PAH. There are few randomized, placebo-controlled trial data to strongly support efficacy of most combination therapy, particularly oral combination therapy.

This article summarizes the current literature regarding surgical interventions in pulmonary hypertension, excluding chronic thromboembolic pulmonary hypertension. The article discusses the use of atrial septostomy in patients meeting criteria as well as single, double, and heart-lung transplantation.

Available targeted therapies for pulmonary arterial hypertension are capable only of slowing progression of the disease and a cure remains elusive. However with the improved understanding of the pulmonary vascular remodeling that characterizes the disease, there is optimism that the disconnect between preclinical and clinical studies may be bridged with some of the newer therapies that are now at different stages of clinical evaluation. This article examines the evidence behind these new candidate treatments that may become part of the arsenal available for clinicians managing this devastating disease.

CLINICS IN CHEST MEDICINE

FORTHCOMING ISSUES

March 2014
Chronic Obstructive Pulmonary Disease
Peter J. Barnes, MD, *Editor*

June 2014
Pulmonary Rehabilitation
Linda Nici, MD and Richard ZuWallack, MD,
Editors

September 2014
**Sleep and Breathing Beyond Obstructive Sleep
Apnea**
Carolyn D'Ambrosio, *Editor*

RECENT ISSUES

September 2013
Interventional Pulmonology
Ali I. Musani, *Editor*

June 2013
HIV and Respiratory Disease
Kristina Crothers, MD, Laurence Huang, MD,
and Alison Morris, MD, MS, *Editors*

March 2013
Pleural Disease
Jonathan Puchalski, MD, MEd, *Editor*

RELATED INTEREST

Medical Clinics, Vol. 96, No. 4 (July 2012)
Chronic Obstructive Pulmonary Disease
Stephen I. Rennard, MD and Bartolome R. Celli, MD, *Editors*

Preface

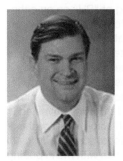

Terence K. Trow, MD
Editor

The specific arteriopathy of pulmonary arterial hypertension (PAH) must be clearly diagnosed and distinguished from other forms of pulmonary hypertension (PH) in order to arrive at the proper therapeutic approach, which has evolved rapidly over the past 15 years. PAH is comprised of idiopathic PAH, heritable PAH, and PAH associated with identified conditions. All of these forms of PH share common features that include an elevated mean pulmonary artery pressure in the setting of a normal left ventricular end-diastolic pressure due to abnormalities in the pulmonary arterial vascular bed that impose increased resistance to blood flow with attendant increased right ventricular workload. All, with the exception of pulmonary veno-occlusive disease and pulmonary capilliary hemangiomatosis, share similar beneficial responses to PAH-specific therapies. By far the most common causes of PH that the practicing clinician will encounter is PH due to left heart disease (pulmonary venous hypertension [PVH], PH due to intrinsic pulmonary disease, and hypoxemia [be it obstructive, restrictive, or sleep-disordered breathing with or without obesity-hypoventilation syndrome]), or PH due to acute or chronic thromboembolic disease. Therapies for these conditions are markedly different and, for most, PAH-specific therapies have not been shown to be beneficial and may even be deleterious.

In this issue of *Clinics in Chest Medicine*, PH experts from throughout the world share their experience and the most recent up-to-date findings from the literature. The value of this is heightened by the significant advances in our understanding of the diseases of the pulmonary vascular bed since the last issue of *Clinics in Chest Medicine* devoted to PAH in 2007.

First, Darren B. Taichman, MD, PhD and Jess Mandel, MD offer an updated discussion of the epidemiology of PAH. This discussion is followed by a review of what is known about the pathology of PAH, including exciting new observations from the Pulmonary Hypertension Breakthrough Initiative offered by Rubin M. Tuder, MD, Elvira Stracher, MD, Jeffrey Robinson, MD, Rahul Kumar, PhD, and Brian B. Graham, MD. Next C. Greg Elliott, MD reviews what is known of the genetics of PAH, including discussion of the newly discovered acid-dependent potassium-gated channel gene KCNK3 and its association with PAH.

The next section of this *Clinics in Chest Medicine* focuses on the important principles underlying proper diagnosis and classification of PH with special detailed discussions of associated forms of PH. Paul Forfia, MD and I discuss the elements required to properly diagnose PAH, with an expanded discussion of nuances of the echocardiogram that can be helpful in distinguishing PAH from PVH. This article also emphasizes the importance ultimately of right heart catheterization in the evaluation of PH. This is followed, in turn, by thorough reviews of PH owing to left heart disease by Michael A. Mathier, MD, PH owing to lung disease and/or hypoxemia by Steven D. Nathan, MD and Paul M. Hassoun, MD, PH associated with congenital heart disease by Usha Krishnan, MD and Erika B. Rosenzweig, MD, portopulmonary hypertension by Nadine Al-Naamani, MD and Kari E. Roberts, MD, PAH associated with chronic hemolytic anemias and blood dyscrasias by Roberto F. Marchado, MD and Harrison W. Farber, MD, and PH with unclear or multifactorial mechanisms (World Health Organization Group 5) by Tim Lahm, MD and Murali M. Chakinala, MD. The

Clin Chest Med 34 (2013) xiii–xiv
http://dx.doi.org/10.1016/j.ccm.2013.10.009
0272-5231/13/$ – see front matter © 2013 Elsevier Inc. All rights reserved.

important topic of potentially curable chronic thromboembolic PH is next discussed by Peter S. Marshall, MD, Kim K. Kerr, MD, and William R. Auger.

The final section of this *Clinics in Chest Medicine* covers the available therapeutics for PAH, both proven and novel potential therapies. Maor Sauler, MD, Wassim H. Fares, MD, and I first review the limited data on standard nonspecific therapies in the management of PAH. Next, Richard Channick, MD, Ioana Preston, MD, and James R. Klinger, MD review the data on oral therapies in the management of PAH, specifically phosphodiesterase-5 inhibitors and endothelin receptor antagonists. Harold I. Palevsky, MD, and Valerie V. McLaughlin, MD next review the use of inhaled and parenteral prostanoid therapies. Meredith E. Pugh, MD, Anna R. Hemnes, MD, and Ivan M. Robbins, MD discuss what is known about combining the aforementioned therapies in attempts to optimize treatment of this fatal disease. When medical therapies fail, options including atrial septostomy and lung transplantation can be employed and Stephanie G. Norfolk, MD, David J. Lederer, MD, MS, and Victor F. Tapson, MD review these important options. Finally, the many exciting novel therapies being explored for the treatment of these unfortunate patients are reviewed by Caroline O'Connell, MD, Dermot S. O'Callaghan, MD, and Marc Humbert, MD.

I do hope that the readers of this issue will find these contributions useful and informative in their daily approach to the finding of "PH" on an echocardiogram. I do trust the information imparted will serve to improve the evaluations and care of our courageous and unfortunate patients diagnosed with PAH, with an ultimate goal of inspiring a cure for this devastating disease. I wish to offer my sincerest gratitude to each contributing author for their thoughtful input and their time invested in the education of others. I also wish to thank Adrianne Brigido of the editorial staff at *Clinics in Chest Medicine* for her patience with me in putting these contributions together. Finally, I wish to thank my incredible wife and son for their support and gracious tolerance of the demands placed on my time during this editorial endeavor.

Terence K. Trow, MD
Director
Yale Pulmonary Vascular Disease Program
Yale University School of Medicine
Department of Internal Medicine
Section of Pulmonary
Critical Care, and Sleep Medicine
333 Cedar Street, PO Box 208057
New Haven, CT 06520-8057, USA

E-mail address:
terence.trow@yale.edu

Epidemiology of Pulmonary Arterial Hypertension

Darren B. Taichman, MD, PhD[a,b,*], Jess Mandel, MD[c]

KEYWORDS

- Pulmonary arterial hypertension • Idiopathic pulmonary arterial hypertension • HIV infection
- Portopulmonary hypertension • Systemic sclerosis • Hemolytic anemia
- Pulmonary veno-occlusive disease • Anorectic drugs

KEY POINTS

- Changes in the epidemiology of pulmonary arterial hypertension (PAH) have resulted in changes in classification schemes and an increased emphasis on diagnosis because of the availability of effective therapies.
- The terms primary pulmonary hypertension and secondary pulmonary hypertension are considered inappropriate, confusing, and should not be used.
- Recent registries of patients with PAH have provided improved data regarding prognosis in the era of advanced therapies.

INTRODUCTION

The last 2 decades have seen an expansion of interest in pulmonary arterial hypertension (PAH) as new treatments have been introduced and new insights into pulmonary vascular biology obtained. Over this period the epidemiology of PAH has evolved as echocardiography became ubiquitous, the availability of treatments promoted clinicians to pursue the diagnosis of PAH with greater vigor, and the classification of PAH underwent several revisions.

Changes in the Classification of the Pulmonary Hypertensive Diseases

An unexplained sclerosis of the pulmonary arteries was first documented in 1891 by Ernst von Romberg,[1] and again described as cardiacos negros in 1901 by Abel Ayerza because of the degree of cyanosis that patients could develop. Thereafter, his colleagues referred to the entity as Ayerza disease, and thought it was a consequence of luetic (syphilitic) vasculitis, although some cases were described in patients with advanced lung disease. Little more was understood until the 1940s when Oscar Brenner reported the histopathologic changes in the arteries of 100 patients with pulmonary hypertension (PH), notably lacking findings that suggested syphilis as a cause. In the 1950s, when the advent of cardiac catheterization allowed an investigation of the disease's hemodynamic abnormalities,[2] Dresdale and colleagues[3] performed cardiac catheterization and described a hypertensive vasculopathy of the pulmonary circulation. It was characterized by vasoconstriction, an increase in pulmonary arterial pressures, and a measurable response to the injection of tolazoline, a vasodilator with both pulmonary and systemic effects. When no cause such as mitral stenosis or emphysema could be identified in these patients, the entity was termed primary PH. Cases of PH for which a cause could be established

[a] Annals of Internal Medicine, American College of Physicians; [b] Penn Presbyterian Medical Center, University of Pennsylvania Perelman School of Medicine, 190 North Independence Mall West, Philadelphia, PA 19104, USA; [c] University of California, San Diego School of Medicine, 9500 Gilman Drive #0606, La Jolla, CA 92093-0606, USA
* Corresponding author. Penn Presbyterian Medical Center, University of Pennsylvania Perelman School of Medicine, 190 North Independence Mall West, Philadelphia, PA 19104.
E-mail address: darren.taichman@uphs.upenn.edu

Clin Chest Med 34 (2013) 619–637
http://dx.doi.org/10.1016/j.ccm.2013.08.010

Box 1
Classification of the pulmonary hypertensive diseases

Group 1: PAH

Idiopathic PAH

Heritable

BMPR2

ALK1, endoglin (with or without hereditary hemorrhagic telangiectasia)

Unknown

Drug and toxin induced

Associated with:

Connective tissue diseases

Human immunodeficiency virus [HIV] infection

Portal hypertension

Congenital heart diseases

Schistosomiasis

Chronic hemolytic anemia

Persistent PH of the newborn

Pulmonary veno-occlusive disease and/or pulmonary capillary hemangiomatosis

Group 2: PH caused by left heart disease

Systolic dysfunction

Diastolic dysfunction

Valvular disease

Group 3: PH caused by lung diseases and/or hypoxia

Chronic obstructive pulmonary disease

Interstitial lung disease

Other pulmonary diseases with mixed restrictive and obstructive pattern

Sleep-disordered breathing

Alveolar hypoventilation disorders

Chronic exposure to high altitude

Developmental abnormalities

Group 4: chronic thromboembolic PH

Group 5: PH with unclear multifactorial mechanisms

Hematologic disorders: myeloproliferative disorders, splenectomy

Systemic disorders: sarcoidosis, pulmonary Langerhans cell

Histiocytosis: lymphangioleiomyomatosis, neurofibromatosis, vasculitis

Metabolic disorders: glycogen storage disease, Gaucher disease, thyroid disorders

Others: tumoral obstruction, fibrosing mediastinitis, chronic renal failure

Adapted from Simonneau G, Robbins IM, Beghetti M, et al. Updated clinical classification of pulmonary hypertension. J Am Coll Cardiol 2009;54(1 Suppl): S43–54; with permission.

were thereafter labeled secondary PH (eg, PH secondary to left ventricular failure, chronic pulmonary diseases, hypoxemia).[4] Later, using acetylcholine, a vasodilator that was cleared exclusively within the pulmonary circulation, Paul Wood showed a pulmonary-specific hemodynamic improvement in patients with primary PH.[2] Intense pathologic evaluation in a series of 156 patients permitted Wagenvoort and Wagenvoort[5] to describe extensive vascular injury and remodeling, which they termed plexogenic pulmonary arteriopathy, thought to be the pathognomonic hallmark of the disease.

Although the terms primary, secondary, and plexogenic PH were used for many years, an appreciation of important similarities and differences in the histopathologic and clinical characteristics of varying patient groups has prompted the adoption of more precise terminology. In part to reach consensus on clinically useful classification schemes for the pulmonary hypertensive disorders, there have been several international working groups under the sponsorship of the World Health Organization (WHO) since 1973. These classification schemes have evolved as new information has emerged regarding both pathophysiologic mechanisms and clinical characteristics. Histologic findings are no longer the cornerstone of clinical classification because few of the pathologic patterns observed are disease specific, biopsies are now rarely performed, and postmortem diagnoses are, by definition, not clinically useful. The current approach to classification (**Box 1**) is based on a hemodynamic definition of PH, coupled with clinical and associated characteristics.

PH is deemed present when the mean pulmonary artery pressure exceeds 25 mm Hg at rest. The presence of PAH further requires normal left heart filling pressures (ie, a normal left ventricular end diastolic pressure directly measured, or indirectly approximated by a pulmonary artery wedge pressure less than or equal to 15 mm Hg). Classification as PAH further requires the absence of significant chronic respiratory disease or thromboembolic disease.

The distinction between the entities classified as PAH and the other known causes of PH (eg,

---

Box 2
Risk factors for the development of PAH

A. Drugs and toxins

1. Definite
   - Aminorex
   - Fenfluramine
   - Dexfenfluramine
   - Toxic rapeseed oil
   - Dasatinib

2. Very likely
   - Amphetamines
   - L-Tryptophan
   - Interferon

3. Possible
   - Meta-amphetamines
   - Cocaine
   - Chemotherapeutic agents
   - Antidepressants

4. Unlikely
   - Oral contraceptives
   - Estrogen therapy
   - Cigarette smoking

B. Demographic and medical conditions

1. Definite
   - Female gender

2. Possible
   - Pregnancy
   - Systemic hypertension

3. Unlikely
   - Obesity

C. Diseases

1. Definite
   - HIV infection

2. Very likely
   - Portal hypertension/liver disease
   - Collagen vascular diseases
   - Congenital systemic-pulmonary-cardiac shunts
   - Splenectomy

3. Possible
   - Thyroid disorders

Adapted and updated from the assessment of risk factors evaluated at the 1998 World Symposium on Pulmonary Hypertension in Evian, France; and

Simonneau G, Galie N, Rubin LJ, et al. Clinical classification of pulmonary hypertension. J Am Coll Cardiol 2004;43(12 Suppl S):5S–12S; with permission.

chronic left heart or chronic respiratory disease) is important because therapy is different. From similarities in histologic and clinical features of patients with various forms of PAH, entities are grouped as WHO group 1 diseases; this includes patients with identifiable genetic causes of PAH (ie, those with heritable PAH) and those with collagen vascular diseases or other conditions known to be associated with PAH (associated PAH). Patients with PAH in whom no known associated disease entity or genetic cause can be found are classified as having idiopathic PAH (IPAH), rather than the previously used term primary PH.

Abandonment of the name primary PH is important as a means of discouraging the confusing and clinically inappropriate term secondary PH. Use of such primary and secondary groupings inappropriately suggests similarities in the pathophysiology and treatment of patients with many different diseases. As an example, patients with chronic obstructive pulmonary disease, chronic thromboembolic disease, and those with congenital heart disease might each be loosely labeled as having secondary PH, although the pathogenesis is distinct in each category and the appropriate therapy is different. Conceptualizing patients as having either primary or secondary disease may also obscure important clinical similarities (including appropriate treatment) between what was previously called primary PH and other entities labeled secondary (eg, patients with congenital heart disease or human immunodeficiency virus [HIV] infection).

Although understanding of the cellular and molecular mechanisms that produce PH remains incomplete, several clearly identifiable risk factors for the development of PAH are recognized. The causal relationship of some risk factors has been firmly established by controlled epidemiologic studies (eg, exposure to fenfluramine-derived anorectic agents), whereas others (eg, thyroid disease) are less well established (**Box 2**).[6–8]

IDIOPATHIC PAH

IPAH is a rare disease with an estimated incidence of 1 to 2 cases per million in industrialized countries.[9–12] The paucity of patients with IPAH and the likelihood that diverse causes might produce similar clinical syndromes have complicated descriptions of the natural history of the disease. To overcome the limitations of sporadic reports, the National Institutes of Health (NIH) established the prospective National Registry for the Characterization of Primary Pulmonary Hypertension in the early 1980s, enrolling 187 patients from 32 centers between 1981 and 1985.[13] The disease affected all ages, both men and women, and many different ethnic groups. The mean age of patients in the registry was 36.4 years and was similar for women and men. However, women were affected more frequently, with a female/male ratio of 1.7:1 (**Fig. 1**). Nine percent of patients were older than 60 years. The race and ethnicity of the cohort were similar to the general population. Similar demographic trends have been reported in series from France, Israel, Japan, Mexico, and China.[11,14–17] Dyspnea was the most common presenting symptom, and the mean time from the onset of symptoms to diagnosis among patients in the NIH registry was approximately 2 years.

In a more recent series, 674 patients referred for treatment of PAH were enrolled in a French national registry over a 1-year period during 2002 and 2003.[12] Both prevalent and incident patients were evaluated, making up 18% and 82% of the study population, respectively. Patients with IPAH accounted for 39% of the registry and, as in prior studies, disease was seen more commonly

in women, with a ratio to men of 1.6:1. The mean age of patients with IPAH was 52 years, older than that seen in prior series. Although data specific to IPAH were not available, one-quarter of patients with PAH of any form were older than 60 years, and some patients were diagnosed in their 80s. However, despite the significant advances in therapy that had occurred in the 20 years since the NIH registry, a significant delay in the diagnosis of IPAH continued; 80% of patients with IPAH had WHO functional class III or IV symptoms (**Box 3**) at the time of diagnosis, which is similar to what was reported in the National Registry for the Characterization of Primary Pulmonary Hypertension in the early 1980s.[13] Exercise capacity was severely impaired in these patients, with a mean 6-minute walk distance of only 328 m, and hemodynamic values were nearly identical to those of the NIH registry population.

Prognostic Factors in IPAH

Although a diagnosis of IPAH has been associated with an invariably dismal prognosis, therapies developed in the last two decades have significantly improved the prognosis of the condition and yielded many long-term survivors. However, no currently available medical treatment is considered curative and lung transplantation continues to be an important therapeutic consideration.

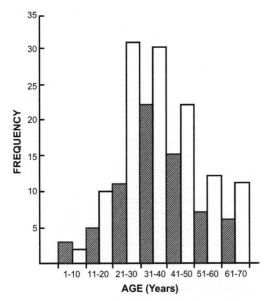

Fig. 1. Distribution of patients with idiopathic PAH entered into the NIH registry. Patients entered into the Registry of the Characterization of Primary Pulmonary Hypertension were most often in their third and fourth decades of life, with a similar ratio of women to men (1.7:1) in all decades. Open bars represent women; shaded bars represent men.

> **Box 3**
> **WHO functional classification**
>
> Class I: patients with PH but without resulting limitation of physical activity. Ordinary physical activity does not cause undue dyspnea or fatigue, chest pain, or near syncope.
>
> Class II: patients with PH resulting in slight limitation of physical activity. They are comfortable at rest. Ordinary physical activity causes undue dyspnea or fatigue, chest pain, or near syncope.
>
> Class III: patients with PH resulting in marked limitation of physical activity. They are comfortable at rest. Less than ordinary activity causes undue dyspnea or fatigue, chest pain, or near syncope.
>
> Class IV: patients with PH with inability to perform any physical activity without symptoms. These patients manifest signs of right heart failure. Dyspnea and/or fatigue may even be present at rest. Discomfort is increased by any physical activity.
>
> *Adapted from* Rubin LJ. Diagnosis and management of pulmonary arterial hypertension: ACCP Evidence-Based Clinical Practice Guidelines. Introduction. Chest 2004;126:7S–10S.

The prognosis of IPAH is poor in the absence of effective therapy. The median survival of patients in the NIH registry was 2.8 years, with estimated survival rates of 68% at 1 year, 48% at 3 years, and 34% at 5 years.[13] Similar outcomes have been reported in other series from various countries,[18,19] with most patients dying of right heart failure.

Although multiple studies have evaluated the outcome of patients with IPAH treated with new therapies and studies have frequently included patients with PAH with the scleroderma spectrum of collagen vascular disease, information on patients with other forms of PAH is sparse. Most subjects in controlled clinical trials of treatment with calcium channel antagonists, prostanoids, endothelin receptor antagonists, or phosphodiesterase inhibitors have had IPAH. Fewer patients with either hereditary or various forms of associated PAH have been studied. It is important to bear in mind this paucity of data when informing patients with some forms of PAH about the expected outcomes of treatment. It is also important to acknowledge the limits in understanding the relative efficacy of available agents. Data from head-to-head comparisons are minimal. Most often, patients treated with intravenous prostanoids have been sicker than those treated with oral therapies, making comparisons between studies problematic.

In the French national registry population from 2002 to 2003, after advanced therapies had become available, the 1-year survival of patients with PAH with either IPAH, familial, or anorexigen-associated PAH was 89.3%. Although information regarding specific treatments involved was not reported, the expected survival from the NIH registry equation was 71.8%.[12]

The multicenter observational Registry to Evaluate Early and Long-Term Pulmonary Arterial Hypertension Disease Management (REVEAL registry) is the largest registry of patients with PAH in the era of advanced PAH therapies.[20] Based on data from 2716 patients, a risk score calculator for newly diagnosed patients with PAH has been developed and validated and is shown in **Fig. 2** and **Table 1**. As can be seen, the strongest contributors to a poor prognosis were a diagnosis of portopulmonary hypertension or heritable PAH, male sex combined with age greater than 60 years, New York Heart Association/WHO functional class IV, and pulmonary vascular resistance (PVR) greater than 32 Wood units.

Objective measurements of exercise capacity also predict survival. Among 43 patients treated predominantly with infused or oral prostanoids, the pretreatment 6-minute walk distance was independently associated with survival, which was significantly better for those who could walk farther than 332 m (**Fig. 3**).[21] In randomized trials of epoprostenol therapy, patients with a lower baseline 6-minute walk distance similarly had poorer survival.[22,23] Maximal oxygen consumption during cardiopulmonary exercise testing also correlates with survival.[24]

Findings on echocardiography, including right atrial enlargement or the presence and size of a pericardial effusion, can be useful in assessing prognosis.[25–27] An index of right ventricular function derived by dividing the combined isovolumetric contraction and relaxation times by the right ventricular ejection time (Tei index) also predicts survival, with a higher index associated with a poorer prognosis.[28] The degree of tricuspid annular displacement during systole was associated with right ventricular function, hemodynamic measurements, as well as survival in a cohort of patients with various forms of PAH, as well as others with PH associated with chronic respiratory or thromboembolic disease (**Fig. 4**).[29] The right ventricular diameter and some measures of right ventricular free wall strain also can also provide prognostic information.[30,31]

Hemodynamic measurements have been predictors of survival in numerous studies, including both observational and clinical trials. Despite isolated differences, overall these studies indicate that values reflecting a declining right ventricular function (eg, an increased right atrial pressure and a decreased cardiac index) are associated with poorer survival.[11,15,16,32,33] Survival is less consistently linked with mean pulmonary artery pressures (mPAPs), and both increasing and decreasing values have been associated with worsened outcomes. This finding reflects the natural history of right heart failure in PAH: mPAP increases progressively as the vascular derangements worsen, only to decrease later as the right heart progressively fails and is no longer able to generate increased pressures (**Fig. 5**).

Many serum markers are increased in patients with IPAH and are associated with a worse prognosis. Uric acid levels are increased in hypoxic states, and the degree of increase correlates with hemodynamic and functional decline in patients with IPAH.[34,35] Levels of B-natriuretic peptide are also increased in patients with IPAH, reflecting right heart failure analogous to that seen in patients with left-sided heart dysfunction. In one series of 60 patients with IPAH, serum brain natriuretic peptide (BNP) concentrations were increased versus control, and inversely correlated with both functional status and survival.[36] BNP levels declined as hemodynamic measures improved with therapy, and a

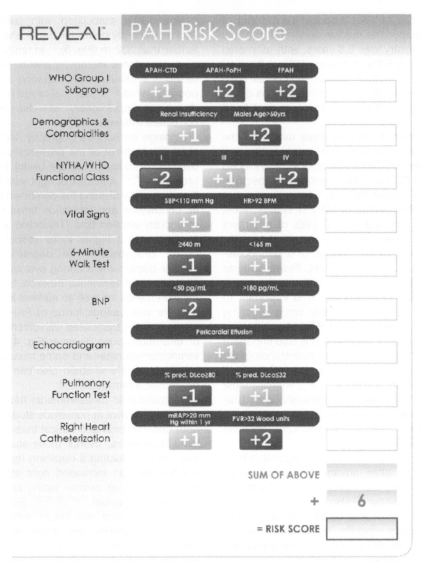

Fig. 2. REVEAL Registry PAH risk score calculator. Calculated risk scores can range from 0 (lowest risk) to 22 (highest risk). If N-terminal proBNP is available and BNP is not, listed cut points are replaced with less than 300 pg/mL and more than 1500 pg/mL. APAH, associated pulmonary arterial hypertension; BNP, brain natriuretic peptide; BPM, beats per minute; CTD, connective tissue disease; DLco, diffusing capacity of lung for carbon monoxide; FPAH, familial PAH; HR, heart rate; mRAP, mean right atrial pressure; NYHA, New York Heart Association; POPH, portopulmonary hypertension; PVR, pulmonary vascular resistance; SBP, systolic blood pressure. (*From* Benza RL, Gomberg-Maitland M, Miller DP, et al. The REVEAL Registry risk score calculator in patients newly diagnosed with pulmonary arterial hypertension. Chest 2012;141(2):354–62; with permission.)

persistently increased BNP (>180 pg/mL) despite therapy predicted a poorer prognosis.

Serum concentrations of endothelin-1,[37] catecholamines,[38] and atrial natriuretic peptide[39] in serum have also been correlated with disease severity. Increases in von Willebrand factor, D-dimer, and troponin-T, or a decrease in the serum albumin level have been individually associated with poorer survival in patients with IPAH.[35,39,40] However, none of these putative prognostic markers are routinely incorporated into clinical decision making.

The prognosis of patients with IPAH who have had cardiac arrest is dismal even when resuscitative efforts are initiated promptly. In one retrospective review of records from more than 3000 patients, 132 episodes of attempted cardiopulmonary resuscitation (CPR) following cardiac arrest

Table 1
Predicted 12-month survival based upon the calculated REVEAL risk score

Score	Risk Group	Predicted 12-mo Survival (%)
0–7	Low	95–100
8	Average	90–<95
9	Moderately high	85–<90
10–11	High	70–<85
>12	Very high	<70

were identified. Survival at 90 days following CPR was only 6%.[41]

The long-term prognosis is good for the small group of patients with IPAH who respond acutely to the administration of short-acting pulmonary vasodilators. Testing is performed at the time of right heart catheterization.[42–48] Although the definition of an acutely responsive patient has varied, a decrease in the mPAP of at least 10 mm Hg to a final value less than 40 mm Hg, with either an increased or unchanged cardiac output, is now generally considered a positive response.[49,50] In one study performed before the availability of other effective treatments, the survival rate of acutely responsive patients treated chronically with oral calcium channel antagonists was 94% at 5 years compared with only 38% among nonresponders.[51] However, only approximately 12% of patients in a 2005 series showed acute vasoreactivity, and of these only about half experienced a sustained clinical response to high-dose oral calcium channel antagonist therapy.[52] For the few acutely vasoreactive patients who do experience

a sustained response to high-dose oral calcium channel antagonists therapy, the prognosis is excellent. In one retrospective study, Sitbon and colleagues[52] found that, among 38 patients with sustained clinical response (defined as being in WHO functional class I or II after 1 year of treatment), survival was 97% in up to 7 years of follow-up. However, oral calcium channel antagonists are of no benefit and can cause considerable harm when administered to patients who do not display acute pulmonary vasoreactivity. Empiric use of high-dose calcium channel antagonists in PAH is never appropriate.

The prognostic significance of acute pulmonary vasoreactivity is less clear in patients treated with therapies other than oral calcium channel antagonists. The magnitude of improvements in mPAP and cardiac index at the time of acute vasodilator testing correlated with survival in one series of patients treated with long-term epoprostenol infusion; such a correlation was not seen in another group of similarly treated patients.[22,53] A retrospective evaluation of survival in patients treated with calcium channel antagonists, prostanoid therapies, bosentan, warfarin, or a combination of these agents found no correlation between survival and acute vasoreactivity at baseline.[40]

Heritable PAH

A genetic basis for the development of PAH has been suspected since a family of patients with IPAH was described by Dresdale and colleagues[3] in 1951. In the NIH registry, 6% of patients reported one or more affected family members.[13] Loyd and colleagues[54] showed that familial PAH has an autosomal dominant pattern of inheritance, an increased tendency for female carriers to manifest clinical disease, and an earlier onset in successive generations (a phenomenon known as genetic anticipation), although more recent data suggest that genetic anticipation may represent an artifact.[55,56] Mutations in the gene for a member of the transforming growth factor beta (TGF-β) superfamily of receptors, the bone morphogenetic protein receptor type II (*BMP-RII*), have been identified as the major cause of familial PAH.[57–60] More than 140 distinct *BMP-RII* mutations have been identified to date, and disease is thought to occur when haploinsufficiency results in inadequate quantities of protein being produced for normal function.[61] The low penetrance of disease observed in familial PAH suggests that environmental factors or other genetic loci likely contribute to disease development in genetically susceptible individuals.[62]

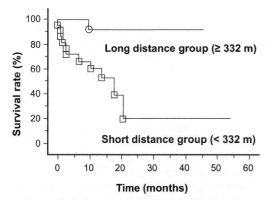

Fig. 3. Survival in IPAH according to 6-minute walk test distance. Kaplan-Meier survival curves according to the median value of distance walked in meters during a 6-minute walk test. Patients unable to walk more than 332 m had a lower survival ($P<.001$).

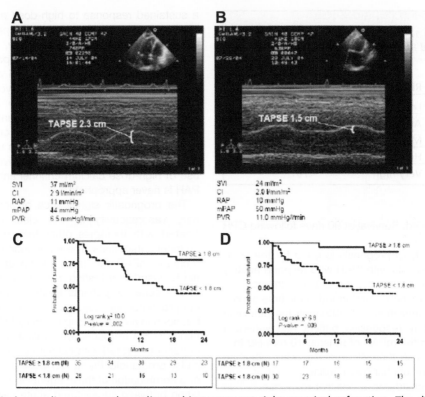

Fig. 4. Survival according to an echocardiographic assessment right ventricular function. The displacement from end diastole to end systole of the lateral tricuspid annulus (tricuspid annular plane excursion [TAPSE]) is shown in M-mode views from 2 patients, one with preserved tricuspid excursion (and right ventricular function) (*A*) compared with a patient with greater impairment (*B*). Kaplan-Meier estimates of survival in a cohort of patients with either PAH (idiopathic or associated with collagen vascular disease) or chronic respiratory or thromboembolic PH (*C* and *D*). (*Adapted from* Forfia P, Fisher MR, Mathei SC, et al. Tricuspid annular displacement predicts survival in pulmonary hypertension. Am J Respir Crit Care Med 2006;174(9):1034–41; with permission.)

Mutations in another member of the TGF-β superfamily, activin receptor-like kinase 1 (*ALK1*), predisposes patients with hereditary hemorrhagic telangiectasia to develop PAH.[63–66]

In 2013, a genomewide association study of 625 individuals with heritable PAH without the *BMP-RII* or *ALK1* mutations and 1525 healthy controls suggested a significant association at the cerebellin 2 (*CBLN2*) locus at 18q22.3, with the risk allele conferring an odds ratio for PAH of 1.97.[67] *CBLN2* codes for a glycoprotein expressed in the lung; its expression is higher in individuals with PAH. New genetic abnormalities specific to PAH have recently been reported at the Fifth World Symposium on Pulmonary Hypertension in Nice, France (see the discussion on the genetics of PH elsewhere in this issue).

Germline mutations in a *BMP-RII* have been identified in up to 80% of patients with heritable PAH.[67,68] Approximately 20% of patients with idiopathic (nonfamilial) and other associated forms of PAH also have *BMPR-II* mutations[59,60,69–73] and common ancestries have been identified in some patients with PAH previously assumed to be sporadic. Mutations in other genes, such as *ACVRL1* (*ALK1*) and *SMAD8*, have also been identified but account for fewer cases of heritable PAH than *BMPR-II* mutations.[74,75]

Heritable cases of PAH might not be recognized on account of incomplete family history taking or reporting, as well as low disease penetrance in small families.[76,77] Carriers of gene mutations may be asymptomatic despite mild PH documented by echocardiography.[78]

Genetic testing of family members can assess the risk of developing PAH. There is a roughly 1 in 5 chance of PAH developing in a first-order relative who carries a disease-causing *BMP-RII* mutation. In the absence of genetic testing results, the risk of disease developing in the first-order relative

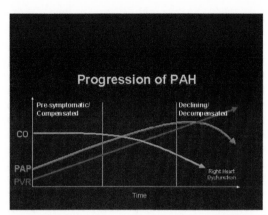

Fig. 5. Hemodynamic changes with progression of PAH. The changes in cardiac output (CO), mean pulmonary artery pressure (PAP), and PVR in the absence of effective therapy. PVR increases progressively as the vascular derangements progress, eventually leading to the development of right heart dysfunction. PAPs initially increase because the right ventricle remains capable of generating the increased pressures required to maintain a given degree of CO. However, with more advanced disease, CO decreases and the PAP decreases because of the inability of the failing right ventricle to generate increased pressures. (*From* Friedman E, Palevsky HI, Taichman DB. Classification and prognosis of pulmonary arterial hypertension. In: Mandel J, Taichman DB, editors. Pulmonary vascular disease. Philadelphia: Elsevier Science; 2006. p. 66–82; with permission.)

of a patient with known familial PAH can be approximated as 1 in 10. When testing shows an absence of disease-causing *BMP-RII* mutations, the risk is the same as in the general population (estimated at 1 in 1 million).[62] Genetic testing should only be performed in conjunction with professional genetic counseling because of the potential interpersonal, psychological, and economic implications of identifying an at-risk genotype.

PAH Associated with Specific Conditions

Collagen vascular diseases

Among the identifiable risk factors for the development of PAH, the presence of systemic sclerosis is the most commonly reported. In the French national registry, 76% of patients with PAH with collagen vascular disease had systemic sclerosis, accounting for 11.6% of all patients enrolled.[12] PAH occurs most often in patients with limited disease or the CREST (calcinosis, Raynaud phenomenon, esophageal dysmotility, sclerodactyly, telangiectasia) syndrome. Estimates vary significantly but, when assessed by right heart catheterization, PAH has been found in between 7% and 29% of patients.[79,80] When screening of symptomatic patients is performed by echocardiogram, approximately 13% of patients with systemic sclerosis had PH in each of 2 large series.[81,82]

The prognosis of patients with systemic sclerosis and PAH is even worse than that of patients with systemic sclerosis who develop severe pulmonary fibrosis. Median survival of patients with systemic sclerosis and PAH is approximately 1 to 3 years, versus 3 years among those with scleroderma and pulmonary fibrosis alone.[83–85] Even when similar therapies are used (including epoprostenol, endothelin receptor antagonists, calcium channel antagonists, and warfarin), survival of patients with PAH associated with systemic sclerosis is generally less favorable than for patients with IPAH (**Fig. 6**).[83] As an example, although hemodynamic values and exercise capacity improve when patients with IPAH are treated with bosentan, the benefit observed among similarly treated patients with systemic sclerosis seems to be primarily a slowing in the rate of deterioration.[86]

PAH also occurs in patients with other forms of collagen vascular disease, including systemic

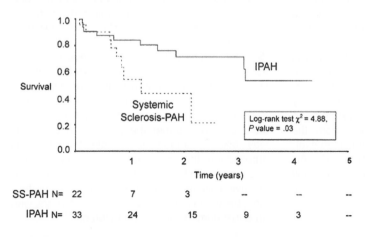

Fig. 6. Survival in PAH associated with systemic sclerosis compared with idiopathic PAH. Kaplan-Meier estimates of survival in patients with PAH associated with the systemic sclerosis (SS) spectrum of diseases (SS-PAH) and IPAH. (*From* Kawut SM, Taichman DB, Archer-Chicko CL, et al. Hemodynamics and survival in patients with pulmonary arterial hypertension related to systemic sclerosis. Chest 2003;123(2):344–50; with permission.)

lupus erythematosis (SLE), rheumatoid arthritis, and Sjögren syndrome. In most studies, pulmonary artery pressures have been estimated by echocardiogram, and thus the prevalence of PAH in these connective tissue disorders is not known. PH has been identified by echocardiogram in approximately 10% of patients with SLE, and up to 43% of patients who are followed prospectively.[87–91] Estimates are similarly broad among patients with mixed connective tissue disease, and again lack confirmation by catheterization in most studies. Regardless of the exact frequency the presence of PH seems to be a significant cause of death in these patients.[89] The possibility of PH patients should therefore be considered in all patients with collagen vascular disease with exertional dyspnea or other symptoms, and early evaluation is warranted.

HIV

Patients infected with HIV are at increased risk for PAH. The mechanisms by which HIV infection leads to PAH are not known. Although direct infection of pulmonary endothelial cells does not seem be involved, indirect mechanisms involving alterations in cytokines, growth factors, and vasoconstrictors have been implicated.[92] Estimates of the incidence of PAH among HIV-infected patients have varied, and although it has been hypothesized that a decrease in incidence followed the introduction of highly active antiretroviral therapy this has not been seen consistently and variation in estimates may be caused by differences in the definitions and modes of evaluation.[93–95] The estimated prevalence of PAH confirmed by right heart catheterization among dyspneic HIV-infected patients since the availability of highly active antiretroviral therapies is 0.5%.[94]

The symptoms, hemodynamic findings, and survival of PAH associated with HIV are similar to those of IPAH.[96] Like IPAH, the prognosis of patients with PAH associated with HIV infection is worse when symptoms are more advanced (eg, WHO functional class III or IV compared with either class I or II) or when cardiac function is depressed.[97] CD4 lymphocyte counts more than approximately 200/mm^3 are associated with a better prognosis.[95,98] Mortality is more often directly attributable to PAH and right heart failure than to infectious complications.[96,98] Survival from the time of diagnostic right heart catheterization evaluated in 48 patients with HIV-associated PAH enrolled in the US-based REVEAL cohort was 93.3% ± 6.2%, 75.1% ± 8.8%, 63.8% ± 9.5%, and 63.8% ± 9.5% at 1, 3, 5, and 7 years, respectively.[99]

Portal hypertension

Patients with chronic liver disease are at risk for the development of pulmonary complications. When portal hypertension and PAH are present, the combination is referred to as portopulmonary hypertension (POPH).[100,101] POPH involves vascular derangements that increase PVR to produce an increased mPAP, as opposed to increased pulmonary pressures caused solely by the increased cardiac output and the volume overloaded state that frequently accompanies chronic liver disease. The cause of PH in these patients may be difficult to identify because the high cardiac output state may precede, or accompany, the development of POPH. Despite similar degrees of clinical impairment, patients with POPH may manifest numerically smaller increases in PVR or smaller decreases in cardiac output than those with IPAH.

The histopathologic changes in patients with POPH are similar to those described in other forms of PAH including both plexiform and thrombotic lesions.[102,103] The pathogenesis is not well understood but seems to involve abnormal proliferative (or other) vascular responses. The inciting causes remain unknown. Portal hypertension might alter the vasoactive mediators to which the pulmonary circulation is exposed because of blood bypassing the liver via portosystemic shunts and returning to the systemic circulation.[104] Alterations in levels of various vasodilators and vasoconstrictors have been observed in patients with POPH as in other forms of PAH.[105,106] Women with portal hypertension seem to be at greater risk for the development of POPH than men, as do patients with autoimmune hepatitis.[107] The severity of portal hypertension does not seem to influence the risk of POPH.[107,108] Predisposing, likely genetic, factors are also thought to determine why only some patients with liver disease develop POPH.[109]

The frequency of PAH in patients with liver disease has not been firmly established. Estimates have ranged from 0.73% in 1241 autopsies from patients with cirrhosis to 16% of 62 patients undergoing catheterization during evaluation for transjugular intrahepatic portosystemic shunting.[105,110] In a prospective study of more than 1200 patients undergoing evaluation for liver transplantation (and thus with advanced liver disease and symptoms) the prevalence of POPH was 5%.[111] Among 2525 patients with PAH enrolled into the US-based REVEAL study cohort of patients with PAH, 136 (5.4%) were categorized as having disease associated with portal hypertension; the mean age at diagnosis was 51 years, with an equal number of men and women.[112]

The prognosis of POPH is poor in the absence of effective treatment. Retrospective series have reported 1-year survival rates less than 50% in the absence of treatment.[113–115] Survival is worse among patients with POPH than IPAH even when available treatments are used.[115] In a large US cohort (REVEAL), the 5-year survival of 174 patients with POPH was significantly worse than that of 1478 patients with idiopathic or heritable PAH (40% vs 64%, respectively), despite less severe hemodynamic derangements among the patients with POPH at the time of enrollment into the study (**Fig. 7**).[116]

Although patients with POPH and advanced hepatic dysfunction often require liver transplantation, the presence of PAH increases the perioperative mortality, and an mPAP more than 35 mm Hg generally is considered a contraindication to liver transplantation.[117,118] Although therapy to lower mPAP has permitted successful orthotopic liver transplantation in some patients,[119–124] the pulmonary vascular abnormalities of PAH are not consistently reversed by liver transplantation. Although some instances of reversal have been reported, in other patients POPH has progressed despite transplantation.[125]

Anorectic agents

The ingestion of certain anorexigens can lead to the development of PAH, possibly by increasing blood levels of the vasoconstrictor serotonin. An epidemic of PAH occurred in Switzerland, Austria, and Germany between 1966 and 1968 when the incidence increased 20-fold following the introduction in those countries of the appetite-depressant, aminorex fumarate.[126] Although only 2% of those exposed to the drug developed PAH, the relative risk compared with unexposed individuals was 52:1.[127] The use of fenfluramine derivatives was similarly associated with the development of PAH both in Europe and North America.[128] In a registry of 95 patients with PAH in Europe, the odds ratio of developing PAH was

6.3 after any anorectic agent use, and 23.8 when anorectic agents were taken for longer than 3 months.[9] Likewise, a North American registry of 579 patients reported that the use of fenfluramine was strongly associated with the development of PAH (odds ratio of 7.5 when taken for more than 6 months). The study also identified a high frequency of anorectic agent use among patients with other associated forms of PAH (eg, collagen vascular disease), suggesting that these drugs might precipitate disease when combined with other risk factors.[129]

In a series of 62 patients evaluated over a 10-year period at a single center in France, the interval between the initial exposure to fenfluramine and the development of dyspnea was approximately 4 years.[130] In the multicenter French national registry from 2002 to 2003, anorexigen-associated PAH was diagnosed within 2 years of drug exposure in 24% of cases, between 2 and 5 years in 32% and after more than 5 years following drug exposure in 44%.[12] In both series, the baseline hemodynamic values were similar to those of patients with IPAH, although patients exposed to anorectic agents were even less likely to show acute vasoreactivity. Among 2525 patients with PAH enrolled into a US-based registry of patients with PAH (REVEAL), 131 (5.3%) had a history of using fenfluramine or fenfluramine derivatives; the mean age at diagnosis was 46 years, and 84% were women.[112]

The prognosis of anorectic agent–associated PAH has not been well established. Data comparing survival with patients with IPAH are conflicting. Survival of patients with aminorex-associated PAH was better than that of patients with IPAH in a retrospective study of 104 patients treated with anticoagulation.[131] With additional therapies, including epoprostenol, survival in fenfluramine-exposed patients with PAH seemed to be similar to that of patients with IPAH in one study[130] but poorer in another series in which patients were matched according to treatments and

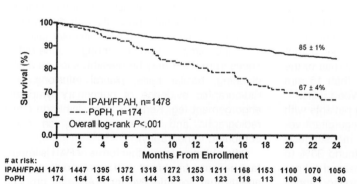

Fig. 7. Survival of patients with IPAH/FPAH compared with POPH from the time of enrollment in a US-based registry. (*From* Krowka MJ, Miller DP, Barst RJ, et al. Portopulmonary hypertension: a report from the US-based REVEAL Registry. Chest 2012;141:4; with permission.)

disease severity.[132] In a cohort of 674 patients with PAH enrolled in a French registry between 2002 and 2003, 9.5% had anorexigen-associated disease; reported survival for this group was similar to that of patients with idiopathic or familial PAH.[133]

Hemoglobinopathies

The risk of developing PH is increased in patients with certain chronic hemolytic disorders.[134] PH in patients with hemolytic anemia in the past has been categorized as group I (PAH); the 2013 Nice Conference reclassified it as group 5 (miscellaneous.) PH caused by difficulty distinguishing between intrinsic pulmonary vascular derangements and increased pulmonary pressures caused by left heart dysfunction in many patients. Hemolytic states might lead to pulmonary vascular derangements by releasing both free hemoglobin and arginase into the plasma where they can reduce the bioavailability of both NO and its substrate, L-arginine.[134–136] Histologic findings consistent with PAH were noted in 15 of 20 autopsies performed on patients with sickle cell anemia.[137]

Prevalence estimates of PH in patients with either sickle cell anemia or thalassemia have ranged significantly, according to the age of the population studied, the severity of symptoms, and the method of pulmonary artery pressure (PAP) assessment used.[138–141] Isolated cases of PH with other chronic hemolytic disorders have been reported, including patients with hereditary spherocytosis and paroxysmal nocturnal hemoglobinuria.[142,143]

Patients with PAH associated with sickle cell anemia tend to have lower mean PAPs and higher cardiac outputs than patients with idiopathic or other forms of associated PAH. Furthermore, patients with PAH associated with hemoglobinopathies also have hemodynamic findings consistent with both intrinsic pulmonary vascular disease (ie, an increased PVR) and increased pulmonary capillary wedge pressures (PCWPs), suggesting the possibility that left ventricular diastolic dysfunction also plays a role. In one study of 20 patients with PAH associated with sickle cell anemia, the mean PAP was 36 mm Hg, cardiac output 8.6 L/min, and PCWP 16 mm Hg; one-half of the patients had PCWP values greater than 15 mm Hg and most had PVR less than 3 Wood units.[144] In another study of 25 adult French patients with sickle cell anemia and a tricuspid regurgitant velocity of greater than or equal to 2.5 m/s suggesting PH, right heart catheterization found 33% to have PAH, whereas 66% had an increased pulmonary artery wedge pressure and pulmonary venous

hypertension.[145] In a prospective study of 398 patients with sickle cell disease, although the prevalence of PH (defined by a tricuspid regurgitant velocity of $\geq$2.0 m/s) was 27%, the prevalence of PH confirmed by right heart catheterization (defined as a mean PAH $\geq$25 mm Hg) was only 6%.[146,147] Similar findings were reported in a prospective study of 80 Brazilian patients with sickle cell anemia.[148]

The presence of PH portends a worse prognosis in patients with sickle cell anemia. Mortality within 2 to 2.5 years of almost 50% of patients with sickle cell with PH has been reported in several series.[144,149,150] In a prospective NIH registry of 195 adult patients with sickle cell anemia followed for a mean of 18 months, Gladwin and colleagues[151] found that mortality increased when the tricuspid regurgitant velocity was greater than 2.5 m/s (relative risk 10.1), compared with death in 2% when the pressures were lower. Markers of hemolysis, such as plasma arginase, correlate not only with the presence of PH but also with an increased risk of death.[135] Whether therapy for PH alters the survival of patients with sickle cell (or other forms of hemolytic anemia) remains incompletely understood. One randomized controlled trial of sildenafil in patients with sickle cell anemia with a tricuspid regurgitant velocity greater than or equal to 2.7 m/s and a 6-minute walk distance between 150 and 500 m was terminated early because of a higher rate of serious adverse events in the active treatment arm (primarily an increased rate of hospitalization for pain).[152]

Pulmonary veno-occlusive disease

Pulmonary veno-occlusive disease (PVOD) is a rare form of PH that is characterized by extensive and diffuse obliteration of small pulmonary veins or venules by cellular proliferation, in situ thrombosis, and fibrous tissue.[153,154] In most patients, pulmonary arteriolar changes accompany the venous changes, although it is unclear whether arteriolar remodeling develops simultaneously with or as a consequence of progressive venous destruction.[155] PVOD usually presents with dyspnea on exertion and findings of right ventricular failure in a manner similar to IPAH, although subtle differences from IPAH may be present, such as digital clubbing, basilar rales, pleural effusions, and radiographic evidence of pulmonary lymphatic engorgement (eg, Kerley B lines visible on chest radiographs and septal thickening on chest computed tomography).[153,156,157]

Differentiation from other forms of PAH is important because treatment with prostanoids or other agents that are effective for IPAH may produce pulmonary edema by increasing cardiac output to postcapillary vessels with obstructing lesions and death in a subset of patients with PVOD.[158] In part because of these difficulties in treatment, the prognosis of PVOD is poor, with most patients dying within 2 years of diagnosis unless long-term treatment with prostanoids is tolerated.[154,156,159] Immediate consideration of lung transplantation is thus encouraged when the diagnosis of PVOD is established, although recurrence of the condition after transplantation has been reported.[160]

The epidemiology of PVOD is not clearly defined. Unlike IPAH, men and women seem equally at risk for PVOD, and the age at diagnosis has ranged from the first weeks through the seventh decade of life.[154,161,162] Because PVOD seems approximately one-tenth as common as IPAH, the annual incidence of PVOD in the general population has been estimated at 0.1 to 0.2 cases per million persons per year.[153] However, this may represent an underestimate because many cases are probably misclassified as IPAH, heart failure, or interstitial lung disease. No well-designed studies have adequately examined the magnitude of this likely misclassification phenomenon. Of 2525 patients with PAH in a multicenter US registry, 0.4% were classified as having PVOD.[112]

The cause of PVOD remains unknown and likely represents a common clinicopathologic pathway that develops in a susceptible host following exposure to one of several different triggers. *BMP-RII* mutation has been reported in patients with PVOD,[73,163] as have epigenetic abnormalities in an effector protein active in the control of specific inflammatory cell populations.[164]

Several factors associated with PVOD have been proposed but none of these epidemiologic hypotheses have been tested by rigorous methods. Conditions theorized to be associated with an increased risk of PVOD include the development of the condition in a sibling, exposure to antineoplastic chemotherapy, infection with HIV or other agents, or the presence of thrombophilia or autoimmune diseases.[153,165–173] Small autopsy series have suggested a high prevalence of PVOD-type pathologic lesions among patients with systemic sclerosis, suggesting that the condition may frequently go unrecognized in patients with PH from this connective tissue disease.[174–176]

SUMMARY

The epidemiology of PAH has changed. Classification schemes have evolved from a focus on histopathology to systems grouping patients according to similarities in hemodynamic and other clinical characteristics. Beyond helping to guide further research and understanding of the causes of PH, study of the epidemiology of PH will inform further refinements in disease classification, the enrollment of patients within clinical trials, and ultimately the care of patients. An accurate understanding of disease epidemiology and classification informs accurate diagnosis, a prerequisite to guiding appropriate therapy.

REFERENCES

1. Romberg E. Uber Sklerose der Lungen Arterie. Dtsch Arch Klin Med 1891;48:197–206.
2. Fishman AP. A century of pulmonary hemodynamics. Am J Respir Crit Care Med 2004;170(2):109–13.
3. Dresdale DT, Schultz M, Michtom RJ. Primary pulmonary hypertension. I. Clinical and hemodynamic study. Am J Med 1951;11(6):686–705.
4. Rubin LJ. Diagnosis and management of pulmonary arterial hypertension: ACCP evidence-based clinical practice guidelines. Chest 2004;126(Suppl 1):7S–10S.
5. Wagenvoort CA, Wagenvoort N. Primary pulmonary hypertension: a pathologic study of the lung vessels in 156 classically diagnosed cases. Circulation 1970;42:1163–84.
6. Curnock A, Dweik R, Higgins B, et al. High prevalence of hypothyroidism in patients with primary pulmonary hypertension. Am J Med Sci 1999;318(5):289–92.
7. Lozano H, Sharma C. Reversible pulmonary hypertension, tricuspid regurgitation and right-sided heart failure associated with hyperthyroidism: case report and review of the literature. Cardiol Rev 2004;12(6):299–305.
8. Chambers CD, Hernandez-Diaz S, Van Marter LJ, et al. Selective serotonin-reuptake inhibitors and risk of persistent pulmonary hypertension of the newborn. N Engl J Med 2006;354(6):579–87.
9. Abenhaim L, Moride Y, Brenot F, et al. Appetite-suppressant drugs and the risk of primary pulmonary hypertension. International Primary Pulmonary Hypertension Study Group. N Engl J Med 1996;335(9):609–16.
10. Group IPPHS. The International Primary Pulmonary Hypertension Study. Chest 1994;105(2):37S–41S.
11. Appelbaum L, Yigla M, Bendayan D, et al. Primary pulmonary hypertension In Israel: a National Survey. Chest 2001;119(6):1801–6.
12. Humbert M, Sitbon O, Chaouat A, et al. Pulmonary arterial hypertension in France: results from a national registry. Am J Respir Crit Care Med 2006;173(9):1023–30.
13. Rich S, Dantzker DR, Ayres SM, et al. Primary pulmonary hypertension. A national prospective study. Ann Intern Med 1987;107(2):216–23.

14. Brenot F. Primary pulmonary hypertension: case series from France. Chest 1994;105(4):33S–6S.

15. Sandoval J, Bauerle O, Palomar A, et al. Survival in primary pulmonary hypertension. Validation of a prognostic equation. Circulation 1994;89(4):1733–44.

16. Okada O, Tanabe N, Yasuda J, et al. Prediction of life expectancy in patients with primary pulmonary hypertension. A retrospective nationwide survey from 1980-1990. Intern Med 1999;38(1):12–6.

17. Jing ZC, Xu XQ, Han ZY, et al. Registry and survival study in Chinese patients with idiopathic and familial pulmonary arterial hypertension. Chest 2007;132(2):373–9.

18. McLaughlin VV, Presberg KW, Doyle RL, et al. Prognosis of pulmonary arterial hypertension: ACCP evidence-based clinical practice guidelines. Chest 2004;126(Suppl 1):78S–92S.

19. Fuster V, Steele PM, Edwards WD, et al. Primary pulmonary hypertension: natural history and the importance of thrombosis. Circulation 1984;70(4):580–7.

20. Benza RL, Gomberg-Maitland M, Miller DP, et al. The REVEAL Registry risk score calculator in patients newly diagnosed with pulmonary arterial hypertension. Chest 2012;141(2):354–62.

21. Miyamoto S, Nagaya N, Satoh T, et al. Clinical correlates and prognostic significance of six-minute walk test in patients with primary pulmonary hypertension. Comparison with cardiopulmonary exercise testing. Am J Respir Crit Care Med 2000;161(2 Pt 1):487–92.

22. Sitbon O, Humbert M, Nunes H, et al. Long-term intravenous epoprostenol infusion in primary pulmonary hypertension: prognostic factors and survival. J Am Coll Cardiol 2002;40(4):780–8.

23. Barst RJ, Rubin LJ, Long WA, et al. A comparison of continuous intravenous epoprostenol (prostacyclin) with conventional therapy for primary pulmonary hypertension. The Primary Pulmonary Hypertension Study Group. N Engl J Med 1996;334(5):296–302.

24. Wensel R, Opitz CF, Anker SD, et al. Assessment of survival in patients with primary pulmonary hypertension: importance of cardiopulmonary exercise testing. Circulation 2002;106(3):319–24.

25. Raymond RJ, Hinderliter AL, Willis I, et al. Echocardiographic predictors of adverse outcomes in primary pulmonary hypertension. J Am Coll Cardiol 2002;39(7):1214–9.

26. Hinderliter AL, Willis PW, Long W, et al. Frequency and prognostic significance of pericardial effusion in primary pulmonary hypertension. PPH Study Group. Primary pulmonary hypertension. Am J Cardiol 1999;84(4):481–4 A410.

27. Eysmann SB, Palevsky HI, Reichek N, et al. Two-dimensional and Doppler-echocardiographic and cardiac catheterization correlates of survival in primary pulmonary hypertension. Circulation 1989;80(2):353–60.

28. Yeo TC, Dujardin KS, Tei C, et al. Value of a Doppler-derived index combining systolic and diastolic time intervals in predicting outcome in primary pulmonary hypertension. Am J Cardiol 1998;81(9):1157–61.

29. Forfia P, Fisher MR, Mathei SC, et al. Tricuspid annular displacement predicts survival in pulmonary hypertension. Am J Respir Crit Care Med 2006;174(9):1034–41.

30. Ghio S, Pazzano AS, Klersy C, et al. Clinical and prognostic relevance of echocardiographic evaluation of right ventricular geometry in patients with idiopathic pulmonary arterial hypertension. Am J Cardiol 2011;107:628–32.

31. Sachdev A, Villarraga HR, Frantz RP, et al. Right ventricular strain for prediction of survival in patients with pulmonary arterial hypertension. Chest 2011;139:1299–309.

32. D'Alonzo GE, Barst RJ, Ayres SM, et al. Survival in patients with primary pulmonary hypertension. Results from a national prospective registry. Ann Intern Med 1991;115(5):343–9.

33. Rajasekhar D, Balakrishnan KG, Venkitachalam CG, et al. Primary pulmonary hypertension: natural history and prognostic factors. Indian Heart J 1994;46(3):165–70.

34. Friedman E, Palevsky HI, Taichman DB. Classification and prognosis of pulmonary arterial hypertension. In: Mandel J, Taichman DB, editors. Pulmonary vascular disease. Philadelphia: Elsevier Science; 2006. p. 66–82.

35. Nagaya N, Uematsu M, Satoh T, et al. Serum uric acid levels correlate with the severity and the mortality of primary pulmonary hypertension. Am J Respir Crit Care Med 1999;160(2):487–92.

36. Nagaya N, Nishikimi T, Uematsu M, et al. Plasma brain natriuretic peptide as a prognostic indicator in patients with primary pulmonary hypertension. Circulation 2000;102(8):865–70.

37. Rubens C, Ewert R, Halank M, et al. Big endothelin-1 and endothelin-1 plasma levels are correlated with the severity of primary pulmonary hypertension. Chest 2001;120(5):1562–9.

38. Nootens M, Kaufmann E, Rector T, et al. Neurohormonal activation in patients with right ventricular failure from pulmonary hypertension: relation to hemodynamic variables and endothelin levels. J Am Coll Cardiol 1995;26(7):1581–5.

39. Nagaya N, Nishikimi T, Uematsu M, et al. Plasma brain natriuretic peptide as a prognostic indicator in patients with primary pulmonary hypertension. J Cardiol 2001;37(2):110–1 [in Japanese].

40. Kawut SM, Horn EM, Berekashvili KK, et al. New predictors of outcome in idiopathic pulmonary

arterial hypertension. Am J Cardiol 2005;95(2): 199–203.

41. Hoeper MM, Galie N, Murali S, et al. Outcome after cardiopulmonary resuscitation in patients with pulmonary arterial hypertension. Am J Respir Crit Care Med 2002;165(3):341–4.

42. Morgan JM, Griffiths M, du Bois RM, et al. Hypoxic pulmonary vasoconstriction in systemic sclerosis and primary pulmonary hypertension. Chest 1991;99(3):551–6.

43. Krasuski RA, Warner JJ, Wang A, et al. Inhaled nitric oxide selectively dilates pulmonary vasculature in adult patients with pulmonary hypertension, irrespective of etiology. J Am Coll Cardiol 2000;36(7): 2204–11.

44. Rubin LJ, Groves BM, Reeves JT, et al. Prostacyclin-induced acute pulmonary vasodilation in primary pulmonary hypertension. Circulation 1982; 66(2):334–8.

45. Sitbon O, Brenot F, Denjean A, et al. Inhaled nitric oxide as a screening vasodilator agent in primary pulmonary hypertension. A dose-response study and comparison with prostacyclin. Am J Respir Crit Care Med 1995;151(2 Pt 1):384–9.

46. Galie N, Ussia G, Passarelli P, et al. Role of pharmacologic tests in the treatment of primary pulmonary hypertension. Am J Cardiol 1995;75: 55A–62A.

47. Nootens M, Schrader B, Kaufmann E, et al. Comparative acute effects of adenosine and prostacyclin in primary pulmonary hypertension. Chest 1995;107(1):54–7.

48. Palevsky HI, Long W, Crow J, et al. Prostacyclin and acetylcholine as screening agents for acute pulmonary vasodilator responsiveness in primary pulmonary hypertension. Circulation 1990;82(6): 2018–26.

49. Barst RJ, McGoon M, Torbicki A, et al. Diagnosis and differential assessment of pulmonary arterial hypertension. J Am Coll Cardiol 2004;43(12 Suppl S): 40S–7S.

50. Badesch DB, Abman SH, Ahearn GS, et al. Medical therapy for pulmonary arterial hypertension: ACCP evidence-based clinical practice guidelines. Chest 2004;126(Suppl 1):35S–62S.

51. Rich S, Kaufmann E, Levy PS. The effect of high doses of calcium-channel blockers on survival in primary pulmonary hypertension. N Engl J Med 1992;327(2):76–81.

52. Sitbon O, Humbert M, Jais X, et al. Long-term response to calcium channel blockers in idiopathic pulmonary arterial hypertension. Circulation 2005; 111(23):3105–11.

53. McLaughlin VV, Shillington A, Rich S. Survival in primary pulmonary hypertension: the impact of epoprostenol therapy. Circulation 2002;106(12): 1477–82.

54. Loyd JE, Primm RK, Newman JH. Familial primary pulmonary hypertension: clinical patterns. Am Rev Respir Dis 1984;129(1):194–7.

55. Loyd JE, Butler MG, Foroud TM, et al. Genetic anticipation and abnormal gender ratio at birth in familial primary pulmonary hypertension. Am J Respir Crit Care Med 1995;152(1):93–7.

56. Larkin EK, Newman JH, Austin ED, et al. Longitudinal analysis casts doubt on the presence of genetic anticipation in heritable pulmonary arterial hypertension. Am J Respir Crit Care Med 2012;186(9): 892–6.

57. Nichols WC, Koller DL, Slovis B, et al. Localization of the gene for familial primary pulmonary hypertension to chromosome 2q31-32. Nat Genet 1997; 15(3):277–80.

58. Morse JH, Jones AC, Barst RJ, et al. Mapping of familial primary pulmonary hypertension locus (PPH1) to chromosome 2q31-q32. Circulation 1997;95(12):2603–6.

59. Deng Z, Morse JH, Slager SL, et al. Familial primary pulmonary hypertension (gene PPH1) is caused by mutations in the bone morphogenetic protein receptor-II gene. Am J Hum Genet 2000; 67(3):737–44.

60. Lane KB, Machado RD, Pauciulo MW, et al. Heterozygous germline mutations in BMPR2, encoding a TGF-beta receptor, cause familial primary pulmonary hypertension. The International PPH Consortium. Nat Genet 2000;26(1):81–4.

61. Machado RD, Aldred MA, James V, et al. Mutations of the TGF-beta type II receptor BMPR2 in pulmonary arterial hypertension. Hum Mutat 2006;27(2): 121–32.

62. Elliott CG. Genetics of pulmonary arterial hypertension. In: Mandel J, Taichman DB, editors. Pulmonary vascular disease. Philadelphia: Elsevier Science; 2006. p. 50–65.

63. Trembath RC, Thomson JR, Machado RD, et al. Clinical and molecular genetic features of pulmonary hypertension in patients with hereditary hemorrhagic telangiectasia. N Engl J Med 2001; 345(5):325–34.

64. Chaouat A, Coulet F, Favre C, et al. Endoglin germline mutation in a patient with hereditary haemorrhagic telangiectasia and dexfenfluramine associated pulmonary arterial hypertension. Thorax 2004;59(5):446–8.

65. Harrison RE, Flanagan JA, Sankelo M, et al. Molecular and functional analysis identifies ALK-1 as the predominant cause of pulmonary hypertension related to hereditary haemorrhagic telangiectasia. J Med Genet 2003;40(12):865–71.

66. Abdalla SA, Gallione CJ, Barst RJ, et al. Primary pulmonary hypertension in families with hereditary haemorrhagic telangiectasia. Eur Respir J 2004; 23(3):373–7.

67. Germain M, Eyries M, Montani D, et al. Genome-wide association analysis identifies a susceptibility locus for pulmonary arterial hypertension. Nat Genet 2013;45(5):518–21.

68. Cogan JD, Pauciulo MW, Batchman AP, et al. High frequency of BMPR2 exonic deletions/duplications in familial pulmonary arterial hypertension. Am J Respir Crit Care Med 2006;174(5):590–8.

69. Thomson JR, Machado RD, Pauciulo MW, et al. Sporadic primary pulmonary hypertension is associated with germline mutations of the gene encoding BMPR-II, a receptor member of the TGF-beta family. J Med Genet 2000;37(10):741–5.

70. Newman JH, Trembath RC, Morse JA, et al. Genetic basis of pulmonary arterial hypertension: current understanding and future directions. J Am Coll Cardiol 2004;43(12 Suppl S):33S–9S.

71. Humbert M, Deng Z, Simonneau G, et al. BMPR2 germline mutations in pulmonary hypertension associated with fenfluramine derivatives. Eur Respir J 2002;20(3):518–23.

72. Roberts KE, McElroy JJ, Wong WP, et al. BMPR2 mutations in pulmonary arterial hypertension with congenital heart disease. Eur Respir J 2004; 24(3):371–4.

73. Runo JR, Vnencak-Jones CL, Prince M, et al. Pulmonary veno-occlusive disease caused by an inherited mutation in bone morphogenetic protein receptor II. Am J Respir Crit Care Med 2003; 167(6):889–94.

74. Girerd B, Montani D, Coulet F, et al. Clinical outcomes of pulmonary arterial hypertension in patients carrying an ACVRL1 (ALK1) mutation. Am J Respir Crit Care Med 2010;181(8):851–61.

75. Shintani M, Yagi H, Nakayama T, et al. A new nonsense mutation of SMAD8 associated with pulmonary arterial hypertension. J Med Genet 2009; 46(5):331–7.

76. Newman JH, Wheeler L, Lane KB, et al. Mutation in the gene for bone morphogenetic protein receptor II as a cause of primary pulmonary hypertension in a large kindred. N Engl J Med 2001; 345(5):319–24.

77. Elliott G, Alexander G, Leppert M, et al. Coancestry in apparently sporadic primary pulmonary hypertension. Chest 1995;108(4):973–7.

78. Grunig E, Janssen B, Mereles D, et al. Abnormal pulmonary artery pressure response in asymptomatic carriers of primary pulmonary hypertension gene. Circulation 2000;102(10):1145–50.

79. Mukerjee D, St George D, Coleiro B, et al. Prevalence and outcome in systemic sclerosis associated pulmonary arterial hypertension: application of a registry approach. Ann Rheum Dis 2003; 62(11):1088–93.

80. Avouac J, Airò P, Meune C, et al. Prevalence of pulmonary hypertension in systemic sclerosis in European Caucasians and metaanalysis of 5 studies. J Rheumatol 2010;37(11):2290–8.

81. Stupi AM, Steen VD, Owens GR, et al. Pulmonary hypertension in the CREST syndrome variant of systemic sclerosis. Arthritis Rheum 1986;29(4): 515–24.

82. MacGregor AJ, Canavan R, Knight C, et al. Pulmonary hypertension in systemic sclerosis: risk factors for progression and consequences for survival. Rheumatology (Oxford) 2001;40(4):453–9.

83. Kawut SM, Taichman DB, Archer-Chicko CL, et al. Hemodynamics and survival in patients with pulmonary arterial hypertension related to systemic sclerosis. Chest 2003;123(2):344–50.

84. Steen VD, Medsger TA Jr. Severe organ involvement in systemic sclerosis with diffuse scleroderma. Arthritis Rheum 2000;43(11):2437–44.

85. Johnson SR, Granton JT. Pulmonary hypertension in systemic sclerosis and systemic lupus erythematosus. Eur Respir Rev 2011;20(122):277–86.

86. Rubin LJ, Badesch DB, Barst RJ, et al. Bosentan therapy for pulmonary arterial hypertension. N Engl J Med 2002;346(12):896–903.

87. Shen JY, Chen SL, Wu YX, et al. Pulmonary hypertension in systemic lupus erythematosus. Rheumatol Int 1999;18(4):147–51.

88. Badui E, Garcia-Rubi D, Robles E, et al. Cardiovascular manifestations in systemic lupus erythematosus. Prospective study of 100 patients. Angiology 1985;36(7):431–41.

89. Li EK, Tam LS. Pulmonary hypertension in systemic lupus erythematosus: clinical association and survival in 18 patients. J Rheumatol 1999;26(9):1923–9.

90. Simonson JS, Schiller NB, Petri M, et al. Pulmonary hypertension in systemic lupus erythematosus. J Rheumatol 1989;16(7):918–25.

91. Winslow TM, Ossipov MA, Fazio GP, et al. Five-year follow-up study of the prevalence and progression of pulmonary hypertension in systemic lupus erythematosus. Am Heart J 1995;129(3):510–5.

92. El Chami H, Hassoun PM. Immune and inflammatory mechanisms in pulmonary arterial hypertension. Prog Cardiovasc Dis 2012;55(2):218–28.

93. Speich R, Jenni R, Opravil M, et al. Primary pulmonary hypertension in HIV infection. Chest 1991; 100(5):1268–71.

94. Sitbon O, Lascoux-Combe C, Delfraissy JF, et al. Prevalence of HIV-related pulmonary arterial hypertension in the current antiretroviral therapy era. Am J Respir Crit Care Med 2008;177:1.

95. Degano B, Guillaume M, Savale L, et al. HIV-associated pulmonary arterial hypertension: survival and prognostic factors in the modern therapeutic era. AIDS 2010;24(1):67–75.

96. Petitpretz P, Brenot F, Azarian R, et al. Pulmonary hypertension in patients with human immunodeficiency virus infection. Comparison with primary

pulmonary hypertension. Circulation 1994;89(6): 2722–7.

97. Pugliese A, Isnardi D, Saini A, et al. Impact of highly active antiretroviral therapy in HIV-positive patients with cardiac involvement. J Infect 2000;40: 282–4.

98. Nunes H, Humbert M, Sitbon O, et al. Prognostic factors for survival in human immunodeficiency virus-associated pulmonary arterial hypertension. Am J Respir Crit Care Med 2003;167(10):1433–9.

99. Benza RL, Miller DP, Barst RJ, et al. An evaluation of long-term survival from time of diagnosis in pulmonary arterial hypertension from the REVEAL Registry. Chest 2012;142(2):448–56.

100. Swanson K, Krowka M. Portopulmonary hypertension. In: Mandel J, Taichman DB, editors. Pulmonary vascular disease. Philadelphia: Elsevier Science; 2006. p. 132–42.

101. Fritz JS, Fallon MB, Kawut SM. Pulmonary vascular complications of liver disease. Am J Respir Crit Care Med 2013;187(2):133–43.

102. Ramsay MA, Simpson BR, Nguyen AT, et al. Severe pulmonary hypertension in liver transplant candidates. Liver Transpl Surg 1997;3:5.

103. Edwards BS, Weir KE, Edwards WD, et al. Coexistent pulmonary and portal hypertension: morphologic and clinical features. J Am Coll Cardiol 1987;10:1233–8.

104. Hoeper MM, Krowka MJ, Strassburg CP. Portopulmonary hypertension and hepatopulmonary syndrome. Lancet 2004;363:1461–8.

105. Benjaminov FS, Prentice M, Sniderman KW, et al. Portopulmonary hypertension in decompensated cirrhosis with refractory ascites. Gut 2003;52(9): 1355–62.

106. Tuder RM, Cool CD, Geraci MW, et al. Prostacyclin synthase expression is decreased in lungs from patients with severe pulmonary hypertension. Am J Respir Crit Care Med 1999;159(6).

107. Kawut SM, Krowka MJ, Trotter JF, et al. Clinical risk factors for portopulmonary hypertension. Hepatology 2008;48(1).

108. Hadengue A, Benhayoun MK, Lebrec D, et al. Pulmonary hypertension complicating portal hypertension: prevalence and relation to splanchnic hemodynamics. Gastroenterology 1991;100(2).

109. Roberts KE, Fallon MB, Krowka MJ, et al. Genetic risk factors for portopulmonary hypertension in patients with advanced liver disease. Am J Respir Crit Care Med 2009;179(9).

110. McDonnell PJ, Toye PA, Hutchins GM. Primary pulmonary hypertension and cirrhosis: are they related? Am Rev Respir Dis 1983;127(4):437–41.

111. Krowka MJ, Swanson KL, Frantz RP, et al. Portopulmonary hypertension: results from a 10-year screening algorithm. Hepatology 2006; 44:1502–10.

112. Badesch DB, Raskob GE, Elliott CG, et al. Pulmonary arterial hypertension: baseline characteristics from the REVEAL registry. Chest 2010; 137(2):376–87.

113. Robalino BD, Moodie DS. Association between primary pulmonary hypertension and portal hypertension: analysis of its pathophysiology and clinical, laboratory and hemodynamic manifestations. J Am Coll Cardiol 1991;17(2):492–8.

114. Swanson KL, Wiesner RH, Nyberg SL, et al. Survival in portopulmonary hypertension: Mayo Clinic experience categorized by treatment subgroups. Am J Transplant 2008;8:2445–53.

115. Kawut SM, Taichman DB, Ahya VN, et al. Hemodynamics and survival of patients with portopulmonary hypertension. Liver Transpl 2005;11(9):1107–11.

116. Krowka MJ, Miller DP, Barst RJ, et al. Portopulmonary hypertension: a report from the US-based REVEAL Registry. Chest 2012;141(4).

117. Krowka MJ, Mandell MS, Ramsay MA, et al. Hepatopulmonary syndrome and portopulmonary hypertension: a report of the multicenter liver transplant database. Liver Transpl 2004;10(2):174–82.

118. Krowka MJ, Plevak DJ, Findlay JY, et al. Pulmonary hemodynamics and perioperative cardiopulmonary-related mortality in patients with portopulmonary hypertension undergoing liver transplantation. Liver Transpl 2000;6(4):443–50.

119. Kuo PC, Johnson LB, Plotkin JS, et al. Continuous intravenous infusion of epoprostenol for the treatment of portopulmonary hypertension. Transplantation 1997;63:604–16.

120. Findlay JY, Plevak DJ, Krowka MJ, et al. Progressive splenomegaly after epoprostenol therapy in portopulmonary hypertension. Liver Transpl Surg 1999;5(5):381–7.

121. Krowka MJ, Frantz RP, McGoon MD, et al. Improvement in pulmonary hemodynamics during intravenous epoprostenol (prostacyclin): a study of 15 patients with moderate to severe portopulmonary hypertension. Hepatology 1999;30(3):641–8.

122. Kahler CM, Graziadei I, Wiedermann CJ, et al. Successful use of continuous intravenous prostacyclin in a patient with severe portopulmonary hypertension. Wien Klin Wochenschr 2000;112(14):637–40.

123. Makisalo H, Koivusalo A, Vakkuri A, et al. Sildenafil for portopulmonary hypertension in a patient undergoing liver transplantation. Liver Transpl 2004; 10(7):945–50.

124. Minder S, Fischler M, Muellhaupt B, et al. Intravenous iloprost bridging to orthotopic liver transplantation in portopulmonary hypertension. Eur Respir J 2004;24(4):703–7.

125. Rodriguez-Roisin R, Krowka MJ, Herve P, et al. Pulmonary-Hepatic Vascular Disorders Scientific Committee ERS Task Force. Eur Respir J 2004;24: 861–80.

126. Gurtner HP. Aminorex pulmonary hypertension. In: AF F, editor. The pulmonary circulation: normal and abnormal. Philadelphia: University of Pennsylvania Press; 1990. p. 397–411.

127. Brenot F. Risk factors for primary pulmonary hypertension. In: Rubin LJ, Rich S, editors. Primary pulmonary hypertension. New York: Marcel Dekker; 1996. p. 131–49.

128. Brenot F, Herve P, Petitpretz P, et al. Primary pulmonary hypertension and fenfluramine use. Br Heart J 1993;70(6):537–41.

129. Rich S, Rubin L, Walker AM, et al. Anorexigens and pulmonary hypertension in the United States: results from the surveillance of North American pulmonary hypertension. Chest 2000;117(3): 870–4.

130. Simonneau G, Fartoukh M, Sitbon O, et al. Primary pulmonary hypertension associated with the use of fenfluramine derivatives. Chest 1998;114(Suppl 3): 195S–9S.

131. Frank H, Mlczoch J, Huber K, et al. The effect of anticoagulant therapy in primary and anorectic drug-induced pulmonary hypertension. Chest 1997;112(3):714–21.

132. Rich S, Shillington A, McLaughlin V. Comparison of survival in patients with pulmonary hypertension associated with fenfluramine to patients with primary pulmonary hypertension. Am J Cardiol 2003;92(11):1366–8.

133. Humbert M, Sitbon O, Yaïci A, et al. Survival in incident and prevalent cohorts of patients with pulmonary arterial hypertension. Eur Respir J 2010;36(3): 549–55.

134. Machado RF, Gladwin MT. Hemolytic anemia associated pulmonary hypertension. In: Mandel J, Taichman DB, editors. Pulmonary vascular disease. Philadelphia: Elsevier; 2006. p. 170–87.

135. Morris CR, Kato GJ, Poljakovic M, et al. Dysregulated arginine metabolism, hemolysis-associated pulmonary hypertension, and mortality in sickle cell disease. JAMA 2005;294(1):81–90.

136. Castro O. Pulmonary hypertension in sickle cell disease and thalassemia. In: Peacock AJ, Rubin L, editors. Pulmonary circulation: diseases and their treatment. London: Arnold Publishers; 2004. p. 237–43.

137. Haque AK, Gokhale S, Rampy BA, et al. Pulmonary hypertension in sickle cell hemoglobinopathy: a clinicopathologic study of 20 cases. Hum Pathol 2002;33(10):1037–43.

138. Jootar P, Fucharoen S. Cardiac involvement in beta-thalassemia/hemoglobin E disease: clinical and hemodynamic findings. Southeast Asian J Trop Med Public Health 1990;21(2):269–73.

139. Du Z, Roguin N, Milgram E, et al. Pulmonary hypertension in patients with thalassemia major. Am Heart J 1997;134(3):532–7.

140. Aessopos A, Farmakis D, Deftereos S, et al. Thalassemia heart disease: a comparative evaluation of thalassemia major and thalassemia intermedia. Chest 2005;127(5):1523–30.

141. Aessopos A, Farmakis D. Pulmonary hypertension in β-thalassemia. Ann N Y Acad Sci 2005;1054: 342–9.

142. Verresen D, De Backer W, Van Meerbeeck J, et al. Spherocytosis and pulmonary hypertension coincidental occurrence or causal relationship? Eur Respir J 1991;4(5):629–31.

143. Heller PG, Grinberg AR, Lencioni M, et al. Pulmonary hypertension in paroxysmal nocturnal hemoglobinuria. Chest 1992;102(2):642–3.

144. Castro O, Hoque M, Brown BD. Pulmonary hypertension in sickle cell disease: cardiac catheterization results and survival. Blood 2003;101(4): 1257–61.

145. Fitzgerald M, Fagan K, Herbert DE, et al. Misclassification of pulmonary hypertension in adults with sickle hemoglobinopathies using Doppler echocardiography. South Med J 2012;105(6):300–5.

146. Simonneau G, Parent F. Pulmonary hypertension in patients with sickle cell disease: not so frequent but so different. Eur Respir J 2012;39(1):3–4.

147. Parent F, Bachir D, Inamo J, et al. A hemodynamic study of pulmonary hypertension in sickle cell disease. N Engl J Med 2011;365(1):44–53.

148. Fonseca GH, Souza R, Salemi VM, et al. Pulmonary hypertension diagnosed by right heart catheterisation in sickle cell disease. Eur Respir J 2012;39(1): 112–8.

149. Powars D, Weidman JA, Odom-Maryon T, et al. Sickle cell chronic lung disease: prior morbidity and the risk of pulmonary failure. Medicine (Baltimore) 1988;67(1):66–76.

150. Sutton LL, Castro O, Cross DJ, et al. Pulmonary hypertension in sickle cell disease. Am J Cardiol 1994;74(6):626–8.

151. Gladwin MT, Sachdev V, Jison ML, et al. Pulmonary hypertension as a risk factor for death in patients with sickle cell disease. N Engl J Med 2004; 350(9):886–95.

152. Machado RF, Barst RJ, Yovetich NA, et al, walk-PHaSST Investigators and Patients. Hospitalization for pain in patients with sickle cell disease treated with sildenafil for elevated TRV and low exercise capacity. Blood 2011;118(4):855–64.

153. Mandel J. Pulmonary veno-occlusive disease. In: Mandel J, Taichman DB, editors. Pulmonary vascular disease. Philadelphia: Elsevier Science; 2006.

154. Mandel J, Mark EJ, Hales CA. Pulmonary veno-occlusive disease. Am J Respir Crit Care Med 2000;162(5):1964–73.

155. Simonneau G, Galie N, Rubin LJ, et al. Clinical classification of pulmonary hypertension. J Am Coll Cardiol 2004;43(12 Suppl S):5S–12S.

156. Holcomb BW Jr, Loyd JE, Ely EW, et al. Pulmonary veno-occlusive disease: a case series and new observations. Chest 2000;118(6):1671–9.

157. Swensen SJ, Tashjian JH, Myers JL, et al. Pulmonary venoocclusive disease: CT findings in eight patients. AJR Am J Roentgenol 1996;167(4): 937–40.

158. Palmer S, Robinson L, Wang A, et al. Massive pulmonary edema and death after prostacyclin infusion in a patient with pulmonary veno-occlusive disease. Chest 1998;113:237.

159. Okumura H, Nagaya N, Kyotani S, et al. Effects of continuous IV prostacyclin in a patient with pulmonary veno-occlusive disease. Chest 2002;122(3): 1096–8.

160. Izbicki G, Shitrit D, Schechtman I, et al. Recurrence of pulmonary veno-occlusive disease after heart-lung transplantation. J Heart Lung Transplant 2005;24(5):635–7.

161. Thadani U, Burrow C, Whitaker W, et al. Pulmonary veno-occlusive disease. Q J Med 1975;44(173): 133–59.

162. Wagenvoort CA. Pulmonary veno-occlusive disease. Entity or syndrome? Chest 1976;69(1): 82–6.

163. Montani D, Achouh L, Dorfmuller P, et al. Pulmonary veno-occlusive disease: clinical, functional, radiologic, and hemodynamic characteristics and outcome of 24 cases confirmed by histology. Medicine (Baltimore) 2008;87(4).

164. Perros F, Cohen-Kaminsky S, Gambaryan N, et al. Cytotoxic cells and granulysin in pulmonary arterial hypertension and pulmonary veno-occlusive disease. Am J Respir Crit Care Med 2013;187(2).

165. Bjornsson J, Edwards WD. Primary pulmonary hypertension: a histopathologic study of 80 cases. Mayo Clin Proc 1985;60(1):16–25.

166. Davies P, Reid L. Pulmonary veno-occlusive disease in siblings: case reports and morphometric study. Hum Pathol 1982;13(10):911–5.

167. Devereux G, Evans MJ, Kerr KM, et al. Pulmonary veno-occlusive disease complicating Felty's syndrome. Respir Med 1998;92(8):1089–91.

168. Hourseau M, Capron F, Nunes H, et al. Pulmonary veno-occlusive disease in a patient with HIV infection. A case report with autopsy findings. Ann Pathol 2002;22(6):472–5 [in French].

169. Joselson R, Warnock M. Pulmonary veno-occlusive disease after chemotherapy. Hum Pathol 1983; 14(1):88–91.

170. Knight BK, Rose AG. Pulmonary veno-occlusive disease after chemotherapy. Thorax 1985;40(11): 874–5.

171. Townend JN, Roberts DH, Jones EL, et al. Fatal pulmonary venoocclusive disease after use of oral contraceptives. Am Heart J 1992;124(6): 1643–4.

172. Voordes C, Kuipers J, Elema J. Familial pulmonary veno-occlusive disease: a case report. Thorax 1977;32(6):763.

173. Williams L, Fussell S, Veith R, et al. Pulmonary veno-occlusive disease in an adult following bone marrow transplantation. Case report and review of the literature. Chest 1996;109(5):1388.

174. Overbeek MJ, Vonk MC, Boonstra A, et al. Pulmonary arterial hypertension in limited cutaneous systemic sclerosis: a distinctive vasculopathy. Eur Respir J 2009;34(2):371–9.

175. Montani D, Bergot E, Günther S, et al. Pulmonary arterial hypertension in patients treated by dasatinib. Circulation 2012;125(17):2128–37.

176. Dhillon S, Kaker A, Dosanjh A, et al. Irreversible pulmonary hypertension associated with the use of interferon alpha for chronic hepatitis C. Dig Dis Sci 2010;55(6):1785–90.

Pathology of Pulmonary Hypertension

Rubin M. Tuder, MD[a,*], Elvira Stacher, MD[b,c],
Jeffrey Robinson, MD[a], Rahul Kumar, PhD[a],
Brian B. Graham, MD[a]

KEYWORDS

- Pulmonary hypertension • Smooth muscle cells • Endothelial cells • Angiogenesis
- Vascular remodeling

KEY POINTS

- Control lungs may have significant disorders in pulmonary arteries that need to be considered when studied in the context of pulmonary vascular or interstitial disease samples.
- Pulmonary arterial hypertension (PAH) lungs show increased pulmonary remodeling compared with control lungs. These parameters correlate with pulmonary hemodynamics.
- The 2 histopathologic patterns, idiopathic PAH (IPAH)–type (seen in IPAH, familial PAH, or PAH associated with congenital heart disease) and PAH associated with collagen vascular disease have:
  o Significant heterogeneity of pulmonary vascular remodeling, both within regions from the same lung and between different lungs of each pattern
  o Pathologic subphenotypes, with significant variation in the severity of intimal and medial remodeling (largely involving smooth muscle cells) and presence of plexiform lesions
  o High correlation and a statistically significant association between perivascular inflammation and pulmonary artery pressures and pulmonary vascular remodeling
- Using the Pulmonary Hypertension Breakthrough Initiative cohort, pulmonary veins did not undergo significant remodeling in the setting of PAH.
- Stringent stereological approaches are lacking in the assessment of the pulmonary vascular remodeling in pulmonary hypertension research.
- Animal models may not reflect the structural abnormalities and the molecular pathways involved in the human disease.

INTRODUCTION

The last 2 generations of physicians and researchers in pulmonary hypertension (PH) have undergone their training, performed investigations, and practiced without a thorough knowledge of the scope of the pathologic alterations underlying PH. Many reasons have contributed to relegating pulmonary vascular pathology to a secondary role in the overall clinical management and classification of the disease. Pathology is not part of the clinical algorithms outlined for diagnosis and

Supported by the Cardiovascular Medical and Research Educational Fund (to R.M. Tuder), Parker B. Francis, NIH K08HL105536, and Pfizer ASPIRE grants (to B.B. Graham).
The authors have nothing to disclose.
[a] Program in Translational Lung Research, Division of Pulmonary Sciences and Critical Care Medicine, Department of Medicine, University of Colorado School of Medicine, 12700 East 19th Avenue, Research Complex 2, Room 9001, Aurora, CO 80045, USA; [b] Institute of Pathology, Medical University of Graz, Universitätsplatz 3, 8010 Graz, Austria; [c] Ludwig Boltzmann Institute for Lung Vascular Research, Universitätsplatz 3, 8010 Graz, Austria
* Corresponding author.
E-mail address: rubin.tuder@ucdenver.edu

monitoring response to therapies, except for a minority of cases with unusual clinical presentation. There is lack of large lung cohorts from well-characterized pulmonary hypertensive patients, and, if available, the samples were obtained by limited and neither systematic nor random (ie, biased) sampling. There has also been reliance on outdated or scope-limited past pathologic studies. The last large comprehensive study was published in 1995, before the implementation of any of the current therapies for the disease.[1] Notwithstanding these important limitations, most of the current translational studies require human tissue analysis. However, lack of understanding regarding the spectrum of pathologic alterations may limit an investigator's ability to appreciate their overall relevance to the understanding of the disease. Most importantly, there have not been insights into the status of pulmonary vascular pathology in lungs subjected to the current therapies, even with the caveats of studying lungs from patients with advanced disease.

The Pulmonary Hypertension Breakthrough Initiative (PHBI), under the sponsorship of the Cardiovascular Medical Research and Educational Fund (CMREF), has undertaken a transforming initiative to affect research in PH. As a result of legal settlements with drug manufacturers and representatives of patients who developed pulmonary arterial hypertension (PAH) caused by the use of anorectic drugs, particularly dexfenfluramine,[2] money was set aside to foster research in PAH. The CMREF then focused on establishing a research network with the goal of accruing diseased PAH lungs from patients undergoing lung transplantation and control lungs incompatible for lung transplantation. The scope and mission of the PHBI is accessible at http://www.ipahresearch.org/.

As of 2013, more than 100 PAH and 30 control lungs have been collected, phenotyped, and studied by the PHBI. In August 2012, we reported the first comprehensive and systematic assessment of the scope of pathologic alterations present in these lungs.[3] The patients with PAH were treated with different combinations of the currently available PAH-specific drugs, which have made a significant impact on survival and well-being of affected patients.[4] This study forms the basis of this article,[3] which expands on the reported findings and highlights pathologic alterations of interest associated with pulmonary hemodynamics. Moreover, it underscores the need for studies using state-of-the-art methodologies to better understand the scope of pathologic alterations seen in patients with PAH. These highlights form the basis of recommendations on how best to use human lung samples for translational studies and how human PAH pathology relates to animal models of PH.

NORMAL PULMONARY CIRCULATION

We have described previously the histology of the normal pulmonary circulation.[5,6] However, it is worth revisiting some important characteristics of the pulmonary circulation because they have important implications in the interpretation of the pulmonary vascular remodeling in PH. Based on a casting study of the left lung of a 43-year-old male donor, it was estimated that the pulmonary artery (PA) branches approximately 15 times from the main PA (largest order) to the precapillary level (smallest order), often in close proximity to accompanying airways (Figs. 1 and 2).[4,5] A preceding similar study found 17 orders of branching (the difference derives from differences in criteria on how to ascribe successive orders to the artery branches; see Fig. 1).[4] These assessments indicated that pulmonary arteries contain 10^8 vascular segments at the level of precapillary arteries (order 1), which measured 20 μm in diameter (see Fig. 2; Fig. 3A). As the diameter progressively increases from orders 1 to 15, the length of each order also increases up to order 13 (see Fig. 3B, C). There are approximately 10^7 and 1.6×10^6 PA segments in the range of 40 μm and 70 μm in diameter, respectively. In the critical segment around 200 μm in diameter, which largely regulates pulmonary vascular tone and may be the key artery diameter range affected by medial and intimal lesions in PH, there are approximately 2.8×10^5 vascular segments.

The muscular wall is usually detectable in normal arteries approximately 40 μm in diameter and, more consistently, in arteries larger than 70 μm in diameter.[6] The predicted volume of the muscular medial layer (derived from the data in Refs.[4,5]) is shown in Fig. 4. It progressively increases with larger segments, from orders 1 to 13, followed by a decrease in the largest orders (ie, right hilar PA). Moreover, after calculating the ratio of volume of PA media in relation to the length of the pulmonary arteries for each branching order, it became apparent that the rate of increase in the volume of media/length of blood vessel segment is more marked in small pulmonary arteries, which are the segments that undergo most of the remodeling in PAH (Fig. 5). The high ratio between volume media/length of vascular segment is accompanied by the largest surface area of the intima (ie, lumen) among all vascular segments, a finding that is predictable because the capillary surface area reaches approximately

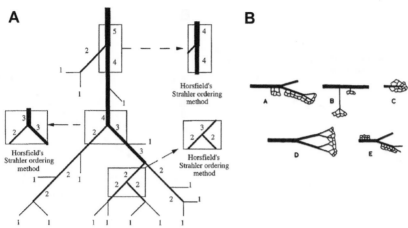

Fig. 1. (*A*) Ordering methods for counting PA branching, detailed in Refs.[4,5] The most distal casted precapillary order is assigned number 1; the convergence of 2 segments of equal diameter form the next order (or n + 1; exemplified in boxed order 2 + 3 = 4). If the parent branch is of the same size as the resulting branch, then the order number is maintained (lower boxed scenario with orders 2 + 2 = 2). Differences in assignment of orders between Huang and colleagues[5] and Horsfield[4] are illustrated as well. (*B*) Patterns of distal capillary formation, sprouting out of terminal segments of pulmonary arteries. (*From* Horsfield K. Morphometry of the small pulmonary arteries in man. Circ Res 1978;42:593–7; with permission.)

17 m², equivalent to an increase in 4 logs of overall surface area (**Fig. 6**).

The appreciation of the magnitude of complexity of the pulmonary vascular tree is critical for estimating the extent of pulmonary vascular lesions required to produce PH. Because the normal pulmonary circulation can accommodate a 5-fold increase in cardiac output without the development of PH, it might be predicted that PH requires 80% of the pulmonary vascular bed to be compromised. However, the number of lesions required to achieve this reduction in cross-sectional area varies depending on the vascular segment primarily affected. Approximately 224,000 lesions are required to restrict flow at pulmonary arteries of 200-μm diameter, whereas a log higher number (2 × 10⁶) of lesions would be required to block vascular segments measuring 40 μm in diameter. At the present time, the distribution and extent of pulmonary vascular involvement in PH remains undetermined (discussed later). Given that the smallest arteries have the highest luminal surface/length ratios, obliterative injuries to these segments have a profound impact on overall pulmonary resistance.

However, localized alterations in PA structure are commonly present in normal pulmonary arteries. These alterations include focal thickening of the intima, probably caused by accumulation of extracellular matrix and myofibroblasts and medial thickening. These alterations are predicted to be not extensive enough to lead to a significant decrease in overall perfusion. As indicated for PAH, the overall impact of these lesions depends on their location, number, and extent to which they restrict luminal blood flow.

In our assessment of the normal pulmonary circulation using the PHBI samples, we investigated the normal range of intima and media remodeling in lungs of young adults, with a mean age of approximately 32 years (**Fig. 7A**). A surprising finding was the degree of pulmonary vascular remodeling in approximately 21% of control lungs (see **Fig. 7B**). Although, the intimal thickness in this abnormal subgroup was in the range seen in

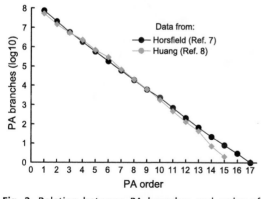

Fig. 2. Relation between PA branches and order of reconstruction based on pulmonary vascular casting. (*Data from* Horsfield K. Morphometry of the small pulmonary arteries in man. Circ Res 1978;42:593–7; and Huang W, Yen RT, McLaurine M, et al. Morphometry of the human pulmonary vasculature. J Appl Physiol 1996;81:2123–33.)

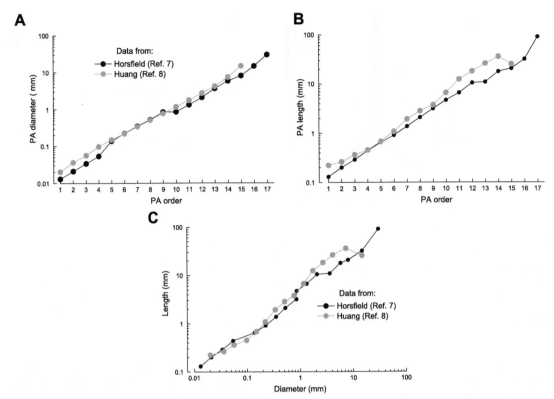

Fig. 3. (*A*) Relation between PA branch diameter (*A*) or length (*B*) and PA order and between PA branch length and diameter (*C*). (*Data from* Horsfield K. Morphometry of the small pulmonary arteries in man. Circ Res 1978;42:593–7; and Huang W, Yen RT, McLaurine M, et al. Morphometry of the human pulmonary vasculature. J Appl Physiol 1996;81:2123–33.)

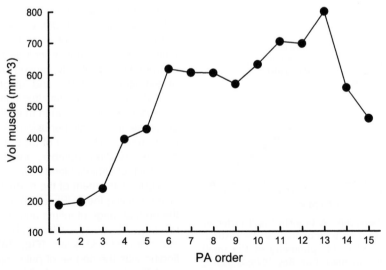

Fig. 4. Relation between volume of muscular media and PA order. (*Data from* Horsfield K. Morphometry of the small pulmonary arteries in man. Circ Res 1978;42:593–7; and Huang W, Yen RT, McLaurine M, et al. Morphometry of the human pulmonary vasculature. J Appl Physiol 1996;81:2123–33.)

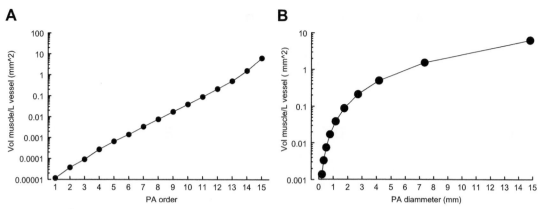

Fig. 5. Rate of increase in volume with PA order (*A*) and diameter (*B*). (*Data from* Horsfield K. Morphometry of the small pulmonary arteries in man. Circ Res 1978;42:593–7; and Huang W, Yen RT, McLaurine M, et al. Morphometry of the human pulmonary vasculature. J Appl Physiol 1996;81:2123–33.)

the normal-appearing lungs, the media, as assessed by the medial fractional thickness (equivalent to the percentage of media in relation to the overall vascular diameter) was significantly thicker in this control group with remodeled pulmonary arteries, within the range seen in patients with PAH.[3]

Were these control patients hypertensive? Because these donor lungs were made available as unsuitable for lung transplantation, no clinical information regarding PA pressures were available (donors were victims of accidents or catastrophic and acute diseases that spared the lungs). Notwithstanding these constraints, demographic information revealed that these control samples were older and predominantly male compared with normal controls and patients with PAH. Age-related pulmonary vascular remodeling could also explain our findings. Furthermore, it is conceivable that these abnormal control samples

with incidental pulmonary vascular remodeling had left heart dysfunction, leading to alterations in their pulmonary circulation. Moreover, many of these lungs had pathologic alterations that indicated smoking, such as respiratory bronchiolitis.[7] Smoking leads to pulmonary vascular remodeling,[8] even in smokers with no clinical evidence of PH. In summary, pulmonary vascular remodeling can occur but its clinical impact and overall significance remain to be better elucidated. For the subsequent comparisons with the PAH group, we used only the control lungs with normal pulmonary arteries.

INTIMAL LESIONS

The reduction of PA luminal area is probably the critical factor in the increase in pulmonary vascular resistance (PVR) in PAH (**Fig. 8**A).[3] We have

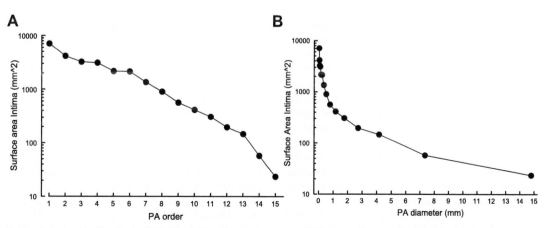

Fig. 6. Relation between surface area of intima and PA order (*A*) or diameter (*B*). (*Data from* Horsfield K. Morphometry of the small pulmonary arteries in man. Circ Res 1978;42:593–7; and Huang W, Yen RT, McLaurine M, et al. Morphometry of the human pulmonary vasculature. J Appl Physiol 1996;81:2123–33.)

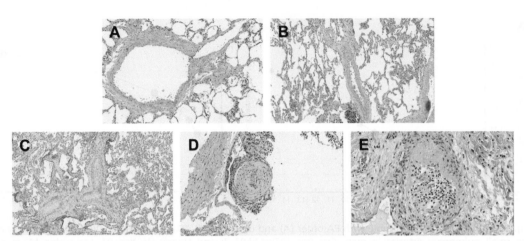

Fig. 7. Control lungs with histologically normal (*A*) or remodeled PA with media thickening (*B*). IPAH lungs with both media and intima thickening (*C*), intima obliteration (*D*), and plexiform lesion with inflammation (*E*). Hematoxylin-eosin; A, B: 10×; C, D: 20×; E: 40× magnification.

previously outlined the range of pathologic alterations involving the intima in lungs of patients with PH.[9] Although these lesions impinge significantly on the normal pulmonary blood flow and account for the increase in PVR, their distribution, cellular nature, and natural history are largely unknown (see **Fig. 7**C). The cellular composition ranges from a preponderance of endothelial cells (forming plexiform or concentric lesions[10,11]) to myofibroblasts; electron microscopic studies highlighted the identification of undifferentiated cells in the plexiform lesions.[12] Whether occlusive intimal lesions require prior endothelial cell proliferation or derive from uncoordinated growth of myofibroblasts remains unclear. However, plexiform lesions are predominantly seen in idiopathic PAH (IPAH); although infrequent, we have also observed plexiform lesions in cases that were associated with collagen vascular disease.[3]

Although plexiform lesions are seen primarily in severe PAH, their importance as a trigger of severe PAH remains unclear. Endothelial cell proliferation, the key event underscoring the process of misguided angiogenesis in plexiform lesions,[13] might precede occlusive intima lesions, obscuring their occurrence and overall frequency. Notwithstanding this potential role for plexiform lesions, we approached the potential pathobiological importance of the plexiform lesion by investigating its occurrence and relation to pulmonary hemodynamics and pulmonary vascular remodeling in the PHBI cohort. Several findings were noteworthy. The number of plexiform lesions seen (ie, profiles, which is largely proportional to size as well as density)[14] varied significantly in the different regions of individual PAH lungs, with an overall coefficient of variation (CV) of approximately 1.2.[3] The CV for plexiform lesions was 3-fold to 6-fold

higher than that for intimal, medial, and adventitial remodeling assessed by fractional thickness.[3] More importantly, we were not able to relate the number of profiles of plexiform lesions to hemodynamics at patient enrollment or with the extent of intimal or medial remodeling. Although all cases of IPAH-like pathology had plexiform lesions, these were present in only 50% of lungs with APAH (associated PAH)-like pathology. These data suggest that the profiles of plexiform lesions are variable and, when present, cannot be related to other parameters of pulmonary vascular remodeling or hemodynamics. This finding casts some degree of uncertainty regarding the relevance of the concept of angioproliferative PH, which predicates that there is a form of PH that requires angioproliferation for its development.[15]

The extent of intimal and medial remodeling was equivalent among IPAH, APAH, and veno-occlusive disease (VOD) patterns.[3] Furthermore, we were able to compare the extent of pulmonary vascular remodeling among forms of PAH presenting with an IPAH-like morphology, including IPAH, congenital heart disease–associated PAH, and VOD-PAH. No significant differences in remodeling of the intima and media were observed among these subtypes.

Perhaps the most novel and potentially important finding was the identification of more severe intimal remodeling in lungs of patients harboring mutations for bone morphogenetic protein receptor II (see **Fig. 8**B).[3] This is the first documentation that bone morphogenetic protein receptor (BMPR) II mutation and associated disorders differ from wild-type BMPR II-IPAH; it supports the finding that silencing BMPR II causes increased endothelial cell apoptosis.[16] The decrease in BMPR II signaling, with

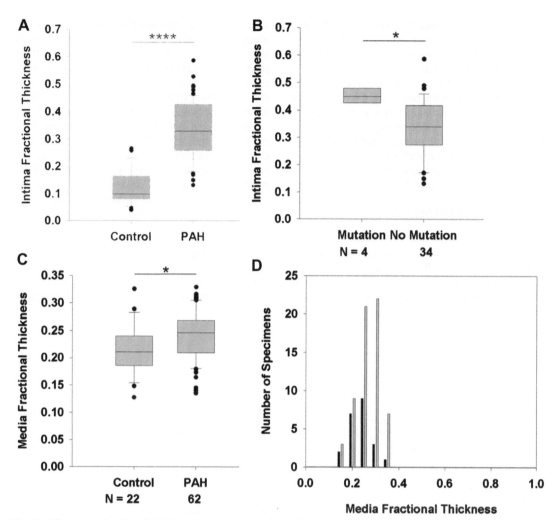

Fig. 8. (A) Intima fractional thickness in control and PAH lungs. (B) Intima fractional thickness in PAH lungs without and with mutations in BMPR2. (C) Media fractional thickness in control and PAH lungs. (D) Distribution of control (black) and PAH (gray) lungs according to medial fractional thickness. (From Stacher E, Graham BB, Hunt JM, et al. Modern age pathology of pulmonary arterial hypertension. Am J Respir Crit Care Med 2012;186:261–72; with permission.)

decreased Smad1/5/8 activity, may result in upregulated transforming growth factor beta (TGF-β) and Smad2/3 signaling, which may be the mechanism for increased remodeling in these patients.[17] These data explain the clinical finding that patients with BMPR II mutations present at a younger age[18] and have more severe clinical disease[19] than those patients without mutations.

MEDIAL REMODELING

Contrary to previously descriptions,[1] pulmonary vascular medial remodeling, although statistically more marked in severe PAH, had a quartile distribution largely within the range seen in normal lungs (see Fig. 8C, D).[3] This finding raises the

possibility that the current treatments for PAH,[20] which extend survival and improve overall morbidity of the disease, may do it by promoting regression of medial remodeling. Given that all patients had advance disease, the lack of pronounced medial remodeling in PAH may suggest that these therapies cannot halt the intimal lesions, and therefore may be unable to prevent the development of severe disease. An alternative explanation consists of a potential effect of therapies in a subgroup of patients with treatment-responsive disease (not on the transplant list). As patients become terminal with advanced disease, the spectrum of pulmonary vascular remodeling becomes more uniform. However, we do not have access to historical lung samples from patients who never received medical treatment of PH and were processed with a similar protocol to ours, to address whether this could be an effect of therapeutic interventions.

Given the unclear impact of medial remodeling, proper elucidation of the potential role for smooth muscle cells in remodeling requires the integration of molecular phenotyping coupled with structural stereological analysis. Notwithstanding these challenges, the combination of intimal and medial remodeling correlated with mean PA pressures (mPAPs) and PVR (**Fig. 9**).

ADVENTITIAL REMODELING

Early studies showed that adventitia thickening was also part of the remodeling spectrum seen in patients with IPAH.[1] It is difficult to define the exact boundaries of the adventitia because it blends with the peribronchiolar connective tissue;

the only clear demarcating landmark is the abrupt interface with the teetered alveolar septa. Using an arbitrary criterion based on the projection of this boundary to the transition region between the vessel and the accompanying airway, we did not find differences in adventitia fractional thickness between controls and PAH lungs.[3]

However, as discussed later, adventitia fibroblasts and the adventitia microenvironment may provide important signaling cues leading to pulmonary vascular remodeling, particularly those involving perivascular inflammation[21] and the potential for formation of tertiary lymphoid follicles in the context of a possible autoimmune component to the disease.[22]

VEINS IN PAH

The understanding of pulmonary vein remodeling in arterial and venous forms of PAH has lagged

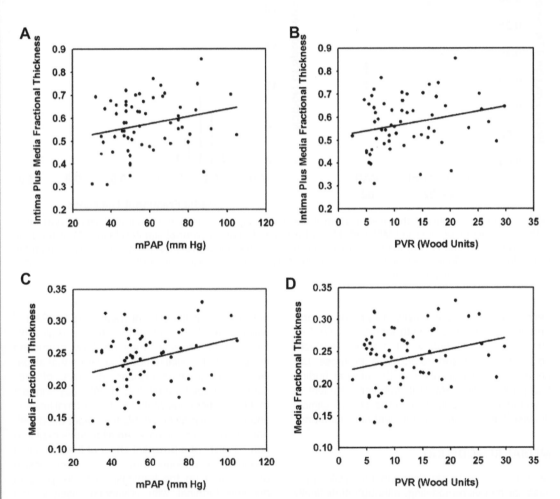

Fig. 9. Correlation between intima plus medial (*A, B*) and medial (*C, D*) fractional thickness with mPAP (*A, C*) and PVR (*B, D*). (*From* Stacher E, Graham BB, Hunt JM, et al. Modern age pathology of pulmonary arterial hypertension. Am J Respir Crit Care Med 2012;186:261–72; with permission.)

behind the focus on pulmonary arterial changes. This limitation is compounded by the lack of specific venous markers, therefore requiring architectural landmarks (ie, location in interlobular septa) for the proper identification of pulmonary veins. Despite these limitations, we investigated the degree of pulmonary vein remodeling when veins were identified in interlobular septa. We did not find any significant evidence of remodeling when comparing PAH and control lungs. Moreover, no significant correlations were found between venous remodeling and parameters of the intima, media, and number of profiles of plexiform lesions.[3] However, pulmonary vascular remodeling may occur in forms of venous PH associated with left heart disease, as we have noted in unpublished ongoing studies.

INFLAMMATION IN PAH

The inflammatory angle in PH has become a promising area of investigation in PAH. Earlier studies have delineated the presence of inflammatory cells around the vascular lesions in PAH.[12,22] These studies identified a mixed population of inflammatory cells, including macrophages, T cells, B cells, and mast cells. The potential importance of lung (interstitial and perivascular) inflammation was recently underscored by our finding that perivascular inflammation is more pronounced in PAH lungs and that it correlates with pulmonary hemodynamics and, more importantly, with intimal, medial, and adventitial remodeling (**Fig. 10**).[3]

More recently, based on a large panel of inflammatory cell markers, a more detailed picture of the types and potential quantities for the different inflammatory cell populations emerged.[23] Higher numbers of cells of the monocyte/macrophage lineage, mast cells, and T-cell and B-cell profiles were detected around IPAH arteries compared with control vessels. Consistent with an exaggerated acquired immunologic response in IPAH, T regulatory cells were decreased around remodeled pulmonary arteries. The aggregate of these findings supports the concept of deregulated immunity or frank autoimmunity in both IPAH and APAH associated with collagen vascular disease.

The concept of an autoimmune[24] and inflammatory component to PH is supported by the presence of autoantibodies in patients with IPAH,[25] the immunologic basis of collagen vascular diseases,[26] and the presence of markers of inflammation systemically in patients with IPAH.[27,28] The recent documentation of the presence of tertiary lymphoid follicles in lungs of patients with IPAH provides further evidence of underlying immune dysregulation in PAH.[22] It is unclear whether the finding of tertiary follicles represents a general feature of PAH because we were not able to find these structures in the PHBI samples, despite some samples having marked interstitial inflammation. Also unresolved is the precise pathogenetic role of innate and acquired immunity in PAH, particularly with regard to whether they play roles in disease initiation and/or progression, rather than representing irrelevant bystanders or even a protective compensatory response.

METHODOLOGICAL APPROACHES TO SAMPLING

More than 100 years after formal recognition of PAH, a stringent stereological analysis of the key lesions in PAH remains lacking. All published pathologic studies in this area have biases: even involuntary biases or the superficially compelling nature of the results does not mitigate the limitations that these errors impose on understanding of the disease. These errors have occurred in multiple stages of the analytical process, most importantly related to sampling. Lung sampling is often not supported by experimental approaches that incorporate designed uniform, random analysis, intended to give all regions or structures an equal chance of being analyzed. Moreover, the extent of sampling is not supported by variability among individuals for a given structural parameter and error of the analytical method, but rather by an arbitrary approach, which is largely validated by the quality of the data. This argument is common but

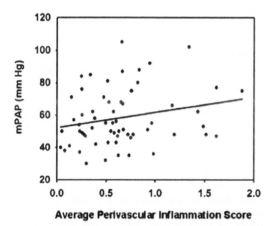

Fig. 10. Correlation between mPAP with average perivascular inflammation score. (*From* Stacher E, Graham BB, Hunt JM, et al. Modern age pathology of pulmonary arterial hypertension. Am J Respir Crit Care Med 2012;186:261–72; with permission.)

flawed, and is used by investigators to avoid complying with recommended stereological guidelines; this is compounded by a lack of understanding of the importance of stereology to measure key events in two-dimensional sections.

Fundamental questions related to distribution of pulmonary vascular lesions along the pulmonary vascular tree, described in detail earlier, their impact on the overall surface area of the lumen of the pulmonary arteries, and the distribution of specific signaling events among the cells involved in PAH cannot be accurately addressed or validated until stringent stereology is applied to the analysis of lungs with the disease. Even our recently reported systematic approach to sampling in the PHBI does not overcome these important limitations.

Recent reviews in lung stereology[29] and societal professional recommendations and guidelines[30] provide a much-needed framework to guide the implementation of these approaches. Rather than parameters of media percent thickness or percentage of muscularized vessels, meaningful end points of volume density of intima lesions in relation to luminal volume or length of vessel segments, blood vessel volume and relation between surface area of intima or media in relation to the length of pulmonary arteries, or total length of pulmonary arteries provide solid parameters of the degree of pulmonary vascular disease. In summary, stereological parameters similar to those that were inferred for the normal lung based on the casting studies described earlier[4,5] are required to better understand the morphologic impact of the different forms of pulmonary vascular remodeling. It is perhaps by the use of standardized stereological approaches that it may be possible to test unambiguously whether there is true vascular dropout in PAH, as suggested by the decrease in peripheral haziness in angiographic studies.

RELEVANCE OF ANIMAL MODELS

A detailed review of animal models in PAH research is beyond the scope of this article. However, the recognition of their strengths and weaknesses depends on the extent that these models are used to answer key questions related to human disease. The phenotype of an ideal animal model would involve integrated intimal and medial remodeling in the setting of almost systemic levels of PA pressures. Moreover, this phenotype would be triggered by causally relevant processes, referenced to human disease. Although mice are amenable to elegant genetic gain and loss of

function manipulations, they do not fulfill these requirements. In the mouse, PH is usually mild and triggered by hypoxia[31] or it develops spontaneously in the setting of transgenic overexpression of a pathologic mediator (eg, interleukin-6[32] or loss of a vasodilator agent, like endothelial-derived nitric oxide[33]). There are clear advantages of using mice lacking key genes (eg, Smad 2 and 3, which mediate TGF-β signaling) in signaling pathways that display close resemblance to key features in humans, like the model of PH caused by the parasite *Schistosoma mansoni*,[34,35] particularly when the key findings are supported by parallel human studies.

In distinction to mice, rats develop more robust pulmonary hemodynamics and remodeling in the setting of PH. Normal pulmonary arteries in rats have similarities to those in the human, but with shorter vascular segments.[36] The muscular arteries extend down to 70 μm in diameter. Between 50 and 150 μm in diameter, pulmonary arteries are partly muscularized; the largest nonmuscular segments are 100 μm in diameter. The percent medial thickness ranges from 6.23 percent in arteries of 0 to 50 μm to 1.36 percent in segments of greater than 1000 μm in diameter.[36] The monocrotaline model is characterized by a predominant medial remodeling allied to interstitial inflammation.[37] These characteristics may explain the numerous reports of reversibility of this model to several pharmacologic interventions. Given that these models do not accurately reproduce the characteristics of human PAH, investigators have explored alternative models that can reflect key aspects of the human disease.

Two rodent models have fulfilled some of these requirements regarding a potential relevance to the human disease. The combination of monocrotaline and pneumectomy introduces the element of enhanced shear stress, which causes a pronounced intimal and medial remodeling when superimposed with cellular injury caused by monocrotaline.[38] However, because of its technical difficulties, this model has been used sparsely, which has resulted in limited insights into the underlying molecular pathophysiology of severe PH in this model. An alternative model that has emerged in the past 10 years combines SU5416 with chronic hypoxia.[39] This model was the first to develop lesions similar to plexiform lesions early in the disease process, with suprasystemic pulmonary hemodynamics in almost 100% of treated rats. The model provided the first documentation that early endothelial cell death contributes mechanistically to the severity of PH and characteristic pulmonary features. The model remained unnoticed until observations were conducted on rats in which the disease was allowed to progress for an additional 4 weeks, revealing the development of intimal lesions closely resembling those in humans.[40] However, like the model combining monocrotaline and pneumectomy, it is still not known whether there is a molecular resemblance between human PAH and rats with severe PH caused by SU5416 and chronic hypoxia. It is therefore predictable that many interventions that may be beneficial in the model may not relate to outcome in the human disease. To overcome these pitfalls, it is critical that modeling studies be validated by concomitant investigations using relevant human tissues and cells.

In addition, experimental evidence revealed that macaques infected with simian immunodeficiency virus develop pulmonary vascular remodeling similar to that seen in patients infected with human immunodeficiency virus.[9,41] Although these are notable observations of potentially high impact, the limitations of using a nonhuman primate experimental system are significant and restrictive to most investigators.

SUMMARY

The ultimate article in detailing the pathology of PH remains to be written. Despite the contributions brought about by initiatives like the PHBI, knowledge of the relationship between pulmonary vascular disorders and human disease remains restricted by a lack of stereological validation. Although insights have been gained into how the integrated intimal and medial remodeling relates to pulmonary hemodynamics in the modern age of PAH-specific therapy, it is not known whether more than 1 lesion per vascular segment occurs in PAH lungs and how this distribution relates to clinical outcome. Moreover, it is unclear how specific pathways (shown by expression studies using diseased human lungs) underlie specific forms and sites of pulmonary vascular remodeling: focal and variable findings tend to be generalized as pertaining to the entire pulmonary circulation. A further investigational goal would be to model three-dimensionally (like an angiogram) the compromised pulmonary circulation in PAH. Computational algorithms that cross over between stereological and structural vascular modeling are needed for a better understanding of the impact of pulmonary vascular remodeling on flow patterns, forming the basis for future functional pulmonary vascular imaging studies.

REFERENCES

1. Chazova I, Loyd JE, Newman JH, et al. Pulmonary artery adventitial changes and venous involvement in primary pulmonary hypertension. Am J Pathol 1995;146:389–97.

2. Voelkel NF, Clarke WR, Higenbottam T. Obesity, dexfenfluramine, and pulmonary hypertension. A lesson not learned. Am J Respir Crit Care Med 1997;155:786–8.

3. Stacher E, Graham BB, Hunt JM, et al. Modern age pathology of pulmonary arterial hypertension. Am J Respir Crit Care Med 2012;186:261–72.

4. Horsfield K. Morphometry of the small pulmonary arteries in man. Circ Res 1978;42:593–7.

5. Huang W, Yen RT, McLaurine M, et al. Morphometry of the human pulmonary vasculature. J Appl Physiol 1996;81:2123–33.

6. Hislop A, Reid L. Intra-pulmonary arterial development during fetal life-branching pattern and structure. J Anat 1972;113:35–48.

7. Tuder RM, Groshong SD, Cool CD. General features of non-neoplastic lung diseases. In: Mason RJ, Broaddus VC, Martin TR, et al, editors. Murray & Nadel's textbook of respiratory medicine. 5th edition. Philadelphia: Saunders; 2009. p. 314–29.

8. Peinado VI, Barbera JA, Abate P, et al. Inflammatory reaction in pulmonary muscular arteries of patients with mild chronic obstructive pulmonary disease. Am J Respir Crit Care Med 1999;159:1605–11.

9. Tuder RM, Marecki JC, Richter A, et al. Pathology of pulmonary hypertension. Clin Chest Med 2007;28:23–42, vii.

10. Tuder RM, Groves BM, Badesch DB, et al. Exuberant endothelial cell growth and elements of inflammation are present in plexiform lesions of pulmonary hypertension. Am J Pathol 1994;144:275–85.

11. Cool CD, Stewart JS, Werahera P, et al. Three-dimensional reconstruction of pulmonary arteries in plexiform pulmonary hypertension using cell specific markers: evidence for a dynamic and heterogeneous process of pulmonary endothelial cell growth. Am J Pathol 1999;155:411–9.

12. Smith P, Heath D. Electron microscopy of the plexiform lesion. Thorax 1979;34:177–86.

13. Tuder RM, Chacon M, Alger LA, et al. Expression of angiogenesis-related molecules in plexiform lesions in severe pulmonary hypertension: evidence for a process of disordered angiogenesis. J Pathol 2001;195:367–74.

14. Howard CV, Reed MG. Unbiased stereology. Liverpool (United Kingdom): QTP Publications; 2010.

15. Nicolls MR, Mizuno S, Taraseviciene-Stewart L, et al. New models of pulmonary hypertension based on

VEGF receptor blockade-induced endothelial cell apoptosis. Pulm Circ 2012;2:434–42.

16. Teichert-Kuliszewska K, Kutryk MJ, Kuliszewski MA, et al. Bone morphogenetic protein receptor-2 signaling promotes pulmonary arterial endothelial cell survival: implications for loss-of-function mutations in the pathogenesis of pulmonary hypertension. Circ Res 2006;98:209–17.

17. Yang X, Long L, Southwood M, et al. Dysfunctional Smad signaling contributes to abnormal smooth muscle cell proliferation in familial pulmonary arterial hypertension. Circ Res 2005;96:1053–63.

18. Austin ED, Phillips JA, Cogan JD, et al. Truncating and missense BMPR2 mutations differentially affect the severity of heritable pulmonary arterial hypertension. Respir Res 2009;10:87.

19. Girerd B, Montani D, Eyries M, et al. Absence of influence of gender and BMPR2 mutation type on clinical phenotypes of pulmonary arterial hypertension. Respir Res 2010;11:73.

20. Humbert M, Sitbon O, Simonneau G. Treatment of pulmonary arterial hypertension. N Engl J Med 2004;351:1425–36.

21. Davie NJ, Gerasimovskaya EV, Hofmeister SE, et al. Pulmonary artery adventitial fibroblasts cooperate with vasa vasorum endothelial cells to regulate vasa vasorum neovascularization–A process mediated by hypoxia and endothelin-1. Am J Pathol 2006;168:1793–807.

22. Perros F, Dorfmuller P, Montani D, et al. Pulmonary lymphoid neogenesis in idiopathic pulmonary arterial hypertension. Am J Respir Crit Care Med 2012; 185:311–21.

23. Savai R, Pullamsetti SS, Kolbe J, et al. Immune and inflammatory cell involvement in the pathology of idiopathic pulmonary arterial hypertension. Am J Respir Crit Care Med 2012;186:897–908.

24. Mouthon L, Guillevin L, Humbert M. Pulmonary arterial hypertension: an autoimmune disease? Eur Respir J 2005;26:986–8.

25. Hassoun PM, Mouthon L, Barbera JA, et al. Inflammation, growth factors, and pulmonary vascular remodeling. J Am Coll Cardiol 2009;54:S10–9.

26. Dib H, Tamby MC, Bussone G, et al. Targets of anti-endothelial cell antibodies in pulmonary hypertension and scleroderma. Eur Respir J 2011;39(6): 1405–14.

27. Dorfmuller P, Perros F, Balabanian K, et al. Inflammation in pulmonary arterial hypertension. Eur Respir J 2003;22:358–63.

28. Soon E, Holmes AM, Treacy CM, et al. Elevated levels of inflammatory cytokines predict survival in idiopathic and familial pulmonary arterial hypertension. Circulation 2010;122:920–7.

29. Muehlfeld C, Ochs M. Quantitative microscopy of the lung-a problem-based approach. Part 2: stereological parameters and study designs in various diseases of the respiratory tract. Am J Physiol Lung Cell Mol Physiol 2013;305(3):L205–21.

30. Hsia CC, Hyde DM, Ochs M, et al. An official research policy statement of the American Thoracic Society/European Respiratory Society: standards for quantitative assessment of lung structure. Am J Respir Crit Care Med 2010;181:394–418.

31. Voelkel NF, Tuder RM. Hypoxia-induced pulmonary vascular remodeling–A model for what human disease? J Clin Invest 2000;106:733–8.

32. Steiner MK, Syrkina OL, Kolliputi N, et al. Interleukin-6 overexpression induces pulmonary hypertension. Circ Res 2009;104:236–44.

33. Fagan KA, Fouty BW, Tyler RC, et al. The pulmonary circulation of mice with either homozygous or heterozygous disruption of endothelial nitric oxide synthase is hyperresponsive to chronic mild hypoxia. J Clin Invest 1998;103:291–9.

34. Crosby A, Jones FM, Southwood M, et al. Pulmonary vascular remodeling correlates with lung eggs and cytokines in murine schistosomiasis. Am J Respir Crit Care Med 2010;181:279–88.

35. Graham BB, Mentink-Kane MM, El-Haddad H, et al. Schistosomiasis-induced experimental pulmonary hypertension: role of interleukin-13 signaling. Am J Pathol 2010;177:1549–61.

36. Hislop A, Reid L. Normal structure and dimensions of the pulmonary arteries in the rat. J Anat 1978; 125:71–83.

37. Carillo L, Aviado DM. Monocrotaline-induced pulmonary hypertension. Lab Invest 1968;20: 243–8.

38. Tanaka Y, Schuster DP, Davis EC, et al. The role of vascular injury and hemodynamics in rat pulmonary artery remodeling. J Clin Invest 1996;98:434–42.

39. Taraseviciene-Stewart L, Kasahara Y, Alger L, et al. Inhibition of the VEGF receptor 2 combined with chronic hypoxia causes cell death-dependent pulmonary endothelial cell proliferation and severe pulmonary hypertension. Faseb J 2001;15:427–38.

40. Abe K, Toba M, Alzoubi A, et al. Formation of plexiform lesions in experimental severe pulmonary arterial hypertension. Circulation 2010;121:2747–54.

41. Marecki JC, Cool CD, Parr JE, et al. HIV-1 Nef is associated with complex pulmonary vascular lesions in SHIV-nef-infected macaques. Am J Respir Crit Care Med 2006;174:437–45.

Genetics of Pulmonary Arterial Hypertension

C. Gregory Elliott, MD[a,b,*]

KEYWORDS

- Genetics • Pulmonary arterial hypertension • Bone morphogenetic protein receptor
- Voltage gated potassium channel • Activin-like kinase receptor • Endoglin • Caveolin • SMAD9

KEY POINTS

- Painstaking research led to the discovery of gene mutations responsible for heritable forms of pulmonary arterial hypertension (PAH).
- Mutations in the gene *BMPR2*, which codes for a cell surface receptor (BMPRII), cause approximately 80% of heritable cases of PAH.
- Less commonly mutations in *ALK1*, *CAV1*, *ENG*, and *SMAD9*, and newly discovered mutations in *KCNK3*, cause heritable PAH.
- Other family members of many patients diagnosed with idiopathic PAH may be diagnosed with PAH.
- Genetic counseling and testing are appropriate for patients diagnosed with heritable or idiopathic PAH.

PULMONARY ARTERIAL HYPERTENSION

Pulmonary arterial hypertension (PAH) is an uncommon disorder with significant morbidity and mortality. The natural history of PAH includes increasing pulmonary vascular resistance (PVR), leading to death from progressive right ventricular failure.[1] Effective treatment of PAH is available, although no therapy provides a cure.

PAH is ultimately a clinical diagnosis that cannot be made accurately without hemodynamic measurements from pulmonary artery catheterization. The current consensus hemodynamic criteria needed to diagnose PAH include mean pulmonary artery pressure (mPAP) of 25 mm Hg or more and pulmonary capillary wedge pressure of 15 mm Hg or less. Some consensus groups have advocated inclusion of PVR greater than 3 Wood units,[2] although the authors of the 4th World Symposium on Pulmonary Hypertension recommended against inclusion of PVR.[3] At the time of pulmonary artery catheterization, a reduction in mPAP of at least 10 mm Hg to an absolute mPAP of 40 mm Hg or less with a preserved or increased cardiac output[4,5] identifies a small subgroup of patients who have an excellent prognosis when treated with high doses of calcium channel blockers, such as nifedipine.[6,7] An article elsewhere in this issue discusses specific therapies for PAH.

The most recent clinical classification of pulmonary hypertension includes 5 major diagnostic groups, with group 1 encompassing PAH. Within

Funding: None.

Disclosure: Dr C.G. Elliott is employed by Intermountain Healthcare (IHC Health Services, Inc.). In the past 12 months IHC Health Services, Inc. has received compensation for clinical trial contracts (on which Dr C.G. Elliott is the Principal Investigator) from Actelion, Gilead, and United Therapeutics. Dr C.G. Elliott is currently the Principal Investigator on an Intermountain Medical and Research Foundation grant.

[a] Department of Medicine, Intermountain Medical Center, 5121 South Cottonwood Street, Suite 307, Murray, UT 84107, USA; [b] Department of Internal Medicine, University of Utah School of Medicine, 30 N. 1900 E, Salt Lake City, UT 84132, USA

* Department of Medicine, Intermountain Medical Center, 5121 South Cottonwood Street, Suite 307, Murray, UT 84107.

E-mail address: greg.elliott@imail.org

group 1 PAH, the diagnoses may include idiopathic PAH (IPAH), formerly referred to as *primary pulmonary hypertension* (PPH); heritable PAH (HPAH); and PAH associated (APAH) with a variety of circumstances (eg, drug and toxin exposures, congenital heart diseases, connective tissue diseases, portal hypertension, or human immunodeficiency virus [HIV] infection).[8] The 4th World Symposium on Pulmonary Hypertension revised group 1 PAH to include the subcategory HPAH. This subcategory includes patients with PAH who have either more than one family member diagnosed with PAH or an identifiable mutation known to cause PAH.[9–11]

FAMILY PEDIGREES
Autosomal Dominant Inheritance

Dresdale and colleagues[12] first described PPH affecting a family in 1954, when they reported PPH in a mother, her sister, and her son. In 1984, Loyd and colleagues[13] described 14 families with 2 or more members affected by PPH (**Fig. 1**). Vertical transmission was seen between generations in 10 of these 14 families. Furthermore, examples were seen of disease transmission from a father to a son, and a grandfather to a granddaughter through a father, which excluded X-linked inheritance. These pedigrees suggested an autosomal dominant mode of inheritance.

Incomplete Penetrance

The transmission of PPH through 9 individuals who were without evidence of PPH was another important observation from the pedigrees assembled by Loyd and colleagues.[13] These obligate carriers of a disease-causing gene suggested that incomplete penetrance also characterized familial PPH. Currently, the lifetime risk of developing PAH seems to be approximately 27% for carriers of disease-causing mutations.[14] The penetrance of HPAH for women (approximately 42%) is much higher than the penetrance of HPAH for men (approximately 14%).

The incomplete penetrance of HPAH is not well understood. The only clear predilection for the development of HPAH within families is female sex. The idea of a second hit is a popular concept that is not unlike that implicated in the development of many malignancies. The concept suggests that interplay between a genetic predisposition and either an environmental stimulus or another genetic factor leads to clinical expression of the disease.

Variable Age of Onset

In 1995, Loyd and colleagues[15] reported genetic anticipation in an analysis of 24 families affected by PPH. The investigators noted earlier onset of more severe disease in successive generations.[13]

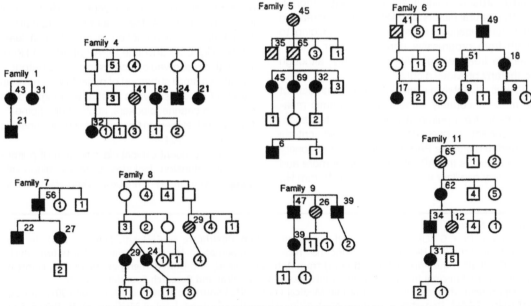

Fig. 1. Drs Jim Loyd and John Newman of Vanderbilt University assembled these family pedigrees. Their careful work showed an autosomal dominant pattern of inheritance, variable age of disease onset, female predominance, and incomplete penetrance of the heritable factor, so that a carrier of a disease-causing mutation did not develop PAH. (*Reprinted* with permission of the American Thoracic Society. Copyright © 2013 American Thoracic Society. *From* Loyd J, Butler M, Foroud T, et al. Genetic anticipation and abnormal gender ratio at birth in familial primary pulmonary hypertension. Am J Respir Crit Care Med 1995;152:93–7. Official journal of the American Thoracic Society.)

It seemed that family members affected with PPH in each successive generation had a life expectancy approximately 10 years shorter than the previous generation. This observation suggested that trinucleotide repeat amplification may occur in familial PPH. However, investigators recently reported a new analysis of 53 families in which they limited the effects of shorter durations of follow-up.[14] They found no evidence of genetic anticipation when they limited cases to those patients with 57 years of follow-up. The age of disease onset can vary widely among those who develop HPAH, although more than 90% of patients with HPAH seem to manifest PAH by age 57 years.

Common Ancestry

Investigators also considered the possibility that many patients diagnosed with sporadic PPH may have unrecognized familial PPH.[13,16] A study of 7 patients with sporadic PPH identified in Utah as part of the National Institutes of Health PPH registry identified coancestry that was unlikely a chance occurrence (**Fig. 2**).[17] A subsequent report uncovered a kindred affected by PPH that spanned 7 generations and involved 5 subfamilies initially not known to be related.[18] The kindred included 12 affected members who were initially thought to have sporadic PPH, and 7 affected members whose conditions were first misdiagnosed as other cardiopulmonary diseases.

DISEASE-CAUSING MUTATIONS
Bone Morphogenetic Protein Receptor Type II Gene Mutations

Investigators at Vanderbilt University and Columbia University assembled familial PPH pedigrees, identified affected and unaffected individuals, and collected DNA samples. By the 1990s these investigators had stored enough DNA samples to provide the power to search for a familial PPH locus. In 1997, 2 independent research teams performed linkage studies using microsatellite DNA probes and identified a PPH gene locus on chromosome 2q31–32 (**Fig. 3**).[19,20] Three years later, the same teams of investigators discovered mutations in a gene within this chromosomal locus among familial cases of PPH. The gene (*BMPR2*) encoded bone morphogenetic protein receptor type II (BMPRII), a member of the transforming growth factor (TGF)-β superfamily of receptors.[9,10] BMPRII consisted of 4 functional domains; an N-terminal ligand binding domain, a single transmembrane region, a serine/threonine kinase, and a cytoplasmic domain (**Fig. 4**). BMPRII functioned as a receptor for a group of cytokines known as bone morphogenetic proteins (BMPs). BMPs have many functions, ranging from facilitating ectopic bone and cartilage formation to regulating mammalian development.[21] BMP signaling pathways impacted cellular function in a tissue-specific manner. Within the pulmonary circulation, the BMPRII pathway seems to inhibit cellular

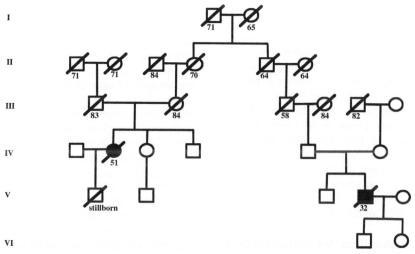

Fig. 2. Many patients diagnosed with idiopathic PAH have heritable PAH when extensive pedigree analysis or genetic testing is available. Both patients with PAH in this pedigree were diagnosed initially with IPAH. Incomplete penetrance and incomplete family histories obscured the heritable nature of their PAH. In an era of effective therapies, genetic counseling and testing of patients diagnosed with IPAH seems justified to detect HPAH and to provide optimal care for other family members who may develop PAH. (*From* Elliott CG, Alexander G, Leppert M, et al. Coancestry in apparently sporadic primary pulmonary hypertension. Chest 1995;108:973–7; with permission.)

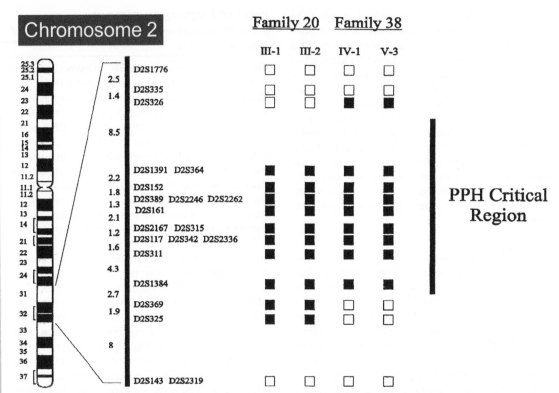

Fig. 3. Linkage data using microsatellite probes and DNA samples from 2 informative families narrowed the search for a gene that caused familial primary pulmonary hypertension (PPH) to an approximate 25 cM region on the long arm of chromosome 2 (2q31–33). (*From* Nichols WC, Koller DL, Foroud T, et al. Localization of the gene for familial primary pulmonary hypertension to chromosome 2q31-32. Nat Genet 1997;15(3):277–80; with permission.)

proliferation, especially within small pulmonary arterioles.[22]

BMPR2 Mutations in IPAH

Soon after the discovery that *BMPR2* mutations caused most familial PPH, investigators discovered novel heterozygous *BMPR2* mutations in 13 of 50 patients diagnosed with sporadic PPH (IPAH), suggesting a common genetic pathway in both familial and many sporadic cases of PPH (now IPAH).[23] Analysis of parental DNA samples showed that some parents were unaffected obligate carriers of *BMPR2* mutations and in other cases the *BMPR2* mutations were spontaneous.[23,24] Currently, 10% to 40% of patients with IPAH reportedly have a detectable *BMPR2* mutation.[23,25,26]

Some BMPR2 Mutations Are Missed by DNA Sequencing

Early studies identified *BMPR2* mutations in only one-half of the families affected by PPH.[24] However these studies were based on gene sequencing methods that were unable to detect *BMPR2* rearrangements and deletions. In 2005, Cogan and colleagues[27] reported that approximately 33% of families with PAH without *BMPR2* mutations detected by sequence analysis had exon deletions or duplications in the *BMPR2* gene. This study illustrated the limitations of solely performing DNA sequencing, and, as a result, mRNA analysis by reverse-transcriptase polymerase chain reaction and analysis of exon dose across the entire gene, using multiplex ligation-dependent probe amplification, were incorporated into PAH genetic testing protocols. Through including this methodology, laboratories were able to detect large gene rearrangements and further increase the sensitivity of the test, such that defects in *BMPR2* accounted for more than 70% of families affected with PAH, making *BMPR2* mutations the major genetic determinant of HPAH. Even with these discoveries, a genetic abnormality could not be identified in approximately 20% of families affected by PAH.[25,28]

BMPR2 Mutations Are Widespread and Diverse, and May Guide Effective Interventions

Investigators around the world have identified more than 500 mutations throughout the *BMPR2*

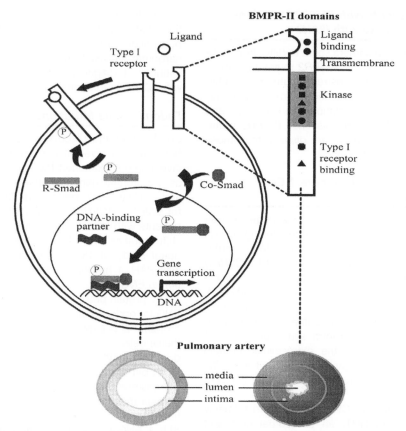

Fig. 4. Bone morphogenetic protein receptor type II (BMPRII), a member of the TGF-β superfamily of receptors, consists of 4 functional domains: (1) an *N*-terminal ligand binding domain, (2) a single transmembrane region, (3) a serine/threonine kinase, and (4) a cytoplasmic domain. BMPRII functioned as a receptor for a group of ligands known as *bone morphogenetic proteins* (BMPs). BMPs have many functions, ranging from facilitating ectopic bone and cartilage formation, to regulating mammalian development. BMP signaling pathways impact cellular function in a tissue-specific manner. Within the pulmonary circulation, the BMPRII pathway seems to inhibit cellular proliferation, especially within small pulmonary arterioles. (*From* Thomson JR, Machado RD, Pauciulo MW, et al. Sporadic primary pulmonary hypertension is associated with germline mutations of the gene encoding BMPR-II, a receptor member of the TGF-beta family. J Med Genet 2000;37:741–5; with permission.)

gene.[22] All types of mutations have been described, with approximately two-thirds of the mutations predicting premature truncation of the protein. In one large survey, Machado[22] reported that 29% of the premature truncation mutations were nonsense mutations, 24% were frame-shift mutations, 9% were splice-site mutations, and 6% were duplication/deletion mutations. In addition, the 5′-untranslated promoter region of *BMPR2*, which regulates transcription, may contain pathogenic mutations.[29] Regardless of the mutation site or the type of mutation, a common end result seems to be haploinsufficiency of the BMPRII signaling pathway through the process of nonsense-mediated decay,[27,28] and failure of antiproliferative effects within the pulmonary vasculature.[24,30] Some *BMPR2* mutations seem to act in a dominant negative manner and impair trafficking of the mutated BMPRII receptor to the cell surface.[31] Understanding these molecular mechanisms may allow the introduction of therapies that are targeted to the molecular pathogenesis of PAH.

BMPR2 Mutations Cause Cellular Dysfunction Beyond the Pulmonary Circulation

Investigators have also suggested that *BMPR2* mutations cause cellular dysfunction beyond the pulmonary vasculature.[32] BMPRII regulates steroid hormone trafficking, and mutations in *BMPR2* may lead to alterations in energy metabolism. For example, *BMPR2* mutant mice are insulin-resistant.[32]

How Do Patients with BMPR2 Mutations Differ from Those with IPAH?

BMPR2 mutation carriers seem to differ from non-carriers with IPAH.[33–35] BMPR2 mutation carriers are less likely to demonstrate acute vasoreactivity.[33,34,36,37] BMPR2 mutation carriers also may have reduced transplantation-free survival,[34] and patients with PAH with missense BMPR2 mutations may have more severe disease than those with truncating mutations.[38]

Activin Receptor–Like Kinase-1 Gene Mutations

In 2001, investigators identified 2 large families affected by hereditary hemorrhagic telangiectasia (HHT) and PAH.[11] The investigators found mutations in a gene on chromosome 12q13 (ACVRL1) that coded for a serine/threonine protein kinase receptor, activin receptor–like kinase 1 (ALK-1). ALK-1 protein is composed of 3 main functional domains: an extracellular domain, a transmembrane domain, and an intracellular domain.[39–41] In the wild-type cell, the extracellular domain mainly functions in ligand binding, but it is also involved in complex formation with type II TGF-β receptor (TRβII).[39,41,42]

Mutations in the ACVRL1 gene were primarily associated with HHT, an autosomal dominant vascular dysplasia characterized by the presence of arteriovenous malformations, recurrent epistaxis, gastrointestinal bleeding, and mucocutaneous telangiectasias.[43,44] Although more than 100 ACVRL1 mutations have been described that result in the development of HHT, only a few ACVRL1 mutations have been associated with PAH.[11,22,44–46] Most ACVRL1 mutations associated with PAH are missense mutations that occur in ALK-1 functional domains (ie, the kinase domain).[22] Functional studies using ALK-1 mutant constructs suggest that disruption of receptor complex trafficking is the primary cause of the vascular phenotype observed in these patients.[44,46]

Although ACVRL1 mutations are relatively rare, the role of ACVRL1 mutations in PAH has been the focus of several studies.[11,44–46] In each of these studies it has been noted that the disease onset in ACVRL1 mutation carriers occurs at a young age and that disease characteristics seem to be severe compared with those in patients with mutation-negative PAH.[11,44–46] Perhaps the most striking findings were reported by Girerd and colleagues[45] who performed ACVRL1 and BMPR2 mutation analysis on 379 of the 388 patients in the French PAH network. They identified 93 patients with PAH with BMPR2 mutations and 9 with ACVRL1 mutations, and 23 additional patients with PAH with ACVRL1 mutations from prior publications. The investigators found that patients harboring ACVRL1 mutations were significantly younger at diagnosis and at death than those with BMPR2 mutations.

Endoglin Gene Mutations

Shortly after the discovery that ACVRL1 mutations were involved in the development of PAH, investigators examined the endoglin gene (ENG) as a potential genetic cause of PAH. Harrison and colleagues[46] performed DNA sequencing for BMPR2, ACVRL1, and ENG in a cohort of 11 patients with HPAH, and showed an ENG frameshift mutation in 2 of the patients.[47] In a subsequent study of 18 children clinically diagnosed with PAH, 1 harbored an intronic splicing mutation in ENG.[44]

The protein produced by ENG is also known as ENG (or endoglin) and is a transmembrane glycoprotein that is expressed predominantly on endothelial cells.[48,49] ENG contains 3 main functional domains: a cytoplasmic domain involved in regulating dimerization and protein trafficking activity, a transmembrane domain, and an extracellular domain that is important in the protein's interactions with other signaling proteins.[48,49] Like ALK-1, ENG is a member of the TGF-β superfamily of receptors that interact with both type I and II TGF-β signaling receptors to control cellular responses to TGF-β.[48] However, unlike many receptors in this superfamily, ENG is not capable of binding a ligand unless it is already bound to a TGF-β signaling receptor.[48] Recently, functional studies have suggested that wild-type ENG is important in angiogenesis, and that ENG mutations likely result in haploinsufficiency. The remaining wild-type protein is not capable of maintaining proper angiogenesis, leading to vascular malformations, inappropriate proliferation of endothelial cells, and the disease phenotype observed in patients with HHT.[50]

Mothers Against Decapentaplegic 9 Gene Mutations

Genes that do not code for TGF-β receptors also cause heritable PAH. Mutations associated with mothers against decapentaplegic 9 (SMAD9) cause a heritable form of PAH.[22,51] The SMAD9 variants are particularly compelling, because these data are supported by the development of clinical and histopathologic features of pulmonary hypertension in a SMAD9 knockout mouse model.[52] Dysfunctional SMAD signaling can affect smooth muscle cell proliferation.[53]

Caveolin Gene Mutations

In 2012 Austin and colleagues[54] used exome sequencing to study a 3-generation family with 6 members affected in an autosomal dominant pattern with PAH, but without known mutations in TGF-β pathway genes. The investigators identified a novel mutation (c.474delA) in a gene, caveolin-1 (CAV1), in 5 of 6 affected family members. An additional CAV1 mutation was identified in a patient diagnosed with IPAH, whereas no mutations were found in 1000 ethnically matched Caucasians. CAV1 encodes a membrane protein of caveolae, which are found in endothelial cells of the lung. Because caveolae are necessary for receptor signaling cascades, such as the TGF-β superfamily, CAV1 mutations may also cause PAH by disrupting TGF-β signals.[55,56]

Acid-Dependent Potassium Channel Gene

In 2013, Ma and colleagues used exome sequencing to study DNA from members of a family affected by PAH who did not have other mutations known to be associated with PAH (eg, BMPR2 mutations).[57] The investigators identified mutations in KCNK3, a gene that codes for an acid-dependent potassium channel (**Fig. 5**). The protein, KCNK3, also called TASK-1, belongs to 2-pore-domain potassium channel family. KCNK3 is expressed in pulmonary artery smooth muscle cells. This channel produces potassium currents that contribute to resting membrane potential. The activity of KCNK3 is strongly dependent on external pH and oxygen tension.

Calcium-activated potassium channels cause vasodilation and activate apoptosis. Dysfunctional potassium channels predictably promote vasoconstriction and cell proliferation.[58]

NEW LOCUS FOR SUSCEPTIBILITY TO PAH IDENTIFIED THROUGH GENOME-WIDE ASSOCIATION ANALYSIS

In 2013, a large consortium of investigators conducted a genome-wide association study on 2 independent populations of patients diagnosed with IPAH or familial PAH (without BMPR2 mutations). These investigators reported an association of PAH with the cerebellin 2 (CBLN2) locus mapping to 18q22.3, with the risk allele conferring an odds ratio for PAH of 1.97.[58] Two single nucleotide polymorphisms, rs2217560 and rs9916909, were in almost complete linkage disequilibrium, and were 52 kB beyond CBLN2. Although CBLN2 encodes a group of secreted neuronal glycoproteins (cerebellin 1–4: CBLN1–CBLN4), the investigators identified increased expression of CBLN2 messenger ribonucleic acid (mRNA) in pulmonary arterial endothelial cells from patients with PAH.[59] This gene locus identifies a new contributor to PAH pathogenesis and a new potential target for therapeutic intervention.

PREVALENCE OF HPAH

The prevalence of HPAH remains unknown. Family histories provide low estimates of the prevalence of HPAH because of small family size, fragmented families, unknown medical histories, incomplete penetrance, and absence of genetic testing.[23,60–62] Twelve of 187 patients (6.4%) had PPH recognized in one or more family members of patients diagnosed with PPH and enrolled in the National

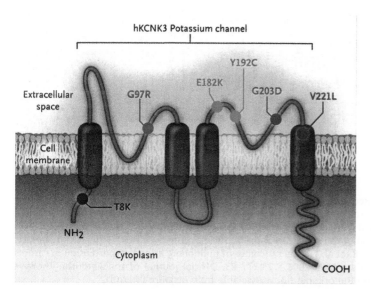

Fig. 5. Mutations in an acid dependent potassium channel gene, KCNK3, represent a newly recognized cause of heritable PAH. Mutations in KCNK3 the substitute amino acids (T8K, G97R, E182K, Y192C, G203D, and V2216) in the hKCNK3 potassium channel. Mutations in genes that regulate TGF-β signaling, especially BMPR2 mutations, cause most cases of HPAH. KCNK3 mutations illustrate the diversity of molecular pathways that may cause the PAH phenotype. (Adapted from Ma L, Roman-Campos D, Austin D, et al. A novel channelopathy in pulmonary arterial hypertension. N Engl J Med 2013;369(4):351–61.)

Institutes of Health PPH registry (ie, they had familial PAH).[60] These results are similar to those found in the French national PAH registry, which reported that 9.0% of 290 enrolled patients without APAH had familial PAH.[61] The REVEAL Registry is the largest registry of World Health Organization diagnostic group 1 PAH patients to date, with 2525 adult patients meeting traditional hemodynamic criteria for PAH. In this registry, investigators identified familial PAH in 5.5% of 1234 patients without APAH.[62] Most (approximately 80%) of patients with HPAH have *BMPR2* mutations.

Many patients with HPAH are misdiagnosed with IPAH in the absence of genetic testing. When genetic tests are performed on patients diagnosed with IPAH, investigators report that 15% to 25% have disease-causing mutations. Sztrymf and colleagues[34] reported that 40 of 195 patients with IPAH had HPAH when they were tested for *BMPR2* mutations (**Fig. 6**). Even this report likely underestimates HPAH prevalence in patients diagnosed with IPAH, because not all causative genes were evaluated (eg, *KCNK3*).

BMPR2 MUTATIONS IN APAH
PAH Associated with Anorexigen Ingestion

The exact mechanism responsible for the development of PAH associated with anorexigen exposure remains unknown. Approximately one in 10,000 people exposed to fenfluramine derivatives developed PAH, leading investigators to hypothesize a link between *BMPR2* mutations and the development of PAH. Humbert and colleagues[63] examined 2 affected sisters and 33 unrelated patients with PAH associated with anorexigen exposure, and found 3 mutations in *BMPR2* that predicted alterations in the BMPRII protein structure in the 33 unrelated cases (9%), and a fourth mutation among the 2 affected sisters. Despite these findings, germline mutations in *BMPR2* did not seem to be sufficiently frequent to confirm that exposure to fenfluramines provided a second hit leading to the development of PAH.

PAH Associated with Congenital Systemic-to-Pulmonary Shunts

TGF-β receptors have pivotal roles in cardiac embryogenesis and vascular development. Roberts and colleagues[64] explored the potential relationship of PAH associated with congenital systemic-to-pulmonary shunts and *BMPR2* mutations in 40 adults and 66 children with PAH associated with congenital heart disease (APAH-CHD), and found *BMPR2* mutations in 6% of these patients. The observed frequency of *BMPR2* mutations in patients with APAH-CHD does not support a causative role for *BMPR2* mutations in APAH-CHD.

PAH Associated with Connective Tissue Diseases, Viral Infection, or Portal Hypertension

PAH is also associated with connective tissue diseases (APAH-CTD), HIV infection, and portal

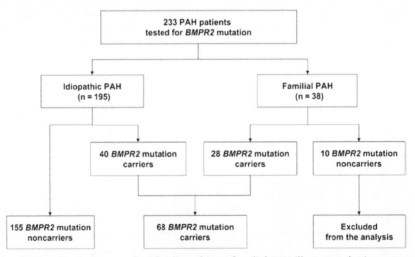

Fig. 6. A study of 233 patients diagnosed with idiopathic or familial PAH illustrates the importance of tests for *BMPR2* point mutations and large gene rearrangements. More patients with heritable disease (*n* = 40) were identified among the 195 patients diagnosed with idiopathic PAH than among patients diagnosed with familial PAH. (*Modified and reprinted* with permission of the American Thoracic Society. Copyright © 2013 American Thoracic Society. *From* Sztrymf B, Coulet F, Girerd B, et al. Clinical outcomes of pulmonary arterial hypertension in carriers of BMPR2 mutation. Am J Respir Crit Care Med 2008;177:1377–83. Official journal of the American Thoracic Society. This modified figure is based on the original figure available from atsjournals.org.)

hypertension. Although approximately 10% of patients with the scleroderma spectrum of disease develop PAH, 2 small studies failed to show *BMPR2* mutations among patients with APAH-CTD.[65,66] Another small study examined PAH associated with HIV infection and also failed to identify *BMPR2* mutations.[67] Furthermore, there are no reports to date of *BMPR2* mutations associated with portopulmonary hypertension. However, investigators have associated portopulmonary hypertension with single nucleotide polymorphisms in genes related to estrogen signaling and cell growth regulation.[68]

Pulmonary Veno-occlusive Disease

Pulmonary veno-occlusive disease (PVOD) is a rare form of pulmonary hypertension characterized by vascular lesions in septal and preseptal pulmonary veins.[69] In 1977 Voordes and colleagues[70] described PVOD in siblings, suggesting the possibility of a heritable disorder. After the discovery that *BMPR2* mutations caused most HPAH, several investigators identified *BMPR2* mutations in patients with PVOD.[22,71,72] As with *BMPR2* mutations in families with PAH, large deletions or gene rearrangements can also be detected in individuals diagnosed with PVOD.[25]

Pulmonary Capillary Hemangiomatosis

Pulmonary capillary hemangiomatosis (PCH) is a rare disease characterized by capillary proliferation.[73] In 1988, Langleben et al described a family affected by PCH.[74] The family pedigree suggested an autosomal recessive pattern of inheritance. In 2013, Best et al used whole exome sequencing to identify novel mutations in Eukaryotic Translation Initiation Factor 2 Alpha Kinase 4 (*EIF2AK4*) in another family affected by PCH as well as 2 of 10 unrelated individuals with sporadic PCH.[75]

GENETIC COUNSELING AND TESTING

Two consensus guidelines recommend that physicians offer professional genetic counseling and genetic testing to patients with a history suggesting HPAH.[2,76] In addition, the authors of these guidelines recommended that patients with IPAH be advised about the availability of genetic testing and counseling because of the possibility that they carry a disease-causing mutation. The guidelines recommend that professionals offer counseling and testing to the affected patient first. The identification of a disease-causing mutation in an affected family member allows less-expensive testing of other family members if they want this testing. Affected individuals and family members

with increased risk for developing PAH may want to know their mutation status for family planning purposes. Prenatal screening is possible, as is preimplantation diagnosis and management.[77]

Physicians and patients with PAH and their family members have not embraced these guidelines for several reasons. First, genetic testing is expensive ($1000–$3000 to analyze the first affected family member; and $300–$500 to test other family members for a known family-specific mutation). Second, the potential psychological impact of either a positive test (anxiety and depression) or a negative test (survivor guilt) dissuades some individuals, and test results may impact other family members who do not wish to know their mutational status. Third, concerns over discrimination remain, despite the passage of the Genetic Information Nondiscrimination Act (GINA, H.R. 493).[78] Although GINA protects against discrimination by insurers and employers, some gaps remain in these protections, such as when applying for life, disability, or long-term insurance, or when employed by a business with fewer than 15 employees.

MONITORING OF ASYMPTOMATIC *BMPR2* MUTATION CARRIERS

Clinical monitoring of asymptomatic *BMPR2* mutation carriers remains an inexact science with respect to which tests to perform and the frequency of testing. The American College of Cardiology Foundation/American Heart Association expert consensus task force on pulmonary hypertension recommended that *BMPR2* mutation carriers undergo annual screening with echocardiography and that a right heart catheterization be performed if an echocardiogram shows evidence of PAH.[2] The American College of Chest Physicians expert consensus group also recommended echocardiography for asymptomatic patients at high risk, without stating at what intervals echocardiography should be repeated.[76]

PHARMACOGENETICS OF PAH

A patient's clinical response to disease-specific therapy is complex, involving the severity of the patient's disease, comorbidities, appropriateness of the prescribed therapy, and patient compliance. For treatment of other disorders, it has been stated that approximately 30% of patients benefit from a given medication, whereas another 30% of patients show no benefit at all. Furthermore, 30% of patients are noncompliant with their medication, and the remaining 10% experience only side effects from the medication.[77] This unpredictable response means that a given therapy has the potential to be ineffective or harmful, or to allow progression of untreated illness. Ideally, medical therapy would be tailored to an individual, with a predictable response that included maximum benefit and no harm.

Pharmacogenetics, the science of effects of single gene variants on drug efficacy and toxicity, and pharmacogenomics, the science of multiple interacting gene variants on drug efficacy and toxicity, both offer the promise of pharmacotherapy uniquely targeted to individual patients.[79] Although physicians have always individualized treatment, physician-investigators hypothesize that knowledge of the patient's genetic characteristics would advance the safety and efficacy of medical therapeutics. An advance such as this would be welcome for physicians who treat PAH, because therapeutic responses and drug toxicities are unpredictable for individual patients.[80]

CALCIUM CHANNEL BLOCKERS AND VASOREACTIVITY

Approximately 10% of patients with IPAH will have a positive acute vasoreactivity test, which predicts a 5-year survival rate of approximately 95% in response to prolonged oral calcium channel blocker therapy.[6,7] Genetic tests may identify patients with HPAH who are not vasoreactive. Elliott and colleagues[36] reported that 3.7% of patients with PAH with a nonsynonymous BMPR2 mutation were vasoreactive compared with 35% of patients without a nonsynonymous BMPR2 mutation. Furthermore, none of the patients with nonsynonymous BMPR2 sequence variations was vasoreactive when the common polymorphism c.2324G>A was excluded. Similar results were found in a cohort of 147 children and adults with IPAH and familial PAH.[37] In addition, Sztrymf and colleagues[34] examined 379 patients with either IPAH or familial PAH. The patients with BMPR2 mutations were unlikely to respond with acute vasoreactivity at diagnostic right heart catheterization. Patients with an ACVRL1 mutation also were not vasoreactive.[45] Thus, the presence of a mutation in the TGF-β superfamily of receptors seems to identify patients with PAH for whom calcium channel blockers would be predicted to be ineffective.

SUMMARY

Over the past 2 decades investigators have identified gene mutations responsible for an inherited predisposition to develop PAH, and characterized HPAH as a disorder typified by earlier onset and more severe hemodynamic impairment. Mutations in BMPR2 and genes that code for other TGF-β receptors cause most instances of HPAH. Recently, using whole exome sequencing, investigators added CAV1 and KCNK3 to the list of genes harboring mutations responsible for HPAH. Investigators also have shown that genetic anticipation is not a feature of HPAH, and that the penetrance of BMPR2 mutations is higher for women than men, suggesting that sex hormones influence the development of this devastating disease.

Finally, opportunities now exist to use knowledge derived from genetic discoveries to advance the management of individuals with HPAH. Soon it may be possible to target the molecular defects that cause HPAH, rather than targeting important pathophysiologic mechanisms such as vasoconstriction.

ACKNOWLEDGMENTS

In the past 12 months, Dr Elliott chaired a steering committee for Ikaria, and served on a Data and Safety Monitoring Board for Actelion.

REFERENCES

1. Rubin LJ. Primary pulmonary hypertension. Chest 1993;104(1):236–50.
2. McLaughlin VV, Archer SL, Badesch DB, et al. ACCF/AHA 2009 expert consensus document on pulmonary hypertension: a report of the American College of Cardiology Foundation Task Force on Expert Consensus Documents and the American Heart Association: developed in collaboration with the American College of Chest Physicians, American Thoracic Society, Inc., and the Pulmonary Hypertension Association. Circulation 2009;119(16):2250–94.
3. Badesch DB, Champion HC, Gomez Sanchez MA, et al. Diagnosis and assessment of pulmonary arterial hypertension. J Am Coll Cardiol 2009;54(Suppl 1):S55–66.
4. Badesch DB, Abman SH, Ahearn GS, et al. Medical therapy for pulmonary arterial hypertension: ACCP evidence-based clinical practice guidelines. Chest 2004;126(Suppl 1):35S–62S.
5. Barst RJ, Gibbs JS, Ghofrani HA, et al. Updated evidence-based treatment algorithm in pulmonary arterial hypertension. J Am Coll Cardiol 2009;54(Suppl 1):S78–84.
6. Rich S, Kaufmann E, Levy PS. The effect of high doses of calcium-channel blockers on survival in primary pulmonary hypertension. N Engl J Med 1992;327(2):76–81.
7. Sitbon O, Humbert M, Jais X, et al. Long-term response to calcium channel blockers in idiopathic pulmonary arterial hypertension. Circulation 2005;111(23):3105–11.

8. Simonneau G, Robbins IM, Beghetti M, et al. Updated clinical classification of pulmonary hypertension. J Am Coll Cardiol 2009;54(Suppl 1):S43–54.

9. Deng Z, Morse JH, Slager SL, et al. Familial primary pulmonary hypertension (gene PPH1) is caused by mutations in the bone morphogenetic protein receptor-II gene. Am J Hum Genet 2000;67(3):737–44.

10. Lane KB, Machado RD, Pauciulo MW, et al. Heterozygous germline mutations in BMPR2, encoding a TGF-beta receptor, cause familial primary pulmonary hypertension. The International PPH Consortium. Nat Genet 2000;26(1):81–4.

11. Trembath RC, Thomson JR, Machado RD, et al. Clinical and molecular genetic features of pulmonary hypertension in patients with hereditary hemorrhagic telangiectasia. N Engl J Med 2001;345(5):325–34.

12. Dresdale DT, Michtom RJ, Schultz M. Recent studies in primary pulmonary hypertension, including pharmacodynamic observations on pulmonary vascular resistance. Bull N Y Acad Med 1954;30(3):195–207.

13. Loyd JE, Primm RK, Newman JH. Familial primary pulmonary hypertension: clinical patterns. Am Rev Respir Dis 1984;129(1):194–7.

14. Larkin EK, Newman JH, Austin ED, et al. Longitudinal analysis casts doubt on the presence of genetic anticipation in heritable pulmonary arterial hypertension. Am J Respir Crit Care Med 2012;186(9):892–6.

15. Loyd J, Butler M, Foroud T, et al. Genetic anticipation and abnormal gender ratio at birth in familial primary pulmonary hypertension. Am J Respir Crit Care Med 1995;152(1):93–7.

16. Newman JH, Loyd JE. Familial pulmonary hypertension. In: Fishman AP, editor. The pulmonary circulation: normal and abnormal. Philadelphia: University of Pennsylvania Press; 1990. p. 301–13.

17. Elliott CG, Alexander G, Leppert M, et al. Coancestry in apparently sporadic primary pulmonary hypertension. Chest 1995;108:973–7.

18. Newman JH, Wheeler L, Lane KB, et al. Mutation in the gene for bone morphogenetic protein receptor ii as a cause of primary pulmonary hypertension in a large kindred. N Engl J Med 2001;345(5):319–24.

19. Nichols WC, Koller DL, Slovis B, et al. Localization of the gene for familial primary pulmonary hypertension to chromosome 2q31-32. Nat Genet 1997;15(3):277–80.

20. Morse JH, Jones AC, Barst RJ, et al. Mapping of familial primary pulmonary hypertension locus (PPH1) to chromosome 2q31-q32. Circulation 1997;95(12):2603–6.

21. De Caestecker M, Meyrick B. Bone morphogenetic proteins, genetics and the pathophysiology of primary pulmonary hypertension. Respir Res 2001;2(4):193–7.

22. Machado RD, Eickelberg O, Elliott CG, et al. Genetics and genomics of pulmonary arterial hypertension. J Am Coll Cardiol 2009;54(Suppl 1):S32–42.

23. Thomson JR, Machado RD, Pauciulo MW, et al. Sporadic primary pulmonary hypertension is associated with germline mutations of the gene encoding BMPR-II, a receptor member of the TGF-beta family. J Med Genet 2000;37(10):741–5.

24. Machado RD, Pauciulo MW, Thomson JR, et al. BMPR2 haploinsufficiency as the inherited molecular mechanism for primary pulmonary hypertension. Am J Hum Genet 2001;68(1):92–102.

25. Aldred MA, Vijayakrishnan J, James V, et al. BMPR2 gene rearrangements account for a significant proportion of mutations in familial and idiopathic pulmonary arterial hypertension. Hum Mutat 2006;27(2):212–3.

26. Machado RD, Aldred MA, James V, et al. Mutations of the TGF-beta type II receptor BMPR2 in pulmonary arterial hypertension. Hum Mutat 2006;27(2):121–32.

27. Cogan JD, Vnencak-Jones CL, Phillips JA 3rd, et al. Gross BMPR2 gene rearrangements constitute a new cause for primary pulmonary hypertension. Genet Med 2005;7(3):169–74.

28. Cogan JD, Pauciulo MW, Batchman AP, et al. High frequency of BMPR2 exonic deletions/duplications in familial pulmonary arterial hypertension. Am J Respir Crit Care Med 2006;174(5):590–8.

29. Aldred MA, Machado RD, James V, et al. Characterization of the BMPR2 5'-untranslated region and a novel mutation in pulmonary hypertension. Am J Respir Crit Care Med 2007;176(8):819–24.

30. Humbert M, Morrell NW, Archer SL, et al. Cellular and molecular pathobiology of pulmonary arterial hypertension. J Am Coll Cardiol 2004;43(12 Suppl S):13S–24S.

31. Li W, Dunmore BJ, Morrell NW. Bone morphogenetic protein type II receptor mutations causing protein misfolding in heritable pulmonary arterial hypertension. Proc Am Thorac Soc 2010;7(6):395–8.

32. West J, Niswender KD, Johnson JA, et al. A potential role for insulin resistance in experimental pulmonary hypertension. Eur Respir J 2013;41(4):861–71.

33. Girerd B, Montani D, Eyries M, et al. Absence of influence of gender and BMPR2 mutation type on clinical phenotypes of pulmonary arterial hypertension. Respir Res 2010;11:73.

34. Sztrymf B, Coulet F, Girerd B, et al. Clinical outcomes of pulmonary arterial hypertension in carriers of BMPR2 mutation. Am J Respir Crit Care Med 2008;177(12):1377–83.

35. Pfarr N, Szamalek-Hoegel J, Fischer C, et al. Hemodynamic and clinical onset in patients with hereditary pulmonary arterial hypertension and BMPR2 mutations. Respir Res 2011;12:99.

36. Elliott CG, Glissmeyer EW, Havlena GT, et al. Relationship of BMPR2 mutations to vasoreactivity in pulmonary arterial hypertension. Circulation 2006; 113(21):2509–15.

37. Rosenzweig EB, Morse JH, Knowles JA, et al. Clinical implications of determining BMPR2 mutation status in a large cohort of children and adults with pulmonary arterial hypertension. J Heart Lung Transplant 2008;27(6):668–74.

38. Austin ED, Phillips JA, Cogan JD, et al. Truncating and missense BMPR2 mutations differentially affect the severity of heritable pulmonary arterial hypertension. Respir Res 2009;10:87.

39. Attisano L, Carcamo J, Ventura F, et al. Identification of human activin and TGF beta type I receptors that form heteromeric kinase complexes with type II receptors. Cell 1993;75(4):671–80.

40. Wu X, Robinson CE, Fong HW, et al. Cloning and characterization of the murine activin receptor like kinase-1 (ALK-1) homolog. Biochem Biophys Res Commun 1995;216(1):78–83.

41. Favaro JP, Wiley K, Blobe GC. Alk1. UCSD-Nature Molecule Pages. 2005. http://dx.doi.org/10.1038/mp.a000254.000201.

42. ten Dijke P, Yamashita H, Ichijo H, et al. Characterization of type I receptors for transforming growth factor-beta and activin. Science 1994;264(5155): 101–4.

43. Abdalla SA, Letarte M. Hereditary haemorrhagic telangiectasia: current views on genetics and mechanisms of disease. J Med Genet 2006;43(2):97–110.

44. Harrison RE, Berger R, Haworth SG, et al. Transforming growth factor-beta receptor mutations and pulmonary arterial hypertension in childhood. Circulation 2005;111(4):435–41.

45. Girerd B, Montani D, Coulet F, et al. Clinical outcomes of pulmonary arterial hypertension in patients carrying an ACVRL1 (ALK1) mutation. Am J Respir Crit Care Med 2010;181(8):851–61.

46. Harrison RE, Flanagan JA, Sankelo M, et al. Molecular and functional analysis identifies ALK-1 as the predominant cause of pulmonary hypertension related to hereditary haemorrhagic telangiectasia. J Med Genet 2003;40(12):865–71.

47. Chaouat A, Coulet F, Favre C, et al. Endoglin germline mutation in a patient with hereditary haemorrhagic telangiectasia and dexfenfluramine associated pulmonary arterial hypertension. Thorax 2004;59(5):446–8.

48. Llorca O, Trujillo A, Blanco FJ, et al. Structural model of human endoglin, a transmembrane receptor responsible for hereditary hemorrhagic telangiectasia. J Mol Biol 2007;365(3):694–705.

49. Ray B, Blobe GC. Endoglin. UCSD-Nature Molecule Pages. 2005. http://dx.doi.org/10.1038/mp.a000048.000001.

50. Shovlin CL. Hereditary haemorrhagic telangiectasia: pathophysiology, diagnosis and treatment. Blood Rev 2010;24(6):203–19.

51. Shintani M, Yagi H, Nakayama T, et al. A new nonsense mutation of SMAD8 associated with pulmonary arterial hypertension. J Med Genet 2009; 46(5):331–7.

52. Chida A, Shintani M, Nakayama T, et al. Missense mutations of the BMPR1B (ALK6) gene in childhood idiopathic pulmonary arterial hypertension. Circ J 2012;76(6):1501–8.

53. Yang X, Long L, Southwood M, et al. Dysfunctional smad signaling contributes to abnormal smooth muscle cell proliferation in familial pulmonary arterial hypertension. Circ Res 2005;96(10):1053–63.

54. Austin ED, Ma L, LeDuc C, et al. Whole exome sequencing to identify a novel gene (caveolin-1) associated with human pulmonary arterial hypertension. Circ Cardiovasc Genet 2012;5(3):336–43.

55. Razani B, Zhang XL, Bitzer M, et al. Caveolin-1 regulates transforming growth factor (TGF)-beta/SMAD signaling through an interaction with the TGF-beta type I receptor. J Biol Chem 2001; 276(9):6727–38.

56. Maniatis NA, Shinin V, Schraufnagel DE, et al. Increased pulmonary vascular resistance and defective pulmonary artery filling in caveolin-1-/-mice. Am J Physiol Lung Cell Mol Physiol 2008; 294(5):L865–73.

57. Ma L, Roman-Campos D, Austin ED, et al. A novel channelopathy in pulmonary arterial hypertension. N Engl J Med 2013;369:351–61.

58. Mandegar M, Yuan JX. Role of K+ channels in pulmonary hypertension. Vascul Pharmacol 2002; 38(1):25–33.

59. Germain M, Eyries M, Montani D, et al. Genome-wide association analysis identifies a susceptibility locus for pulmonary arterial hypertension. Nat Genet 2013;45(5):518–21.

60. Rich S, Dantzker DR, Ayres SM, et al. Primary pulmonary hypertension: a national prospective study. Ann Intern Med 1987;107(2):216–23.

61. Humbert M, Sitbon O, Chaouat A, et al. Pulmonary arterial hypertension in France: results from a National Registry. Am J Respir Crit Care Med 2006; 173(9):1023–30.

62. Badesch DB, Raskob GE, Elliott CG, et al. Pulmonary arterial hypertension: baseline characteristics from the REVEAL Registry. Chest 2010;137(2): 376–87.

63. Humbert M, Deng Z, Simonneau G, et al. BMPR2 germline mutations in pulmonary hypertension associated with fenfluramine derivatives. Eur Respir J 2002;20(3):518–23.

64. Roberts KE, McElroy JJ, Wong WP, et al. BMPR2 mutations in pulmonary arterial hypertension with congenital heart disease. Eur Respir J 2004; 24(3):371–4.

65. Morse J, Barst R, Horn E, et al. Pulmonary hypertension in scleroderma spectrum of disease: lack of bone morphogenetic protein receptor 2 mutations. J Rheumatol 2002;29(11):2379–81.

66. Tew MB, Arnett FC, Reveille JD, et al. Mutations of bone morphogenetic protein receptor type II are not found in patients with pulmonary hypertension and underlying connective tissue diseases. Arthritis Rheum 2002;46(10):2829–30.

67. Nunes H, Humbert M, Sitbon O, et al. Prognostic factors for survival in human immunodeficiency virus-associated pulmonary arterial hypertension. Am J Respir Crit Care Med 2003;167(10):1433–9.

68. Roberts KE, Fallon MB, Krowka MJ, et al. Genetic risk factors for portopulmonary hypertension in patients with advanced liver disease. Am J Respir Crit Care Med 2009;179(9):835–42.

69. Montani D, Price LC, Dorfmuller P, et al. Pulmonary veno-occlusive disease. Eur Respir J 2009;33(1): 189–200.

70. Voordes CG, Kuipers JR, Elema JD. Familial pulmonary veno-occlusive disease: a case report. Thorax 1977;32(6):763–6.

71. Montani D, Achouh L, Dorfmuller P, et al. Pulmonary veno-occlusive disease: clinical, functional, radiologic, and hemodynamic characteristics and outcome of 24 cases confirmed by histology. Medicine (Baltimore) 2008;87(4):220–33.

72. Runo JR, Vnencak-Jones CL, Prince M, et al. Pulmonary veno-occlusive disease caused by an inherited mutation in bone morphogenetic protein receptor II. Am J Respir Crit Care Med 2003; 167(6):889–94.

73. Wagenvoort CA, Beetstra A, Spijker J. Capillary haemangiomatosis of the lungs. Histopathology 1978;2(6):401–6.

74. Langleben D, Heneghan JM, Batten AP, et al. Familial pulmonary capillary hemangiomatosis resulting in primary pulmonary hypertension. Ann Intern Med Jul 15 1988;109(2):106–9.

75. Best DH, Sumner KL, Austin ED, et al. *EIF2AK4* mutations in pulmonary capillary hemangiomatosis. CHEST 2013. [Epub ahead of print].

76. Badesch DB, Abman SH, Simonneau G, et al. Medical therapy for pulmonary arterial hypertension: updated ACCP evidence-based clinical practice guidelines. Chest 2007;131(6):1917–28.

77. Frydman N, Steffann J, Girerd B, et al. Pre-implantation genetic diagnosis in pulmonary arterial hypertension due to BMPR2 mutation. Eur Respir J 2012;39(6):1534–5.

78. An act to prohibit discrimination on the basis of genetic information with respect to health insurance and employment: Wikipedia, 2008; Public Law enacted by the 110th United States Congress. Available at http://en.wikipedia.org/wiki/Genetic_Information_Nondiscrimination_Act. Accessed October 10, 2013.

79. Maitland-van der Zee AH, de Boer A, Leufkens HG. The interface between pharmacoepidemiology and pharmacogenetics. Eur J Pharmacol 2000; 410(2–3):121–30.

80. Murali S. Pulmonary arterial hypertension. Curr Opin Crit Care 2006;12(3):228–34.

Diagnosis of Pulmonary Arterial Hypertension

Paul R. Forfia, MD[a],*, Terence K. Trow, MD[b,c]

KEYWORDS

- Diagnosis • Pulmonary • Arterial • Hypertension • Echocardiography • Doppler • Catheterization

KEY POINTS

- Diagnosing pulmonary arterial hypertension requires a high index of clinical suspicion and the ability to identify clinical clues of pulmonary vascular disease.
- The astute clinician should suspect the presence of pulmonary arterial hypertension before performing a right heart catheterization.
- The echo-Doppler examination is used in part to screen for the presence of increased pulmonary artery pressure. However, this examination provides a great deal more physiologic information about pulmonary hypertension than just pulmonary pressure estimation.
- The presence of pulmonary vascular disease, and thus high right ventricular afterload, leads to several findings that are unique to these conditions, including right ventricular dilatation, systolic dysfunction, septal flattening and Doppler notching. Patients with pulmonary hypertension not caused by pulmonary vascular disease do not possess these echo-Doppler findings.
- Right heart catheterization is necessary to establish the hemodynamic criteria of pulmonary arterial hypertension. However, right heart catheterization is subject to pitfalls and thus should be scrutinized carefully to ensure the accuracy of hemodynamic data.

INTRODUCTION

The accurate diagnosis of pulmonary arterial hypertension (PAH) can be a challenging and complex process that requires a high index of clinical suspicion from even the most astute clinician. Because pulmonary vascular disease (PVD) is not the exclusive domain of any given medical discipline, general internists and a broad range of medical specialists alike must be aware of the potential presentations of this disorder[1] as well as the limitations and vagaries of noninvasive tests used to define patients in whom invasive testing is warranted. Right, and sometimes left, heart catheterization is required to establish the diagnosis and to characterize the PAH phenotype before proper treatment can be initiated. This article reviews the evidence supporting the detection and diagnosis of PAH in patients at risk for this disorder.

Disclosures: T.K. Trow has served on speaker's bureaus for Actelion, Gilead, Lung Rx, and United Therapeutic pharmaceutical (not in the past 12 months). He has also served on advisory boards for Bayer, Actelion, United Therapeutics, Gilead (not in past 12 months). He received funding support as the principal investigator at Yale on the COMPASS II study from Actelion and received funding support as principal investigator on the RESPIRE registry from Actelion. P.R. Forfia has served on speaker's bureaus for Actelion, Gilead, and United Therapeutic pharmaceutical (not in past 24 months). He has also served as a consultant or member of advisory boards for Bayer, Actelion, United Therapeutics, and Gilead.

a Division of Cardiovascular Medicine, Pulmonary Hypertension and Right Heart Failure Program, Temple University Hospital, 3401 North Broad Street, 9th Floor, Parkinson Pavillion, Philadelphia, PA 19140, USA; b Section of Pulmonary and Critical Care Medicine, Yale University School of Medicine, 333 Cedar Street, PO Box 208057, LLCI 105D, New Haven, CT 06520, USA; c Pulmonary Vascular Disease Program, Yale University School of Medicine, 333 Cedar Street, PO Box 208057, LLCI 105D, New Haven, CT 06520, USA
* Corresponding author.
E-mail address: paul.forfia@temple.edu

PATIENT HISTORY

The symptoms associated with PAH are nonspecific and are often confounded by the presence of comorbid conditions that might explain them. The National Institutes of Health (NIH) registry found that there was a median of 2 years before the correct diagnosis of PAH was established.[2] Dyspnea was the most common initial complaint (60%), followed by syncope, near-syncope or lightheadedness (34%), fatigue (21%), chest pain (8%), and leg edema (7%).[2] In the authors' experience, a classic presentation of PAH occurs when a patient presents with 2 or more complaints within the triad of dyspnea, exertional angina, and exertional near-syncope or syncope. Idiopathic PAH (IPAH) presentations occur more often in young women, often with normal examinations early in their course,[3] making reassurance the most common initial intervention. A complaint of exertional angina also may not be sufficiently appreciated by the interviewing physician in this context. Patients often discount their symptoms, often increasing the time before medical attention is sought.[3] For this reason, a high index of clinical suspicion should be maintained when an explanation for such symptoms is not readily evident. In addition, conditions with an increased incidence of associated PAH, such as connective tissue disease,[4–8] cirrhosis of the liver,[9–12] human immunodeficiency virus (HIV) infection, or current or prior history of systemic-to-pulmonary shunt conditions warrant increased concern on the part of the frontline practitioner.

PHYSICAL EXAMINATION

Because the number of conditions associated with the development of PAH is extensive, a variety of examination clues may be present and should be looked for. These clues are often subtle and may be overlooked.[13] Cardiac auscultation may reveal an accentuated pulmonic component to the second heart sound and delayed closure of the pulmonic valve (split P2) in up to 90% of patients with IPAH.[3] This is characteristically fixed without variation during inspiration and expiration in cases of atrial septal defect–associated PAH.[14–16] Other signs may include a palpable left parasternal heave, a right ventricular S3 or S4 gallop, prominence of the jugular a wave or v wave, hepatojugular reflux, and lower extremity edema.[3] A variety of murmurs may also be encountered on cardiac auscultation, including the high-pitched holosystolic murmur of tricuspid regurgitation (TR) heard best at the left sternal border or the early diastolic high-pitched murmur of pulmonic regurgitation (PR).[15,16] The high pitch of the TR or PR murmur is not typical, and relates to the high velocity of regurgitant flow imparted by high pulmonary artery pressure.

Aside from cardiac auscultation, cyanosis is seen in 20% of IPAH cases[3] and suggests right-to-left shunting and severe reduction of cardiac output. The sequelae of liver disease, such as testicular atrophy, palmar erythema, and spider telangiectasias, should also be sought. Oral mucosal telangiectasias may suggest a diagnosis of hereditary hemorrhagic telangiectasia (HHT) syndrome, now known to be associated with a mutation in the activin receptor–like kinase-1 (ALK-1) gene in a minority of cases.[17] Calcinosis, sclerodactyly, telangiectasias, Raynaud phenomenon, and digital ulcerations may all be seen in scleroderma-associated PAH.[14] Because many women with telangiectasias are self-conscious about the skin telangiectasias that appear on their faces, the examiner may need to ask for the removal of facial make-up to appreciate this finding. Digital clubbing is rare in IPAH[3] and when present should raise the possibility of congenital heart disease or pulmonary veno-occlusive disease (PVOD).[18] A sternotomy scar should alert the clinician to prior chest surgery in a patient with congenital heart disease.

ELECTROCARDIOGRAPHY

Although electrocardiography (ECG) lacks sufficient sensitivity and specificity to serve as an effective screening tool[19,20] it can contribute important diagnostic and prognostic information and should be performed. Right ventricular hypertrophy (RVH) and right-axis deviation (RAD) can be detected 87% and 79% of the time, respectively, in PAH.[3] Features of RVH suggesting PAH include a tall R wave and small S wave (R/S ratio of >1) in lead V1, a large S wave and small R wave (R/S ratio<1) in lead V5 or V6, a qR complex in V1, and a rSR pattern in V1 (**Fig. 1**).[20] However, absence of these findings does not exclude PAH, with one study of 61 patients with PAH showing 8 patients with normal ECG despite severe PAH by catheterization.[20] When ECG findings are present, they may be helpful prognostically because the presence of right atrial enlargement has been associated with a 2.8-fold greater risk of death over a 6-year period of observation, and RVH by World Health Organization (WHO) diagnostic criteria portended a 4.3-fold greater risk of death.[21] Greater degrees of RAD have also correlated with decreased survival, as did S1Q3 pattern in one retrospective study of patients with IPAH.[22]

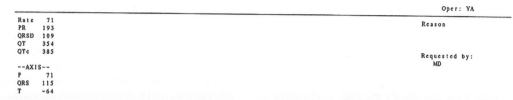

Oper: YA

Reason

Requested by:
MD

Rate   71
PR   193
QRSD   109
QT   354
QTc   385

--AXIS--
P   71
QRS   115
T   -64

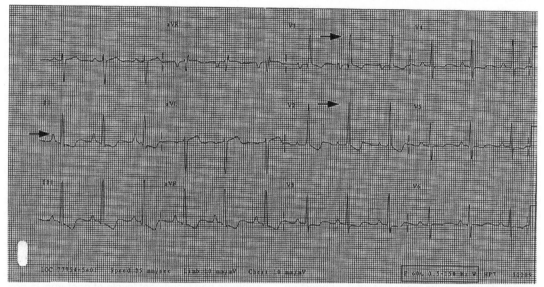

Fig. 1. An ECG from a patient with severe PAH. Note the prominent R wave magnitude in leads V1 and V2 (*arrow*) indicating RVH. Vector forces for the QRS complex are 115° indicating RAD. The presence of P wave magnitude of greater than 2.5 mm in lead II (*arrow*) indicates significant right atrial enlargement.

CHEST RADIOGRAPHY

Like the ECG, a chest radiograph (CXR) should be obtained in all patients with suspected PAH even though it lacks sensitivity and specificity to establish the diagnosis.[19,23] Radiographic features of attenuated peripheral vascular markings, enlarged main and hilar pulmonary artery shadows, and obscuration of the retrosternal clear space on a lateral view caused by enlargement of the right ventricle (RV) may be noted (**Fig. 2**). An increase in the hilar thoracic index (defined as the ratio of the summed horizontal measurements of the pulmonary artery from the midline to their first division

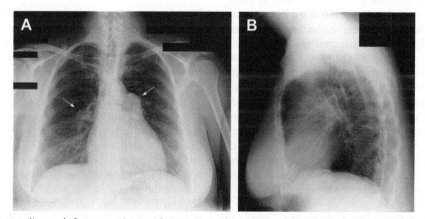

Fig. 2. A chest radiograph from a patient with PAH. Note the prominently enlarged right descending pulmonary artery (*arrow*) and left main pulmonary artery (*arrow*) seen on the posterior-anterior projection (*A*). Peripheral vasculature is attenuated. The lateral view (*B*) shows encroachment of the right ventricle on the retrosternal airspace (*arrow*).

divided by the maximum transverse thorax diameter) of greater than 38% strongly suggested PAH in one study of 50 patients[23] but this finding did not correlate well with the extent of pulmonary artery pressure (PAP) increase seen. When patients with chronic obstructive pulmonary disease (COPD) were specifically studied, an increase in the right descending pulmonary artery (RDPA) diameter greater than 16 mm on a posterior-anterior projection and greater than 18 mm for the left descending pulmonary artery (LDPA) also on a posterior-anterior film permitted the correct diagnosis of pulmonary hypertension (PH) in most of these patients when right heart catheterization was used to define PAP.[24] Chetty and colleagues[25] combined the hilar thoracic index, RDPA branch diameter, hilar width, and cardiothoracic ratio in 34 patients with COPD and 19 of 20 (95%) with increased mean PAP (mPAP) had a hilar thoracic index of 36 or more versus none of the 14 patients with COPD with normal mean PAP. Nineteen of 20 patients with increased mPAP also had RDPA diameters of 20 mm versus 3 of the 14 patients with normal mPAP; however, the CXR could not be used to accurately predict the PAP.[26]

The CXR may also define concomitant parenchymal disease, pulmonary vascular congestion seen in PVOD,[27] hyperinflation changes of COPD, kyphosis, or findings suggesting chronic thromboembolic disease such as mosaic oligemia, RVH, or an enlarged RDPA.[28,29]

PULMONARY FUNCTION TESTING AND HYPOXEMIA ASSESSMENT

All patients with known or suspected PAH should have pulmonary function testing as a part of their initial evaluation. In IPAH, Rich and colleagues[3] found mild reductions in total lung capacity (TLC) and forced vital capacity (FVC) in both male and female subjects. Diffusing capacity for carbon monoxide (DLco) also measured significantly less than predicted in the NIH registry trial,[3] a finding confirmed by Sun and colleagues[30] in patients with IPAH. Patients with chronic thromboembolic PH (CTEPH) also show mild to moderate restrictive defects,[31] a finding thought to be caused by parenchymal scarring from prior infarcts.[31,32] They also often have mild DLco reductions (60%–80% of the time) largely caused by pulmonary membrane diffusing capacity abnormalities rather than pulmonary capillary blood volume alterations.[31,32]

When other phenotypes of PH are examined, DLco impairments are commonly seen in portopulmonary-associated PAH[33] as well as in sarcoidosis-related PH.[34] The latter study also showed more significant forced expiratory volume

in the first second and FVC reductions in patients with PH compared with patients with sarcoidosis without PH.[34] Patients with systemic sclerosis also frequently have DLco abnormalities, with 20% having such findings in one study of 88 patients with progressive systemic sclerosis.[35] Compared with patients with scleroderma with calcinosis, Raynaud phenomenon, esophageal dysmotility, sclerodactyly, and telangiectasia (CREST), the latter had lower mean DLco values despite a higher mean vital capacity. When isolated DLco impairments are seen in the limited cutaneous form of scleroderma, the likelihood of PH development is high.[36,37] Scorza and colleagues[38] found that over 15 years of follow-up in a cohort of patients with systemic sclerosis and baseline DLco less than 45% of predicted, 75% went on to develop PH defined by echocardiographic systolic PAPs of greater than 40 mm Hg, and in these patients DLco was inversely correlated with PAPs measured by right heart catheterization.

Measures of oxygen saturation with exercise are important to include in the work-up even when resting measures of oxygenation are normal, because supplemental oxygen may assist in control of vasoconstriction with exertion.[13] In a relatively small study of patients with IPAH, 10 of 13 subjects had significant levels of nocturnal hypoxemia even in the absence of sleep-disordered breathing[39] and therefore, it is recommended that patients with all forms of PAH be assessed with overnight oximetry testing even when suspicion of sleep apnea is not high. Schulz and colleagues[40] discovered periodic (Cheyne-Stokes) breathing patterns in 30% in one study of 20 patients with IPAH, which seemed reversible with nocturnal oxygen supplementation.

DOPPLER ECHOCARDIOGRAPHY

The transthoracic Doppler echocardiographic (DE) examination consists of both a two-dimensional examination of cardiac structure, size, and function, as well as Doppler techniques that inform the clinician about blood flow, valve function, flow velocity, and wave shape, as well as pressure estimations. The most emphasized part of the DE examination in the assessment of PH is Doppler estimation of pulmonary artery systolic pressure (PASP$_{Doppler}$). Used as a screening tool, PASP$_{Doppler}$ serves an important role and has led to an increased recognition of PH. However, the usefulness of Doppler echocardiography in the work-up of PH extends beyond PASP$_{Doppler}$ estimation or as a screening tool, with the integration of relevant DE parameters providing insight into the hemodynamic basis of PH before invasive cardiac catheterization. Moreover, changes in the DE examination occurring in response to PAH medical therapy are associated with the efficacy of medical therapy. The DE examination can reliably distinguish between PH related to PVD (PH$_{PVD}$; herein defined as mPAP greater than 25 mm Hg, pulmonary arterial wedge pressure [PAWP] <15 mm Hg, and pulmonary vascular resistance [PVR] >3 mm Hg/L/min) versus pulmonary venous hypertension (PVH; mPAP>25 mm Hg, PAWP>15 mm Hg, and PVR<3 mm Hg/L/min). The DE examination also can detect the mixed phenotype of left heart congestion combined with a high PVR.[41]

The PASP$_{Doppler}$ estimate is achieved by using continuous wave Doppler to determine the peak tricuspid regurgitant jet velocity, which when applied to the modified Bernoulli equation (4 v^2) and added to the estimated right atrial pressure (RAP) provides an estimate for PASP.[42] A cutoff of 40 mm Hg or higher is typically consistent with an mPAP greater than 25 mm Hg, and thus a diagnosis of PH. However, in order for the PASP$_{Doppler}$ estimate to provide a reliable measure of pressure, there are several requisites: (1) the Doppler probe needs to be as close to parallel to the regurgitant jet as possible in order to obtain the optimal quality and maximal velocity Doppler envelope; (2) the peak jet velocity measurement should not be overestimated or underestimated; (3) the RAP estimate obtained by vena cava diameter must accurately reflect RAP. In addition, some patients do not have tricuspid regurgitation, thus precluding TR velocity assessment. The absence of TR does not preclude even severe PH, although this scenario is most typically seen when the RV is well compensated to the pulmonary vascular load.[43–45]

Under optimal conditions, the PASP$_{Doppler}$ estimation correlates well with invasive measures.[46] However, the presence of one or all of the limitations discussed earlier often results in significant discrepancies between PASP$_{Doppler}$ and invasive measurements; several studies have shown that in nearly 50% of cases PASP$_{Doppler}$ estimates differ by more than 10 mm Hg from invasive values, with a relative balance of overestimation and underestimation.[45,47,48] However, the remainder of the Doppler echocardiography examination often provides additional insight that may improve the diagnostic yield from Doppler echocardiography. For example, 75% of patients with significantly underestimated PASP$_{Doppler}$ have right ventricular dysfunction or dilatation on their remaining examination.[45] Thus, the PASP$_{Doppler}$ should not be viewed in isolation, but rather integrated into the overall two-dimensional and Doppler examination of the heart.

The two-dimensional examination provides critical insight into PH pathophysiology, given that an increased right ventricular afterload alters right ventricular function, size, shape, and septal position in a manner that is characteristic of high afterload states. An increased RV afterload arises from an increased PVR and decreased pulmonary artery compliance. An increase in PAP without an increase in PVR and loss of pulmonary artery compliance (ie, PVH without PVD or high pulmonary flow without PVD) only mildly affects RV afterload and does not produce these characteristic changes in RV structure and function. As a result, the presence or absence of the characteristic triad (RV dilatation, systolic dysfunction, and leftward interventricular septal displacement during systole) provides a crucial differentiation between a diagnosis of PH$_{PVD}$ from normal physiology or non-PVD causes of PH.[41,49]

As an example, note the differences in RV size, shape, and septal position between 2 patients with the same mPAP (45 mm Hg); one subject has PAH and the other has PVH (**Fig. 3**). **Fig. 3** panel A depicts the typical morphology of the right ventricular in the setting of PH$_{PVD}$. The RV/left ventricle (LV) dimension ratio is approximately 1.5 (normal 0.6–0.8), consistent with severe RV dilatation. The RV apical angle is open because of high afterload, often leading to the RV and LV sharing the cardiac apex. In contrast, patients with PVH without an increased PVR (see **Fig. 3** panel B) lack these findings even at the same degree of PAP increase. As a result, the heart appears fundamentally different in the apical 4-chamber view in the patient with PH$_{PVD}$ versus PVH.

Right ventricular contraction is a complex and coordinated event occurring because of shortening of longitudinal and circumferential muscle fibers, along with the assistance of physical connections between the LV and right ventricular free wall (ie, moderator band). Longitudinal shortening represents a larger percentage of total shortening in the RV compared with the LV.[50] At present, the most common approach to right ventricular systolic function is to assess right ventricular performance along the longitudinal plane. The tricuspid annular plane systolic excursion (TAPSE) is the most common and validated of the methods of longitudinal RV function assessment, measuring the total displacement of the heart from the right ventricular base toward the apex in systole.[51–53] Measured in two-dimensional or M-mode echocardiography, TAPSE correlates well with right ventricular ejection fraction and is a simple, reproducible method for estimating right ventricular function. A normal TAPSE ranges from 2.3 to 2.7 cm.[52] A TAPSE less than 1.8 cm accurately predicts a depressed, invasively measured stroke volume index. TAPSE is strongly associated with other measures of right

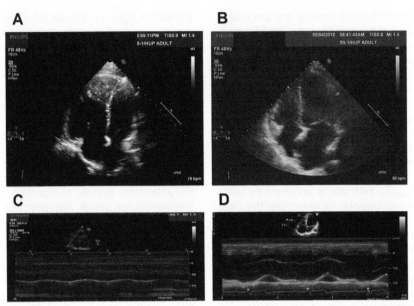

Fig. 3. (A) Representative apical 4-chamber view of a patient with PH$_{PVD}$. Note that the end-diastolic RV dimension obtained 1 cm apical of the tricuspid annulus is greater than the left ventricle (LV) diastolic dimension. Hence, the RV/LV dimension ratio is greater than 1.0. The RV apical angle is open or rounded, and the RV and LV form the apex of the heart. (B) Representative apical 4-chamber view of a patient with PVH. Note the RV/LV ratio of less than 1.0, closed RV apical angle, and that the LV alone forms the cardiac apex. This patient has a similar degree of PH to the subject in (A). (C, D) Tricuspid annular plane systolic excursion (TAPSE) by M-mode, obtained in the apical 4-chamber view. The distance between the end-diastolic and end-systolic points represents TAPSE. In (C), the TAPSE is severely depressed (1.4 cm). In (D), TAPSE is normal (2.6 cm).

ventricular dysfunction, and has been correlated with increased hospitalization rates and death in patients with PAH.[51,54] A TAPSE of 1.5 cm or less (severe right ventricular dysfunction) was associated with a 3-fold higher event rate (death or emergent lung transplant) in a PAH cohort.[55]

Tissue Doppler of the tricuspid annular velocity (S′) can also be used to evaluate right ventricular longitudinal systolic motion. An S′ of less than 10 cm/s reflects right ventricular dysfunction and reliably predicts a cardiac index less than 2.2.[56]

On a practical level, depressed right ventricular systolic function strongly suggests PH$_{PVD}$, given

that increased right ventricular afterload is the most common cause of right ventricular systolic dysfunction (see **Fig. 3**, panel A and C), particularly when the LV systolic function is normal. As such, significant right ventricular dysfunction should alert the clinician to PH$_{PVD}$, even if the PASP$_{Doppler}$ is reported as normal.

Systolic septal flattening occurs in response to mechanical dyssynchrony between the RV and LV, most commonly caused by afterload-dependent RV dysfunction.[41,57] Thus, when PH is present without evidence of interventricular septal flattening, PVH is the most likely cause (**Fig. 4**).

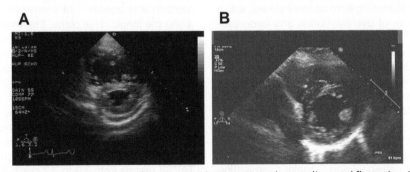

Fig. 4. (A) Representative short-axis view of a patient with PH$_{PVD}$. Note the systolic septal flattening. The small pericardial effusion is another important finding, often resulting from chronically increased RAP. (B) Representative short-axis view of a patient with PVH. In the presence of PH, the lack of interventricular sepal flattening provides key evidence of the lack of PVD.

A pericardial effusion is seen in 20% to 50% of patients with PAH on initial presentation, likely because of transudation of fluid into the pericardial space caused by right atrial hypertension and right heart decompensation.[58,59] Treatment should be directed at reducing right ventricular afterload to alleviate right ventricular failure (diuretics, pulmonary artery vasodilators), and not pericardial drainage, because the effusion is the result (not the cause) of right ventricular decompensation and is associated with high periprocedure mortality.[60]

A simple Doppler-based approach to detecting PVD exploits the effect of differences in right ventricular afterload on the manner and timing with which pressure and flow waves travel within the pulmonary circulation. As a result, differences in RV afterload impart distinct differences in the shape of the pulsed-wave RVOT$_{Doppler}$.[61–64] In the setting of an increased PVR and decreased pulmonary artery compliance, the RVOT$_{Doppler}$ profile show a pattern of late-systolic (late-systolic notching [LSN]) or midsystolic (midsystolic notching [MSN]) flow deceleration (**Figs. 5** and **6**). These distinct patterns of RVOT$_{Doppler}$ notching provide immediate and reliable qualitative evidence of increased pulmonary artery load. The LSN pattern typically coincides with a PVR between 3 and 6 Wood units (WU), and thus moderate PVD. In contrast, the MSN pattern is specific for a PVR more than 5 WU (average PVR, 9 WU) and coincides with moderate or greater degrees of right ventricular dilation, septal displacement, and systolic dysfunction.[64] The presence of a notched RVOT$_{Doppler}$ profile is strongly associated with a PVR of more than 3WU (odds ratio, 29:1). RVOT$_{Doppler}$ notching (MSN or LSN) was present in 100% of patients with incident PAH, and is also highly prevalent in PH related to acute or chronic pulmonary emboli.[62,64] The acceleration time (AcT) obtained from the RVOT$_{Doppler}$ profile similarly reflects right ventricular afterload, and correlates with the shape of the RVOT$_{Doppler}$ profile (MSN mean AcT, 67 milliseconds; LSN mean AcT, 79 milliseconds; no notch (NN) mean AcT, 113 milliseconds). When PH occurs without Doppler notching (see **Fig. 5** panel C), it strongly predicts a PVR less than 3 WU and a pulmonary artery wedge pressure more than 15 mm Hg (odds ratio, 33:1), thus implicating left-sided dysfunction as the cause of PH.[64] Thus, visual assessment of the shape of the RVOT$_{Doppler}$ profile represents a simple, reproducible measure on routine Doppler echocardiography that can help distinguish an increased PVR versus a normal PVR as the underlying hemodynamic cause of PH.[64]

Recent work shows that a DE prediction rule can be applied to patients with PH to help identify the underlying hemodynamic mechanism and distinguish PH$_{PVD}$ from PVH.[41] Using simple measures including left atrial size, the ratio of early transmitral filling to early diastolic tissue Doppler velocity (E/e'; the most common method of left atrial pressure estimation by Doppler), and the RVOT$_{Doppler}$ profile, a score is derived (range -2 to $+2$; higher scores suggesting PH$_{PVD}$, with lower scores suggesting PVH). The echo score detects PH$_{PVD}$ with an area under the curve (AUC) of 0.92, and

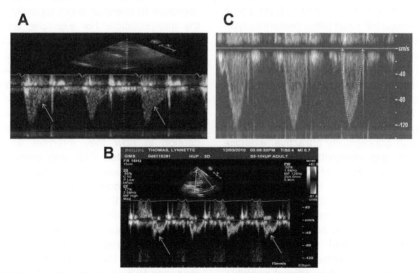

Fig. 5. Late-systolic notching (*arrows, panel A*) and midsystolic notching (*arrows, panel B*) of the RVOT$_{Doppler}$ flow velocity profile. Midsystolic notching is associated with more severe PVD and should immediately raise suspicion for a markedly increased PVR. (*C*) A parabolic, non-notched RVOT$_{Doppler}$ profile, strongly suggesting a lack of PVD. PH in the absence of Doppler notching strongly suggests PVH.

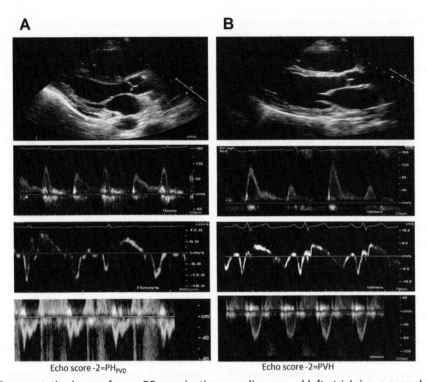

A

Echo score -2=PH$_{PVD}$

B

Echo score -2=PVH

Fig. 6. (*A*) Representative images from a DE examination revealing normal left atrial size, a normal diastolic left ventricular filling pattern (ratio of early transmitral filling to early diastolic tissue Doppler velocity [E/e']<10), and midsystolic notching of the RVOT$_{Doppler}$ profile. The echo score is −2, strongly suggesting PH$_{PVD}$. (*B*) Representative images from a DE examination revealing increased left atrial size, an increased E/e' ratio (denoting high left atrial pressure) and a parabolic, non-notched RVOT$_{Doppler}$ profile. This constellation of findings strongly favors PVH without PVD.

differentiated WHO group I PH from group II PH with an AUC of 0.97. No patients with an echo score less than 0 met the hemodynamic definition of PH$_{PVD}$. Patients with PH related to both a high PVR and increased left heart filling pressures typically had a score between −1 and +1, owing to the varying balance of two-dimensional and Doppler features that are consistent with this physiology.

The role of stress echocardiography in identifying PAH remains controversial. No clear consensus exists in the literature regarding the best exercise technique (eg, treadmill vs cycle ergometry) or protocols. Although conceptually attractive, exercise DE assessment and interpretation has multiple important limitations. First, at peak exertion in normal healthy subjects, 30% to 40% of subjects can show an mPAP greater than 30 mm Hg; in one study, the pressure-flow relationship and pulmonary resistance remained normal.[65] Also, cardiac output and left atrial pressure are not accounted for on the exercise DE examination, thus neglecting the two most significant contributors to an increase in PAP with exercise.[66,67] Exercise-induced pulmonary vasoconstriction is uncommon; Laskey and colleagues[68] showed that

the PVR of patients with IPAH remained increased during exercise, but unchanged from resting values. In addition, the systemic blood pressure response to exercise is not typically factored into the interpretation. For example, an increase in PASP from 35 to 70 mm Hg in the context of an increase in systemic systolic pressure from 120 to 210 mm Hg indicates that the relative proportion of pulmonary to systemic blood pressure has remained similar from rest to exercise, thus questioning the clinical significance of the increase in PAP in this context. Clinicians should exercise caution in how they interpret an increase in Doppler-estimated PAP with exercise, because, even when accurate, an increase in PAP with exercise does not necessarily implicate the pulmonary vasculature as the source of PH, that the PH is appropriate for PH specific therapies, or whether the PH is the source of dyspnea in a patient.

An alternative approach to exercise DE may be to focus on the right ventricular functional response to exercise, especially considering that impaired RV functional reserve is the mechanism of exercise limitation in PAH and other forms of PVD. This approach may provide a more direct and clinically relevant answer as to whether a patient has clinically significant latent PVD or PH as the cause of dyspnea. If the RV function augments normally with exercise, the increase in PAP is likely flow mediated and of less clinical significance. In contrast, a dilating and nonaugmenting RV in response to exercise indicates an impedance-mediated process of greater clinical significance. Preliminary evidence suggests that the RV functional response to exercise (change in TAPSE) is linked to clinical outcome. In a small cohort of patients with stable PAH, subjects either maintained a TAPSE similar to their resting TAPSE following graded supine ergometry, or had a decrease in TAPSE with exercise. A decrease in TAPSE with exercise was strongly associated with adverse clinical events within 1 year of follow-up.[69] An increase in the peak TR jet velocity following exercise was associated with better exercise-induced RV function and better clinical outcome. More evidence will probably arise in the near future supporting the notion that the focus of exercise echocardiography should be placed primarily on the RV functional response to exercise.

EXCLUDING THROMBOEMBOLIC DISEASE

The presentation of CTEPH can mimic that of IPAH and often is not associated with an awareness of the original pulmonary embolus on the part of the patient or caregiver.[70] Although previous reports of CTEPH complicating acute pulmonary embolism (PE) suggested rates of 0.1% to 0.5 %,[70] more recent prospective evaluation suggests that up to 4% of patients surviving their acute PE develop PH, usually within the first 2 years.[71] Because this form of PH is potentially curable by surgical intervention, all patients should undergo evaluation for this before being assigned an IPAH diagnosis.[13] A normal or low-probability ventilation-perfusion (V/Q)scan effectively excludes the diagnosis of CTEPH[72–75] with sensitivities of 90% to 100% and a specificity of 94% to 100% and therefore the V/Q scan is the screening method of choice for CTEPH (**Fig. 7**).[76] However, perfusion scans alone tend to underestimate the degree of severity of large-vessel obstruction.[77] Pulmonary angiography remains the diagnostic procedure of choice to evaluate suspected CTEPH and to define potential surgical candidates.[13] Although both contrast-enhanced computerized tomography pulmonary angiography (CTPA)[78–80] and magnetic resonance imaging (MRI)[81–84] have usefulness in CTEPH and in defining alternative diagnoses (eg, sarcoma, vasculitis, mediastinal fibrosis) and are complementary with V/Q scanning, these techniques are not applied with consistent algorithms

and equipment at the current time in all centers and are not generally recommended as stand-alone techniques to exclude CTEPH.[13] Cases of false-negative CTPA in our own institution (see **Fig. 7**) and others (Richard Channick MD, May 12, 2004, and Harold Palevsky, MD, April 21, 2006, personal communications) have underscored the dangers of substituting these for V/Q scans in the screening assessment for CTEPH. CTPA has been shown to be less sensitive than angiography for defining vascular distortions, stenoses, and webs in chronic PE.[77]

SEROLOGIC TESTING

Selective testing of blood samples is appropriate in known or suspected PAH.[13,85] The specific tests ordered depend on clinical suspicion as assessed by the history and physical examination, as well as by the absence of other clear causes of PAH in a patient. Although serologic tests may help focus diagnostic efforts aimed at connective tissue disease–associated PAH, up to 40% of patients with IPAH have increased antinuclear antibodies.[86] Because the most common connective tissue disease associated with PAH, limited scleroderma, typically does not manifest interstitial lung disease on examination or CXR, patients with perceived IPAH should be carefully assessed for features of systemic sclerosis. Anticentromere antibodies are typically positive in limited scleroderma,[87] as are positive antinuclear antibodies including U3-RNP, B23, Th/To, and U1-RNP.[88–90] When PAH is associated with diffuse forms of scleroderma, U3-RNP is usually positive.[91] Anticardiolipin antibodies have been associated with PAH in systemic lupus erythemotosus.[92,93] HIV testing is advised because PAH is associated with HIV infection in up to 0.5% of cases[94]; it is common for a new diagnosis of HIV to be established in parallel with the diagnosis of PAH. It is equally important to assess for cirrhotic liver disease because 5% to 6% of these patients manifest PAH.[9] As such, measures of aminotransferases, alkaline phosphatase, bilirubin levels, and measures of synthetic function such as the activated partial thromboplastin time and prothrombin time are advisable. Even when blood testing is unremarkable, hepatic Doppler ultrasound imaging and liver-spleen scanning may still suggest portal hypertension and should be considered when suspicion is high. Thyroid disease has been implicated as a risk factor for PAH,[95–98] although its exact relationship to PAH awaits definition. Disorders of the thyroid gland should be sought and treated in PAH because case reports of PAH reversal with treatment have been offered.[99,100]

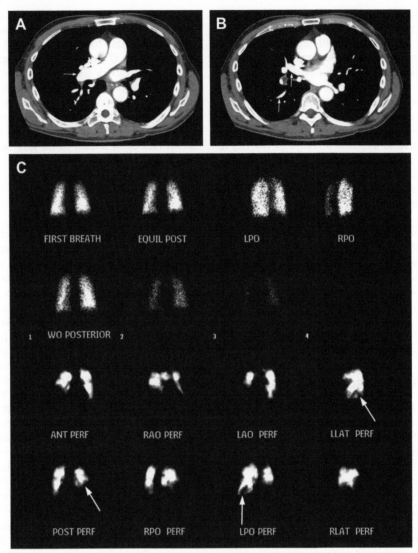

Fig. 7. CTEPH. This patient presented to the Yale Pulmonary Hypertension Center with 8 months of slowly increasing dyspnea with exertion without chest pain, pleurisy, or any recollection of an acute event. Computerized tomography pulmonary angiography done at an outside institution was interpreted as normal without evidence of thromboemboli. Representative images are shown in (A) and (B) with arrows in A and B indicating areas of consistent with chronic pulmonary embolism. Subsequent ventilation-perfusion scanning revealed multiple segmental and subsegmental unmatched defects (C). Pulmonary angiography confirmed interlobar embolic occlusions (*arrows* in D and E).

MRI

MRI is being used with increasing frequency for the diagnosis of PAH and related conditions, as well as for the evaluation of right ventricular morphology and function.[101] In CTEPH, reports suggest that good correlations with V/Q results can be expected with MRI with experienced clinicians[81,83] and, with proper breath holding, it may be useful in identifying typical findings of CTEPH.[83] Noninvasive measures of right ventricular chamber size, shape, thickness, and mass can all be offered by MRI, and mPAP has been shown to correlate with MRI measurement of right ventricular thickness, main pulmonary artery diameter, and right ventricular mass.[102–107] In a more recent study, on follow-up assessment of patients with PAH on PH medical therapy, an MRI-derived RV ejection fraction greater than 35% predicted survival, whereas baseline or follow-up PVR by cardiac catheterization did not.[108] Moreover, RV dysfunction could progress despite a decrease in PVR. This study and others have set the stage for future studies to show that serial assessment

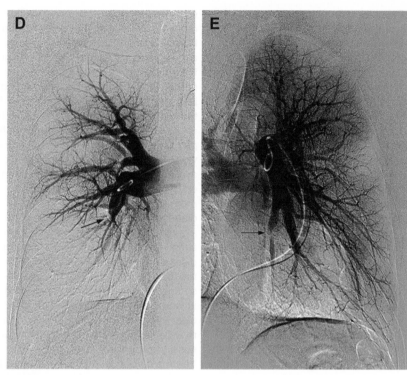

Fig. 7. (*continued*)

EXERCISE TESTING

of RV function will be the most important and innovative way to both monitor patients with PAH on therapy and to alter therapy in order to reach specific RV function goals.[108,109]

EXERCISE TESTING

Measures of exercise intolerance may be helpful in the diagnosis of early PAH (before it is present at rest) as well as in predicting survival and response to therapy.[110,111] Reductions in maximum oxygen consumption (Vo_2 max), anaerobic threshold, and ventilatory efficiency as assessed by cycle ergometry cardiopulmonary exercise testing (CPET) correlate well with New York Heart Association (NYHA) functional class.[112] In addition end-tidal pressure of carbon dioxide (P_{ETco2}) in patients with IPAH is significantly reduced at rest and with exercise in proportion to physiologic disease severity, and this finding on CPET when accompanied by arterial hypoxemia should trigger consideration of pulmonary vasculopathy.[113] CPET is reproducible and safe without complications or fatalities even in the most severely exercise-intolerant patient with PH.[114] Peak Vo_2 measures and ventilatory efficiency by CPET also show progressive improvement in CTEPH patients in response to surgical thromboendarterectomy.[115]

A simple and practical substitute for full CPET is the 6-minute walk test (6MWT). This validated test shows strong correlation between distance ambulated and peak Vo_2 seen on CPET,[116] as well as with total PVR, mean RAP, baseline cardiac output, and NYHA functional class.[117] The 6MWT can also predict disease progression as well as patient response to therapy.[118]

Measures of 6MWT and CPET also predict survival, with 6MWT distance of less than 380 m after 3 months of therapy[119] and peak oxygen uptake of less than 10.4 mL/min/kg showing significantly worse survival outcomes.[120] Combining these two measures to determine when to add new therapies in an algorithm for combination therapy has recently been proposed.[121]

CARDIAC CATHETERIZATION

The diagnosis of PAH (as opposed to PH) requires right, and often left, heart catheterization,[122] which allows for complete hemodynamic assessment, including measurement of PAP, transpulmonary and diastolic pressure gradients, and PVR. In addition, left heart filling pressures are measured, thus confirming or excluding pulmonary venous congestion as the explanation or contributor to PH.[122] At times, right heart catheterization is paired with exercise provocation or volume loading in order to reveal the dominant physiology in PH, such as in revealing increased left heart filling pressures not apparent at rest but manifest with mild physiologic stress.[123–125] It also allows oxygen saturation determinations that may be the only clue in diagnosing atrial septal defects with left-to-right shunting, especially of the sinus venosus type, which are more likely to be missed on the initial echo-Doppler evaluation.[122] Vasodilator testing should be done in all cases of IPAH without evidence of right heart failure,[126,127] although its role in other forms of PAH is controversial.[122] Positive response has prognostic implications,[128,129] and although recent work suggests that only 6.8% of patients with IPAH may be long-term responders to calcium channel blockers typically used for treatment in this group,[127] this group should be aggressively sought out and treated with these agents.[13]

Right heart catheterization represents a snapshot in time in a resting, supine patient and thus should not be viewed in isolation but instead integrated into the overall clinical context, and, most importantly, with the information obtained by cardiac imaging. For example, if a right heart catheterization reports a wedge pressure of 10 mm Hg in a patient with multiple risk factors and stigmata for left heart disease, careful review of the primary data should be undertaken, because such information is inconsistent with the overall assessment and there are known pitfalls of the hemodynamic assessment (in particular, accurate assessment of left heart filling pressures). The most common source of left atrial pressure underestimation occurs when the pressure (typically pulmonary arterial wedge pressure) measurement is not obtained at end expiration, thus allowing the influence of negative pleural pressure with inspiration to lower the pressure measurement. This occurrence is especially common when pleural pressure swings are exaggerated, as occurs in the obese supine patient or in patients with significant pulmonary disease.[125] Pulmonary arterial wedge pressure overestimation occurs when balloon occlusion of the segmental pulmonary artery is incomplete, allowing the wedge pressure estimation to represent a hybrid pressure, falling in between mPAP and wedge pressure. This problem can be avoided by careful observation of the hemodynamic tracings, sequential balloon deflation to obtain full artery occlusion, and confirmation of wedge position by wedge oximetry.[125,130]

SUMMARY

The accurate diagnosis of PAH is a complex process. Initial clues from the history and physical examinations can be nonspecific and subtle, requiring heightened acumen on the part of the front-line practitioner. With increased awareness and experience on the part of the diagnostician, these findings become more obvious clues to the presence of PAH. Noninvasive testing that should be ordered in all cases of suspected PAH include the ECG, CXR, pulmonary function tests (PFTs), and nocturnal oximetry. Doppler echocardiography plays a vital role in the PH work-up, with a wealth of diagnostic and physiologic information available on a routine study when interpreted properly. Ventilation-perfusion scanning is the best method to exclude CTEPH.[76] The incremental diagnostic and prognostic value of MRI is warranting increasing attention in the PH work-up and on serial assessment of PAH. Collagen vascular disease serologies, liver function testing, thyroid function testing, HIV testing, and nocturnal polysomnography should be considered in all cases in which they are clinically warranted and when a clear cause of PH is not readily apparent. CPET may be helpful in clarifying a diagnosis of PVD, assessing prognosis, and determining response to treatment, but is generally reserved for use in specialized centers with expertise. The 6MWT is a simple and reproducible validated test that correlates well with CPET measures and should be used to assess exercise capacity at diagnosis as well as serially with treatment of the patient with PH. Cardiac catheterization is required for full hemodynamic assessment and diagnostic confirmation of PAH, to exclude left heart disease and systemic-to-pulmonary shunt conditions. Right heart catheterization can also be useful in acquisition of prognostic information that may temper treatment decisions.

REFERENCES

1. Rubin LJ. Diagnosis and management of pulmonary arterial hypertension: ACCP evidence-based clinical practice guidelines. Chest 2004;126(1): 7S–10S.

2. Elliott CG, Barst RJ, Seeger W, et al. Worldwide physician education and training in pulmonary hypertension: pulmonary vascular disease: the global perspective. Chest 2010;137(6 Suppl):85S–94S.

3. Rich S, Dantzker DR, Ayres SM, et al. Primary pulmonary hypertension. A national prospective study. Ann Intern Med 1987;107(2):216–23.

4. Wigley FM, Lima JA, Mayes M, et al. The prevalence of undiagnosed pulmonary arterial hypertension in subjects with connective tissue disease at the secondary health care level of community-based rheumatologists (the UNCOVER study). Arthritis Rheum 2005;52(7):2125–32.

5. MacGregor AJ, Canavan R, Knight C, et al. Pulmonary hypertension in systemic sclerosis: risk factors for progression and consequences for survival. Rheumatology 2001;40:453–9.

6. Chang B, Schachna L, White B, et al. Natural history of mild-moderate pulmonary hypertension and the risk factors for severe pulmonary hypertension in scleroderma. J Rheumatol 2006;33(2):269–74.

7. Pan TL, Thumboo J, Boey ML. Primary and secondary pulmonary hypertension in systemic lupus erythematosus. Lupus 2000;9:338–42.

8. Johnson SR, Gladman DD, Urowitz MB, et al. Pulmonary hypertension in systemic lupus. Lupus 2004;13:506–9.

9. Roberts KE, Fallon MB, Krowka MJ, et al. Genetic risk factors for portopulmonary hypertension in patients with advanced liver disease. Am J Respir Crit Care Med 2009;179(9):835–42.

10. Ramsay MA, Simpson BR, Nguyen AT, et al. Severe pulmonary hypertension in liver transplant candidates. Liver Transpl Surg 1997;3(5):494–500.

11. Starkel P, Vera A, Gunson B, et al. Outcome of liver transplantation for patients with pulmonary hypertension. Liver Transpl 2002;8(4):382–8.

12. Krowka MJ. Hepatopulmonary syndrome and portopulmonary hypertension: implications for liver transplantation. Clin Chest Med 2005;26(4):587–97.

13. McGoon M, Gutterman D, Steen V, et al. Screening, early detection, and diagnosis of pulmonary arterial hypertension. ACCP evidence-based clinical practice guidelines. Chest 2004;126(1):14S–34S.

14. Bull TM. Physical examination in pulmonary arterial hypertension. Advance Pulmonary Hypertension 2005;4(3):6–10.

15. Rios JC, Massumi RA, Breesman WT, et al. Auscultatory features of acute tricuspid regurgitation. Am J Cardiol 1969;23(1):4–11.

16. Braunwald E, editor. Heart disease: a textbook of cardiovascular medicine. New York: WB Saunders Company; 1997.

17. Trembath RC, Thomson JR, Machado RD, et al. Clinical and molecular genetic features of pulmonary hypertension in patients with hereditary hemorrhagic telangiectasia. N Engl J Med 2001;345(5):325–34.

18. Holcomb BW, Loyd JE, Ely EW, et al. Pulmonary veno-occlusive disease. A case series and new observations. Chest 2000;118(6):1671–9.

19. Alegro S, Morrison D, Ovitt T, et al. Noninvasive detection of pulmonary hypertension. Clin Cardiol 1984;7:148–56.

20. Ahern GS, Tapson VF, Rebetz A, et al. Electrocardiography to define clinical status of primary pulmonary hypertension and pulmonary arterial hypertension secondary to collagen vascular disease. Chest 2002;122(2):524–7.

21. Bossone E, Pacioco G, Iarussi D, et al. The role prognostic role of the ECG in primary pulmonary hypertension. Chest 2002;121(2):513–8.

22. Kanemoto N. Electrocardiogram in primary pulmonary hypertension. Eur J Cardiol 1980;12:181–93.

23. Lupi E, Dumont C, Tejada VM, et al. A radiologic index of pulmonary arterial hypertension. Chest 1975;68:28–31.

24. Matthay RA, Schwarz MI, Ellis JH, et al. Pulmonary artery hypertension in chronic obstructive pulmonary disease: determination by chest radiography. Invest Radiol 1981;16(2):95–100.

25. Chetty KG, Brown SE, Light RW. Identification of pulmonary hypertension in chronic obstructive pulmonary disease from routine chest radiographs. Am Rev Respir Dis 1982;126(2):338–41.

26. Rich S, Pietra GG, Kieras K, et al. Primary pulmonary hypertension: radiographic and scintigraphic patterns of histologic subtypes. Ann Intern Med 1986;105(4):449–502.

27. Woodruff WW, Hoeck BE, Chitwood WR, et al. Radiographic findings in pulmonary hypertension from unresolved embolism. AJR Am J Roentgenol 1985;144:681–6.

28. Schmidt HC, Kauczor HU, Schild HH, et al. Pulmonary hypertension in patients with chronic pulmonary thromboembolism: chest radiograph and CT evaluation before and after surgery. Eur Radiol 1996;6:817–25.

29. Stein PD, Anthanasoulis C, Greenspan RH, et al. Relation of plain chest radiographic findings to pulmonary arterial pressure and arterial blood oxygen levels in patients with acute pulmonary embolism. Am J Cardiol 1992;69:394–6.

30. Sun XG, Hansen JE, Oudiz RJ, et al. Pulmonary function in primary pulmonary hypertension. J Am Coll Cardiol 2003;41:1028–35.

31. Morris TA, Auger WR, Ysrael MZ, et al. Parenchymal scarring is associated with restrictive spirometric defects in patients with chronic thromboembolic pulmonary hypertension. Chest 1996;110(2):399–403.

32. Steenhius LH, Groen HJ, Koeter GH, et al. Diffusion capacity and haemodynamics in primary and chronic thromboembolic pulmonary hypertension. Eur Respir J 2000;16:276–81.

33. Mohamed R, Freeman JW, Guest PJ, et al. Pulmonary gas exchange in liver transplant candidates. Liver Transpl 2002;8(9):802–8.

34. Sulica R, Teirstein AS, Kakarla S, et al. Distinctive clinical, radiographic, and functional characteristics of patients with sarcoidosis-related pulmonary hypertension. Chest 2005;128(3):1483–9.

35. Owens GR, Fino GJ, Herbert DL, et al. Pulmonary function in progressive systemic sclerosis. Comparison of CREST syndrome variant with diffuse scleroderma. Chest 1984;84(5):546–50.

36. Steen VD, Graham G, Conte C, et al. Isolated diffusing capacity reduction in systemic sclerosis. Arthritis Rheum 1992;35(7):765–70.

37. Stupi AM, Steen VD, Owens GR, et al. Pulmonary hypertension in the CREST syndrome variant of systemic sclerosis. Arthritis Rheum 1986;29(4):515–24.

38. Scorza R, Caronni M, Bassi S, et al. Post-menopause is the main risk factor for developing isolated pulmonary hypertension in systemic sclerosis. Ann N Y Acad Sci 2002;966:238–46.

39. Rafanan AL, Golish JA, Dinner DS, et al. Nocturnal hypoxemia is common in primary pulmonary hypertension. Chest 2001;120(3):894–9.

40. Schulz R, Baseler G, Ghofrani HA, et al. Nocturnal periodic breathing in primary pulmonary hypertension. Eur Respir J 2002;19:658–63.

41. Alexander R, Opotowsky AR, Ojeda J, et al. A simple echocardiographic prediction rule for hemodynamics in pulmonary hypertension. Circ Cardiovasc Imaging 2012;5:765–75.

42. Berger M, Haimowitz A, Van Tosh A, et al. Quantitative assessment of pulmonary hypertension in patients with tricuspid regurgitation using continuous wave Doppler ultrasound. J Am Coll Cardiol 1985;6:359–65.

43. Imanishi T, Nakatani S, Yamada S, et al. Validation of continuous wave Doppler-determined right ventricular peak positive and negative dP/dt: effect of right atrial pressure on measurement. J Am Coll Cardiol 1994;23:1638–43.

44. Lopez-Candales A, Rajagopalan N, Gulyasy B, et al. A delayed time of the peak tricuspid regurgitation signal: marker of right ventricular dysfunction. Am J Med Sci 2008;336:224–9.

45. Fisher MR, Forfia PR, Chamera E, et al. Accuracy of Doppler echocardiography in the hemodynamic assessment of pulmonary hypertension. Am J Respir Crit Care Med 2009;179:615–21.

46. Currie PJ, Seward JB, Chan KL, et al. Continuous wave Doppler determination of right ventricular pressure: a simultaneous Doppler-catheterization study in 127 patients. J Am Coll Cardiol 1985;6:750–6.

47. Rich JD, Shah SJ, Swamy RS, et al. Inaccuracy of Doppler echocardiographic estimates of pulmonary artery pressures in patients with pulmonary hypertension. Chest 2011;139:988–93.

48. Testani JM, St John Sutton MG, Wiegers SE, et al. Accuracy of noninvasively determined pulmonary artery systolic pressure. Am J Cardiol 2010;105:1192–7.

49. Bossone E, Duong-Wagner TH, Paciocco G, et al. Echocardiographic features of primary pulmonary hypertension. J Am Soc Echocardiogr 1999;12(8):655–62.

50. Rushmer RF, Crystal DK, Wagner C. The functional anatomy of ventricular contraction. Circ Res 1953;1:162–70.

51. Forfia PR, Fisher MR, Mathai SC, et al. Tricuspid annular displacement predicts survival in pulmonary hypertension. Am J Respir Crit Care Med 2006;174:1034–41.

52. Brown SB, Rania A, Katz D, et al. Longitudinal shortening accounts for the majority of right ventricular contraction in normal subjects and in pulmonary arterial hypertension and improves after pulmonary vasodilator therapy. Chest 2011;140:27–33.

53. Kaul S, Tei C, Hopkins JM, et al. Assessment of right ventricular function using two-dimensional echocardiography. Am Heart J 1984;107:526–31.

54. Lee CY, Chang SM, Hsiao SH, et al. Right heart function and scleroderma: insights from tricuspid annular plane systolic excursion. Echocardiography 2007;24:118–25.

55. Ghio S, Klersy C, Magrini G, et al. Prognostic relevance of the echocardiographic assessment of right ventricular function in patients with idiopathic pulmonary arterial hypertension. Int J Cardiol 2010;140:272–8.

56. Saxena N, Rajagopalan N, Edelman K, et al. Tricuspid annular systolic velocity: a useful measurement in determining right ventricular systolic function regardless of pulmonary artery pressures. Echocardiography 2006;23:750–5.

57. Mauritz GJ, Marcus JT, Westerhof N, et al. Prolonged right ventricular post-systolic isovolumic period in pulmonary arterial hypertension is not a reflection of diastolic dysfunction. Heart 2011;97(6):473–8.

58. Hinderliter AL, Willis PW 4th, Long W, et al. Frequency and prognostic significance of pericardial effusion in primary pulmonary hypertension. PPH Study Group. Primary pulmonary hypertension. Am J Cardiol 1999;84:481–4.

59. Miller AJ. Some observations concerning pericardial effusions and their relationship to the venous and lymphatic circulation of the heart. Lymphology 1970;3:76–8.

60. Hemnes AR, Gaine SP, Wiener CM. Poor outcomes associated with drainage of pericardial effusions in patients with pulmonary arterial hypertension. South Med J 2008;101:490–4.

61. Furuno Y, Nagamoto Y, Fujita M, et al. Reflection as a cause of midsystolic deceleration of pulmonary flow wave in dogs with acute pulmonary hypertension: comparison of pulmonary artery constriction with pulmonary embolisation. Cardiovasc Res 1991;25:118–24.

62. Castelain V, Hervé P, Lecarpentier Y, et al. Pulmonary artery pulse pressure and wave reflection in chronic pulmonary thromboembolism and primary pulmonary hypertension. J Am Coll Cardiol 2001;37:1085–92.

63. Torbicki A, Kurzyna M, Ciurzynski M, et al. Proximal pulmonary emboli modify right ventricular ejection pattern. Eur Respir J 1999;13:616–21.

64. Arkles JS, Opotowsky AR, Ojeda J, et al. Shape of the right ventricular Doppler envelope predicts hemodynamics and right heart function in pulmonary hypertension. Am J Respir Crit Care Med 2011; 183:268–76.

65. Damato AN, Galante JG, Smith WM. Hemodynamic response to treadmill exercise in normal subjects. J Appl Physiol 1966;21:959–66.

66. Bossone E, Rubenfire M, Bach DS, et al. Range of tricuspid regurgitation velocity at rest and during exercise in normal adult men: Implications for the diagnosis of pulmonary hypertension. J Am Coll Cardiol 1999;33:1662–6.

67. West JB. Left ventricular filling pressures during exercise: a cardiological blind spot? Chest 1998; 113:1695–7.

68. Laskey WK, Ferrari VA, Palevsky HI, et al. Pulmonary artery hemodynamics in primary pulmonary hypertension. J Am Coll Cardiol 1993;21: 406–12.

69. Hacobian M, Cohen MC, Atherton D, et al. Right ventricular exercise echocardiographic predictors of worsened clinical status in patients with pulmonary arterial hypertension. Am J Respir Crit Care Med 2011;183:A4996.

70. Fedullo PF, Auger WR, Kerr KM, et al. Chronic thromboembolic pulmonary hypertension. N Engl J Med 2001;345(20):1465–72.

71. Pengo V, Lensing AW, Prins MH, et al. Incidence of chronic thromboembolic pulmonary hypertension after pulmonary embolism. N Engl J Med 2004; 350(22):2257–64.

72. Fishman AJ, Moser KM, Fedullo PF. Perfusion lung scans vs. pulmonary angiography in evaluation of suspected primary pulmonary hypertension. Chest 1983;84(6):679–83.

73. D'Alonzo GE, Bower JS, Dantzker DR. Differentiation of patients with primary and thromboembolic pulmonary hypertension. Chest 1984;85(4):457–61.

74. Chapman PJ, Bateman ED, Benatar SR. Primary pulmonary hypertension and thromboembolic pulmonary hypertension – similarities and differences. Respir Med 1990;84(6):485–8.

75. Worsley DF, Palevsky HI, Alavi A. Ventilation-perfusion lung scanning in the evaluation of pulmonary hypertension. J Nucl Med 1994;35(5):793–6.

76. Tunariu N, Gibbs SJ, Win Z, et al. Ventilation-perfusion scintigraphy is more sensitive than multidetector CTPA in detecting chronic thromboembolic pulmonary disease as a treatable cause of pulmonary hypertension. J Nucl Med 2007;48(5):680–4.

77. Ryan KL, Fedullo PF, Davis GB, et al. Perfusion scan findings understate the severity of angiographic and hemodynamic compromise in chronic thromboembolic pulmonary hypertension. Chest 1988;93(6):1180–5.

78. Tardivon AA, Musset D, Maitre S, et al. Role of CT in chronic pulmonary embolism: comparison with pulmonary angiography. J Comput Assist Tomogr 1993;17(3):345–51.

79. Remy-Jardin M, Duhamel A, Deken V, et al. Systemic collateral supply in patients with chronic thromboembolic and primary pulmonary hypertension: assessment with multi-detector row helical CT angiography. Radiology 2005;235:274–81.

80. Heinrich M, Uder M, Tscholl D, et al. CT findings in chronic thromboembolic pulmonary hypertension. Predictors of hemodynamic improvement after pulmonary thromboendarterectomy. Chest 2005; 127(5):1606–13.

81. Bergin CJ, Hauschildt J, Rios G, et al. Accuracy of MR angiography compared with radionuclide scanning in identifying the cause of pulmonary arterial hypertension. AJR Am J Roentgenol 1997; 168:1549–55.

82. Ley S, Kauczor HU, Heussel CP, et al. Value of contrast-enhanced MR angiography and helical CT angiography in chronic thromboembolic pulmonary hypertension. Eur Radiol 2003;13:2365–71.

83. Kreitner KF, Ley S, Kauczor HU, et al. Chronic thromboembolic pulmonary hypertension: pre- and postoperative assessment with breath-hold MR imaging techniques. Radiology 2004;232: 535–43.

84. Nikolaou K, Schoenberg SO, Attenberger U, et al. Pulmonary arterial hypertension: diagnosis with fast perfusion MR imaging and high-spatial-resolution MR angiography- preliminary experience. Radiology 2005;236:694–703.

85. McLauglin VV, Channick R, Robbins IM, et al. Integrating current strategies for continuing assessment of pulmonary arterial hypertension. Advance Pulmonary Hypertension 2005;4(3):26–30.

86. Rich S, Kieras K, Hart K, et al. Antinuclear antibodies in primary pulmonary hypertension. J Am Coll Cardiol 1986;8(6):1307–11.

87. Steen VD, Ziegler GL, Rodnan GP, et al. Clinical and laboratory associations of anticentromere antibody in patients with progressive systemic sclerosis. Arthritis Rheum 1984;27(2):125–31.

88. Okano Y, Steen VD, Medsger TA. Autoantibody to U3 nucleolar ribonucleoprotein (fibrillarin) in patients with systemic sclerosis. Arthritis Rheum 1992;35(1):95–100.

89. Mitri GM, Lucas M, Fertig N, et al. A comparison between anti-Th/To and anticentromere antibody-positive systemic sclerosis patients with limited cutaneous involvement. Arthritis Rheum 2003; 48(1):203–9.

90. Ulanet DB, Wigley FM, Gelber AC, et al. Autoantibodies against B23, a nucleolar phosphoprotein,

occur in scleroderma and are associated with pulmonary hypertension. Arthritis Rheum 2003; 49(1):85–92.

91. Sacks DG, Okano Y, Steen VD, et al. Isolated pulmonary hypertension in systemic sclerosis with diffuse cutaneous involvement: association with serum anti-U3RNP antibody. J Rheumatol 1996; 23(4):639–42.

92. Falcao CA, Alves IC, Chahade WH, et al. Echocardiographic abnormalities and antiphospholipid antibodies in patients with systemic lupus erythematosus. Arq Bras Cardiol 2002;79(3):285–91.

93. Asherson RA, Higgenbottam TM, Dinh Xuan AT, et al. Pulmonary hypertension in a lupus clinic: experience with twenty-four patients. J Rheumatol 1990;17(10):1292–8.

94. Petitpretz P, Brenot F, Azarian R, et al. Pulmonary hypertension in patients with human immunodeficiency virus infection. Comparison with primary pulmonary hypertension. Circulation 1994;89(6): 2722–7.

95. Ma RC, Chow CC. Thyrotoxicosis as a risk factor for pulmonary arterial hypertension. Ann Intern Med 2005;143(4):282–92.

96. Roberts KE, Barst RJ, McElroy JJ, et al. Bone morphogenetic protein receptor 2 mutations in adults and children with idiopathic pulmonary arterial hypertension: association with thyroid disease. Chest 2005;128(Suppl 6):618S.

97. Chu JW, Kao PN, Faul JL, et al. High prevalence of autoimmune thyroid disease in pulmonary hypertension. Chest 2002;122(5):1668–73.

98. Curnock AL, Dweik RA, Higgins BH, et al. High prevalence of hypothyroidism in patients with primary pulmonary hypertension. Am J Med Sci 1999;318(5):289–92.

99. Nakchbandi IA, Wirth JA, Inzucchi SE. Pulmonary hypertension caused by Graves' thyrotoxicosis: normal pulmonary hemodynamics restored by (131) I treatment. Chest 1999;116(5):1483–5.

100. Lozano HF, Sharma CN. Reversible pulmonary hypertension, tricuspid regurgitation and right-sided heart failure associated with hyperthyroidism: case report and review of the literature. Cardiol Rev 2004;12(6):299–305.

101. Benza R, Biederman R, Murali S, et al. Role of cardiac magnetic resonance imaging in the management of patients with pulmonary arterial hypertension. J Am Coll Cardiol 2008;52(21):1683–92.

102. Laffon E, Vallet C, Bernard V, et al. A computed method for noninvasive MRI assessment of pulmonary arterial hypertension. J Appl Physiol 2004;96: 463–8.

103. Saba TS, Foster J, Cockburn M, et al. Ventricular mass index using magnetic resonance imaging accurately estimates pulmonary artery pressure. Eur Respir J 2002;20:1519–24.

104. Boxt LM, Katz J, Kolb T, et al. Direct quantification of right and left ventricular volumes with nuclear magnetic resonance imaging in patients with primary pulmonary hypertension. J Am Coll Cardiol 1992;19(7):1508–15.

105. Frank H, Globits S, Glogar D, et al. Detection and quantification of pulmonary hypertension with MR imaging: results in 23 patients. AJR Am J Roentgenol 1993;161:27–31.

106. Katz J, Whang J, Boxt LM, et al. Estimation of right ventricular mass in normal subjects and in patients with primary pulmonary hypertension by nuclear magnetic resonance imaging. J Am Coll Cardiol 1993;21(6):1475–81.

107. Roeleveld RJ, Marcus JT, Boonstra A, et al. A comparison of noninvasive MRI-based methods of estimating pulmonary artery pressure in pulmonary hypertension. J Magn Reson Imaging 2005; 22:67–72.

108. van de Veerdonk MC, Kind T, Marcus JT, et al. Progressive right ventricular dysfunction in patients with pulmonary arterial hypertension responding to therapy. J Am Coll Cardiol 2011; 58(24):2511–9.

109. Nickel N, Golpon H, Greer M, et al. The prognostic impact of follow-up assessments in patients with idiopathic pulmonary arterial hypertension. Eur Respir J 2012;39(3):589–96.

110. Waxman AB. Pulmonary function test abnormalities in pulmonary vascular disease and chronic heart failure. Clin Chest Med 2001;22(4):751–8.

111. Janicki JS, Weber KT, Likoff MJ, et al. Exercise testing to evaluate patients with primary vascular disease. Am Rev Respir Dis 1984;129(2):S93–5.

112. Sun XG, Hansen JE, Oudiz RJ, et al. Exercise pathophysiology in patients with primary pulmonary hypertension. Circulation 2001;104:429–35.

113. Yasunobu Y, Oudiz RJ, Sun XG, et al. End-tidal Pco_2 abnormality in patients with primary pulmonary hypertension. Chest 2005;127(5):1637–46.

114. Hansen JE, Sun XG, Yasunobu Y, et al. Reproducibility of cardiopulmonary exercise measurements in patients with pulmonary arterial hypertension. Chest 2004;126(3):816–24.

115. Iwase T, Nagaya N, Ando M, et al. Acute and chronic effects of surgical thromboendarterectomy on exercise capacity and ventilatory efficiency in patients with chronic thromboembolic pulmonary hypertension. Heart 2001;86:188–92.

116. Cahalin LP, Mathier MA, Semigran MJ, et al. The six-minute walk test predicts peak oxygen uptake and survival in patients with advanced heart failure. Chest 1996;110(2):325–32.

117. Miyamoto S, Nagaya N, Satoh T, et al. Clinical correlates and prognostic significance of six-minute walk test in patients with primary pulmonary hypertension. Comparison with cardiopulmonary

exercise testing. Am J Respir Crit Care Med 2000; 161:487–92.

118. Wax D, Garofano R, Barst RJ. Effects of long-term infusion of prostacyclin on exercise performance in patients with primary pulmonary hypertension. Chest 1999;116(4):914–20.

119. Sitbon O, Humbert M, Nunes H, et al. Long-term intravenous epoprostenol infusion in primary pulmonary hypertension. Prognostic factors and survival. J Am Coll Cardiol 2002;40(4):780–8.

120. Wensel R, Opitz CF, Anker SD, et al. Assessment in patients with primary pulmonary hypertension. Importance of cardiopulmonary exercise testing. Circulation 2002;106:319–24.

121. Hoeper MM, Markevych I, Spiekerkoetter E, et al. Goal-oriented treatment and combination therapy for pulmonary arterial hypertension. Eur Respir J 2005;26(5):858–63.

122. Oudiz RJ, Langleben D. Cardiac catheterization in pulmonary arterial hypertension: an updated guide to proper use. Advance Pulmonary Hypertension 2005;4(3):15–25.

123. Nootens M, Wolfkiel CJ, Chomka EV, et al. Understanding right and left ventricular systolic function and interactions at rest and exercise in primary pulmonary hypertension. Am J Cardiol 1995;75:374–7.

124. Shapiro BP, Nishimura RA, McGoon M, et al. Diagnostic dilemmas: diastolic heart failure causing pulmonary hypertension and pulmonary hypertension causing diastolic dysfunction. Advance Pulmonary Hypertension 2006;5(1):13–20.

125. Hemnes AR, Forfia PR, Champion HC. Assessment of pulmonary vasculature and right heart by invasive haemodynamics and echocardiography. Int J Clin Pract 2009;(162):4–19.

126. D'Alonzo GE, Barst RJ, Ayres SM, et al. Survival in patients with primary pulmonary hypertension. Results from a national prospective registry. Ann Intern Med 1991;115(5):343–9.

127. Rich S, Brundage BH. High-dose calcium channel-blocking therapy for primary pulmonary hypertension: evidence for long-term reduction in pulmonary arterial pressure and regression of right ventricular hypertrophy. Circulation 1987; 76(1):135–41.

128. Sitbon O, Humber M, Jais X, et al. Long-term response to calcium channel blockers in idiopathic pulmonary hypertension. Circulation 2005;111: 3105–11.

129. McLaughlin VV, Shillington A, Rich S. Survival in primary pulmonary hypertension. The impact of epoprostenol therapy. Circulation 2002;106:1477–82.

130. Leatherman JW, Shapiro RS. Overestimation of pulmonary artery occlusion pressure in pulmonary hypertension due to partial occlusion. Crit Care Med 2003;31(1):93–7.

Pulmonary Hypertension Owing to Left Heart Disease

Michael A. Mathier, MD

KEYWORDS

- Pulmonary hypertension • Heart failure • Hemodynamics • Echocardiography
- Cardiac catheterization

KEY POINTS

- It is critical to distinguish pulmonary arterial hypertension (PAH) from pulmonary hypertension (PH) owing to left heart disease (LHD).
- Clues to this distinction can be found in the history, physical examination, and routine testing.
- Cardiac catheterization is required for the distinction between PAH and PH owing to LHD.
- Treatment of PH owing to LHD should focus on optimally managing the underlying LHD.
- It is unclear if PAH-specific therapies can be used safely and effectively in patients with PH owing to LHD but based on limited studies conducted to date they cannot be recommended.

INTRODUCTION: NATURE OF THE PROBLEM

There is a complex relationship between PH and LHD: the two may exist independent of each other or in combination; when they exist in combination, the PH may be entirely and passively a product of the LHD, or it may have an additional component intrinsic to the pulmonary vasculature (mixed PH). PH can be seen in any form of LHD, as long as the LHD raises the left atrial pressure sufficiently and for long enough duration. Thus, PH can be seen in systolic and diastolic left heart failure (LHF), in left-sided valvular disease, and during and after cardiac surgery. PH owing to LHD is classified as World Health Organization group 2 PH or pulmonary venous hypertension. This article reviews the epidemiology, diagnostic strategies, and treatment options for PH owing to LHD. Throughout, contrasts with PAH are drawn to illustrate important differences between these two often-confused diagnoses.

EPIDEMIOLOGY

With the widespread use of diagnostic screening modalities, such as echocardiography and brain natriuretic peptide (BNP), the remarkable prevalence of PH owing to LHD has come into clearer focus. It has long been recognized that PH is common in advanced systolic LHF and that its development confers a poor prognosis.[1] Additionally, the presence of PH in patients with advanced LHF may remove the possibility of cardiac transplantation as a treatment option.[2] More recently, population-based studies have suggested that PH may be even more prevalent in patients with diastolic LHF. Lam and colleagues[3] found that 83% of predominantly elderly patients with diastolic LHF had echocardiographic evidence of PH. Furthermore, longitudinal assessment of a population with similar demographics but no LHF showed that increasing age was associated with echocardiographic evidence of increasing pulmonary and left heart pressures.[4] This suggests that the relationship between PH and diastolic LHF begins early in the course of LHF. PH has also been reported to be fairly common in patients with left-sided valve disease, including aortic stenosis and mitral stenosis and regurgitation.[5,6] The reported impact of surgical or percutaneous correction of the valve lesion on PH has been variable,

No relevant disclosures.
Pulmonary Hypertension Program, University of Pittsburgh Medical Center, University of Pittsburgh School of Medicine, Scaife Hall S559, 200 Lothrop Street, Pittsburgh, PA 15213, USA
E-mail address: mathierm@upmc.edu

Clin Chest Med 34 (2013) 683–694
http://dx.doi.org/10.1016/j.ccm.2013.09.004

with some studies suggesting improvement and others showing none or even PH progression.[5,7]

DIAGNOSIS

The importance of an accurate diagnosis of PH is obvious: PH is a heterogeneous group of diseases that differ substantially in pathophysiology, presentation, and, most critically, treatment. Arguably the most challenging diagnostic distinction is that between PAH and PH owing to LHD. By pursuing and carefully analyzing a standard set of diagnostic modalities, however, clinicians can usually have a strong sense of the true diagnosis even before the gold standard of cardiac catheterization is performed. Coming to this strong sense (a qualitative equivalent of the prior probability) of the diagnosis is important for several reasons: it can influence treatment strategy before the diagnostic assessment is complete; it can determine specifics of the diagnostic studies pursued (especially cardiac catheterization); and it can guide the counseling provided to patients as an accurate diagnosis is sought. Diagnostic modalities are discussed in the context of how they influence the prior probability of an eventual diagnosis of PAH versus PH owing to LHD.

HISTORY AND PHYSICAL EXAMINATION

There are many aspects of the history and physical examination that can point in the direction of PAH versus PH owing to LHD. From the history, a diagnosis of PAH is more likely in patients who are younger, female, and nonobese; have specific risk factors for PAH (connective tissue disease, HIV, portal hypertension, prior anorexigen or stimulant use, or a family history of PAH); and an absence of risk factors for LHD.[8,9] A diagnosis of PH owing to LHD is more likely in patients who are older, male, obese, and have risk factors for LHD (systemic hypertension, diabetes, tobacco use, dyslipidemia, family history of coronary artery disease, or prior rheumatic heart disease). Both PAH and PH owing to LHD can present with complaints of resting or exertional dyspnea, chest pain, fatigue, edema, palpitations, and presyncope or syncope. Complaints of orthopnea or paroxysmal nocturnal dyspnea, however, point strongly to LHD. On physical examination, both PAH and PH owing to LHD can feature a range of vital signs, findings of right heart failure (elevated jugular venous pressure, hepatomegaly, ascites, and edema), a loud pulmonic closure sound, a right ventricular (RV) lift, and right-sided extra heart sounds (including regurgitant murmurs). Pulmonary rales, left-sided third and fourth heart sounds, left-sided murmurs, and an irregular heartbeat indicative of atrial fibrillation strongly suggest LHD. Findings on history and physical examination alone, however, are insufficient to differentiate between these two diagnoses.

LABORATORY TESTING/IMAGING

Although the history and physical examination can raise the possibility of a diagnosis of PAH versus PH owing to LHD, a series of diagnostic studies is necessary to refine the differential and eventually lead to a final diagnosis.

Electrocardiogram

ECG is often of little help in distinguishing between PAH and PH owing to LHD. A pattern of RV hypertrophy (with the attendant repolarization abnormalities, or strain), right axis deviation, and right atrial enlargement favors a diagnosis of PAH. Findings more indicative of LHD include left ventricular (LV) hypertrophy (with strain), left axis deviation, left atrial enlargement, patterns consistent with prior infarction, and atrial fibrillation. An ECG may be normal or have only nonspecific abnormalities in both PAH and PH owing to LHD.[8,9]

Brain Natriuretic Peptide

Both PAH and PH owing to LHD may cause elevation in serum BNP levels. In general, the magnitude of the elevation seen in LHD exceeds that seen in PAH. Typically, patients with even advanced degrees of PAH have BNP levels under 300 pg/mL,[10] whereas patients with PH owing to LHD may have levels far greater.[11] Many factors influence the BNP level, including age, gender, obesity, renal function, and other poorly defined individual factors.

Chest Radiography

Chest radiography (chest x-ray and chest CT) is rarely a sensitive enough tool in differentiating reliably between PAH and PH owing to LHD.[9,12] Its primary role in this population is in documenting or excluding clinically important parenchymal lung or airway disease. On chest x-ray, a finding of pulmonary artery (PA) enlargement, pulmonary vascular pruning, and/or isolated RV enlargement (seen best on the lateral film as loss of the retrosternal airspace) favors a diagnosis of PAH.[9] The presence of global cardiac enlargement, left atrial enlargement, valvular or coronary calcification, or pulmonary edema favors a diagnosis of LHD. On chest CT, these same findings (and their impact on diagnosis) may be present. Additionally, CT technology is increasingly used to specifically look at cardiac structure and function. Especially when contrast is administered and special cardiac gating protocols are used, details of coronary anatomy and myocardial and valvular structure and function can be seen on CT scanning.[13] It is uncertain whether these advances will ever supplant more specific cardiac imaging studies, including echocardiography, MRI, and angiography.

Pulmonary Function Testing

Pulmonary function testing (PFT) is rarely helpful in differentiating between PAH and PH owing to LHD. Like chest radiography, its greatest value is in screening for intrinsic lung disease. In PAH, the PFT often shows a disproportionate decrease in diffusing capacity with relatively preserved flow volume loops.[14] In PH owing to LHD, however, this same pattern may be present.

Echocardiography

Transthoracic echocardiography has emerged as a critical diagnostic tool in the evaluation of patients suspected of having PH.[15,16] From its inception as simple M-mode, echocardiography has evolved into providing remarkably detailed 2-D and 3-D images as well as physiologic data from traditional and tissue Doppler techniques. These advances have allowed for a fuller understanding of right and left heart myocardial and valvular structure and function and reasonably accurate estimates of pulmonary artery, right atrial, and potentially left atrial pressures. Although cardiac catheterization is still necessary for the proper diagnosis of PH, the remarkable evolution of echocardiography has greatly improved decision making regarding catheterization. Qualitative estimates of pretest probability of PAH versus PH owing to LHD have also improved with advances in echocardiography.[17]

Echocardiography in pulmonary hypertension
The development and widespread utilization of echocardiography has arguably revolutionized the field of PH. As a widely available, noninvasive, and inexpensive modality, echocardiography has emerged as the primary screening tool for PH among at-risk populations and in patients suspected of having the disease. The widespread use of echocardiography for this purpose has undoubtedly contributed to the changing epidemiology of PH: the disease seems more prevalent, to be diagnosed at an earlier stage, and to have a better outcome compared to the era before its routine use.[18] The primary echo technique used to detect PH starts with a Doppler-derived measure of the peak velocity of the tricuspid valve insufficiency

jet (V). An estimate is then made of the right atrial pressure (RAP). These values are then entered into the modified Bernoulli equation to yield the estimated RV systolic pressure ($ERVSP$):

$$ERVSP = 4V^2 + RAP$$

Assuming there is no RV outflow obstruction (including pulmonic stenosis), the ERVSP is a good surrogate for PA systolic pressure (PASP). Although PH is traditionally defined as a catheter-derived PA mean pressure greater than 25 mm Hg, an echo-derived ERVSP greater than 35–40 mm Hg is generally considered abnormal.[16]

Although this technique for estimating PASP is the most commonly used, other techniques have been described.[16] More important to the optimal use of echocardiography in the diagnosis of PH, however, is the incorporation of markers of right heart pressure overload and performance. The pressure loaded right heart undergoes fairly predictable changes in structure and function. Structural changes include RV, RA, and inferior vena cava dilation; RV hypertrophy; and flattening of the interventricular septum. Functional changes include qualitative RV hypokinesis, a decrease in RV fractional area change, and a decrease in the tricuspid annular plane systolic excursion. This latter marker has gained popularity because it is straightforward and reproducible and has been shown to correlate with outcomes in PH.[19] Combining the ERVSP with these measures of right heart structure and function can yield excellent accuracy in the diagnosis of PH. Despite this, right heart catheterization (RHC) is still considered a mandatory part of the diagnostic work-up of PH because it provides greater accuracy and information not available even with modern echocardiographic techniques.

Echocardiography in left heart disease
Echocardiography arguably first gained popularity because of its ability to elucidate LHD. The evolution of echocardiography to the current technology has only enhanced its value in this regard. 2-D echocardiography yields important regarding LV size, wall thickness, and systolic performance. It also can be used to measure left atrial size, which is a critical parameter in predicting a diagnosis of PAH versus PH owing to LHD (discussed later). Application of standard and tissue Doppler analysis can yield insights into LV diastolic function. The use of these techniques in the assessment of diastole is described in detail by Khouri and colleagues.[20] The development and widespread use of echocardiography has allowed for recognition of the high prevalence of diastolic dysfunction and diastolic LHF.[21] Lastly, the combination of

2-D and Doppler echocardiography techniques can provide information regarding mitral and aortic valve disease, both of which frequently result in the development of PH.[5,6]

Echocardiography in pulmonary hypertension owing to left heart disease

Although RHC is necessary for the proper diagnosis of PH in general, it is especially important in differentiating PAH from PH owing to LHD. Nevertheless, careful use of echocardiography can substantially improve the qualitative pretest probability for either of these conditions. In general terms, an echocardiogram showing clear evidence of LHD and PH substantially increases the probability of an eventual diagnosis of pulmonary venous hypertension. Conversely, an echocardiogram showing an absence of LHD and clear evidence of PH increases the probability of a diagnosis of PAH. It is much more challenging when the echocardiogram shows only subtle signs of PH or LHD. Recent studies have put forward more quantitative approaches to using echocardiography to distinguish between PAH and PH owing to LHD.[17] **Fig. 1** shows a representative echocardiogram from a patient with PH owing to LHD.

MRI

MRI is an emerging imaging modality in the assessment of a variety of cardiovascular diseases, including heart failure and PH.[22] It provides an unrivaled degree of anatomic detail, including information about tissue characteristics that cannot be obtained with other modalities. Increasingly it is used to obtain physiologic information, including pressure and flow estimates.[23] These advantages have begun to outweigh the disadvantages of the technology: its limited availability, cost, and technical demands. Because of its unique ability to detect and quantify alterations in RV structure and function, many PH specialists believe it will emerge as the critical imaging tool in the evaluation and management of patients with PH.

MRI in pulmonary hypertension

MRI has evolved to where it can provide detailed information regarding the right heart and the pulmonary circulation. Given the traditional limitations of echocardiography in providing detail about the right heart, it is no surprise that MRI has emerged as an important diagnostic modality in patients with PH. MRI can provide quantitative measures

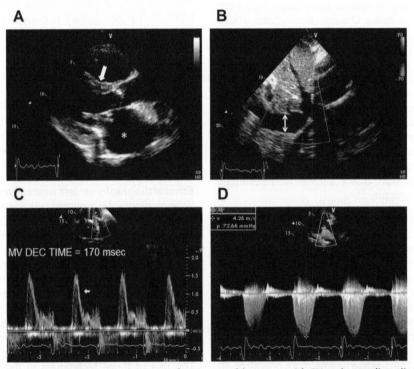

Fig. 1. Transthoracic echocardiographic imaging of a 70-year-old woman with PH owing to diastolic heart failure. (*A*) Parasternal long axis view showing LV hypertrophy (*solid arrow*) and left atrial enlargement (*asterisk*). RV enlargement and aortic valve thickening are also seen. (*B*) Shows a dilated inferior vena cava (*double-headed arrow*) at 3 cm, indicating elevated central venous pressure. (*C*) Shows a short mitral valve deceleration time (*arrow*) indicating elevated left atrial pressure. (*D*) Shows a tricuspid valve regurgitation velocity of 4.26 m/s, which, assuming an RAP of 15 mm Hg, yields an estimated RV systolic pressure of approximately 88 mm Hg.

of RV size and function in PH,[22] and these measures can be repeated after initiation of therapy to assess response. Several studies have demonstrated the prognostic importance of changes in RV size and function with therapy in patients with PH.[24] These changes seem more important prognostically than changes in pulmonary hemodynamics.[25] Emerging MRI techniques can also shed light on PA and pulmonic valve structure and blood flow characteristics through the right heart and pulmonary circulation.[26]

MRI in left heart disease

Similar to its capabilities in PH and right heart disease, MRI provides remarkably detailed images of left heart structure and function. This include LV dimensions and wall thickness and left atrial dimensions. Detail is sufficient to allow for accurate determination of chamber volumes as well. Additionally, MRI can provide functional measures, including systolic wall thickening and chamber shortening (and consequently fractional shortening and ejection fraction) of the LV. Furthermore, MRI allows for characterization of the myocardium, including the presence of prior infarction and collagen deposition. This latter finding, often detected by the presence of late gadolinium enhancement or an increase in extracellular volume fraction of fibrosis, can be an indicator of LHD and dysfunction. Lastly, cardiac MRI can provide detailed information regarding the pulmonary veins, the aorta, the aortic valve, and the mitral valve.[27]

MRI in pulmonary hypertension owing to left heart disease

Just as echocardiography can help differentiate PAH from PH owing to LHD, MRI can be useful for this as well. The two modalities should be thought of as complementary: echocardiography is more appropriate for broad and initial screening purposes whereas MRI provides more detailed information in properly selected cases. Although again it is important to emphasize the crucial role of catheterization in the diagnosis of PH, MRI, like echocardiography, can substantially improve estimates of the pretest probability of PAH versus PH owing to LHD. **Fig. 2** shows an example of an MRI in a patient with PH owing to LHD.

INTEGRATING THE DATA PRIOR TO CATHETERIZATION

When considering patients with apparent PH based on history, physical examination, and noninvasive diagnostics, it is important to establish a pretest probability of the diagnosis being PAH versus PH owing to LHD. When the suspicion

is strongly in favor of PH owing to LHD, it may be prudent to initiate and adjust medications (diuretics, antihypertensives, and rate-controlling agents) prior to catheterization in an effort to optimize left heart filling pressures. Additionally, a suspicion of PH owing to LHD should strongly prompt the performance of a full right and left heart catheterization to fully evaluate the presence and extent of LHD. Conversely, when the suspicion is for PAH, an RHC alone may be sufficient. If it is truly unclear whether the diagnosis is PAH or PH owing to LHD, a full right and left heart catheterization is recommended. **Table 1** summarizes features of the history, physical examination, and diagnostic testing that favor a diagnosis of PAH versus PH owing to LHD.

CARDIAC CATHETERIZATION

Cardiac catheterization is critical in the diagnosis of PH and in differentiating between PAH and PH owing to LHD. The procedure almost always allows for a definitive diagnosis to be made. Furthermore, catheterization allows for a more refined diagnosis of PH owing to LHD, identifying clinically important subsets. All of this requires, however, a full understanding of the proper performance and interpretation of cardiac catheterization as well as the potential pitfalls that can limit the utility of the procedure.

Importance of Cardiac Catheterization

The definitions of PAH and of PH owing to LHD help illustrate why cardiac catheterization is critical in the differentiation of these conditions. PAH is defined by a PA mean pressure greater than 25 mm Hg whereas the left heart filling pressure (either the PA wedge pressure [PAWP] or LV end-diastolic pressure [LVEDP]) is less than 15 mm Hg. Many PH specialists also believe that a pulmonary vascular resistance (PVR) greater than 3 Wood units is necessary for the diagnosis.[8] In contrast, PH owing to LHD is defined by a PA mean pressure greater than 25 mm Hg whereas the PAWP or LVEDP is greater than 15 mm Hg. Further analysis of catheterization data can yield 4 distinct types of PH owing to LHD: passive, mixed, reactive, and nonreactive.[28] Passive PH owing to LHD exists when the PVR is normal. Mixed PH owing to LHD exists if the PVR is elevated. Reactive and nonreactive are determined by whether or not the PVR can be normalized with acute or subacute interventions (such as the administration of a vasodilator). The precise subset of PH owing to LHD may be important in determining treatment strategy, including eligibility for cardiac transplantation.

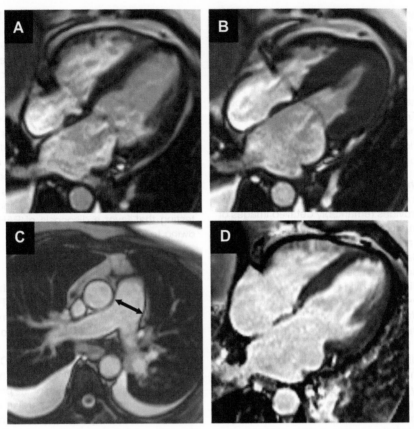

Fig. 2. MRI of a 73-year-old man with PH owing to diastolic heart failure. Imaging demonstrates preserved systolic function and mild LV hypertrophy (1.3 cm) in the 4-chamber view at end diastole (*A*) and end systole (*B*). Also demonstrated is an enlarged main pulmonary artery—the black line measures 3.3 cm (*C*). Late gadolinium enhancement imaging 15 minutes postgadolinium contrast administration does not reveal any hyperintense signal to suggest focal fibrosis (*D*), although a cardiac magnetic resonance measure of diffuse myocardial fibrosis (extracellular volume fraction) was abnormal, a common finding in LHD.

Basics of Cardiac Catheterization

The technique of cardiac catheterization has been described in detail in textbooks devoted to the subject.[29] Although RHC alone is often sufficient for the correct diagnosis of PH, left heart catheterization if often indicated in patients where the diagnosis of PH owing to LHD is being entertained (to assess coronary anatomy and valve function and to confirm left heart filling pressure). RHC is safe, as documented in a study of more than 7000 such procedures performed over a 5-year period at 20 PH centers by experienced operators.[30] In this study, there was a 1.1% significant complication rate (mostly related to venous access) and a 0.05% procedural mortality. Left heart catheterization carries a somewhat higher risk,[29] but it is generally agreed that the benefits of catheterization in these patients outweigh the risks in almost all cases and should be performed unless clearly contraindicated.

Waveforms and Interpretation

An example of normal RHC pressure waveforms is shown in **Fig. 3**. Many catheterization laboratories report computer-generated mean pressures for the RA, PA, and PAW pressures. These are arguably acceptable in most patients but can yield erroneous values in certain situations where dramatic respiratory variation in pressure is present (discussed later). Considering the critical importance in deriving accurate hemodynamics, it is recommended that pressure measurements be read at end expiration and end diastole (**Fig. 4**).

Cardiac Output Measurement

Cardiac output (CO) is measured often by both thermodilution and modified Fick techniques, which require oxygen saturation measurements from the pulmonary and systemic arteries (the

Table 1
Diagnostic clues to the etiology of PH: PAH vs PH owing to LHD

Favors PAH	Modality	Favors PH Owing to LHD
Younger Female Nonobese PAH risk factors Absence of LHD risk factors	History	Older Male Obese LHD risk factors Absence of PAH risk factors Orthopnea PND
—	Physical	Rales Left-sided S3, S4 Left-sided murmurs
RAD RVH RAE	ECG	Atrial fibrillation LAD LAE LVH Q waves
>80, rarely >300 pg/mL	BNP	>80, often >300 pg/mL
PA enlargement Vascular pruning Isolated RVE (loss of retrosternal airspace)	CXR/CT	Pulmonary edema LAE Global cardiac enlargement Coronary/valve calcification
Isolated low DLCO	PFT	—
Elevated ERVSP RAE, RVE, RVH RV dysfunction Absence of left-sided abnormalities	Echocardiography	Elevated ERVSP RAE, RVE, RVH RV dysfunction Presence of left-sided abnormalities: LAE, LVE, LVH LV dysfunction Mitral, aortic valve disease
Similar to echo	CMR	Similar to echo Presence of LV fibrosis
PA mean >25 mm Hg PAWP/LVEDP <15 mm Hg	Catheterization	PA mean >25 mm Hg PAWP/LVEDP >15 mm Hg

Abbreviations: CMR, cardiac magnetic resonance; CXR, chest X ray; DLCO, diffusion capacity for carbon monoxide; LAD, left axis deviation; LAE, left atrial enlargement; LHD risk factors, systemic hypertension, diabetes, tobacco use, dyslipidemia, family history of coronary artery disease, or prior rheumatic heart disease; LVE, LV enlargement; LVH, LV hypertrophy; PAH risk factors, connective tissue disease, HIV, portal hypertension, prior anorexigen or stimulant use, or a family history of PAH; PNE, paroxysmal nocturnal dyspnea; RAD, right axis deviation; RAE, right atrial enlargement; RVE, RV enlargement; RVH, RV hypertrophy.

latter is often done noninvasively with oximetry). If the PA oxygen saturation is high, oxygen saturation measurements should also be made throughout the right heart, including the central veins, to rule out a left-to-right shunt. Thermodilution CO is thought particularly subject to error in patients with severe tricuspid insufficiency, intracardiac shunts, and extremely high or low CO.[31] Accordingly, with a patient in the resting state, and with no physiologic issues (such as metabolic derangements or general anesthesia) that render the assumed oxygen consumption erroneous, the modified Fick method is likely the more accurate measurement. When the assumed oxygen consumption is not valid, such as with exercise,

however, the Fick method cannot be used unless a direct measure of oxygen consumption is made. Even in the best of circumstances, there can be significant disagreement in the CO values obtained by these 2 techniques[32]; which method is entered into calculations may come down to operator preference and sense of which is more accurate, and the chosen methodology should be documented.

Provocative Maneuvers

Provocative maneuvers, including acute vasodilator testing, volume loading, and exercise, may be performed during RHC to confirm a

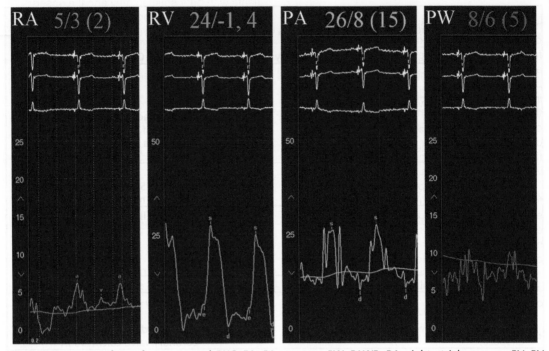

Fig. 3. Pressure waveforms from a normal RHC. PA, PA pressure; PW, PAWP; RA, right atrial pressure; RV, RV pressure.

diagnosis of LHD not apparent on the resting hemodynamic data. These results can help refine the diagnosis, provide prognostic and therapeutic information, and yield insights into the mechanisms underlying a patient's functional limitation. Although consensus guidelines recommend that acute vasodilator testing be performed at the time of RHC in patients diagnosed with PAH,[8] administering one of the commonly used selective pulmonary vasodilators in patients with PH owing to LHD risks precipitating pulmonary edema and thus should be avoided. If it is thought that acute vasodilator testing may be valuable for such patients, a balanced systemic and pulmonary vasodilator (such as nitroprusside or nitroglycerine) is a safer choice. In patients with low CO, an inotropic and vasodilating agent, such as milrinone, is sometimes preferred.[33]

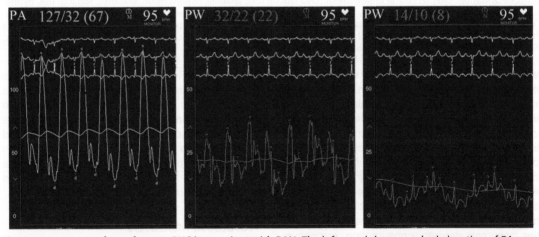

Fig. 4. Pressure waveforms from an RHC in a patient with PAH. The left panel shows marked elevation of PA pressure. The middle panel shows a PA wedge (PW) pressure with the catheter in an underwedged position. Note the waveform retains elements of the PA pressure waveform, and the mean pressure is falsely elevated. The right panel shows the true PW pressure.

Occasionally, acute administration of intravenous fluid may help elucidate a patient's underlying pathophysiology. An example of this maneuver is for a patient with a high probability of LHD and an RHC showing elevated pulmonary pressures but with low cardiac filling pressures. In this instance, rapid acute administration of intravenous fluid may unmask underlying LHD. In this scenario, care should be taken that only enough fluid to demonstrate a clinically significant rise in left heart filling pressures be administered so as not to provoke pulmonary edema.

Frequently, patients present with cardiorespiratory symptoms predominantly or exclusively with exercise. If resting RHC data do not elucidate an explanation for the symptoms, repeating measurements can be considered while the patient is exercising. A variety of protocols are used with as yet no consensus on the best methodology.[34,35] An abrupt rise in PAWP with exercise is a reliable indicator of LHD.

Pitfalls of Cardiac Catheterization

The pitfalls of cardiac catheterization fall into 2 general categories: errors in data acquisition and errors in data interpretation. Errors in data acquisition may be related to improperly flushed catheters or calibrated manometers. They also may relate to operator errors in catheter placement. The most common examples of these result from an improperly wedged catheter. Overwedging occurs with excessive inflation pressure in the catheter balloon, usually producing a dampened waveform, and can lead to artificially high or low values. A more common error is underwedging (see **Fig. 4**). Underwedging results from the catheter balloon incompletely occluding the branch PA, producing a hybrid waveform composed of elements of both the PA tracing and the PAWP tracing. As a rule this artificially increases the PAWP value. Underwedging is a frequent problem in patients with very high PA pressures, likely related to the poor compliance of their pulmonary arteries. Given that the PAWP is the main hemodynamic discriminator between PAH and PH owing to LHD, it is clear why an accurate PAWP is so crucial. Proper wedge position should be confirmed by fluoroscopy, waveform inspection, and, if possible, by confirming that the oxygen saturation of the blood withdrawn from the distal port while in the wedge position is in the systemic arterial range. If there is any doubt about the PAWP being accurate, a left heart catheterization should be performed to directly measure the LVEDP.[36] The entire clinical picture of patients should be considered when judging the need for a left heart catheterization.

Even when accurate RHC data are acquired, errors can be made in the interpretation of these data. Among the conditions that can lead to errors in the interpretation of RHC data are advanced lung disease, morbid obesity, severe mitral regurgitation, and LHD in patients with volume depletion. With advanced lung disease, intrathoracic pressure fluctuation is exaggerated, and the PAWP at end expiration can differ considerably from the mean PAWP.[37] Relying on the mean in this circumstance significantly underestimates the true PAWP. Morbid obesity often produces the same phenomenon and can have the added confounding influences of elevated PAWP from LHD and elevated CO. Severe mitral regurgitation usually results in large v waves in the PAWP tracing. These v waves drive the mean PAWP up significantly; many PH specialists advocate reading the PAWP at the a wave to account for this expected change.[29] In volume-depleted patients with LHD, elevated PA pressures may be misinterpreted as PAH because intracardiac filling pressures are low. As described previously, volume loading in this instance may bring out the true pathophysiology.

Despite the caveats listed previously, a well-performed and interpreted cardiac catheterization usually allows for an accurate diagnosis of PH owing to LHD and its differentiation from PAH.

TREATMENT OF PH OWING TO LHD

Once a diagnosis of PH owing to LHD is made, targeted treatments can be instituted with the goal of improving symptoms and functional status. The first step in therapy is to optimally treat the underlying LHD. This often entails instituting and adjusting medications but may also include an intervention, such as coronary revascularization, cardiac rate or rhythm control, valve repair or replacement, or insertion of a biventricular pacer.[38] Once the LHD is optimized, treatment of the PH that accompanies it falls into one of two categories: either the LHD is dominant and the PH is a lesser component, or the PH is more dominant and the LHD is a lesser component. An example of the former is in patients with longstanding severe LHF with superimposed PH. In this case, progressive efforts to treat the LHF, such as with chronic inotropic and vasodilator therapy or placement of a ventricular assist device, may improve the PH, potentially even allowing for cardiac transplantation.[39] Recent case reports suggest that PAH-specific therapies may have a limited adjunctive role in this scenario.[40,41] They should be used with great caution, however, because prior larger-scale studies in advanced LHF have shown ineffectiveness or clinical worsening.[42,43]

The more common scenario is when the PH is more dominant and the LHD is a lesser component. This pattern is usually seen in patients with more mild systolic LHF, diastolic LHF, or valvular disease. In this scenario, once the underlying LHD is optimally treated, a trial of PAH-specific therapy may be considered. Several reports have suggested that the phosphodiesterase type 5 inhibitors may be useful in these situations. Lewis and colleagues[44] studied the effects of sildenafil versus placebo in 32 patients with mild systolic LHF and PH. They found that sildenafil was well tolerated and improved exercise capacity, hemodynamics, and quality of life. Guazzi and colleagues[45] studied the effects of sildenafil versus placebo in 44 patients with diastolic LHF and PH. They found that sildenafil was again well tolerated and improved hemodynamics and RV function. Enthusiasm for the use of sildenafil in patients with diastolic LHF has diminished, however, with the results of the recent RELAX study.[46] This larger study (216 patients) found that sildenafil did not improve exercise capacity or clinical status in patients with diastolic LHF. It must be emphasized that none of the PAH-specific therapies is approved for use in any patients with PH owing to LHD. Furthermore, if these agents are used in such patients, great care must be taken because their safety has not been fully established and they may provoke clinical compromise in the form of hypotension, pulmonary venous congestion, or even frank pulmonary edema.

SUMMARY

PH owing to LHD is a common problem that carries significant morbidity. The principal diagnostic challenge is in differentiating it from PAH. This can be readily done, however, with the use and proper interpretation of a series of diagnostic studies. A qualitative pretest probability prior to catheterization can be made based on the noninvasive diagnostics and may aid in counseling, formulation of a treatment strategy, and choice of RHC alone versus combined right and left heart catheterization. Once a diagnosis of PH owing to LHD is made, targeted treatments can be instituted in the hopes of improving symptoms.

REFERENCES

1. Voelkel NF, Quaife RA, Leinwand LA, et al. Right ventricular function and failure: report of a National Heart, Lung, and Blood Institute working group on cellular and molecular mechanisms of right heart failure. Circulation 2006;114:1883–91.

2. Teuteberg JJ, Mathier MA, Shullo MA. Cardiac transplantation and circulatory support devices. In: Antman EM, Sabatine MS, editors. Cardiovascular therapeutics. Philadelphia: Elsevier; 2013. p. 307–21.

3. Lam CS, Roger VL, Rodeheffer RJ, et al. Pulmonary hypertension in heart failure with preserved ejection fraction: a community-based study. J Am Coll Cardiol 2009;53:1119–26.

4. Lam CS, Borlaug BA, Kane GC, et al. Age-associated increases in pulmonary artery systolic pressure in the general population. Circulation 2009;119:2663–70.

5. Malouf JF, Enriquez-Sarano M, Pellikka PA, et al. Severe pulmonary hypertension in patients with severe aortic valve stenosis: clinical profile and prognostic implications. J Am Coll Cardiol 2002;40:789–95.

6. Vincens JJ, Temizer D, Post JR, et al. Long-term outcome of cardiac surgery in patients with mitral stenosis and severe pulmonary hypertension. Circulation 1995;92:II137–42.

7. Umesan CV, Kapoor A, Sinha N, et al. Effect of Inoue balloon mitral valvotomy on severe pulmonary arterial hypertension in 315 patients with rheumatic mitral stenosis: immediate and long-term results. J Heart Valve Dis 2000;9:609–15.

8. McLaughlin VV, Archer SL, Badesch DB, et al. ACCF/AHA 2009 expert consensus document on pulmonary hypertension. J Am Coll Cardiol 2009; 53:1573–619.

9. Trow TK, McArdle JR. Diagnosis of pulmonary arterial hypertension. Clin Chest Med 2007;28:59–73.

10. Nagaya N, Nishikimi T, Uematsu M, et al. Plasma brain natriuretic peptide as a prognostic indicator in patients with primary pulmonary hypertension. Circulation 2000;102:865–70.

11. Silver MA, Maisel A, Yancy CW, et al. BNP Consensus Panel 2004: a clinical approach for the diagnostic, prognostic, screening, treatment monitoring, and therapeutic roles of natriuretic peptides in cardiovascular diseases. Congest Heart Fail 2004;10:1–30.

12. Alegro S, Morrison D, Ovitt T, et al. Noninvasive detection of pulmonary hypertension. Clin Cardiol 1984;7:148–56.

13. Nasis A, Mottram PM, Cameron JD, et al. Current and evolving clinical applications of multidetector cardiac CT in assessment of structural heart disease. Radiology 2013;267:11–25.

14. Jing ZC, Xu XQ, Badesch DB, et al. Pulmonary function testing in patients with pulmonary arterial hypertension. Respir Med 2009;103:1136–42.

15. Bossone E, D'Andrea A, D'Alto M, et al. Echocardiography in pulmonary arterial hypertension: from diagnosis to prognosis. J Am Soc Echocardiogr 2013;26:1–14.

16. Forfia PR, Vachiéry JL. Echocardiography in pulmonary arterial hypertension. Am J Cardiol 2012; 110(Suppl 6):16S–24S.

17. Opotowsky AR, Ojeda J, Rogers F, et al. A simple echocardiographic prediction rule for hemodynamics in pulmonary hypertension. Circ Cardiovasc Imaging 2012;5:765–75.

18. Badesch DB, Raskob GE, Elliott CG, et al. Pulmonary arterial hypertension: baseline characteristics from the REVEAL Registry. Chest 2010;137:376–87.

19. Forfia PR, Fisher MR, Mathai SC, et al. Tricuspid annular displacement predicts survival in pulmonary hypertension. Am J Respir Crit Care Med 2006;174: 1034–41.

20. Khouri SJ, Maly GT, Suh DD, et al. A practical approach to the echocardiographic evaluation of diastolic function. J Am Soc Echocardiogr 2004;17: 290–7.

21. Owan TE, Redfield MM. Epidemiology of diastolic heart failure. Prog Cardiovasc Dis 2005;47:320–32.

22. Benza R, Biederman R, Murali S, et al. Role of cardiac magnetic resonance imaging in the management of patients with pulmonary arterial hypertension. J Am Coll Cardiol 2008;52:1683–92.

23. Roeleveld RJ, Marcus JT, Boonstra A, et al. A comparison of noninvasive MRI-based methods of estimating pulmonary artery pressure in pulmonary hypertension. J Magn Reson Imaging 2005;22:67–72.

24. van Wolferen SA, Marcus JT, Boonstra A, et al. Prognostic value of right ventricular mass, volume, and function in idiopathic pulmonary arterial hypertension. Eur Heart J 2007;28:1250–7.

25. van de Veerdonk MC, Kind T, Marcus JT, et al. Progressive right ventricular dysfunction in patients with pulmonary arterial hypertension responding to therapy. J Am Coll Cardiol 2011;58:2511–9.

26. Kuehne T, Yilmaz S, Steendijk P, et al. Magnetic resonance imaging analysis of right ventricular pressure-volume loops: in vivo validation and clinical application in patients with pulmonary hypertension. Circulation 2004;110:2010–6.

27. Bogaert J, Dymarkowski S, Taylor AM, editors. Clinical cardiac MRI. Berlin Heidelberg: Springer-Verlag; 2005.

28. Fang JC, DeMarco T, Givertz MM, et al. World Health Organization Pulmonary Hypertension group 2: pulmonary hypertension due to left heart disease in the adult–a summary statement from the Pulmonary Hypertension Council of the International Society for Heart and Lung Transplantation. J Heart Lung Transplant 2012;31:913–33.

29. Baim DS, editor. Grossman's cardiac catheterization, angiography, and intervention. 7th edition. Philadelphia: Lippincott Williams & Wilkins; 2005.

30. Hoeper MM, Lee SH, Voswinckel R. Complications of right heart catheterization procedures in patients with pulmonary hypertension in experienced centers. J Am Coll Cardiol 2006;48:2546–52.

31. Hoeper MM, Maier R, Tongers J. Determination of cardiac output by the Fick method, thermodilution, and acetylene rebreathing in pulmonary hypertension. Am J Respir Crit Care Med 1999;160:535–41.

32. Fares WH, Blanchard SK, Stouffer GA, et al. Thermodilution and Fick cardiac outputs differ: impact on pulmonary hypertension evaluation. Can Respir J 2012;19:261–6.

33. Givertz MM, Hare JM, Loh E, et al. Effect of bolus milrinone on hemodynamic variables and pulmonary vascular resistance in patients with severe left ventricular dysfunction: a rapid test for reversibility of pulmonary hypertension. J Am Coll Cardiol 1996; 28:1775–80.

34. Kovacs G, Berghold A, Scheidl S, et al. Pulmonary arterial pressure during rest and exercise in healthy subjects: a systematic review. Eur Respir J 2009;34: 888–94.

35. Naeije R, Vanderpool R, Dhakal BP, et al. Exercise-induced pulmonary hypertension: physiological basis and methodological concerns. Am J Respir Crit Care Med 2013;187:576–83.

36. Halpern SD, Taichman DB. Misclassification of pulmonary hypertension due to reliance on pulmonary capillary wedge pressure rather than left ventricular end-diastolic pressure. Chest 2009;136:37–43.

37. Ryan JJ, Rich JD, Thiruvoipati T, et al. Current practice for determining pulmonary capillary wedge pressure predisposes to serious errors in the classification of patients with pulmonary hypertension. Am Heart J 2012;163:589–94.

38. Hunt SA, Abraham WT, Chin MH, et al. 2009 Focused update incorporated into the ACC/AHA 2005 guidelines for the diagnosis and management of heart failure in Adults. A report of the American College of Cardiology Foundation/American Heart Association Task Force on practice guidelines developed in collaboration with the International Society for heart and lung transplantation. J Am Coll Cardiol 2009;53:e1–90.

39. Mikus E, Stepanenko A, Krabatsch T, et al. Reversibility of fixed pulmonary hypertension in left ventricular assist device support recipients. Eur J Cardiothorac Surg 2011;40:971–7.

40. Zakliczynski M, Maruszewski M, Pyka L, et al. Effectiveness and safety of treatment with sildenafil for secondary pulmonary hypertension in heart transplant candidates. Transplant Proc 2007;39(9): 2856–8.

41. Perez-Villa F, Farrero M, Cardona M, et al. Bosentan in heart transplantation candidates with severe pulmonary hypertension: efficacy, safety and outcome after transplantation. Clin Transplant 2013;27:25–31.

42. Califf RM, Adams KF, McKenna WJ, et al. A randomized controlled trial of epoprostenol therapy for severe congestive heart failure: the Flolan International Randomized Survival Trial (FIRST). Am Heart J 1997;134:44–54.

43. Teerlink JR. Recent heart failure trials of neurohormonal modulation (OVERTURE and ENABLE): approaching the asymptote of efficacy? J Card Fail 2002;8:124–7.

44. Lewis GD, Shah R, Shahzad K, et al. Sildenafil improves exercise capacity and quality of life in patients with systolic heart failure and secondary pulmonary hypertension. Circulation 2007;116:1555–62.

45. Guazzi M, Vicenzi M, Arena R, et al. Pulmonary hypertension in heart failure with preserved ejection fraction: a target of phosphodiesterase-5 inhibition in a 1-year study. Circulation 2011;124:164–74.

46. Redfield MM, Chen HH, Borlaug BA, et al. Effect of phosphodiesterase-5 inhibition on exercise capacity and clinical status in heart failure with preserved ejection fraction: a randomized clinical trial. JAMA 2013;309:1268–77.

Pulmonary Hypertension due to Lung Disease and/or Hypoxia

Steven D. Nathan, MD[a],*, Paul M. Hassoun, MD[b]

KEYWORDS

- Obstructive lung disease • Interstitial lung disease • Pulmonary hypertension • Sarcoidosis
- Prognosis • Respiratory function tests • Echocardiography

KEY POINTS

- Pulmonary hypertension frequently complicates the course of patients with diffuse parenchymal lung disease.
- The presence of pulmonary hypertension does not always correlate with the severity of the underlying parenchymal lung disease, attesting to other factors likely playing a role in the pathogenesis.
- The presence of pulmonary hypertension is invariably associated with reduced functional status, greater supplemental oxygen needs, and increased mortality.
- There are many unknowns and areas ripe for further research including in whom and how best to screen for pulmonary hypertension and the role, if any, for vasoactive therapies.

INTRODUCTION

Pulmonary hypertension (PH) may complicate the course of many forms of diffuse parenchymal lung disease.[1,2] There is a growing appreciation for this interceding complication and its association with functional impairment, greater oxygen needs, quality of life, and prognosis. PH due to lung disease, most commonly interstitial lung disease (ILD) and chronic obstructive pulmonary disease (COPD), as well as hypoxia are classified within the World Health Organization (WHO) group 3.[3] Other forms of diffuse parenchymal lung disease such as sarcoidosis, lymphangioleiomyomatosis, and pulmonary Langerhans cell histiocytosis are more complex in their etiology and are currently classified as WHO group 5 with other miscellaneous disorders. The severity of PH in the context of lung disease tends to be mild to moderate, but there are cases where it may be severe. There is an interplay of many factors in the pathogenesis of WHO group 3 PH, which is evidently more complex than the simple concept of loss of lung units and pulmonary vascular bed. Some of the multifactorial contributors are common to many forms of parenchymal lung disease and others are unique to the specific disease entities.

The focus of this article is to describe the prevalence and impact of PH in diffuse parenchymal lung disease (DPLD) and the role of hypoxia. The pathogenesis is discussed, highlighting commonalities and disease-specific nuances as well as areas for future research into the pathogenesis. The hemodynamic impact and whether the currently held definition of PH is appropriate in the context of lung disease are discussed as well as the concept of disproportionate PH. The

Disclosures: S.D. Nathan has been a consultant and is on the speakers' bureau for Actelion, Gilead Sciences and United Therapeutics. He has also received research funding from these companies. P.M. Hassoun serves on advisory boards for Merck, Gilead, and Novartis and has received research funding from Actelion/United Therapeutics for the REVEAL Registry, and from the NIH/NHLBI (P01HL84946 and R01 HL114910).
[a] Advanced Lung Disease and Transplant Program, Department of Medicine, Inova Fairfax Hospital, 3300 Gallows Road, Falls Church, VA 22042, USA; [b] Division of Pulmonary and Critical Care Medicine, Johns Hopkins University, 1830 East Monument Street, Baltimore, MD 21287, USA
* Corresponding author.
E-mail address: steven.nathan@inova.org

Clin Chest Med 34 (2013) 695–705
http://dx.doi.org/10.1016/j.ccm.2013.08.004
0272-5231/13/$ – see front matter © 2013 Elsevier Inc. All rights reserved.

chestmed.theclinics.com

groundswell of interest in group 3 and 5 PH stems largely from the availability and effectiveness of vasoactive agents in modulating the course of disease in patients with group 1 PH. The data, or paucity thereof, supporting the use of these agents in PH due to lung disease are discussed, as well as the caveats and potential pitfalls to instituting such therapies in the absence of the necessary prospective trials. Whether PH is an adaptive or maladaptive phenomenon remains unknown. It is possible that there is a spectrum where initially PH might be an adaptive phenomenon, but with time may transform to a maladaptive one. Whether and when such a transition occurs is integral to the concept of disproportionate or severe PH, as is identifying the patient phenotype best suited for enrollment in future clinical trials of vasoactive therapies.

EPIDEMIOLOGY AND PREVALENCE OF PH

The prevalence of PH in the various forms of DPLD spans a wide spectrum. In COPD, there have been prevalence rates reported between 5% and 90%.[2,4–12] In idiopathic pulmonary fibrosis (IPF), there is a similarly wide reported range of 10% to 86%.[13–20] These wide ranges attest to the issue of when the presence of PH is addressed. It makes intuitive sense that the earlier in the disease course it is sought, the lower the prevalence, whereas a late look results in a higher prevalence. What is clear and common to all the different parenchymal lung disorders, is that the presence of PH does portend a worse outcome. Although the accepted hemodynamic definition of a mean pulmonary artery pressure (mPAP) greater than 25 mm Hg has been used to delineate PH, there is also evidence to suggest that mPAP cutoffs as low as 17 mm Hg do discern groups with differing prognoses.[19] Whether lower pressure increases should be used to define an abnormal pulmonary vascular response in parenchymal lung disease is an issue that warrants further study and debate. Whether it is the mPAP itself that should define an aberrant vasculopathic response also merits further discussion. An interesting and noteworthy observation is the excellent prognostic discrimination provided by echocardiographic (echo) estimates of the right ventricular systolic pressure (RVSP), specifically in IPF.[14,21] Although it is well recognized that echo-derived estimates tend to be inexact, especially in patients with advanced lung disease, this does raise the notion that it is perhaps the pulmonary artery (PA) systolic pressure that is most important.[22,23] The pressure generated during systolic excursion is influenced by the available cross-sectional area, afterload, and capacitance of the pulmonary circulation, which then raises the notion that the PA systolic pressure might reflect the severity of the associated parenchymal disease. Therefore, whether it is the PH itself that determines outcomes or the increased pressures that are a surrogate for the parenchymal aspects of the disease remains uncertain. One may speculate that both might be true; specifically that PH is the passenger to the parenchymal process, with evolution over time becoming the driver of outcomes, especially when right ventricular decompensation ensues.

There are certain risk factors that are common to all the parenchymal lung disorders. As a general rule, the more severe the disease, the greater the risk of intervening PH. In parallel with this, hypoxia is a risk factor, but it remains unclear if the hypoxemia is causing the PH or vice versa. Whichever occurred first might be immaterial because it seems likely that they are interdependent and perpetuate each other in an inexorable feedback loop mechanism.

IDIOPATHIC PULMONARY FIBROSIS

In IPF, it seems that complicating PH is a relatively common occurrence, even in patients with early or mild disease.[16,24] Most of the studies evaluating the presence of PH have been in patients with more advanced disease, specifically patients who are being evaluated as potential lung transplant candidates. On the upper end of the prevalence spectrum, an 86% prevalence estimate was documented in a study of patients who received right heart catheterizations (RHC) at the time of their lung transplant.[18] An approximate 10% prevalence was found in a prospective cohort of patients with mild or early disease, who had a mean disease duration of less than 1 year and a mean value of forced vital capacity (FVC) of 70% of predicted.[16] In addition, approximately 5% of enrolled patients in this study had hemodynamic evidence of group II PH with increased pulmonary capillary wedge pressures (PCWP). This attests to the potential multifactorial cause of PH, especially when dealing with diseases such as IPF and COPD, which tend to afflict the elderly in whom systolic and heart failure with preserved ejection fraction (HF-pEF) are common. PH in IPF is generally associated with more advanced age, a greater need for supplemental oxygen therapy, reduced exercise tolerance, worse lung function, and a longer duration of disease. The hemodynamic severity of PH tends to be mild with ~50% of patients having mPAPs of 30 mm Hg or less.[13] Nonetheless, severe PH can occur and an mPAP greater than 40 mm Hg has been described in

2% to 9% of patients with IPF listed for lung transplantation.[13,15]

The evolution of PH in the setting of IPF tends to be progressive with some cases demonstrating an accelerated trajectory. This progressive course has been evaluated in 1 study in which serial RHCs were evaluated from the time of workup for lung transplantation and at the time of actual transplant.[18] In some of these patients the second RHC did demonstrate PA pressures that were almost systemic in severity.

IPF can occur in combination with comorbidities that can contribute to the underlying PH. Common comorbidities that seem to have an increased prevalence in IPF and may contribute to PH include congestive heart failure, obstructive sleep apnea (OSA), and COPD. Combined pulmonary fibrosis and emphysema (CPFE) has been described as a distinct IPF phenotype, with evidence of emphysematous changes noted in approximately one-third of patients with IPF.[25] In cases of CPFE, the prevalence of PH tends to be high at ~50%. Clues to the presence of coexistent emphysema are well-preserved lung volumes with a markedly reduced single-breath diffusing capacity for carbon monoxide (DLco) and marked hypoxemia. The lung volumes tend to be well preserved due to the opposing restrictive and obstructive mechanical forces, and the DLco is markedly reduced due to destruction of the pulmonary vascular bed by both disease processes.

COPD

The prevalence of PH in COPD has been reported at between 5% and 90%.[2,4–12] These estimates are difficult to compare because the methodology and cutoff points to define PH have differed, as have the patient populations studied. These have spanned the spectrum from primary care–based community cohorts to patients being considered for surgical intervention in the form of either lung volume reduction surgery (LVRS) or lung transplantation. PH is generally associated with a lower forced expiratory volume in the first second of expiration (FEV$_1$) and more severe hypoxemia. There seems to be an association between age and the likelihood of PH in COPD, but whether this is attributable to age alone or an increased propensity for other comorbidities remains uncertain.[26] Gender might also have a role to play with 1 study reporting that PH is more common in women exposed to smoke from biomass fuels.[27]

Similar to IPF, PH associated with COPD tends to be mostly mild in its severity. However, there does seem to be a distinct clinical COPD phenotype with moderate to severe PH, usually seen in the context of moderate airflow obstruction. A clue to the presence of PH in this patient population is a markedly reduced DLco in conjunction with severe hypoxemia and exercise desaturation. In 1 study of patients with COPD referred for LVRS or transplant, 7.4% had a modest decrement in FEV$_1$ (mean 48% of predicted) in association with significant PH (mean mPAP of 39.8 mm Hg).[2]

SARCOIDOSIS

PH is an increasingly recognized complication of sarcoidosis with a reported prevalence of between 1% and 74%.[28–33] PH is most commonly detected in patients with stage IV fibrocystic disease, but can also occur in the context of relatively normal lung function and preserved parenchymal architecture. The presence of PH should be considered in any patient with recalcitrant dyspnea and in those with disease and symptoms severe enough to warrant consideration for lung transplantation. It is in these latter patients that the higher end of the prevalence range has been defined (~74%).[32]

A distinguishing epidemiologic feature of the PH complicating sarcoidosis is the distribution in the mPAPs, which is interesting to contrast with that of patients with COPD and IPF. Whereas the latter 2 groups of patients tend to have a Gaussian distribution, the histogram distribution of the mPAP in sarcoidosis tends to demonstrate a tail of patients with more severe PH. **Fig. 1** shows the difference in distribution among these 3 patient groups (COPD, IPF, and sarcoidosis) from the Inova Fairfax Advanced Lung Disease Program.

NONSPECIFIC INTERSTITIAL PNEUMONITIS

There is a paucity of literature on PH complicating nonspecific interstitial pneumonia (NSIP). It is the second most common of the idiopathic interstitial pneumonias and although it does portend a better prognosis than IPF, there is a subgroup of patients who develop advanced disease and succumb from this condition. There are data to suggest that the course of NSIP parallels that of IPF once the DLco breaches 35% of the predicted threshold.[34] It is possible that this marks the subgroup of patients who have developed PH, which one can speculate is then the driver of outcomes in both groups.

LYMPHANGIOLEIOMYOMATOSIS

Lymphangioleiomyomatosis (LAM) is a rare disease that is classified as group 5 PH. It occurs almost exclusively in women of reproductive age and is characterized by abnormal smooth muscle proliferation affecting the thoracic lymphatics,

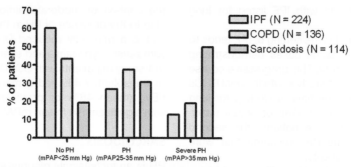

Fig. 1. Distribution of mPAPs of patients with IPF, COPD, and sarcoidosis referred to a large tertiary care center (Advanced Lung Disease Program, Inova Fairfax Hospital) and who underwent right heart catheterization. The prevalence and distribution of pressures depicted does not reflect that of the general population with these diseases, because there is likely bias introduced by referral patterns as well as patient selection for catheterization.

bronchioles, and vasculature. PH is rare in this population, but an increase in RVSP with low-level exercise may be seen fairly commonly, which attests to some degree of pulmonary vascular involvement.[35–37]

PULMONARY LANGERHANS CELL HISTIOCYTOSIS

Pulmonary Langerhans cell histiocytosis (PLCH) is another rare ILD related to tobacco use, which may regress spontaneously with smoking cessation. However, irreversible airflow obstruction may ensue and 20% to 30% of cases do progress to chronic respiratory insufficiency.[38–41] PH, which may be severe, is frequently seen in these advanced cases with a reported prevalence as high as 92% to 100%.[38–41] Purported mechanisms involved in the pathogenesis of PH include chronic hypoxia, abnormal pulmonary parenchymal mechanics, vascular remodeling, and the abnormal production of inflammatory cytokines and growth factors. Similar to other parenchymal lung diseases, pulmonary pressures do not correlate with spirometry and PH may also occur in the absence of significant parenchymal disease.[38]

PH COMPLICATING SLEEP APNEA

The reported prevalence of PH in OSA has varied from 17% to 40% depending on the method of diagnosis (RHC vs echocardiography) and the pulmonary arterial pressure cutoff used to define PH.[42–44] PH in OSA is usually mild to moderate, can be multifactorial, and related to precapillary or postcapillary causes.[43–46] The presence of comorbid conditions including cardiopulmonary diseases is associated with an increased likelihood of PH in these patients.[46,47] Among cardiovascular diseases, diastolic dysfunction is often associated with OSA.[48] In a study of 83 patients in whom RHC

was available within 6 months of OSA diagnosis, 70% of patients had PH including 31% with pulmonary capillary wedge pressures greater than 15 mm Hg.[49] PH correlated with female gender, nocturnal desaturation, FEV_1 less than 70% and a body mass index greater than 26 kg/m^2.

The pathophysiologic mechanisms involved in the development of vascular disease, and by inference PH, in OSA have included endothelial dysfunction related to intermittent hypoxia leading to oxidative stress, systemic inflammation, increased sympathetic activity, as well as intrathoracic pressure swings causing direct vascular damage.[50–56] A comprehensive review of these complex mechanisms and their putative actions can be found elsewhere.[57]

As for other diseases of the lung causing PH, effective treatment of PH related to OSA relies essentially on proper diagnosis of the underlying disease (ie, polysomnogram), continuous positive airway pressure (CPAP) titration when indicated, and other appropriate treatment (nutritional counseling and weight loss, or tracheostomy and bariatric surgery in extreme cases), to prevent nocturnal apneas and oxygen desaturation. When PH is suspected, a screening echocardiogram is warranted followed by RHC if suspicion is high (eg, increased RVSP >40 mm Hg in particular in the presence of a dilated right ventricle). However, if the echocardiographic changes are mild, it is reasonable to institute treatment of OSA first and then obtain a repeat echocardiogram after 6 months of adequate therapy. Adherence to CPAP therapy has been shown to improve hemodynamics in patients with OSA.[58,59]

OVERLAP SYNDROMES

It is not uncommon that patients may have more than 1 cause of their PH that may be within the same WHO PH grouping (eg, OSA and COPD) or from different WHO groups in the case of parenchymal lung disease with associated cardiac abnormalities, such as HF-pEF. HF-pEF may be found in as many as 15% to 17% of patients with parenchymal lung disease.[6,24,33] Similarly, patients with connective tissue disease (CTD) complicated by PH are usually classified in group 1 (pulmonary arterial hypertension [PAH]). However, certain CTDs such as scleroderma can be complicated by ILD, which, when moderate or severe, can also be complicated by PH.[60] In the latter case, patients may be categorized as having group 3 PH. In up to 25% of these patients, the mPAP can be greater than 35 mm Hg and is believed to be out of proportion to ILD and likely related to intrinsic vascular disease in addition to the alveolar disruption.[3,61,62] Several studies have now suggested that the combination of PH and ILD in these patients with scleroderma significantly worsens their prognosis as suggested by a median survival of less than 2 years compared with 4 years in patients with scleroderma-associated PAH.[62–64] PAH-specific therapies did not seem to have a beneficial effect on WHO functional class, 6-minute walk distances, hemodynamic measures, or survival in 1 cohort of patients with combined PH and ILD studied retrospectively in the context of the scleroderma spectrum of disease.[64]

PATHOGENESIS OF PH IN LUNG DISEASE/HYPOXIA

Increased pulmonary vascular load characteristic of PH results from remodeling of the pulmonary vasculature involving, to various degrees, all layers of the vasculature (intima, media, and adventitia). Pulmonary vascular remodeling in chronic hypoxia and lung parenchymal diseases is believed to be multifactorial in its cause. Contributory factors include endothelial dysfunction, excessive vasoconstriction, proliferation of various cells (including endothelial, smooth muscle cells, and fibroblasts) and thrombosis, all of which contribute to narrowing of the vasculature.[65] Whereas plexiform lesions (resulting from uncontrolled proliferation of endothelial cells and fibroblasts at the branching sites of medium size arteries) are characteristic of PAH, medial hypertrophy of small muscular arteries and neomuscularization of more distal arterioles are often the hallmark of hypoxic lung diseases (and animal models of PH induced by chronic hypoxia), with lesser degrees of intimal and adventitial remodeling. In addition, influx of inflammatory cells (eg, macrophages, dendritic cells, and B and T lymphocytes) has been

increasingly recognized.[66] In the case of chronic pulmonary parenchymal diseases, excessive fibrosis (eg, in ILD) and loss of parenchymal tissue (eg, COPD) contribute to disruption and loss of small vessels of the pulmonary vascular bed.

Imbalances between ventilation and perfusion (V/Q) matching, characteristic of chronic parenchymal lung diseases, cause precapillary pulmonary vasoconstriction through mechanisms that remain poorly understood but include changes in nitric oxide balance, release of vasoconstrictors, and metabolic alterations (potassium and calcium flux in smooth muscle cells).[67,68] At high altitude with chronic continuous hypoxia (Monge disease), and in some diseases characterized by chronic intermittent hypoxia (such as sleep apnea syndrome), release of catecholamines and changes in acid-base status may, in addition, cause pulmonary venoconstriction, further exacerbating the increase in pulmonary vascular pressure.[69] Thromboembolic lesions can further impede pulmonary vascular flow, and frequently may complicate chronic lung diseases such as COPD, sarcoidosis, and IPF.[70–74]

In COPD, pulmonary vascular remodeling correlates with the degree and severity of inflammatory cell infiltrates in small airways and is characterized, in smokers, by inflammatory cells infiltrating the adventitia of muscular PAs, largely constituted by activated T lymphocytes with a predominance of the CD8+ T-cell subset.[75] Several growth factors, including vascular endothelial growth factor and transforming growth factor β (TGF-β), and occasionally their receptors (eg, TGF-β RII) have increased expression in remodeled pulmonary arteries of smokers with mild-to-moderate COPD, suggesting that these mediators may play a role in the pulmonary vascular remodeling of COPD.[76–78]

SCREENING FOR PH IN PATIENTS WITH PARENCHYMAL LUNG DISEASES

Screening for parenchymal lung disease should be routine in the evaluation of patients referred for PH. A thorough history should inquire about symptoms suggestive of COPD, ILD, and sleep apnea. Baseline tests should include pulmonary function tests (spirometry, lung volumes, and DLCO), resting, exercise, and nocturnal oxygen saturation, a plain chest film, a high-resolution chest computerized tomogram (CT) scan, a ventilation-perfusion scan, appropriate serologies to rule out CTD, and a polysomnogram when indicated. Lung volume measurements do not tend to correlate with underlying PH.[2,24] However, a low DLCO (<40% of predicted) might be an important clue to the presence of complicating PH.[13] Significant desaturation and a short walk distance have also been associated with the presence of PH as has a low pulse rate recovery. The latter is a relatively simple measure that is calculated by the difference between the pulse rate at the end of the 6-minute walk test and after 1 minute of recovery. A pulse rate recovery of less than 13 beats/min has been shown to correlate with underlying PH in patients with IPF.[79] Biomarkers, including brain natriuretic peptide (BNP) and pro-N terminal brain natriuretic peptide (NT pro-BNP), might also have a role in screening for underlying PH, although these can be increased in heart failure as well.[21]

A two-dimensional Doppler echocardiogram is the best screening tool for PH although it can be technically challenging and inaccurate in patients with advanced lung disease, especially COPD.[22] If PH is suspected from the echocardiogram, RHC is indicated after appropriate initial therapy for the underlying lung disease. In the case of underlying sleep apnea, it is not unreasonable to delay performance of the RHC until after adequate therapy (eg, CPAP) is provided for a certain length of time (eg, 6–9 months). A suggested screening algorithm for PH in parenchymal lung disease is shown in **Fig. 2**.

TREATMENT

Although there has been significant progress made in the past 2 decades in the treatment of PAH, with drugs targeting 3 distinct pathways (ie, the endothelin, nitric oxide/guanylate cyclase signaling, and prostacyclin pathways), there is no currently approved or effective therapy for group 3 PH.[80] Treatment of the underlying condition is key; thus improving alveolar oxygenation, minimizing V/Q mismatch, and treatment of underlying bronchospasm should be achieved as a primary therapeutic goal before considering the use of PAH-specific vasodilators that may prove to do more harm than good in these patients. When OSA is present, appropriate measures such as weight loss and treatment with CPAP ventilation should be attempted first. Nasal CPAP, the treatment of choice for severe OSA, has been shown to result in reductions in pulmonary vascular pressures and

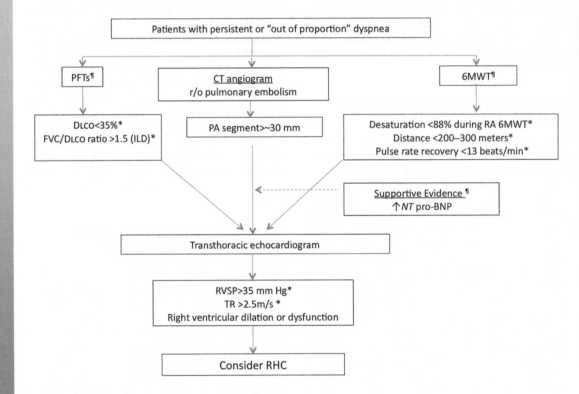

¶ Assessment of parameters are complementary and should be made in parallel
* All of these thresholds have not been validated as indicators
of PH in DPLD and represent the opinion of the authors

Fig. 2. Suggested screening algorithm for PH in patients with parenchymal lung disease. 6MWT, 6-minute walk test; PFT, pulmonary function test.

pulmonary vascular resistance over a period of 4 months compared with pretreatment baseline measures.[58] Surgically induced weight loss has also been associated with significant improvement in pulmonary hemodynamics in patients with obesity-hypoventilation syndrome.[81]

There are no effective therapies currently available for ILD-associated PH. Limited data suggest that corticosteroids may improve hemodynamics in diseases such as sarcoidosis and anecdotally in PLCH.[82,83] Hemodynamic improvements may be related to a potential effect on a vasculitic component of these disorders because there is usually no parallel radiographic improvement. More recently, in the largest publication to date, PAH-specific therapies have been found to be effective in treating PLCH-associated PH hemodynamics without worsening oxygenation.[84] There are no data to help us know the impact of these retrospective observations on outcomes in PLCH.

Inhaled nitric oxide (NO), a selective pulmonary vasodilator, may improve pulmonary vascular resistance and V/Q mismatch during exercise in patients with COPD.[85,86] However, the mode of delivery is currently cumbersome because NO has to be delivered separately from supplemental oxygen to prevent the formation of toxic reactive nitrogen species.

Inhibition of phosphodiesterase 5 (PDE-5), the main isoform of this enzyme in the lung, can be achieved with sildenafil and is one of the primary therapeutic options in PAH. The PDE-5 inhibitor sildenafil causes acute reduction in resting and exercise-induced mean PA pressure and increased cardiac output during exercise, but this may be at the cost of a significant reduction in the partial pressure of arterial oxygen (Pao_2) caused by V/Q mismatching.[87] However, long-term benefits of sildenafil in patients with COPD with PH have not yet been demonstrated. A recent double-blind, randomized, controlled trial of sildenafil in patients with severe COPD and moderately increased PAP undergoing pulmonary rehabilitation, failed to demonstrate improvement in cycle endurance time, 6-minute walk distance, and quality of life. Fortunately, however, there was no effect of this therapy on arterial oxygenation.[88] Likewise, use of sildenafil in a small series of patients with COPD failed to improve the 6-minute walk distance, exercise tolerance as measured by cardiopulmonary testing, or stroke volume as measured by magnetic resonance imaging.[89]

In ILD, an initial open-label trial of sildenafil in patients with IPF with PH did demonstrate improvements in the 6-minute walk distance after 12 weeks of therapy.[90] However, a more recent randomized, placebo-controlled clinical trial in patients with IPF (in whom PH was not documented) was negative based on the primary end point of a categorical change in the 6-minute walk distance.[91] However, in response to therapy, patients with severe IPF reported less dyspnea and had improved oxygenation, D_{LCO}, and quality of life compared with placebo.[91]

Endothelin-1 is produced by endothelial cells and has direct vasoconstrictor and mitogenic effects on vascular smooth muscle cells. Endothelin's vasoconstrictive effects are mediated by 2 receptors: endothelin receptor A (ERA) and endothelin receptor B (ERB) on pulmonary arterial smooth muscle cells. ERB activation stimulates NO release from endothelial cells resulting in vasodilatation. Currently, US Food and Drug Administration (FDA)-approved endothelin receptor antagonists target both receptors (bosentan), or selectively target ERA (ambrisentan). In a randomized, controlled, 12-week trial, bosentan therapy resulted in no improvement in 6-minute walk distance or pulmonary hemodynamics in patients with severe or very severe COPD complicated by PH.[92] Bosentan-treated patients experienced a reduction in Pao_2 with a widened alveolar-arterial oxygen gradient, and a reduced quality of life compared with patients on placebo.[92] Similarly, the selective ERA antagonist ambrisentan did not improve the 6-minute walk distance in patients with COPD or ILD with PH in the ARIES-3 trial.[93] Furthermore, a phase 3 study of ambrisentan therapy for IPF patients with PH was interrupted early because of lack of clinical efficacy.[16] The novel dual endothelin receptor antagonist macitentan failed to delay reduction in FVC in a prospective, randomized, double-blind, multicenter, parallel-group, placebo-controlled phase 2 trial.[94]

Prostacyclin, produced by endothelial cells, is a potent vasodilator that inhibits platelet aggregation and the release of growth factors from endothelial cells, platelets, and macrophages. FDA-approved prostacyclin analogues are available for delivery via intravenous (epoprostenol and treprostinil), subcutaneous (treprostinil), and inhaled (iloprost and treprostinil) routes. Acutely, intravenous prostacyclin analogues have been shown to improve mean PA pressure, pulmonary vascular resistance, and cardiac output in patients with COPD-associated PH.[95] Similar to ERA antagonists, prostacyclin analogues can worsen V/Q matching in COPD and patients with ILD with PH.[87,96,97] These agents can also cause pulmonary edema in some patients with ILD as pulmonary venoocclusive lesions have been described in several pulmonary disorders, including IPF, sarcoidosis, PLCH, and systemic sclerosis–associated ILD.[1] Inhaled prostacyclin analogues may have less effect on V/Q mismatch and oxygenation. In this regard, patients with COPD (n = 10) with PH were recently shown to have improved V/Q matching, a reduced alveolar-arterial oxygen gradient, and longer 6-minute walk distances after an acute treatment with inhaled iloprost.[98] Longer-term effects of iloprost for the treatment of COPD-associated PAH are not known.

SUMMARY AND FUTURE DIRECTIONS

There is a growing appreciation that PH complicates the course of most forms of parenchymal lung disease. In all the lung diseases in which it has been described, an association with more functional impairment and worse outcomes has been found. Although there has been an explosion of information on PAH, there has been a paucity of research specific to groups 3 and 5 PH. Understandably, the focus of interest in group 1 PAH has emanated from the fact that this is a primary phenomenon that is at the forefront of patients' presentation, symptoms, and outcomes. Further interest in group 1 has been fueled by the discovery and development of effective and approved therapies. In the context of lung disease, PH is generally a secondary phenomenon that frequently exists and remains undiscovered as well as poorly understood in the shadows of the underlying parenchymal disease. If only COPD was to be considered, a disease with a worldwide prevalence of ~6 to 12 million, and the lowest estimate of PH prevalence (~1%) extrapolated to the lower end of this range, then this alone translates to ~60,000 patients with COPD-related PH. The worldwide estimate of IPF prevalence is about 200,000 and the low end of the prevalence estimates (~10%) would equate to a further ~20,000 patients with associated PH. This underscores the health care burden and consequences of PH related to lung disease, which, by these estimates of 2 of the more common group 3 conditions, overwhelm that of PAH due to the cumulative prevalence of these diseases.

Studies into all aspects of PH related to lung disease, including further characterization of the prevalence and the pathogenesis, are needed. Which patients should be screened, when, and by which modality remain unclear. Which hemodynamic parameter and which cutoff point best define pulmonary vascular involvement, and most importantly the role of therapy, remain unanswered questions. At this time, empirical therapy is commonly used without adequate studies to support this approach. It may seem to make intuitive sense in many cases, especially in those patients with very high pressures and evidence of hemodynamic decompensation. However, the field of medicine is replete with medical reversals where new studies have refuted the commonly accepted standard of care. This has included pathophysiologically plausible therapeutic interventions with supportive evidence from small case series or inadequately powered studies that have not proved to be beneficial and, in some cases, have proved more harmful than helpful.

REFERENCES

1. Shlobin OA, Nathan SD. Pulmonary hypertension secondary to interstitial lung disease. Expert Rev Respir Med 2011;5:179–89.
2. Thabut G, Dauriat G, Stern JB, et al. Pulmonary hemodynamics in advanced COPD candidates for lung volume reduction surgery or lung transplantation. Chest 2005;127:1531–6.
3. Simonneau G, Robbins IM, Beghetti M, et al. Updated clinical classification of pulmonary hypertension. J Am Coll Cardiol 2009;54:S43–54.
4. Chaouat A, Naeije R, Weitzenblum E. Pulmonary hypertension in COPD. Eur Respir J 2008;32: 1371–85.
5. Chaouat A, Bugnet AS, Kadaoui N, et al. Severe pulmonary hypertension and chronic obstructive pulmonary disease. Am J Respir Crit Care Med 2005;172:189–94.
6. Cuttica MJ, Kalhan R, Shlobin OA, et al. Functional impact of pulmonary hypertension in patients with COPD listed for lung transplant. Respir Med 2010;104:1877–82.
7. Chatila WM, Thomashow BM, Minai OA, et al. Comorbidities in chronic obstructive pulmonary disease. Proc Am Thorac Soc 2008;5:549–55.
8. Falk JA, Kadiev S, Criner GJ, et al. Cardiac disease in chronic obstructive pulmonary disease. Proc Am Thorac Soc 2008;5:543–8.
9. Scharf SM, Iqbal M, Keller C, et al. Hemodynamic characterization of patients with severe emphysema. Am J Respir Crit Care Med 2002; 166:314–22.
10. Weitzenblum E, Hirth C, Ducolone A, et al. Prognostic value of pulmonary artery pressure in chronic obstructive pulmonary disease. Thorax 1981;36:752–8.
11. Mykland Hilde J, Skjorten I, Hansteen V, et al. Hemodynamic responses to exercise in patients with COPD. Eur Respir J 2013;41:1031–41.
12. Gartman EJ, Blundin M, Klinger JR, et al. Initial risk assessment for pulmonary hypertension in patients with COPD. Lung 2012;190:83–9.
13. Lettieri CJ, Nathan SD, Barnett S, et al. Prevalence and outcomes of pulmonary arterial hypertension in idiopathic pulmonary fibrosis. Chest 2006;129: 746–52.

14. Nadrous HF, Pellikka PA, Krowka MJ, et al. Pulmonary hypertension in patients with idiopathic pulmonary fibrosis. Chest 2005;128:2393–9.

15. Shorr AF, Wainright JL, Cors CS, et al. Pulmonary hypertension in patients with pulmonary fibrosis awaiting transplant. Eur Respir J 2007;30:715–21.

16. Raghu G, Behr J, Brown KK, et al. Artemis-IPF: treatment of idiopathic pulmonary fibrosis with ambrisentan, a selective antagonist of the Endothelin A receptor: a randomized trial. Ann Intern Med 2013;158:641–9.

17. Swanson KL, Utz JP, Krowka MJ. Doppler echocardiography-right heart catheterization relationships in patients with idiopathic pulmonary fibrosis and suspected pulmonary hypertension. Med Sci Monit 2008;14:177–82.

18. Nathan SD, Shlobin OA, Ahmad S, et al. Serial development of pulmonary hypertension in patients with idiopathic pulmonary fibrosis. Respiration 2008;76:288–94.

19. Hamada K, Nagai S, Tanaka S, et al. Significance of pulmonary arterial pressure and diffusion capacity of the lung as prognosticator in patients with idiopathic pulmonary fibrosis. Chest 2007;131:650–6.

20. Zisman DA, Karlamangla AS, Ross DJ, et al. High-resolution chest CT findings do not predict the presence of pulmonary hypertension in advanced idiopathic pulmonary fibrosis. Chest 2007;132:773–9.

21. Song JW, Song JK, Kim DS. Echocardiography and brain natriuretic peptide as prognostic indicators in idiopathic pulmonary fibrosis. Respir Med 2009;103:180–6.

22. Arcasoy SM, Christie JD, Ferrari VA, et al. Echocardiographic assessment of pulmonary hypertension in patients with advanced lung disease. Am J Respir Crit Care Med 2003;167:735–40.

23. Nathan SD, Barnett SD, Saggar R, et al. Right ventricular systolic pressure by echocardiography as a predictor of pulmonary hypertension in patients with idiopathic pulmonary fibrosis. Respir Med 2008;102:1305–10.

24. Nathan SD, Shlobin OA, Ahmad S, et al. Pulmonary hypertension and pulmonary function testing in idiopathic pulmonary fibrosis. Chest 2007;131:657–63.

25. Jankowich MD, Rounds SI. Combined pulmonary fibrosis and emphysema syndrome. Chest 2012;141:222–31.

26. Oswald-Mammosser M, Weitzenblum E, Quoix E, et al. Prognostic factors in COPD patients receiving long-term oxygen therapy. Importance of pulmonary artery pressure. Chest 1995;107:1193–8.

27. Sertogullarindan B, Gumrukcuoglu HA, Sezgi C, et al. Frequency of pulmonary hypertension in patients with COPD due to biomass smoke and tobacco smoke. Int J Med Sci 2012;9:406–12.

28. Sulica R, Teirstein AS, Kakarla S, et al. Distinctive clinical, radiographic and functional characteristics of patients with sarcoidosis-related pulmonary hypertension. Chest 2005;128:1483–9.

29. Handa T, Nagai S, Miki S, et al. Incidence of pulmonary hypertension and its clinical relevance in patients with sarcoidosis. Chest 2006;129:1246–52.

30. Gluskowski J, Hawrylkiewicz I, Zych D, et al. Pulmonary haemodynamics at rest and during exercise in patients with sarcoidosis. Respiration 1984;46:26–32.

31. Baughman RP, Engel PJ, Meyer CA, et al. Pulmonary hypertension in sarcoidosis. Sarcoidosis Vasc Diffuse Lung Dis 2006;23:108–16.

32. Shorr AF, Helman DL, Davies DB, et al. Pulmonary hypertension in advanced sarcoidosis: epidemiology and clinical characteristics. Eur Respir J 2005;25:783–8.

33. Baughman RP, Engel PJ, Taylor L, et al. Survival in sarcoidosis-associated pulmonary hypertension:the importance of hemodynamic evaluation. Chest 2010;138:1078–85.

34. Latsi PI, du Bois RM, Nicholson AG, et al. Fibrotic idiopathic interstitial pneumonia: the prognostic value of longitudinal functional trends. Am J Respir Crit Care Med 2003;168:531–7.

35. Kawahara Y, Taniguchi T, Kadou T, et al. Elevated pulmonary arterial pressure in pulmonary lymphangiomyomatosis. Jpn J Med 1989;28:520–2.

36. Taveira-DaSilva AM, Hathaway OM, Sachdev V, et al. Pulmonary artery pressure in lymphangioleiomyomatosis: an echocardiographic study. Chest 2007;132:1573–8.

37. Taveira-DaSilva AM, Stylianou MP, Hedin CJ, et al. Maximal oxygen uptake and severity of disease in lymphangioleiomyomatosis. Am J Respir Crit Care Med 2003;168:1427–31.

38. Kiakouama L, Cottin V, Etienne-Mastroianni B, et al. Severe pulmonary hypertension in histiocytosis X: long-term improvement with bosentan. Eur Respir J 2010;36:202–4.

39. Lazor R, Etienne-Mastroianni B, Khouatra C, et al. Progressive diffuse pulmonary Langerhans cell histiocytosis improved by cladribine chemotherapy. Thorax 2009;64:274–5.

40. Dauriat G, Mal H, Thabut G, et al. Lung transplantation for pulmonary Langerhans' cell histiocytosis: a multicenter analysis. Transplantation 2006;81:746–50.

41. Fartoukh M, Humbert M, Capron F, et al. Severe pulmonary hypertension in histiocytosis X. Am J Respir Crit Care Med 2000;161:216–23.

42. Chaouat A, Weitzenblum E, Krieger J, et al. Pulmonary hemodynamics in the obstructive sleep apnea syndrome. Results in 220 consecutive patients. Chest 1996;109:380–6.

43. Sajkov D, McEvoy RD. Obstructive sleep apnea and pulmonary hypertension. Prog Cardiovasc Dis 2009;51:363–70.

44. Sajkov D, Cowie RJ, Thornton AT, et al. Pulmonary hypertension and hypoxemia in obstructive sleep apnea syndrome. Am J Respir Crit Care Med 1994;149:416–22.

45. Sanner BM, Doberauer C, Konermann M, et al. Pulmonary hypertension in patients with obstructive sleep apnea syndrome. Arch Intern Med 1997; 157:2483–7.

46. Bady E, Achkar A, Pascal S, et al. Pulmonary arterial hypertension in patients with sleep apnoea syndrome. Thorax 2000;55:934–9.

47. Laaban JP, Cassuto D, Orvoen-Frija E, et al. Cardiorespiratory consequences of sleep apnoea syndrome in patients with massive obesity. Eur Respir J 1998;11:20–7.

48. Usui Y, Takata Y, Inoue Y, et al. Severe obstructive sleep apnea impairs left ventricular diastolic function in non-obese men. Sleep Med 2013;14: 155–9.

49. Minai OA, Ricaurte B, Kaw R, et al. Frequency and impact of pulmonary hypertension in patients with obstructive sleep apnea syndrome. Am J Cardiol 2009;104:1300–6.

50. Garvey JF, Taylor CT, McNicholas WT. Cardiovascular disease in obstructive sleep apnoea syndrome: the role of intermittent hypoxia and inflammation. Eur Respir J 2009;33:1195–205.

51. Lavie L, Lavie P. Molecular mechanisms of cardiovascular disease in OSAHS: the oxidative stress link. Eur Respir J 2009;33:1467–84.

52. Ryan S, Taylor CT, McNicholas WT. Predictors of elevated nuclear factor-kappab-dependent genes in obstructive sleep apnea syndrome. Am J Respir Crit Care Med 2006;174:824–30.

53. Somers VK, Dyken ME, Clary MP, et al. Sympathetic neural mechanisms in obstructive sleep apnea. J Clin Invest 1995;96:1897–904.

54. Eisenberg E, Zimlichman R, Lavie P. Plasma norepinephrine levels in patients with sleep apnea syndrome. N Engl J Med 1990;322:932–3.

55. Marrone O, Bellia V, Ferrara G, et al. Transmural pressure measurements. Importance in the assessment of pulmonary hypertension in obstructive sleep apneas. Chest 1989;95:338–42.

56. Tilkian AG, Guilleminault C, Schroeder JS, et al. Hemodynamics in sleep-induced apnea. Studies during wakefulness and sleep. Ann Intern Med 1976;85:714–9.

57. Kohler M, Stradling JR. Mechanisms of vascular damage in obstructive sleep apnea. Nat Rev Cardiol 2010;7:677–85.

58. Sajkov D, Wang T, Saunders NA, et al. Continuous positive airway pressure treatment improves pulmonary hemodynamics in patients with obstructive sleep apnea. Am J Respir Crit Care Med 2002;165: 152–8.

59. Arias MA, Garcia-Rio F, Alonso-Fernandez A, et al. Pulmonary hypertension in obstructive sleep apnoea: effects of continuous positive airway pressure: a randomized, controlled cross-over study. Eur Heart J 2006;27:1106–13.

60. MacGregor AJ, Canavan R, Knight C, et al. Pulmonary hypertension in systemic sclerosis: risk factors for progression and consequences for survival. Rheumatology 2001;40:453–9.

61. Mukerjee D, St George D, Coleiro B, et al. Prevalence and outcome in systemic sclerosis associated pulmonary arterial hypertension: application of a registry approach. Ann Rheum Dis 2003;62: 1088–93.

62. Mathai SC, Hummers LK, Champion HC, et al. Survival in pulmonary hypertension associated with the scleroderma spectrum of diseases: impact of interstitial lung disease. Arthritis Rheum 2009;60: 569–77.

63. Le Pavec J, Girgis RE, Lechtzin N, et al. Systemic sclerosis-related pulmonary hypertension associated with interstitial lung disease: impact of pulmonary arterial hypertension therapies. Arthritis Rheum 2011;63:2456–64.

64. Campo A, Mathai SC, Le Pavec J, et al. Hemodynamic predictors of survival in scleroderma-related pulmonary arterial hypertension. Am J Respir Crit Care Med 2010;182:252–60.

65. Budhiraja R, Tuder RM, Hassoun PM. Endothelial dysfunction in pulmonary hypertension. Circulation 2004;109:159–65.

66. Hassoun PM, Mouthon L, Barbera JA, et al. Inflammation, growth factors, and pulmonary vascular remodeling. J Am Coll Cardiol 2009;54:S10–9.

67. Archer S, Michelakis E. The mechanism(s) of hypoxic pulmonary vasoconstriction: potassium channels, redox O(2) sensors, and controversies. News Physiol Sci 2002;17:131–7.

68. Enson Y, Giuntini C, Lewis ML, et al. The influence of hydrogen ion concentration and hypoxia on the pulmonary circulation. J Clin Invest 1964;43:1146–62.

69. Cruz JC, Grover RF, Reeves JT, et al. Sustained venoconstriction in man supplemented with CO_2 at high altitude. J Appl Physiol 1976;40:96–100.

70. Tillie-Leblond I, Marquette CH, Perez T, et al. Pulmonary embolism in patients with unexplained exacerbation of chronic obstructive pulmonary disease: prevalence and risk factors. Ann Intern Med 2006;144:390–6.

71. Rizkallah J, Man SF, Sin DD. Prevalence of pulmonary embolism in acute exacerbations of COPD: a systematic review and metaanalysis. Chest 2009; 135:786–93.

72. Swigris JJ, Olson AL, Huie TJ, et al. Increased risk of pulmonary embolism among us decedents with

sarcoidosis from 1988 to 2007. Chest 2011;140: 1261–6.

73. Panos RJ, Mortenson RL, Niccoli SA, et al. Clinical deterioration in patients with idiopathic pulmonary fibrosis: causes and assessment. Am J Med 1990;88:396–404.

74. Barbera JA, Riverola A, Roca J, et al. Pulmonary vascular abnormalities and ventilation-perfusion relationships in mild chronic obstructive pulmonary disease. Am J Respir Crit Care Med 1994;149: 423–9.

75. Peinado VI, Barbera JA, Abate P, et al. Inflammatory reaction in pulmonary muscular arteries of patients with mild chronic obstructive pulmonary disease. Am J Respir Crit Care Med 1999;159: 1605–11.

76. Santos S, Peinado VI, Ramirez J, et al. Enhanced expression of vascular endothelial growth factor in pulmonary arteries of smokers and patients with moderate chronic obstructive pulmonary disease. Am J Respir Crit Care Med 2003;167:1250–6.

77. Vignola AM, Chanez P, Chiappara G, et al. Transforming growth factor-beta expression in mucosal biopsies in asthma and chronic bronchitis. Am J Respir Crit Care Med 1997;156:591–9.

78. Beghe B, Bazzan E, Baraldo S, et al. Transforming growth factor-beta type ii receptor in pulmonary arteries of patients with very severe COPD. Eur Respir J 2006;28:556–62.

79. Swigris JJ, Olson A, Shlobin OA, et al. Heart rate recovery after 6MWT predicts pulmonary hypertension in patients with IPF. Respirology 2011; 16:439–45.

80. Humbert M, Sitbon O, Simonneau G. Treatment of pulmonary arterial hypertension. N Engl J Med 2004;351:1425–36.

81. Sugerman HJ, Baron PL, Fairman RP, et al. Hemodynamic dysfunction in obesity hypoventilation syndrome and the effects of treatment with surgically induced weight loss. Ann Surg 1988;207: 604–13.

82. Nunes H, Humbert M, Capron F, et al. Pulmonary hypertension associated with sarcoidosis: mechanisms, haemodynamics and prognosis. Thorax 2006;61:68–74.

83. Gluskowski J, Hawrylkiewicz I, Zych D, et al. Effects of corticosteroid treatment on pulmonary haemodynamics in patients with sarcoidosis. Eur Respir J 1990;3:403–7.

84. Le Pavec J, Lorillon G, Jais X, et al. Pulmonary Langerhans cell histiocytosis-associated pulmonary hypertension: clinical characteristics and impact of pulmonary arterial hypertension therapies. Chest 2012;142:1150–7.

85. Vonbank K, Ziesche R, Higenbottam TW, et al. Controlled prospective randomised trial on the effects on pulmonary haemodynamics of the ambulatory long term use of nitric oxide and oxygen in patients with severe COPD. Thorax 2003;58:289–93.

86. Roger N, Barbera JA, Roca J, et al. Nitric oxide inhalation during exercise in chronic obstructive pulmonary disease. Am J Respir Crit Care Med 1997;156:800–6.

87. Blanco I, Gimeno E, Munoz PA, et al. Hemodynamic and gas exchange effects of sildenafil in patients with chronic obstructive pulmonary disease and pulmonary hypertension. Am J Respir Crit Care Med 2010;181:270–8.

88. Blanco I, Santos S, Gea J, et al. Sildenafil to improve respiratory rehabilitation outcomes in COPD: a controlled trial. Eur Respir J 2013. Available at: http://www.ncbi.nlm.nih.gov/pubmed/23429918. Accessed September 10, 2013.

89. Rietema H, Holverda S, Bogaard HJ, et al. Sildenafil treatment in COPD does not affect stroke volume or exercise capacity. Eur Respir J 2008;31: 759–64.

90. Collard HR, Anstrom KJ, Schwarz MI, et al. Sildenafil improves walk distance in idiopathic pulmonary fibrosis. Chest 2007;131:897–9.

91. Zisman DA, Schwarz M, Anstrom KJ, et al. A controlled trial of sildenafil in advanced idiopathic pulmonary fibrosis. N Engl J Med 2010; 363:620–8.

92. Stolz D, Rasch H, Linka A, et al. A randomised, controlled trial of bosentan in severe COPD. Eur Respir J 2008;32:619–28.

93. Badesch DB, Feldman J, Keogh A, et al. Aries-3: ambrisentan therapy in a diverse population of patients with pulmonary hypertension. Cardiovasc Ther 2012;30:93–9.

94. Raghu G, Million-Rousseau R, Morganti A, et al. Macitentan for the treatment of idiopathic pulmonary fibrosis: the randomised controlled music trial. Eur Respir J 2013. Available at: http://www.ncbi.nlm.nih.gov/pubmed/23682110. Accessed September 10, 2013.

95. Naeije R, Melot C, Mols P, et al. Reduction in pulmonary hypertension by prostaglandin E1 in decompensated chronic obstructive pulmonary disease. Am Rev Respir Dis 1982;125:1–5.

96. Archer SL, Mike D, Crow J, et al. A placebo-controlled trial of prostacyclin in acute respiratory failure in COPD. Chest 1996;109:750–5.

97. Ghofrani HA, Wiedemann R, Rose F, et al. Sildenafil for treatment of lung fibrosis and pulmonary hypertension: a randomised controlled trial. Lancet 2002; 360:895–900.

98. Dernaika TA, Beavin M, Kinasewitz GT. Iloprost improves gas exchange and exercise tolerance in patients with pulmonary hypertension and chronic obstructive pulmonary disease. Respiration 2010; 79:377–82.

Pulmonary Arterial Hypertension Associated with Congenital Heart Disease

Usha Krishnan, MD, Erika B. Rosenzweig, MD*

KEYWORDS

- Pulmonary arterial hypertension • Congenital heart disease • Eisenmenger syndrome • Operability
- Fontan

KEY POINTS

- Pulmonary arterial hypertension (PAH) is a frequent complication of congenital heart disease (CHD), most commonly occurring with systemic-to-pulmonary shunt lesions.
- Given similar histopathologic changes, clinical presentation, and response to targeted therapy, PAH associated with CHD is classified with other forms of PAH in World Health Organization group 1.
- Prognosis varies depending on the type of congenital heart defect, and the timing of the manifestation of PAH.
- PAH associated with univentricular heart (both before and after total cavo-pulmonary connection), forms a unique and challenging subgroup of APAH-CHD, with different diagnostic and prognostic criteria and therapeutic indications.

INTRODUCTION

In the modern era, with increasing survival of patients with congenital heart disease (CHD), pulmonary arterial hypertension (PAH) associated with CHD (APAH-CHD) is more commonly encountered.[1,2] This increased prevalence has been seen despite significant advances in early diagnosis and surgical correction of patients with structural heart disease. PAH is the cause of significant morbidity and mortality in these patients and comes in many forms. In comparison with patients with idiopathic PAH (IPAH), the pathophysiology of PAH with CHD varies with the underlying anatomy of the defect, presence and size of shunt, and status of the right ventricle (RV). In patients with unoperated large systemic to pulmonary shunts and subsequent development of classic Eisenmenger physiology with shunt reversal, PAH results from pulmonary vascular remodeling due to initial increased pulmonary blood flow (PBF) and shear stress.[3] Despite differences in pathophysiologic triggers, the histopathologic and pathobiologic changes at the level of the pulmonary arterioles in APAH-CHD are remarkably similar to IPAH. Thus these conditions have been grouped together into World Health Organization (WHO) group 1 PAH according to the Dana point classification system.[4] Further, there are similarities as well as differences in the clinical presentation, disease progression, and management strategies

Disclosures: Dr Erika B. Rosenzweig has received honoraria from Actelion, Gilead, and United Therapeutics for advice at scientific advisory board meetings. Dr Rosenzweig's institution also receives research grant support for clinical trials from Actelion, Bayer, Gilead, GSK, Eli Lilly, and United Therapeutics. Dr Usha Krishnan has received honoraria for CME balanced lectures from Actelion and Gilead.
Columbia University Medical Center, Pulmonary Hypertension Center, Division of Pediatric Cardiology, 3959 Broadway, CH-2N, New York, NY 10032, USA
* Corresponding author.
E-mail address: esb14@columbia.edu

between APAH-CHD and other forms of group 1 PAH. With availability of targeted therapies for PAH, there is hope for improved hemodynamics, exercise capacity, quality of life, and possibly survival in these patients.

EPIDEMIOLOGY AND PATHOPHYSIOLOGY OF APAH-CHD

Data from the Registry to Evaluate Early and Long-Term Pulmonary Arterial Hypertension Disease Management (REVEAL) registry and the French registry estimate the prevalence of APAH-CHD to be between 10% and 11% of all patients with pulmonary hypertension.[5,6] This number is likely to continue to grow as the number of patients with CHD surviving to adulthood rises. In the pediatric age group, CHD forms a much larger proportion of patients with PAH.[7] PAH is a type of PH characterized by having mean pulmonary artery pressure greater than or equal to 25 mmHg at rest, with mean pulmonary artery wedge pressure (PAWP) 15 mm Hg or less. In patients with CHD, it is important to differentiate between PAH with low pulmonary vascular resistance (PVR) versus high PVR, which implies vasoconstriction and changes at the arteriolar level. For example, patients with large post tricuspid shunts can have elevated pulmonary arterial pressures (PAPs) without elevation of PVR, due to increased PBF from large systemic to pulmonary shunts. However, with prolonged exposure of the pulmonary circulation to increased flow, vasoconstriction, intimal proliferation, in situ thrombosis, impaired apoptosis, vascular remodeling, and inflammation ensue, all of which contribute to increasing PVR and irreversible vascular disease.[8] These histopathologic changes are very similar to those seen in the lungs of patients with IPAH. However, there are important differences in the clinical presentation, physiology, and outcome of the 2 conditions. Despite similar changes at the level of the lung microvasculature and the endothelium, the effect of these changes on the RV are different in APAH-CHD versus IPAH. Despite hypertrophy and dilatation, the RV systolic function can remain normal for decades in the patient with classic Eisenmenger syndrome (ES). This is due to the ability of the RV to unload itself with a right to left shunt, reducing the pressure overload on the RV at the cost of cyanosis. Another hypothesis proposed in these patients to account for the relatively preserved RV function is that these RVs are subjected to systemic pressures from fetal life, and have never undergone the postnatal regression that normally occurs in other forms of PAH. This RV phenotype

may be better able to work against higher resistances for a longer time.[9]

ANATOMIC AND PHYSIOLOGIC CLASSIFICATION

Even among patients with APAH-CHD, there are several clinical subtypes with significant differences in clinical manifestations and outcome, leading to investigators further classifying this group.

Simonneau and colleagues[4] in 2009 proposed an important classification to better describe the anatomy and physiology of patients with APAH-CHD. The classification describes 5 anatomic features, including (1) defect type (including simple or complex defects), (2) defect size hemodynamically speaking (by amount of shunting) and anatomic size (by dimensions), (3) direction of shunt, (4) associated cardiac or extracardiac anomalies, and (5) repair status (Box 1). Unrestrictive post tricuspid shunts, for example, large ventricular septal defects (VSD) and aortopulmonary shunts begin developing pulmonary vascular disease in early childhood as compared with pretricuspid defects, such as atrial septal defects (ASD). Directionality of the shunt can be determined by echocardiography, as well as clinically by oximetry at rest and during exercise. In patients with a patent ductus arteriosus (PDA), preductal and postductal saturations[10] should be checked to look for right to left shunting at rest and with exertion. The repair status of the defect is also important, as patients with severe residual PAH after closure of shunts may have more rapid progression of disease and worse outcome, similar to IPAH, than those with unrepaired shunts and ES physiology.

CLINICAL CLASSIFICATION

Simonneau and colleagues[4] also proposed a clinical classification of APAH-CHD, which best describes their physiologic and clinical subtype. These 4 physiologic subtypes of patients with APAH-CHD, are described in Box 2:

- Subgroup 1, patients with classic ES (inoperable with reversal of shunt)
- Subgroup 2, patients with large systemic to pulmonary shunts but low PVR that are operable
- Subgroup 3, patients with severe PAH in the setting of small restrictive CHD with physiology and course similar to IPAH patients; these patients are at increased risk for more rapidly progressive RV failure and have worse

Box 1
Anatomic classification of congenital systemic-to-pulmonary shunts

1.	Type
1.1.	Simple pretricuspid shunts
1.1.1.	Atrial septal defect (ASD)
1.1.1.1.	Ostium secundum
1.1.1.2.	Sinus venosus
1.1.1.3.	Ostium primum
1.1.2.	Total or partial unobstructed anomalous pulmonary venous return
1.2	Simple post-tricuspid shunts
1.2.1.	Ventricular septal defect (VSD)
1.2.2.	Patent ductus arteriosus (PDA)
1.3	Combined shunts (describe combination and predominant defect)
1.4	Complex congenital heart disease
1.4.1.	Complete atrioventricular septal defect
1.4.2.	Truncus arteriosus
1.4.3.	Single-ventricle physiology with unobstructed pulmonary blood flow
1.4.4.	Transposition of the great arteries with VSD (without pulmonary stenosis) and/or PDA
1.4.5.	Other
2.	Dimension (specify for each defect if more than 1)
2.1.	Hemodynamic (specify ratio of pulmonary-to-systemic blood flow)
2.1.1.	Restrictive (pressure gradient across the defect)
2.1.2.	Nonrestrictive
2.2.	Anatomic
2.2.1.	Small to moderate (ASD ≤2 cm and VSD ≤1 cm)
2.2.2.	Large (ASD >2 cm and VSD >1 cm)
3.	Direction of shunt
3.1	Predominantly systemic-to-pulmonary
3.2	Predominantly pulmonary-to-systemic
3.3	Bidirectional
4.	Associated cardiac and extracardiac abnormalities
5.	Repair status
5.1.	Unoperated
5.2.	Palliated (specify type of operation(s), age at surgery)
5.3.	Repaired (specify type of operation(s), age at surgery)

From Simonneau G, Robbins IM, Beghetti M, et al. Updated clinical classification of pulmonary hypertension. J Am Coll Cardiol 2009;54(Suppl 1):S43–54; with permission.

Box 2
Clinical classification of congenital systemic-to-pulmonary shunts associated with PAH

Eisenmenger syndrome	Patients with unrepaired systemic-to-pulmonary shunts resulting from large, nonrestrictive defects leading to a severe, progressive increase in PVR, bidirectional shunting, and ultimately reversed shunting with central cyanosis
PAH with moderate to large defects	PVR is mildly to moderately increased, systemic-to-pulmonary shunt is still present, and no cyanosis is present at rest
PAH with small defects	Smaller defects generally include VSD ≤1 cm and ASD ≤2 cm, and clinical picture is similar to IPAH
PAH following corrective cardiac surgery	CHD has been corrected, but PAH is present either immediately after surgery or recurs several months or years after surgery in the absence of significant residual shunts

Abbreviations: ASD, atrial septal defect; CHD, congenital heart disease; IPAH, idiopathic pulmonary arterial hypertension; PAH, pulmonary arterial hypertension; PVR, pulmonary vascular resistance; VSD, ventricular septal defect.
From Simonneau G, Robbins IM, Beghetti M, et al. Updated Clinical classification of pulmonary hypertension. J Am Coll Cardiol 2009;54(Suppl 1):S43–54; with permission.

outcomes than patients with ES, as there is no pop-off mechanism to unload the RV
• Subgroup 4, postoperative residual or recurrent PAH

Some patients develop PAH months or even years following surgery, despite shunt closure being performed at an appropriate age. Although genetic factors may play a role in their predisposition to develop PAH, it is not completely understood why some patients develop PAH even with timely repair of a systemic to pulmonary shunt. Patients with postoperative PAH also act physiologically like IPAH, and need to be treated more aggressively, with strategies similar to those used for IPAH.

Manes and colleagues[10] analyzed data from 192 patients with APAH-CHD collected over 13 years, and compared the outcomes of different subtypes of APAH-CHD with patients with IPAH. The investigators demonstrated that patients with ES had the highest baseline PVR and lowest exercise capacity. However, they also found a 20-year Kaplan-Meier survival estimate of 87% for ES compared with 36% in postoperative APAH-CHD. Other studies have also shown a favorable prognosis for patients with APAH-CHD as compared with IPAH.[9,11,12] However, in 2010, when the long-term outcomes data from the REVEAL study were analyzed, survival in patients with APAH-CHD was not significantly different from that in patients with IPAH.[13] This is probably because this study included all 4 subgroups of patients with APAH-CHD and not just the patients with type 1 ES, who appear to have a survival advantage over IPAH and postoperative APAH-CHD.[10] Management of patients within the first 2 categories, those with Eisenmenger physiology and those with PAH in the setting of unrepaired moderate to large defects, poses added challenges, and is the focus of the remainder of this article. Management of groups 3 and 4 is similar to the management of patients with IPAH.

PAH ASSOCIATED WITH UNRESTRICTIVE SYSTEMIC TO PULMONARY SHUNTS

The clinical presentation of APAH-CHD depends on the status of pulmonary vascular disease at the time of evaluation. In patients with large shunts and normal PVR, such as the infant with a large, nonrestrictive VSD, increased PBF, and congestive heart failure, the presentation is usually of failure to thrive, feeding intolerance, resting tachypnea, and recurrent respiratory infections. In these patients, surgical therapy after medical stabilization is the treatment of choice. Even within this group, in about 2% of children with large systemic to pulmonary shunts present, postoperative PAH occurs, with approximately 0.75% suffering PH crises.[14] In these patients, mortality remains relatively high at 20% to 30%.[14–17] Children at risk for postoperative PAH crises are often those with Down syndrome, complex CHD (atrioventricular canal defects, aortopulmonary window, transposition of great arteries, and truncus arteriosus), and children with very reactive PAH with PH crises in the preoperative period.[15]

In patients with large systemic to pulmonary shunts presenting at an older age, careful evaluation to determine operability is critical before repair. Patients with APAH-CHD (see **Box 2**) with modestly elevated PVR and moderate systemic to pulmonary shunts (type 2) are also quite challenging to manage.[18] Determining whether the patient is operable, and if the patient would benefit with pretreatment with targeted therapies is essential, although there are no evidence-based guidelines available. Closing a defect should not be performed just because it can be, but rather only when the PAH is likely to improve after surgical intervention. This is an important point, particularly now that we have data that show that patients with postoperative APAH-CHD fare worse than other forms of APAH-CHD. Cardiac catheterization and acute vasodilator testing remain important tools to help determine safe operability in these patients. Although no validated criteria exist for predicting long-term postsurgical morbidity and mortality, a complete set of hemodynamics should be obtained; vasodilator testing and temporary balloon occlusion of the defect may also be helpful. Obtaining resting room air oxygen saturations and then oxygen saturation following exertion can be helpful in the assessment of operability. For a patient with resting cyanosis or even cyanosis with exertion, closing the defect can lead to worsening right heart failure by removing the pressure/volume "pop-off" that the defect affords the right ventricle. Other important elements of the history include age at diagnosis, current age, and type and size of CHD. The importance of the type of CHD has been previously discussed, and, in general, the earlier a shunt lesion is diagnosed, the more likely the patient is operable. A history suggestive of initial congestive heart failure, including recurrent respiratory infection and effort intolerance, which improves over time to a "honeymoon period" of symptomatic relief, is suspicious of the development of irreversible pulmonary vascular disease with less net left to right shunting. In this situation, exercise testing may reveal latent cyanosis. Elevated hemoglobin in an iron replete patient, suggesting erythrocytosis in response to hypoxia, may also indicate intermittent right to left shunting through the course of the day.

INTERPRETATION OF HEMODYNAMIC DATA

Indices of right heart function, including right atrial pressure and cardiac index, are important determinants of prognosis in IPAH.[15] In patients with APAH-CHD, PVR also becomes an important tool for the assessment of the patient. It is essential to understand that PAH in patients with large systemic to pulmonary shunts can be due to an increase in PBF or due to an increase in the PVR. In patients with a large unrestrictive VSD or PDA, PAP will be at systemic levels regardless of the PVR because of the increase in PBF (PBF [Qp]:systemic blood flow [Qs]). In contrast, elevation in the PVR is determined by the extent of pulmonary vascular obstructive disease (PVD). Therefore, in patients with APAH-CHD, calculation of the PVR is clinically important as well. In a patient with a large shunt and normal PVR index (PVRi) less than $3 \, U \times M^2$, complete repair of the defect is usually not associated with residual PAH. However, when there is elevation of PVR above $6 \, U \times M^2$, completely repairing the defect can be dangerous and associated with residual PAH and postoperative PH crises and RV strain. During the hemodynamic evaluation of a systemic-to-pulmonary shunt, baseline room air hemodynamics should include 3 complete oxygen saturation runs and pressure measurements in the superior vena cava, right atrium (RA), RV, pulmonary artery (PA), and pulmonary capillary wedge pressures (PCWP). Once baseline data are collected, if there is no elevation of PAWP and PVRi is greater than $3 \, U \times M^2$, acute vasodilator testing should be performed and another full assessment should be performed. Data should be obtained in the absence of respiratory or metabolic acidosis, anemia, or agitation.

Nevertheless, the issue of determining operability is not straightforward and has been highlighted in several recent articles.[19–21] Lopes and O'Leary[21] proposed the following hemodynamic criteria for operability, based on existing literature and surveying centers of excellence with experience in the treatment of pulmonary hypertensive patients: baseline PVRi less than $6 \, WU \times M^2$ and PVR-SVR ratio less than 0.3. Acute vasodilator testing (AVT) was suggested if PVR at baseline was 6 to $9 \, WU \times M^2$ with a PVR-SVR ratio of 0.3 to 0.5. In these patients, a favorable outcome is considered likely if with AVT, the following criteria are met: (1) a decrease of PVRi by greater than 20%, (2) a decrease in PVR-SVR ratio by 20%, (3) a final PVR less than $6 \, WU \times M^2$, and (4) a final PVR-SVR ratio less than 0.3. Other centers have reported higher baseline PVRi values for operability PVRi less than or equal to 7 to $8 \, WU \times M^2$ and PVR-SVR ratios of less than or equal to 0.4.[22,23] None of these studies report long-term outcomes following closure of the defects, and the question of the benefits of pretreating with targeted PAH therapies before surgical repair remains unanswered.

Cardiac catheterization alone, however, is usually not sufficient to determine operability. The hemodynamic findings must be taken in the context of the medical history, physical examination, and results of all invasive and noninvasive testing. For example, in a case of borderline PVR at rest in the catheterization laboratory, but with significant exertional cyanosis, shunt repair may be more harmful than beneficial.

In patients with "borderline" hemodynamics (eg, PVRi 3 to $6 \, U \times M^2$), there may be an evolving role for a combined medical-surgical approach. Although this has not been proven to provide long-term benefit, there have been anecdotal cases, including at our own institution, of being able to partially repair after using targeted PAH therapy in borderline cases (**Fig. 1**). It may be reasonable to treat with targeted PAH therapies for a period of months, and serially reevaluate by catheterization to determine operability or partial operability with intentional creation of a small residual defect as a "pop-off."[18–20] In rare borderline patients, medical therapy may drop the PVR enough to increase the left to right shunt to such an extent that there is significantly elevated PBF and the patient develops signs and symptoms of high-output failure.[20] As a result, surgical shunt closure should be expeditiously performed to protect the pulmonary vasculature from high flow-related damage.

Surgery on a patient with borderline PAH should be undertaken after careful consideration of all these factors and there should be a multidisciplinary team approach involving the cardiologist, surgeon, intensivists, anesthesiologists, and the postoperative intensive care unit team. Care should be taken to anticipate and avoid PA pressure swings during induction of anesthesia and during recovery. Circulating vasoactive factors from blood products (like platelets) are known to precipitate PAH crises and should be avoided if possible. In the postoperative period, use of pulmonary vasodilators, including inhaled nitric oxide (iNO) and adequate oxygenation, as well as avoidance of respiratory acidosis, is essential. Some patients may require sedation (and/or paralysis) and mechanical ventilation for several days if they have labile PH in the postoperative period. The use of sildenafil while weaning iNO has been found to be effective in preventing rebound PH in some cases.[24]

EISENMENGER SYNDROME

The term "Eisenmenger syndrome" (ES) was coined by Paul Hamilton Wood in 1958 to define the condition of increased PAP and PVR in relation to a VSD with resultant shunt reversal and cyanosis. Currently, the term Eisenmenger physiology has been expanded to include any reversed shunt secondary to elevated PVR, including shunts associated with complex

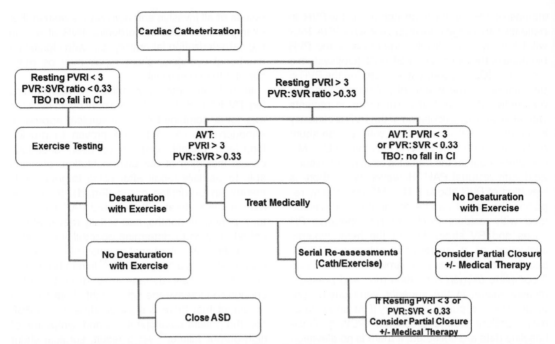

Fig. 1. APAH-CHD (ASD) clinical management algorithm: individualized case approach. ASD, atrial septal defect; AVT, acute vasodilator testing; PVR:SVR ratio, ratio of pulmonary vascular resistance to systemic vascular resistance; PVRI, pulmonary vascular resistance indexed to body surface area; TBO, temporary balloon occlusion. (*From* Rosenzweig EB, Barst RJ. Congenital heart disease and pulmonary hypertension: pharmacology and feasibility of late surgery. Prog Cardiovasc Dis 2012;55(2):128–33; with permission.)

CHD.[25] With timely CHD diagnosis and cardiac surgery, especially during infancy, survival of patients into adulthood is commonplace, and the worldwide incidence of ES has declined by 50%.[26,27] However, ES still remains a significant problem in the developing world, where patients with large shunts are unable to undergo repair before the development of PVD. The worldwide prevalence of PAH in adults with CHD has recently been estimated at between 1.6 and 12.5 million, with 25% to 50% presenting with ES.[28]

Although life expectancy is reduced in ES, it is significantly better than IPAH, with many patients with ES surviving into their third and fourth decades, and even some into their seventh decade.[26,27] More than 40% of subjects are expected to be alive 25 years after diagnosis. **Fig. 2** shows the Kaplan-Meier curves of life expectancy in simple versus complex lesions leading to ES.[29] Patients with complex lesions have a much worse prognosis than those with simple shunts. However, with advances in targeted therapies, the outlook for patients with ES may improve, as a recent study predicted Kaplan-Meier survival estimate at 20 years of 87% in patients with ES.[10]

The presentation and clinical course of ES are a result of chronic hypoxia and are different from those of IPAH. Patients with ES often have objective evidence of significant effort intolerance, but may not perceive their limitation because of the chronicity of their disease. Their symptoms and complications are secondary to the cyanosis, erythrocytosis, and end-organ damage. On physical examination, central cyanosis with clubbing

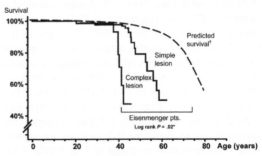

Fig. 2. Survival prospects of patients with Eisenmenger physiology when compared with an age- and gender-matched healthy population showing reduced life expectancy in patients with ES. †, Predicted survival is based on the life tables for UK and Wales (2001–2003 interim life tables) published by the Government Actuary's Department. *, Comparison between Eisenmenger patients with simple and complex lesions. Patients with complex lesions had a significantly worse outcome compared with those with simple lesions.

may be present, RV heave and a prominent second heart sound are often present, and hepatomegaly and peripheral edema may be appreciated in more advanced cases. Patients may also present with serious complications, such as cerebral abscess or stroke, pulmonary arterial thrombosis, massive hemoptysis due to rupture of thin-walled pulmonary vessels, bacterial endocarditis, or severe myocardial dysfunction with low cardiac output.

MANAGEMENT STRATEGIES FOR ES

In the past, treatment options for patients with ES had been limited to palliative therapies and heart-lung transplantation or lung transplantation with repair of the CHD. However, over the past decade, there has been growing experience using both conventional and targeted PAH therapies in patients with ES. Commonly used conventional therapies include digoxin, diuretics, anticoagulation, and antiarrhythmics, although none of these have been shown to improve survival in ES. Anticoagulation in patients with ES remains controversial because of increased risks of pulmonary artery thrombosis, as well as hemoptysis, stroke, and hemorrhage. Although the benefit of anticoagulation in patients with IPAH has been demonstrated, no such data exist for patients with ES, and, given the potential complications, the decision to anticoagulate should be made carefully on an individual case basis. Oxygen is often used long term in patients with ES, and although it may be associated with improvement in subjective status, no survival benefit has been seen. Maternal mortality in patients with ES is reported at approximately 50%, with death usually occurring during delivery or the first postpartum week due to hypervolemia, thromboembolism, or preeclampsia. In addition, spontaneous abortion rates are quite high, and for infants carried to term, there are high rates of intrauterine growth retardation and perinatal mortality.[29–31] As a result, pregnancy is contraindicated in ES.

TARGETED THERAPIES FOR ES

There are 3 main classes of targeted PAH therapies initially used in patients with group 1 PAH, and currently, all have been used in the treatment of patients with ES. These include prostanoids, endothelin receptor antagonists (ERAs), and phosphodiesterase-5 (PDE5) inhibitors. The aim of targeted therapies in patients with ES is to improve exercise tolerance by improving PBF, hypoxemia, physical capacity, and, ultimately, survival.

Prostanoids

The use of intravenous epoprostenol in ES was first described by Rosenzweig and colleagues[32] in 1999, with subjects showing improvements in functional capacity, hemodynamics, and survival. Because epoprostenol is chemically unstable at neutral pH/room temperature, and has a short half-life (1–2 minutes), a continuous intravenous delivery system with cold packs is needed to maintain stability. An indwelling central venous line is necessary, with associated complications, including thrombosis and line occlusion, local and systemic infection, and catheter breakage. The risk of thromboembolism is of particular concern in patients with ES with right to left shunts. In addition, pump malfunction may rarely lead to administration of a sudden bolus of epoprostenol (leading to systemic hypotension) or interruption of the medication, which can cause severe rebound PAH. Therefore, a search for alternate routes of drug delivery has led to the approval of inhaled (iloprost, treprostinil), subcutaneous (treprostinil), and more stable and longer-acting intravenous prostacyclin analogues (treprostinil, veletri). Treprostinil sodium is a prostacyclin analogue with a neutral pH, longer half-life, which is stable at room temperature, and shares the same pharmacologic actions as epoprostenol with potential advantages by being able to deliver the agent via inhalation or subcutaneous infusion, thus eliminating the risk of thromboembolic events in patients with ES.[33]

ERAs

Endothelin (ET)-1 is one of the most potent vasoconstrictors implicated in the pathobiology of PAH and plasma ET-1 levels are increased in patients with IPAH (and other forms of PAH) and correlate inversely with prognosis. The first randomized, double-blinded, placebo-controlled study in patients with ES was the Bosentan Randomized Trial of Endothelin Antagonist Therapy-5 (BREATHE-5) trial investigating the efficacy and safety of the dual ERA bosentan in patients with ES.[34,35] During the 16-week study, bosentan significantly reduced PVR, and improved PAP and exercise capacity compared with placebo without worsening oxygenation, and longer-term data from the follow-up portion of the study demonstrated continued improvements in exercise capacity over an additional 24 weeks.[35] The study also demonstrated a worsening of PVR in the placebo group, which underscores the progressive nature of untreated ES. Risks associated with ERAs include acute hepatotoxicity (bosentan), teratogenicity, and possibly male infertility. The selective ERA ambrisentan may offer potential advantages over bosentan, given its selectivity for the ET-A receptor, which demonstrates vasoconstrictor effects, although this remains controversial. Ambrisentan, which can be administered once a day, was also found to be efficacious in a series of patients with ES with an acceptable safety profile.[36]

PDE5 Inhibitors

PDE5 inhibitors prevent the inactivation of cyclic guanosine monophosphate (GMP), thereby raising cyclic GMP levels. Oral sildenafil is the most widely used of the PDE5 inhibitors in the treatment of PAH, and has been used in children with APAH-CHD, with benefits on exercise capacity and hemodynamics.[37] In a recent prospective, open-label, multicenter study, using sildenafil, patients with ES demonstrated an acceptable safety profile and improved exercise capacity, oxygen saturation, and hemodynamics after 12 months of therapy.[38] A recent randomized, placebo-controlled, double-blinded crossover study using tadalafil in patients with ES also demonstrated safety and short-term improvements in exercise capacity, functional class, oxygen saturation, and hemodynamics after 6 weeks of therapy.[39]

Lung and Heart Lung Transplantation

Currently, the overall 1-year, 5-year, and 10-year survival for lung transplantation for patients with PAH is 64%, 44%, and 20%, respectively.[40–42] For patients with untreated ES, the 5-year and 25-year survival is greater than 80% and 40%, respectively as opposed to following lung transplantation (52% and 39%).[40–42] Thus, lung transplantation should be reserved for patients with WHO functional class IV symptoms with an estimated likelihood of survival of less than 50% at 5 years. Although lung and heart/lung transplantation are imperfect therapies for pulmonary arterial hypertension, when offered to an appropriately selected population, transplantation may improve survival with an improved quality of life. The use of extracorporeal membrane oxygenation as a bridge to recovery (in acutely decompensated patients), as well as a bridge to transplantation, may also be a viable option in selected patients.[42]

PULMONARY HYPERTENSION IN THE UNIVENTRICULAR HEART: THE FAILING FONTAN

The Fontan (total cavopulmonary connection) circulation, which is surgically created for hypoplastic left heart syndrome, lacks a pumping subpulmonary ventricle, and is dependent on the central venous pressure to perfuse the pulmonary circulation. Thus, changes in the PVR can have a tremendous impact on forward flow in this circulation. For patients with a single ventricle, the hemodynamic criteria used for shunt closure do not apply for predicting operability. Pre-Fontan PVRi should be normal in these patients, to sustain the cavopulmonary circulation (ie, <3 WU $\times$ M^2). In these patients, a preoperative mean PAP of only 15 to 18 mm Hg is a risk factor for poor outcome after Fontan repair.[20,21] Postoperatively, even small increases in PAP can lead to low cardiac output syndrome, even in the setting of a technically successful operation. Current medical management of Fontan failure aims mostly at treating manifestations such as ventricular dysfunction and protein-losing enteropathy (PLE). Most of the complications of failing Fontan circulation are attributed to structural changes (stenosis) in the pulmonary vascular tree or to pulmonary vascular disease. Late complications include ventricular dysfunction and low cardiac output syndrome, PLE, hypoxemia, and decreased exercise intolerance, and all of these are ultimately related to elevated PVR.[43,44] There are isolated small case series reporting benefit of therapies, such as subcutaneous heparin, oral budesonide, spironolactone, bosentan, and sildenafil, in the treatment of PLE.[45–48] Because elevated PVR is implicated in failure of the Fontan circulation, targeted PAH therapies, including iNO, are sometimes used. In the immediate postoperative period, iNO in combination with milrinone, has been found to be beneficial in improving hemodynamics.[49] Although prostacyclins are rarely used in the perioperative period, epoprostenol has been shown to prevent the rebound effects of NO cessation.[50] There is scant literature on the effects of targeted PAH therapies in patients with failing Fontan; however, sildenafil and bosentan have been used in the treatment of PLE and plastic bronchitis, and to improve hemodynamic response to exercise.[51–55] Due to the liver toxicity associated with nonselective ERAs and the potential for liver complications in patients with Fontan failure, there may be great hesitation to use bosentan in these patients. Postmarketing surveillance of bosentan found transaminase elevation to be less of a problem in patients with APAH-CHD than other types of PAH; however, these studies do not specifically discuss the Fontan subgroups. Currently, there are several ongoing clinical trials investigating the role of targeted therapies in patients with univentricular circulation.[44]

SUMMARY

Although PAH associated with CHD has common histopathologic and pathobiologic findings as other disorders clustered together under WHO group 1 pulmonary hypertension, this group is very heterogeneous in terms of anatomic, physiologic, and clinical features, as well as outcomes. With improved survival of patients with CHD, the number of patients with CHD and PAH seen in adult CHD clinics is increasing. This subgroup of patients has unique clinical features and potential complications compared with patients with other forms of WHO group 1 PAH. Targeted PAH therapies have clear short-term benefits in these patients, and their use in patients with borderline hemodynamics may pave the way for a combined medical-surgical approach to management in borderline cases in the future. However, further large studies are required to evaluate the long-term outcome using these strategies. A subpopulation of APAH-CHD that is growing rapidly includes those patients with complex single-ventricle anatomy, and large multicenter studies are required to better understand the Fontan physiology and evaluate potential benefits of targeted PAH therapies in these patients.

REFERENCES

1. Rose ML, Strange G, King I, et al. Congenital heart disease-associated pulmonary arterial hypertension: preliminary results from a novel registry. Intern Med J 2012;42:874–9.

2. Gatzoulis MA, Alonso-Gonzalez R, Beghetti M. Pulmonary arterial hypertension in paediatric and adult patients with congenital heart disease. Eur Respir Rev 2009;18:154–61.

3. Fratz S, Geiger R, Kresse H, et al. Pulmonary blood pressure, not flow, is associated with net endothelin-1 production in the lungs of patients with congenital heart disease and normal pulmonary vascular resistance. J Thorac Cardiovasc Surg 2003;126:1724–9.

4. Simonneau G, Robbins IM, Beghetti M, et al. Updated clinical classification of pulmonary hypertension. J Am Coll Cardiol 2009;54(Suppl 1): S43–54.

5. Humbert M, Sitbon O, Chaouat A, et al. Pulmonary arterial hypertension in France: results from a national registry. Am J Respir Crit Care Med 2006; 173:1023–30.

6. Badesch DB, Raskob GE, Elliott CG, et al. Pulmonary arterial hypertension: baseline characteristics from the REVEAL registry. Chest 2009;137: 376–87.

7. Haworth SG, Hislop AA. Treatment and survival in children with pulmonary arterial hypertension: the UK Pulmonary Hypertension Service for Children 2001-2006. Heart 2009;95:312–7.

8. Durmowicz AG, Stenmark KR. Mechanisms of structural remodeling in chronic pulmonary hypertension. Pediatr Rev 1999;20:e9–102.

9. Hopkins WE, Ochoa LL, Richardson GW, et al. Comparison of the hemodynamics and survival of adults with severe primary pulmonary hypertension or Eisenmenger syndrome. J Heart Lung Transplant 1996;15:100–5.

10. Manes A, Palazzini M, Leci E, et al. Current era survival of patients with pulmonary arterial hypertension associated with congenital heart disease: a comparison between clinical subgroups. Eur Heart J 2013. [Epub ahead of print].

11. Engelfriet PM, Duffels MG, Moller T, et al. Pulmonary arterial hypertension in adults born with a heart septal defect: the Euro Heart Survey on adult congenital heart disease. Heart 2007;93: 682–7.

12. McLaughlin VV, Archer SL, Badesch DB, et al. ACCF/AHA 2009 expert consensus document on pulmonary hypertension. A report of the American College of Cardiology Foundation Task Force on Expert Consensus Documents and the American Heart Association developed in collaboration with the American College of Chest Physicians; American Thoracic Society, Inc.; and the Pulmonary Hypertension Association. J Am Coll Cardiol 2009;53: 1573–619.

13. Benza RL, Miller DP, Gomberg-Maitland M, et al. Predicting survival in pulmonary arterial hypertension: insights from the Registry to Evaluate Early and Long-Term Pulmonary Arterial Hypertension Disease Management (REVEAL). Circulation 2010;122:164–72.

14. Lindberg L, Olsson AK, Jogi P, et al. How common is severe pulmonary hypertension after pediatric cardiac surgery? J Thorac Cardiovasc Surg 2002; 123:1155–63.

15. Bando K, Turrentine MW, Sharp TG, et al. Pulmonary hypertension after operations for congenital heart disease: analysis of risk factors and management. J Thorac Cardiovasc Surg 1996;112(6): 1600–7 [discussion: 1607–9].

16. Matsumoto M, Naitoh H, Higashi T, et al. Risk factors for pulmonary hypertensive crisis (PHC) following VSD repair in infants. Masui 1995;44: 1208–12.

17. Adatia I, Beghetti M. Early postoperative care of patients with pulmonary hypertension associated with congenital cardiac disease. Cardiol Young 2009;19:315–9.

18. Rosenzweig EB, Barst RJ. Congenital heart disease and pulmonary hypertension: pharmacology

and feasibility of late surgery. Prog Cardiovasc Dis 2012;55(2):128–33.

19. Beghetti M, Tissot C. Pulmonary hypertension in congenital shunts. Rev Esp Cardiol 2010;63: 1179–93.

20. Beghetti M, Galie' N, Bonnet D. Can inoperable congenital heart defects become operable in patients with pulmonary arterial hypertension? Dream or reality? Congenit Heart Dis 2012;7:3–11.

21. Lopes AA, O'Leary PW. Measurement, interpretation and use of haemodynamic parameters in pulmonary hypertension associated with congenital cardiac disease. Cardiol Young 2009;19:431–5.

22. Viswanathan S, Kumar RK. Assessment of operability of congenital cardiac shunts with increased pulmonary vascular resistance. Catheter Cardiovasc Interv 2008;71:665–70.

23. Giglia TM, Humpl T. Preoperative pulmonary hemodynamics and assessment of operability: is there a pulmonary vascular resistance that precludes cardiac operation? Pediatr Crit Care Med 2010; 11(Suppl 2):S57–69.

24. Matamis D, Pampori S, Papathanasiou A, et al. Inhaled NO and sildenafil combination in cardiac surgery patients with out-of-proportion pulmonary hypertension: acute effects on postoperative gas exchange and hemodynamics. Circ Heart Fail 2012;5:47–53.

25. Galie N, Hoeper MM, Humbert M, et al. Guidelines for the diagnosis and treatment of pulmonary hypertension: the Task Force for the Diagnosis and Treatment of Pulmonary Hypertension of the European Society of Cardiology (ESC) and the European Respiratory Society (ERS), endorsed by the International Society of Heart and Lung Transplantation (ISHLT). Eur Heart J 2009;30:2493–537.

26. Dimopoulos K, Inuzuka R, Goletto S, et al. Improved survival among patients with Eisenmenger syndrome receiving advanced therapy for pulmonary arterial hypertension. Circulation 2010;121:20–5.

27. Galie N, Manes A, Palazzini M, et al. Management of pulmonary arterial hypertension associated with congenital systemic-to-pulmonary shunts and Eisenmenger's syndrome. Drugs 2008;68:1049–66.

28. Lopes AA, Bandeira AP, Flores PC, et al. Pulmonary hypertension in Latin America: pulmonary vascular disease: the global perspective. Chest 2010;137(Suppl 6):78S–84S.

29. Diller GP, Dimopoulos K, Broberg CS, et al. Presentation, survival prospects, and predictors of death in Eisenmenger syndrome: a combined retrospective and case-control study. Eur Heart J 2006;27: 1737–42.

30. Swan L, Lupton M, Anthony J, et al. Controversies in pregnancy and congenital heart disease. Congenit Heart Dis 2006;1:27–34.

31. Bedard E, Dimopoulos K, Gatzoulis MA. Has there been any progress made on pregnancy outcomes among women with pulmonary arterial hypertension? Eur Heart J 2009;30:256–65.

32. Rosenzweig EB, Kerstein D, Barst RJ. Long-term prostacyclin for pulmonary hypertension with associated congenital heart defects. Circulation 1999; 99:1858–65.

33. Barst RJ, Simonneau G, Rich S, et al, for the Uniprost PAH Study Group. Efficacy and safety of chronic subcutaneous infusion of UT-15 (Uniprost) in pulmonary arterial hypertension (PAH). Circulation 2000;102:100–1.

34. Galie N, Beghetti M, Gatzoulis MA, et al. Bosentan therapy in patients with Eisenmenger syndrome: a multicenter, double-blind, randomized, placebo-controlled study. Circulation 2006;114:48–54.

35. Gatzoulis MA, Beghetti M, Galie N, et al. Longer-term bosentan therapy improves functional capacity in Eisenmenger syndrome: results of the BREATHE-5 open-label extension study. Int J Cardiol 2008;127(1):27–32.

36. Zuckerman WA, Leaderer D, Rowan CA, et al. Ambrisentan for pulmonary arterial hypertension due to congenital heart disease. Am J Cardiol 2011; 107(9):1381–5.

37. Schulze-Neick I, Hartenstein P, Li J. Intravenous Sildenafil is a potent pulmonary vasodilator in children with congenital heart disease. Circulation 2003;108:II167–73.

38. Zhang ZN, Jiang X, Zhang R, et al. Oral sildenafil treatment for Eisenmenger syndrome: a prospective, open-label, multicentre study. Heart 2011; 97(22):1876–81.

39. Mukhopadhyay S, Nathani S, Yusuf J, et al. Clinical efficacy of phosphodiesterase-5 inhibitor tadalafil in Eisenmenger syndrome—a randomized, placebo-controlled, double-blind crossover study. Congenit Heart Dis 2011;6(5):424–31.

40. Ofori-Amanfo G, Hsu D, Lamour JM, et al. Heart transplantation in children with markedly elevated pulmonary vascular resistance: impact of right ventricular failure on outcome. J Heart Lung Transplant 2011;30(6):659–66.

41. Lang G, Taghavi S, Aigner C. Primary lung transplantation after bridge with extracorporeal membrane oxygenation: a plea for a shift in our paradigms for indications. Transplantation 2012;93:729–36.

42. Trulock EP, Edwards LB, Taylor DO, et al. The Registry of the International Society for Heart and Lung Transplantation: Twentieth Official Adult Lung and Heart-Lung transplant report—2003. J Heart Lung Transplant 2003;22:625–35.

43. Khambadkone S, Li J, de Leval MR, et al. Basal pulmonary vascular resistance and nitric oxide responsiveness late after Fontan-type operation. Circulation 2003;107(25):3204–8.

44. Beghetti M. Fontan and the pulmonary circulation: a potential role for new pulmonary hypertension therapies. Heart 2010;96(12):911–6.

45. Goldberg DJ, Shaddy RE, Ravishankar C, et al. The failing Fontan: etiology, diagnosis and management. Expert Rev Cardiovasc Ther 2011;9(6):785–93.

46. Ryerson L, Goldberg C, Rosenthal A, et al. Usefulness of heparin therapy in protein-losing enteropathy associated with single ventricle palliation. Am J Cardiol 2008;101:248–51.

47. Ringel RE, Peddy SB. Effect of high-dose spironolactone on protein-losing enteropathy in patients with Fontan palliation of complex congenital heart disease. Am J Cardiol 2003;91:1031–2 A1039.

48. Yoshimura N, Yamaguchi M, Oka S, et al. Inhaled nitric oxide therapy after Fontan-type operations. Surg Today 2005;35:31–5.

49. Cai J, Su Z, Shi Z, et al. Nitric oxide and milrinone: combined effect on pulmonary circulation after Fontan-type procedure: a prospective, randomized study. Ann Thorac Surg 2008;86:882–8.

50. Miyaji K, Nagata N, Miyamoto T, et al. Combined therapy with inhaled nitric oxide and intravenous epoprostenol (prostacyclin) for critical pulmonary perfusion after the Fontan procedure. J Thorac Cardiovasc Surg 2003;125:437–9.

51. Trachte AL, Lobato EB, Urdaneta F, et al. Oral sildenafil reduces pulmonary hypertension after cardiac surgery. Ann Thorac Surg 2005;79:194–7.

52. Haseyama K, Satomi G, Yasukochi S, et al. Pulmonary vasodilation therapy with sildenafil citrate in a patient with plastic bronchitis after the Fontan procedure for hypoplastic left heart syndrome. J Thorac Cardiovasc Surg 2006;132(5):1232–3.

53. Giardini A, Balducci A, Specchia S, et al. Effect of sildenafil on haemodynamic response to exercise and exercise capacity in Fontan patients. Eur Heart J 2008;29:1681–7.

54. Apostolopoulou SC, Papagiannis J, Rammos S. Bosentan induces clinical, exercise and hemodynamic improvement in a pre-transplant patient with plastic bronchitis after Fontan operation. J Heart Lung Transplant 2005;24:1174–6.

55. Ovaert C, Thijs D, Dewolf D, et al. The effect of bosentan in patients with a failing Fontan circulation. Cardiol Young 2009;19:331–9.

Portopulmonary Hypertension

Nadine Al-Naamani, MD, Kari E. Roberts, MD*

KEYWORDS

- Hypertension, portal • Hypertension, pulmonary • Liver transplantation

KEY POINTS

- Portopulmonary hypertension (PoPH) describes the presence of group I pulmonary arterial hypertension (PAH) in patients with portal hypertension caused by cirrhotic or noncirrhotic liver disease.
- PoPH should be considered in the differential diagnosis of any patient with advanced liver disease and unexplained dyspnea or refractory ascites and edema.
- Transthoracic echocardiography is the screening test of choice, although it has a low positive predictive value because of the systemic hemodynamic consequences of portal hypertension.
- Right heart catheterization is required for the diagnosis of PoPH.
- PAH-specific therapies, including prostacyclins, endothelial receptor antagonists, and phosphodiesterase inhibitors, can be safely and effectively used for patients with PoPH.
- Liver transplantation should be considered for patients with mild or moderate PoPH, although the impact of transplantation on the natural history of PAH is uncertain.

INTRODUCTION

Advanced liver disease can be associated with significant pulmonary and pulmonary vascular dysfunction. Portopulmonary hypertension (PoPH) is defined as pulmonary arterial hypertension (PAH) that occurs in the context of portal hypertension. Portal hypertension, with or without cirrhosis, is the third most common clinical entity associated with PAH. Occurring in up to 6% of patients with advanced liver disease, PoPH is a rare, but life-threatening, complication of portal hypertension. Recognition of PoPH can be delayed because of the common clinical presentations of liver disease and right ventricular (RV) failure, and accurate diagnosis can be challenging because of the complex systemic hemodynamic effects of portal hypertension. PoPH must also be distinguished from hepatopulmonary syndrome (HPS), a more prevalent but less morbid pulmonary vascular complication of liver disease. Prompt recognition is critical because the cosegregation of pulmonary arterial and portal hypertension carries important implications for prognosis, medical therapy, and liver transplantation (LT). This article reviews the epidemiology, pathogenesis, clinical features, diagnostic evaluation, and management of PoPH.

DEFINITION OF POPH

Using the Dana Point classification of pulmonary hypertension, PoPH is group 1.4.3 PAH (**Table 1**).[1] Portal hypertension, caused by hepatic or extrahepatic disease, is sufficient to cause the pulmonary arteriopathy classically associated with PAH. The presence of portal hypertension is typically confirmed by direct measurement of the portal pressure gradient and the presence of esophageal and gastric varices or liver biopsy confirming cirrhosis.[2–4]

Intrinsic liver disease and portal hypertension are often accompanied by endothelial dysfunction and a hyperdynamic circulatory state. These systemic changes lead to impaired sodium and water handling, which are reflected clinically as volume overload. Approximately 20% of patients with liver

Disclosures: The authors have no disclosures relevant to this article.
Tufts Medical Center, 800 Washington Street, #257, Boston, MA 02111, USA
* Corresponding author. Tufts Medical Center, 800 Washington Street, #257, Boston, MA 02111.
E-mail address: kroberts@tuftsmedicalcenter.org

Table 1
Dana Point classification of pulmonary hypertension

1.		PAH
1.1.		Idiopathic PAH
1.2.		Heritable
	1.2.1.	BMPR2
	1.2.2.	ALK1, endoglin
	1.2.3.	Unknown
1.3.		Drug-associated and toxin-associated
1.4.		Associated with
	1.4.1.	Connective tissue diseases
	1.4.2.	HIV infection
	1.4.3.	Portal hypertension
	1.4.4.	Congenital heart diseases
	1.4.5.	Schistosomiasis
	1.4.6.	Chronic hemolytic anemia
1.5.		Persistent pulmonary hypertension of the newborn
1′.		Pulmonary veno-occlusive disease or pulmonary capillary hemangiomatosis
2.		**Pulmonary hypertension caused by left heart disease**
2.1.		Systolic dysfunction
2.2.		Diastolic dysfunction
2.3.		Valvular disease
3.		**Pulmonary hypertension caused by lung diseases or hypoxia**
3.1.		Chronic obstructive pulmonary disease
3.2.		Interstitial lung disease
3.3.		Other pulmonary diseases with mixed restrictive and obstructive pattern
3.4.		Sleep-disordered breathing
3.5.		Alveolar hypoventilation disorders
3.6.		Chronic exposure to high altitude
3.7.		Developmental abnormalities
4.		**Chronic thromboembolic pulmonary hypertension**
5.		**Pulmonary hypertension with unclear multifactorial mechanisms**
5.1.		Hematologic disorders: myeloproliferative disorders, splenectomy
5.2.		Systemic disorders: sarcoidosis, pulmonary Langerhans cell histiocytosis
5.3.		Others: tumoral obstruction, fibrosing mediastinitis, chronic renal failure on dialysis

Abbreviations: ALK1, activin receptorlike kinase 1; BMPR2, bone morphogenetic protein receptor 2; HIV, human immunodeficiency virus.

cirrhosis have a moderate increase in pulmonary pressures that is evident at the time of echocardiography[5]; however, a few of these are diagnosed with PoPH. The 2 most common causes for pulmonary hypertension are increased cardiac output (CO)[5–7] and increased left-sided filling pressures. In both of these circumstances, the transpulmonary gradient (mean pulmonary artery pressure [mPAP]–pulmonary capillary wedge pressure [PCWP]) and pulmonary vascular resistance (PVR) are normal or even low.[8]

$$PVR = [(mPAP - PCWP)/CO] \times 80$$

It is critical to distinguish these patients from true PoPH because they not only enjoy a significantly better prognosis, but in addition, they require a different therapeutic approach. The standard hemodynamic definition for PAH is applied for PoPH[9,10]:

1. mPAP of 25 mm Hg or greater (at rest), *and*
2. PCWP of 15 mm Hg or less

The spectrum of systemic and pulmonary hemodynamic changes documented in patients with portal hypertension has created some ambiguity in defining the pulmonary vascular phenotype in this population using conventional PAH hemodynamic criteria. Clinical syndromes consistent with PAH are recognized in patients with portal hypertension and PCWP >15 mm Hg or PVR 120 to 240 dyn s/cm^5 (1.5–3 Wood units).[11] Previous definitions for PAH have included a PVR greater than 240 dyn s/cm^5 (>3 Wood units) as part of the hemodynamic definition of PAH. The usefulness of a PVR threshold to patients with portal hypertension may help to distinguish between increased pulmonary artery pressure in the setting of a hyperdynamic circulation as a result of liver disease from the presence of pulmonary arteriopathy consistent with PAH or PoPH. An increased transpulmonary gradient (>12 mm Hg) may also be helpful in making the distinction between the different forms of pulmonary vascular disease associated with liver disease. Although some experts advocate for flexibility in the hemodynamic definition for patients with portal hypertension, there are insufficient data to validate alternative diagnostic criteria.

PoPH is classified as mild, moderate, or severe, as outlined in **Table 2**.[6,12] Right heart catheterization (RHC), with direct measurement of mPAP, PCWP, and CO is required in order to distinguish PoPH from these other forms of pulmonary hypertension. **Table 3** shows the 3 common pulmonary hemodynamic patterns seen in portal hypertension.[13]

EPIDEMIOLOGY AND OUTCOMES

The association between portal hypertension and PAH was first described by Mantz and Craige in 1951,[14] who presented the case of a 53-year-old woman with portal vein stenosis and cor pulmonale. At autopsy the patient's pulmonary microcirculation showed endothelial proliferation, intimal thickening, and thrombosis. This initial observation was later confirmed in a study of more than 17,000 autopsies,[15] which reported a higher prevalence of PAH among patients with portal hypertension or cirrhosis than in unselected patients (0.73% vs 0.13%, respectively). Among patients with chronic liver disease, the prevalence of PoPH is estimated to be 2%,[16] increasing to 4% to 6% among individuals undergoing LT evaluation.[5,11,17] PoPH may be more prevalent (5%–10%) among individuals with extrahepatic portal hypertension such as that associated with extrahepatic obstruction of the portal vein, biliary atresia, or idiopathic portal hypertension.[18,19] PoPH accounts for 7% to 10% of all group 1 PAH, and it is the third most common clinical subtype after idiopathic PAH and PAH associated with connective tissue diseases.[20,21] Pediatric PoPH has been less well defined, although a recent review[19] reported a prevalence of 5.2% among children with portal hypertension.

Adults with PoPH typically present in the fifth decade of life, likely a reflection of the demographics of liver disease,[5,22] with the diagnosis of portal hypertension preceding PAH by 4 to 7 years.[16,23–25] Defining the at-risk minority amongst those with portal hypertension has led to several observations. First, similar to PAH associated with idiopathic and connective tissue disease, female sex is now an accepted risk factor for PoPH. Women with portal hypertension have nearly 3 times the risk of men; this skewed sex ratio is apparent despite the male predominance of portal hypertension.[26–28] Second, individuals with autoimmune liver disease have a 4-fold increased risk for PoPH compared with other causes of liver disease. This finding also mirrors the pattern in other types of PAH, in which autoimmunity represents a risk factor for PAH (ie, scleroderma) or manifests itself in other organ systems (autoimmune thyroid disease in PAH). Third, among those with advanced liver disease, hepatitis C infection is associated with a lower risk for PoPH (odds ratio 0.24, 95% confidence interval [CI] 0.09-0.56, P = .005).[29] Last, there is no demonstrable correlation between risk of PoPH and portal hemodynamics.[16,29]

PoPH is a morbid and mortal disease. Historically, mean and median survivals of patients with PoPH were 15 and 6 months, respectively, with a 5-year survival less than 10%.[30] More contemporary data from the United States show improved outcomes, yet there remains a nearly 4-fold increased risk of death in PoPH relative to idiopathic PAH (hazard ratio 3.6, 95% CI 2.4–5.4).[31] Of all subtypes of group I PAH, patients with PoPH have the worst outcomes, with 2-year and 5-year survivals of 67% and 40% (**Fig. 1**). This finding is despite the fact that patients with

Table 2 Staging of severity of PoPH			
	Mild	**Moderate**	**Severe**
NYHA FC	I, II	II, III	III, IV
mPAP (mm Hg)	25–34	35–44	>45
CI (L/min/m^2)	>2.5	>2.5	<2.5
PVR (dyn s/cm^5)	240–500	500–800	>800
RAP (mm Hg)	0–5	5–8	>8

Abbreviations: CI, cardiac index; NYHA FC, New York Heart Association functional class; RAP, right atrial pressure.

From Hoeper MM, Krowka MJ, Strassburg CP. Portopulmonary hypertension and hepatopulmonary syndrome. Lancet 2004;363(9419):1463; with permission.

Table 3
Patterns of hemodynamics in portal hypertension

	mPAP	PCWP	CO	PVR
Normal values	<25 mm Hg	<15 mm Hg	5–8 L/min	<240 dyn s/cm^5
Hyperdynamic	↑	Normal	↑	Normal/↓
Volume overload	↑	↑	↑	Normal/↓
PoPH	↑	Normal	↑↓	↑

Adapted from Krowka MJ. Hepatopulmonary syndrome versus portopulmonary hypertension: distinctions and dilemmas. Hepatology 1997;25(5):1283; with permission.

PoPH have more favorable hemodynamics at the time of PAH diagnosis.[28,29] In France, PoPH survival is equivalent to idiopathic PAH (1-year, 3-year, and 5-year survival of 88%, 75%, and 68%, respectively) (**Fig. 2**).[26] It is hypothesized that this situation may be attributable to a smaller lead time bias in France as a result of aggressive screening of the population at risk for PoPH or the absence of severity of illness data in the registry format of REVEAL (Registry to Evaluate Early and Long-Term Pulmonary Arterial Hypertension Disease Management). Independent predictors for death include cirrhotic (vs noncirrhotic) liver disease, Child B or C class, and lower cardiac index at the time of diagnostic catheterization.[26] As expected, the cause of death for patients with PoPH is evenly distributed between the underlying liver disease and heart failure caused by PAH.[32]

PATHOLOGY

The pulmonary arteriopathy in PoPH is indistinguishable from other forms of group I PAH. Typical findings include muscularization of the small pulmonary arterioles, neointimal formation, medial smooth muscle cell hypertrophy, fibrinoid necrosis, and in situ thrombosis.[33] Plexiform lesions, intraluminal proliferations of endothelial cells within dilated pulmonary arteries, have also been described in PoPH.[34–38]

PATHOPHYSIOLOGY AND PATHOGENESIS

PoPH, as with all group I PAH, results from the combination of a proliferative vasculopathy, imbalanced vasoactive signaling, and in situ thrombosis. The pathogenesis of these processes in PAH and portal hypertension is incompletely understood but is believed to be caused by dysregulated signaling in growth, inflammation, and vasoactive signaling cascades.[39] The paradigm for PoPH pathogenesis supports a role for aberrant vasoactive and angiogenic signaling coupled with increased shear/mechanical stress caused by the hyperdynamic circulatory state. In order to understand these influences, it is instructive to examine the relationship between the hepatic and pulmonary circulatory beds, and the unique alterations that characterize the hyperdynamic circulatory state found in portal hypertension.

Portal hypertension is unique among PAH-associated clinical entities in that it is often accompanied by dramatic systemic circulatory disruptions. Up to 50% of patients with portal hypertension experience a progressive vasodilatory syndrome, characterized by decreased systemic vascular resistance, increased CO, recruitment of portosystemic collateral vascular beds, and formation of neovascular structures such as telangectasias and angiomata (reviewed in Ref.[40]).[5,41,42] Hypertension within the portal circulation creates portosystemic shunts, which

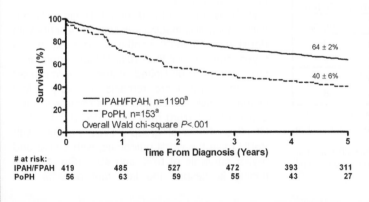

Fig. 1. Five-year survival from diagnosis for PoPH, idiopathic PAH (IPAH), and familial PAH (FPAH) in the REVEAL registry.[a] Only patients enrolled within 5 years of diagnosis were included in the 5-year survival from diagnosis curve. (*From* Krowka MJ, Miller DP, Barst RJ, et al. Portopulmonary hypertension: a report from the US-based REVEAL Registry. Chest 2012;141(4): 909; with permission.)

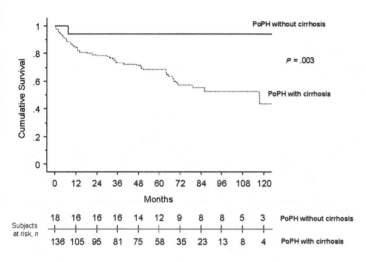

Fig. 2. Survival in cirrhotic and non-cirrhotic PoPH in France. Survival rates were 85%, 73%, and 68% at 1, 3, and 5 years, respectively, in patients with cirrhosis, and 94% at 1, 3, and 5 years in patients without cirrhosis (*P* = .003, log-rank test). (*Data from* Le Pavec J, Souza R, Herve P, et al. Portopulmonary hypertension: survival and prognostic factors. Am J Respir Crit Care Med 2008;178(6):640.)

enable venous blood to return to the right ventricle and pulmonary circulation without passing through the metabolically active liver sinusoids. The stigmata of liver disease, which include ascites, edema, palmar erythema, and esophageal varices, represent overt manifestations of these systemic vascular changes.

Normal hepatopulmonary blood flow is required for pulmonary vascular homeostasis. This requirement became apparent with the advent of corrective surgeries for children born with congenital heart disease characterized by single-ventricle physiology. The creation of a cavopulmonary shunt as part of staged palliation for these children was observed to result in de novo formation of pulmonary arteriovenous malformations (PAVMs).[43,44] After reestablishment of normal flow from the liver to the lungs, PAVMs have been observed to regress.[45] It is therefore hypothesized that, in the presence of portal hypertension, vasoactive or angiogenic substances produced in the splanchnic circulation escape hepatic metabolism, traveling directly to the pulmonary vasculature, where they exert influence on the pulmonary vascular phenotype.[16,19,46] A recent retrospective study[47] reported an association between large portosystemic shunts (define as >10 mm in diameter) and severe PoPH, the first clinical evidence in support of this theory. The role of splanchnic-derived mediators is further supported by the association of PoPH with noncirrhotic portal hypertension, indicating that hepatic synthetic function is not a critical determinant of the pulmonary vascular phenotype.

Dramatic alterations in circulating growth factors, neurohormone levels, and cytokine levels accompany portal hypertension, providing a plethora of candidate mediators for the development of PoPH. Increases in circulating angiogenic growth factors such as vascular endothelial growth factor (VEGF), platelet derived growth factor, and placental growth factor have been documented.[48–51] Similarly, the level of adrenomedullin, an endogenous peptide with vasodilator and angiogenic effects, has been correlated with increased portal and pulmonary pressures.[52–54] Endothelin (ET-1) and serotonin (5HT), neurohormones with effects on vascular tone and growth, have been extensively studied in PAH.[55–57] In portal hypertension, circulating ET-1 level increases, and 5HT biology is altered as platelet levels and function fluctuate.[56,58] Patients with PoPH have recently been found to have higher ET-1 levels than patients with portal hypertension, with or without a hyperdynamic circulation.[59] **Fig. 3** reviews some of the alterations in vasoactive and proliferative signals that occur in portal hypertension.

In addition to vasoactive mediators, there is substantial evidence supporting a pathogenetic role for inflammatory cytokines in PAH (reviewed in Ref.[60]). One particularly well-studied cytokine is interleukin 6 (IL-6). Increased serum and tissue levels of IL-6 have been associated with PAH in both human and animal models of disease,[61–64] and levels of IL-6 predict survival in idiopathic and familial PAH.[65] IL-6 is believed to mediate vascular smooth muscle cell proliferation in PAH.[66] Although portal hypertension alone is characterized by increases in inflammatory mediators such as tumor necrosis factor α, nitric oxide, and endotoxin,[67] Pellicelli and colleagues[59] have shown that increased IL-6 levels are exclusive to patients with liver disease with PoPH (not in those with cirrhosis with or without hyperdynamic circulation).[68] More recently, investigators have reported an accumulation of macrophages in the pulmonary microcirculation of experimental models of portal hypertension, suggesting a role for phagocyte-mediated signaling in the development of local

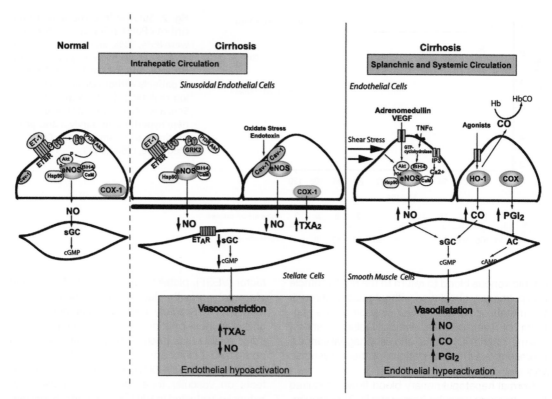

Fig. 3. Endothelial dysfunction in portal hypertension. Early in liver disease, liver sinusoidal endothelial cells adopt a vasoconstricted phenotype, which leads to the development of portal hypertension. In response to increased shear stress caused by high portal vascular resistance, the splanchnic vascular bed adopts a hyperactive and vasodilated phenotype, increasing production of vasoactive mediators including nitric oxide (NO), carbon monoxide (CO), ET-1, and prostacyclin (PGI$_2$). Additional mediators believed to play a role in the vascular dysregulation of portal hypertension are VEGF, adrenomedullin, and tumor necrosis factor α (TNF-α). These mediators are believed to act in a paracrine fashion in the pulmonary circulation, modulating endothelial and smooth muscle cell phenotype, thus contributing to the development of PoPH. AC, adenylate cyclase; BH$_4$, tetrahdrobiopterin; cAMP, cyclic adenosine monophosphate; Ca^{2+}, calcium; CaM, calmodulin; Cav-1, caveolin-1; cGMP, cyclic guanosine monophosphate; CO, carbon monoxide; COX, cyclooxygenase; eNOS, endothelial nitric oxide (NO) synthase; ET-1, endothelin-1; ET$_A$R, endothelin A receptor; ET$_B$R, endothelin B receptor; GRK2, G-protein-coupled receptor kinase-2; HO-1, heme oxygenase; Hsp90, heat shock protein 90; PGI$_2$, prostacyclin; ROS, reactive oxygen species; SEC, sinusoidal endothelial cell; sGC, soluble guanylate cyclase; TNFα, tumor necrosis factor α; TXA$_2$, thromboxane A2; VEGF, vascular endothelial growth factor. (*From* Iwakiri Y, Groszmann RJ. Vascular endothelial dysfunction in cirrhosis. J Hepatol 2007;46(5):929; with permission.)

vascular dysfunction.[69,70] The clinical association between PoPH and autoimmune liver disease further implicates inflammatory signaling in the development of PAH in this population.[27] These data in aggregate show our evolving appreciation of the role of inflammation in PoPH and PAH pathogenesis.

Sex hormone–mediated regulation of vascular growth may also be important, because increased circulating estradiol has been associated with the risk for PoPH among patients with advanced liver disease.[71]

Because clinical-epidemiologic and hemodynamic factors do not completely explain the risk for (or protection against) the development of PoPH in the portal hypertension population,

cryptic genetic risk factors may also be important in pathogenesis. The 2 most studied genetic risk factors for PAH, bone morphogenetic protein receptor 2 (BMPR2)[2] and the 5HT transporter,[57] have not been found to affect risk of PoPH.[72] Most recently, a candidate gene study reported that the risk of PoPH was associated with polymorphisms in several genes, including the estrogen receptor α, aromatase, and phosphodiesterase 5.[71]

The pulmonary vascular remodeling characteristic of PoPH likely results from the disruption of normal hepatopulmonary circulation, which results in altered vasoactive and angiogenic signaling. Along with increased flow and shear stress energy of the hyperdynamic circulation and as yet cryptic genetic risk factors, these signals drive the vascular remodeling that typifies PoPH.

CLINICAL PRESENTATION AND EVALUATION

Dyspnea at rest or with exercise is the most common presenting symptom of patients with PoPH. Additional symptoms include palpitations, fatigue, chest pain, and syncope. Physical examination findings that are suggestive of the presence of PoPH include an accentuated P2 component of the second heart sound and a RV heave.[73,74] These signs and symptoms, along with the presence of refractory ascites or increasing lower extremity edema, should prompt an evaluation for PoPH.[75]

General Considerations

Dyspnea is a common complaint in patients with advanced liver disease, reported by up to 70% of patients evaluated for LT.[76,77] In this patient population, dyspnea can be associated with a myriad of diagnoses, including volume overload states, anemia, cardiomyopathy, myocardial ischemia, chronic obstructive pulmonary disease, hepatic hydrothorax, and the 2 pulmonary vascular complications of liver disease, PoPH and HPS. In order to investigate the potential diagnoses, evaluation of the dyspneic patient with portal hypertension should include the following general cardiopulmonary assessments: chest imaging, electrocardiography, pulmonary function testing, and arterial blood gas testing. Additional testing should include a complete blood count, thyroid function tests, and a nocturnal polysomnogram when indicated, because anemia, thyroid dysfunction, and obstructive sleep apnea (respectively) may contribute to dyspnea.

In patients with PoPH, chest radiography may show cardiomegaly, enlargement of the right heart chambers, or increased pulmonary artery size.[78,79] Electrocardiography may show right atrial hypertrophy, right axis deviation, or right bundle branch block.[73,79] At the time of pulmonary function testing, patients with advanced liver disease often show a mild restrictive ventilatory defect (caused by displacement of the diaphragm by increased abdominal pressure and ascites) and a mild reduction of single-breath diffusing capacity for carbon monoxide (DLCO).[6,80] Similarly, mild hypoxemia and hypocarbia are commonly found on room air arterial blood gas analysis in patients with liver disease.[27,79,81] Therefore, moderate to severe DLCO reductions or moderate hypoxemia should raise concern for PoPH.[27,79,81,82] Severe hypoxemia is more characteristic of HPS.[83] Overall, these general assessments are insensitive for PoPH and

may not allow for discrimination between PoPH and HPS.

Evaluation Specific to PoPH

The diagnosis of PoPH can be made only by RHC. In order to appropriately select patients for this invasive and costly procedure, transthoracic echocardiography (TTE) is the most efficient screening tool. TTE noninvasively estimates the systolic pulmonary artery pressure (sPAP), using the peak tricuspid regurgitant (TR) jet velocity and an estimate of central venous pressure. In the absence of pulmonic stenosis or RV outflow tract obstruction, the RV systolic pressure (RVSP) is considered to be equivalent to the sPAP. Measurement of the velocity of regurgitant blood flow across the tricuspid valve (v) allows for an approximation of the RVSP using the modified Bernoulli equation (RVSP = right atrial pressure + $4v^2$). Right atrial pressure is typically estimated using echocardiographic appearance of the inferior vena cava, or using the jugular venous pressure from physical examination, and as a result, it is subject to significant variability. When using TTE for the assessment of possible pulmonary hypertension in patients with portal hypertension, it is important to consider the following. First, clinically significant PAH can occur in the absence of a measurable TR jet. Second, the hyperdynamic circulatory state characteristic of portal hypertension leads to overestimates of RVSP because of the high prevalence of increased filling pressures or high CO states. On the other hand, the echocardiogram is useful in assessing RV size and function as well as interventricular interaction, which are hallmark signs of pulmonary hypertension, even in the absence of an increased RVSP.[84]

The performance characteristics of screening TTE for PoPH include a high specificity (>82%) and negative predictive value (>92%), but variable sensitivity (54.5%–100%) and a low positive predictive value (18%–60%).[17,85,86] Compared with the standard cutoff of 40 mm Hg, using a threshold of sPAP 50 mm Hg or greater is associated with a higher sensitivity; however, even at this threshold, one-third of patients have a normal PVR at time of RHC.[87] A recent study of TTE in patients with portal hypertension attempted to refine TTE criteria for PoPH. The presence of RV dilatation (defined as RV end diastolic diameter >3.3 cm) raises suspicion for PoPH and should lead to RHC. It has been recently proposed that individuals with sPAP 38 mm Hg or greater should undergo RHC for definitive diagnosis.[88] This cutoff is 100% sensitive and 82% specific. When combined with the presence of RV dysfunction, the specificity is increased to 93%. Alternative echocardiographic indices of RV function such as the tricuspid annular plane systolic excursion, Tei index, or longitudinal shortening have not been studied in the portal hypertension population.[89–91]

TTE should be performed in all patients with suspected PoPH as well as anyone undergoing LT evaluation.[2,23,92–95] In addition to assessment of the right ventricle and pulmonary pressures, it allows visualization of the left-sided valves, atrium, and ventricle. The presence of left-sided heart disease makes PoPH unlikely. Contrast TTE should be strongly considered in this population, because it facilitates the identification of HPS, which is 3 times more prevalent than PoPH.[4,13,96] The clinical and diagnostic distinctions between PoPH and HPS are outlined in **Table 4**.

Current guidelines recommend that finding of any of the following in a patient with portal hypertension should prompt RHC: RVSP 50 mm Hg or higher or the presence of: right atrial enlargement, RV enlargement, or reduced RV systolic function.[11,22] Emerging data suggest that a more aggressive approach may be indicated in order to start treatment with PAH-specific therapy earlier as well as to improve pretransplant risk-benefit assessment. As a result, some transplant centers consider RHC in patients with RVSP greater than 40 mm Hg or RV dilatation. Once a diagnosis of pulmonary hypertension is contemplated, a ventilation-perfusion scan should be performed to rule out the presence of chronic thromboembolic disease, because the treatment of this condition is different from that of PoPH.

RHC remains the gold standard for the diagnosis of PoPH. Careful measurement of right atrial pressure, PAP, PCWP, and CO is critical for a thoughtful appraisal of the hemodynamics seen in advanced liver disease and portal hypertension (see **Table 3**). Acute vasodilator challenge with inhaled nitric oxide or intravenous epoprostenol is also recommended at the time of diagnostic catheterization, even though fewer than 2% of patients with PoPH have an acute vasodilator response.[97,98] The presence of an acute vasodilator response is helpful in staging severity and therapeutic expectations of the disease, and may indicate a better hemodynamic tolerance at the time of LT. Unlike idiopathic PAH, vasodilator response in PoPH should not be used to assess for the ability to respond to calcium channel blockers, because their use is contraindicated in portal hypertension.[22,74,99]

Dyspnea as well as refractory ascites or lower extremity edema should prompt an assessment for the presence of PoPH. History and physical findings can be nonspecific, and therefore accurate diagnosis requires a high clinical suspicion and careful interpretation of diagnostic testing. TTE is the screening test of choice. Because of the inability of TTE to distinguish between alternative causes of pulmonary hypertension in patients with portal hypertension (specifically volume overload or hyperdynamic circulation), RHC is recommended for patients with sPAP greater than 50 mm Hg or evidence of RV/atrial volume or pressure overload. Other causes of pulmonary hypertension should be excluded using history, laboratory, and imaging data as per consensus guidelines. **Fig. 4** outlines the diagnostic approach to patients with suspected PoPH.

Table 4
A comparison of PoPH and HPS

	PoPH	HPS
Symptoms	Dyspnea Chest pain Syncope	Dyspnea Platypnea
Signs	Loud P2 RV heave Lower extremity edema	Cyanosis
Arterial blood gas	Normal to mild hypoxemia	Moderate to severe hypoxemia A-a gradient >20
Contrast TTE	Negative or + intracardiac shunt (positive within <3 cardiac cycles)	Positive for intrapulmonary shunting (3–6 cardiac cycles)
Hemodynamics	PVR >240 dyn s/cm^5	Normal or low PVR
Role of LT	Relatively contraindicated; consider in selected patients if mPAP <35 mm Hg	Indicated; exception points granted if room air Pao$_2$ <60 mm Hg

Abbreviations: A-a gradient, alveolar-arterial oxygen gradient; Pao$_2$, partial pressure of oxygen in arterial blood.

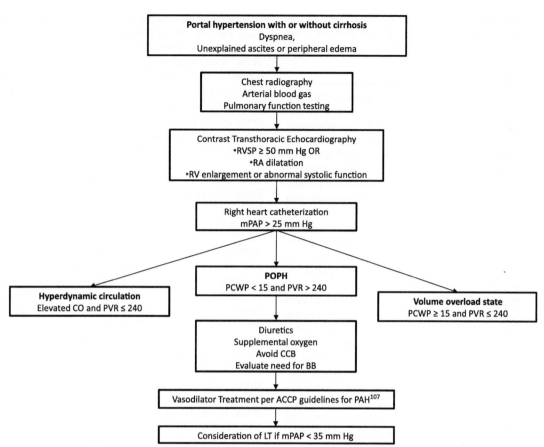

Fig. 4. Diagnostic algorithm for suspected PoPH. ACCP, American College of Chest Physicians; BB, β-blockers; CCB, calcium channel blockers; CO, cardiac output; LT, liver transplantation; mPAP, mean pulmonary artery pressure; PAH, pulmonary arterial hypertension; PCWP, pulmonary capillary wedge pressure; PVR, pulmonary vascular resistance; RA, right atrium; RV, right ventricle; RVSP, right ventricular systolic pressure.

TREATMENT

Treatment approaches for PoPH fall into 2 broad categories: conventional and PAH-specific therapy. When considering therapy for PoPH, the clinician must always be cognizant of the interrelated portal and pulmonary vascular systems, and must balance the potential risks and benefits that interventions may have for each.

Conventional Therapy

Conventional therapy for PoPH follows the standard guidelines for PAH, with some important exceptions. The treatment of fluid overload with diuretic therapy is a mainstay of therapy, although often a particularly vexing management issue in portal hypertension. Supplementary oxygen is also recommended to patients who are hypoxemic on room air. Achieving a target oxygen saturation greater than 90% protects against any contribution of hypoxic pulmonary vasoconstriction.[100] There are 4 unique considerations in the care of patients with portal hypertension and PAH. First, calcium channel blockers should be avoided in PoPH, regardless of the response to vasodilator challenge, because they can promote mesenteric vasodilatation, leading to an increase in hepatic venous pressure gradient, thereby exacerbating portal hypertension.[101] Second, anticoagulation is not advised in patients with PoPH, because they may harbor additional risk of hemorrhagic complications caused by acquired coagulopathy or thrombocytopenia.[2] Third, use of β-blockers as primary prophylaxis against variceal hemorrhage is not recommended because of the adverse cardiopulmonary impact of chronotropic suppression in patients with RV failure and a fixed stroke volume.[102] The use of β-blockers as secondary prevention may be warranted at the discretion of individual patient providers. Transjugular intrahepatic portosystemic shunt should be avoided in patients with PoPH, because placement of the shunt can acutely increase cardiac preload, with the potential to precipitate RV failure.[103]

PAH-Specific Therapies

The use of vasodilator therapy in portal hypertension presents a theoretic risk, because nonspecific vasodilation could exacerbate the hyperdynamic circulatory state via direct action on the splanchnic circulation.[104] In addition, patients with PoPH have been historically excluded from clinical trials of vasodilators for PAH because of perceived excess mortality risk from underlying portal hypertension as well as concerns about hepatotoxicity.[105,106] As a result, current practices and recommendations for the medical management of PoPH represent the combination of expert opinion and extrapolation from clinical trials, which predominately comprise PAH associated with idiopathic, connective tissue disease, and congenital heart disease. The approach to use of PAH-specific therapies in PoPH varies by clinical center, with some treating as per current evidence-based guidelines for PAH,[107] and others treating only if mPAP is greater than 35 mm Hg (the threshold cutoff for LT). This section reviews PAH treatment considerations that are unique to the portal hypertensive population. **Table 5** provides an overview of published experience with vasodilators in PoPH.

Prostacyclin analogues

Prostacyclin analogues, both inhaled and infused, are the best-studied PAH-specific therapy in PoPH, with published data on 50 patients. In one of the few prospective studies of vasodilator therapy in PoPH, Krowka and colleagues[108] found that intravenous epoprostenol (Flolan) resulted in a significant improvement in pulmonary hemodynamics after both acute and long-term administration. Iloprost (Ventavis) has also been associated with sustained improvement in symptoms and New York Heart Association (NYHA) functional class (FC) in some patients with PoPH.[109,110] Treprostinil (Remodulin) has not been studied in PoPH, although there is an ongoing observational, open-label, multicenter trial studying the safety and efficacy profile of treprostinil in patients with PoPH (ClinicalTrials.gov identifier: NCT01028651).

Although they are generally well tolerated, there is a concern that prostacyclins may exacerbate the hyperdynamic circulation seen in portal hypertension.[111] Circulating levels of endogenous prostacyclin are increased in patients with liver cirrhosis, and the administration of exogenous prostacyclin carries the potential for an overdosed state.[112,113] Although the published experience with prostacyclins shows appropriate (not pathologic) improvement in CO, there have been case reports of progressive splenomegaly in 4 patients with severe PoPH treated with continuous epoprostenol infusion.[111] In 3 of these patients, the splenomegaly progressed in the absence of liver disease progression, and was suggested to result from increased portal flow while on epoprostenol. Clinicians should consider this potentially serious complication of epoprostenol treatment of PoPH.

Endothelin receptor antagonists

Bosentan (Tracleer) and ambrisentan (Letaris) can be well tolerated and efficacious in PoPH. In a retrospective review of 11 patients with NYHA FC III to IV PoPH, Hoeper and colleagues[114] reported significant improvements in 6-minute walk distance (6MWD), peak oxygen uptake on cardiopulmonary testing, and PVR. There was no evidence of drug-induced hepatotoxicity in these patients, although the investigators noted that the patients had mild (Child class A) liver disease. In a retrospective study of 34 patients with PoPH, Savale and colleagues[115] reported a significant hemodynamic response (increase in cardiac index, decrease in PVR) to bosentan therapy with more advanced liver disease (Child-Pugh class B vs A). These investigators went on to show that serum levels of bosentan and its metabolites were higher in patients with Child-Pugh B compared with idiopathic PAH controls, raising the possibility that patients with more impaired liver function may gain clinical benefit from exposure to higher levels of drug. In 2 observational studies of moderate to severe PoPH, ambrisentan was associated with significant improvements in 6MWD, NYHA FC, and hemodynamics, without changes in liver function testing.[116,117] There is an ongoing open-label trial of ambrisentan in PoPH (ClinicalTrials.gov identifier: NCT01224210).

Endothelin receptor antagonists (ERAs) have been safely and effectively used in a few patients with PoPH. Although there is no evidence to suggest that the occurrence of hepatotoxicity with this class of medication is greater in PoPH than PAH, the risk is real,[118] and therefore the risk/benefit ratio of treatment with an ERA in a patient with PoPH should be evaluated on an individual patient basis. Monthly monitoring of liver function testing for patients on bosentan is mandated and strongly encouraged for those on ambrisentan.

Phosphodiesterase-5 inhibitors

Of the 2 phosphodiesterase-5 inhibitors (PDI) approved by the US Food and Drug Administration, only sildenafil (Revatio) has been studied

Table 5
Selected experience with PAH-specific therapies in PoPH

Study	Study Size	Inclusion	Treatment	Duration (mo)	6MWD (m) Baseline	Follow-up	PVR (Wood Units) Baseline	Follow-up	Adverse Events
Krowka et al,[108] 1999	11	Child-Pugh A–C	Epoprostenol	8 d–30 m	NA	—	5.1	2.0^a (n = 8)	Splenomegaly (n = 1)
Hoeper et al,[112] 2005	11	Child-Pugh A NYHA FC 3–4	Bosentan	12	310	388^a	12	7.9^a	Significant decrease in Pao2 without clinical change
Reichenberger et al,[129] 2006	20	Child-Pugh B, C NYHA FC 3–4	Sildenafil ± ERA or inh	12	312	407^a	13	7.3^a	None
Hoeper et al,[108] 2007	13	Child-Pugh A, B NYHA FC 2–3	Iloprost	6–18	367	406 (n = 10)	10	11 (n = 11)	None
Hoeper et al,[108] 2007	18	Child-Pugh A NYHA FC 3–4	Bosentan	6–18	377	448^a (n = 17)	12	7.2^a (n = 13)	LFT >3 × ULN (n = 1), dose reduced
Fix et al,[130] 2007	19	Child-Pugh A–C	Epoprostenol ± sildenafil (n = 7)	15	NA	—	7.9	3.5^a	Thrombocytopenia (n = 2), drug discontinued
Gough & White,[117] 2009	9	Child-Pugh B, C NYHA FC 1–3	Sildenafil	3–23	NA	—	7.2	4^a	None
Hemnes & Robbins,[118] 2009	10	MELD 14 NYHA FC 3	Sildenafil	12	369	408	NA	NA	None
Melgosa et al,[107] 2010	12	MELD 15 NYHA FC 2–3	Iloprost	12	396	463^a	10	NA	None
Cartin-Ceba et al,[115] 2011	13	Child-Pugh A (62%) NYHA FC 2–3	Ambrisentan	3–18	NA	—	5.6	2.2^a	Bleeding (n = 1), drug discontinued
Halank et al,[114] 2011	14	NA	Ambrisentan	12	376	413^a	NA	—	None
Hollatz et al,[151] 2012	11	NYHA FC 1–3	Sildenafil + treprostinil	NA	289	351	5.4	2.2^a	None
Savale et al,[113] 2012	34	Child-Pugh A, B NYHA FC 2–4	Bosentan ± sildenafil	4–12	352	403^a	8.7	5.7^a	LFT >3 × ULN (n = 7), drug discontinued

Abbreviations: 6MWD, 6-minute walk distance; ERA, endothelin receptor antagonist; inh, inhaled prostacyclin; LFT, liver function test; MELD, Model for End-Stage Liver Disease; NA, data not available; NYHA FC, New York Heart Association Functional Class; ULN, upper limit of normal.
^a Change from baseline to follow-up was significant.

in PoPH. In 2 retrospective studies of patients,[119,120] investigators at the University of Rochester and Vanderbilt University successfully used sildenafil as a bridge to LT. There was no increased risk of adverse effects compared with patients with other forms of PAH treated with PDI. The impact of PDI therapy on portal hemodynamics is variable, with both improvement[121,122] and worsening[123] of portal pressures reported. Overall PDI are a viable therapeutic option for patients with PoPH.

Combination therapy

The benefit of combination therapy in PAH is unclear, although it is common practice to add additional vasodilator agents when patients are clinically progressing.[124–129] Published series in PoPH include all potential combinations of the 3 vasodilator classes, with no evidence that outcomes are different when compared with other clinical subtypes of PAH.[130–132] Nevertheless this experience is limited (<30 patients), and therefore, validation by larger clinical trials is needed.

Novel Therapeutic Approaches

In recent years, there has been a shift in emphasis in PAH-specific therapy from vasodilator to antiproliferative agents. Imatinib, a tyrosine kinase inhibitor, and rapamycin, a mammalian target of rapamycin inhibitor with immunosuppressant and antiangiogenic activity, have recently emerged as potential therapeutic agents for PAH.[133–136] Two case reports have documented successful use of each on a compassionate care basis in patients with decompensated PoPH.[137,138] Nevertheless, the true potential of these agents for PAH (and PoPH) therapy remains to be seen, and clinical trials are ongoing.

Summary

PAH-specific vasodilators have been used safely and effectively in patients with PoPH. Exclusion of patients with PoPH from trials of vasodilators means that evidence is limited. Furthermore, this precedent may have led to the systematic undertreatment of PoPH, with a possible detrimental impact on survival.[28] In light of these data, we support the use of PAH-specific vasodilator therapy in PoPH, but with the stipulation that it be undertaken with caution, preferably at referral centers with experience in this population, or as part of a clinical trial.

LIVER TRANSPLANTATION

The role of LT in the management of patients with PoPH remains uncertain, because of the perioperative risk of LT in patients with impaired RV function, uncertainty surrounding the natural history of PoPH, and the emerging benefit of PAH-specific therapies in this population. LT is the only known treatment of the other pulmonary vascular complication of liver disease, HPS, with most patients normalizing their gas exchange within 6 to 12 months after transplant (reviewed in Ref.[4]). These observations led to the hypothesis that correction of portal hypertension through transplantation might lead to regression of the PAH that afflicted those with PoPH. Early transplant outcomes were disastrous, with perioperative mortality as high as 36%, increasing to 100% in those with severe PoPH (mPAP >50 mm Hg).[139–141] A period of reflection on the risk/benefit of LT for PoPH followed.

Patients with PAH represent one of the highest risk groups for major surgery, general anesthesia, and positive pressure ventilation, because of a limited capacity for the right ventricle in these patients to handle insults to its contractility, or changes in preload or afterload.[142] LT creates a challenging hemodynamic environment for any patient. This situation is especially relevant at the time of reperfusion of the new liver, a transition point that is characterized by an abrupt increase in preload and a decrease in systemic vascular resistance accompanied by significant shifts in hydrogen ion and potassium levels (reviewed in Ref.[143]). In the setting of the fixed pulmonary vascular remodeling and chronic RV dysfunction characteristic of PoPH, LT can prove fatal, because of dramatic swings in preload and CO as well as marked increases in pulmonary arterial pressures. The resultant RV failure, which can develop at the time of reperfusion or up to a week after transplant, is a well-described phenomenon in patients with PoPH and it is often refractory to intervention.[144–147]

Contemporary liver transplant outcomes in PoPH (with the advent of earlier diagnosis, better risk assessment and the use of PAH-specific therapies) are more encouraging. Carefully selected patients with mild PoPH (mPAP <35 mm Hg) can be safely managed through the acute period of LT, enjoying excellent long-term outcomes, with 1-year and 5-year posttransplant survival rates as high as 91% and 67%.[137] Successful transplantation seems to depend on the ability of the right ventricle to handle the hemodynamic and metabolic demands at the time of transplantation. Recently, Bandara and colleagues[148] reported that RV function and pulmonary arterial capacitance (expressed as CO reserve and stroke volume/pulmonary artery pulse pressure, respectively) predict outcome in PoPH.

The emergence of a postliver transplant PoPH population has shifted the focus to defining the impact of LT on the natural history of PoPH. Unlike HPS, in which most patients are considered cured after transplant, PAH in patients with portal hypertension behaves unpredictably. Several case series show that some individuals with PoPH improve or regress their pulmonary vascular disease after transplant, with variable need for continuation of PAH-specific therapies.[32,149–152] There are also reports of de novo PAH in posttransplant patients.[153–158] One potential explanation for these new cases of PAH is that the hyperdynamic circulation of advanced liver disease (also referred to as a progressive vasodilatory state) may mask or offset precapillary pulmonary hypertension.[157,159] These disparate outcomes indicate that the relationship between portal hypertension and PAH is complex, and they suggest that there is significant phenotypic variability among those with PoPH.

Because the bulk of these data support a benefit for transplantation, patients with successfully treated PoPH are considered eligible for LT. The standard of care for transplant candidates with moderate to severe PoPH is medical therapy with PAH-specific medication. Because of the prohibitive risk of surgery in patients with decompensated RV failure, consideration for LT eligibility is reserved for those patients in whom sustained improvements in hemodynamics, defined as mPAP less than 35 mm Hg and a PVR less than 5 Wood units, can be achieved.[140,160,161] In the United States, some regional transplant boards have gone further, granting a MELD (Model for End-Stage Liver Disease) exception to patients with stable mild PoPH (mPAP <35 mm Hg). This policy is outlined in the Organ Procurement and Transplantation Network policy 3.6.4.5.6, which states that "candidates will be eligible for MELD exception with a 10% mortality equivalent increase every three months if the mean pulmonary artery pressure stays below 35 mm Hg and PVR <400 dyn s/cm^5 (confirmed by right heart catheterization)."[162]

A potential alternative to those eligible (and possibly those ineligible) for orthotopic LT is living-related LT (LRLT), which has the advantages of being electively scheduled as well as allowing for coordination with hemodynamic optimization. Several case reports of patients with moderate to severe PoPH who underwent LRLT had favorable outcomes with preoperative vasodilator therapy and optimization of fluid status, with long-term improvement in mPAP.[163–165]

For those patients on vasodilator therapy with sustained mPAP greater than 50 mm Hg, LT continues to be contraindicated because of high perioperative mortality and considerations regarding the allocation of a scarce organ resource.[140,166] For this population, there may be some hope in combined lung and LT (CLLT) or heart, lung, and LT (CHLLT).[167–171] The 4 reported CHLLT cases had favorable outcomes; however, 2 of the patients who received CLLT died within 24 hours of the combined transplant because of acute heart failure. These data, although scant, indicate that although these procedures may be considered life saving to a highly selected group of patients, they should be attempted only by highly experienced multiorgan transplant centers.

The role of LT for PoPH remains uncertain, although it is considered a potentially beneficial intervention in a highly selected group of patients. Although use of mPAP threshold may exclude some patients with pulmonary hypertension caused by either a hyperdynamic circulatory state or volume overload, there is insufficient evidence to support a more liberal policy. Optimal selection of patients with PoPH for LT remains to be defined.

SUMMARY

PoPH is a serious complication of portal hypertension, which contributes significantly to poor functional status and early mortality in this population. Although the pathogenetic mechanisms linking these 2 clinical entities remain enigmatic, there is clear evidence that the pulmonary vasculature responds dramatically to alterations in blood flow and paracrine factors produced as a consequence of the hyperdynamic circulatory state characteristic of portal hypertension.

When evaluating patients with advanced liver disease, with or without cirrhosis, clinicians must be vigilant for signs and symptoms of PoPH. Distinguishing between PoPH and the other pulmonary vascular complication of liver disease, HPS, is also critical, because they require vastly different management approaches. TTE is the screening test of choice, and verification of noninvasive testing with RHC is required.

Although systematically understudied, judicious use of pulmonary vasodilator therapy has been associated with improved clinical outcomes. LT represents a real risk to patients with PoPH, and thus careful planning and coordination between pulmonary hypertension providers and hepatologists is required.

REFERENCES

1. Simonneau G, Robbins IM, Beghetti M, et al. Updated clinical classification of pulmonary hypertension. J Am Coll Cardiol 2009;54(Suppl 1):S43–54.

2. Rodriguez-Roisin R, Krowka MJ, Herve P, et al. Pulmonary-hepatic vascular disorders (PHD). Eur Respir J 2004;24(5):861–80.

3. Berzigotti A, Seijo S, Reverter E, et al. Assessing portal hypertension in liver diseases. Expert Rev Gastroenterol Hepatol 2013;7(2):141–55.

4. Fritz JS, Fallon MB, Kawut SM. Pulmonary vascular complications of liver disease. Am J Respir Crit Care Med 2013;187(2):133–43.

5. Castro M, Krowka MJ, Schroeder DR, et al. Frequency and clinical implications of increased pulmonary artery pressures in liver transplant patients. Mayo Clin Proc 1996;71(6):543–51.

6. Huffmyer JL, Nemergut EC. Respiratory dysfunction and pulmonary disease in cirrhosis and other hepatic disorders. Respir Care 2007;52(8): 1030–6.

7. Kuo PC, Schroeder RA, Vagelos RH, et al. Volume-mediated pulmonary responses in liver transplant candidates. Clin Transplant 1996;10(6 Pt 1):521–7.

8. Troy PJ, Waxman AB. Portopulmonary hypertension: challenges in diagnosis and management. Therap Adv Gastroenterol 2009;2(5):281–6.

9. McGoon M, Gutterman D, Steen V, et al. Screening, early detection, and diagnosis of pulmonary arterial hypertension: ACCP evidence-based clinical practice guidelines. Chest 2004;126(Suppl 1): 14S–34S.

10. Barst RJ, McGoon M, Torbicki A, et al. Diagnosis and differential assessment of pulmonary arterial hypertension. J Am Coll Cardiol 2004;43(12 Suppl S): 40S–7S.

11. Krowka MJ, Swanson KL, Frantz RP, et al. Portopulmonary hypertension: results from a 10-year screening algorithm. Hepatology 2006;44(6):1502–10.

12. Hoeper MM, Krowka MJ, Strassburg CP. Portopulmonary hypertension and hepatopulmonary syndrome. Lancet 2004;363(9419):1461–8.

13. Krowka MJ. Hepatopulmonary syndrome versus portopulmonary hypertension: distinctions and dilemmas. Hepatology 1997;25(5):1282–4.

14. Mantz FA Jr, Craige E. Portal axis thrombosis with spontaneous portacaval shunt and resultant cor pulmonale. AMA Arch Pathol 1951;52(1):91–7.

15. McDonnell PJ, Toye PA, Hutchins GM. Primary pulmonary hypertension and cirrhosis: are they related? Am Rev Respir Dis 1983;127(4): 437–41.

16. Hadengue A, Benhayoun MK, Lebrec D, et al. Pulmonary hypertension complicating portal hypertension: prevalence and relation to splanchnic hemodynamics. Gastroenterology 1991;100(2): 520–8.

17. Colle IO, Moreau R, Godinho E, et al. Diagnosis of portopulmonary hypertension in candidates for liver transplantation: a prospective study. Hepatology 2003;37(2):401–9.

18. Lebrec D, Capron JP, Dhumeaux D, et al. Pulmonary hypertension complicating portal hypertension. Am Rev Respir Dis 1979;120(4):849–56.

19. Ridaura-Sanz C, Mejia-Hernandez C, Lopez-Corella E. Portopulmonary hypertension in children. A study in pediatric autopsies. Arch Med Res 2009; 40(7):635–9.

20. Humbert M, Sitbon O, Chaouat A, et al. Pulmonary arterial hypertension in France: results from a national registry. Am J Respir Crit Care Med 2006; 173(9):1023–30.

21. Badesch DB, Raskob GE, Elliott CG, et al. Pulmonary arterial hypertension: baseline characteristics from the REVEAL Registry. Chest 2010;137(2): 376–87.

22. Porres-Aguilar M, Zuckerman MJ, Figueroa-Casas JB, et al. Portopulmonary hypertension: state of the art. Ann Hepatol 2008;7(4):321–30.

23. Budhiraja R, Hassoun PM. Portopulmonary hypertension: a tale of two circulations. Chest 2003; 123(2):562–76.

24. Molden D, Abraham JL. Pulmonary hypertension. Its association with hepatic cirrhosis and iron accumulation. Arch Pathol Lab Med 1982;106(7): 328–31.

25. Tasaka S, Kanazawa M, Nakamura H, et al. An autopsied case of primary pulmonary hypertension complicated by hepatopulmonary syndrome. Nihon Kyobu Shikkan Gakkai Zasshi 1995;33(1): 90–4 [in Japanese].

26. Le Pavec J, Souza R, Herve P, et al. Portopulmonary hypertension: survival and prognostic factors. Am J Respir Crit Care Med 2008;178(6):637–43.

27. Kawut SM, Krowka MJ, Trotter JF, et al. Clinical risk factors for portopulmonary hypertension. Hepatology 2008;48(1):196–203.

28. Krowka MJ, Miller DP, Barst RJ, et al. Portopulmonary hypertension: a report from the US-based REVEAL Registry. Chest 2012;141(4):906–15.

29. Kawut SM, Taichman DB, Ahya VN, et al. Hemodynamics and survival of patients with portopulmonary hypertension. Liver Transpl 2005;11(9): 1107–11.

30. Robalino BD, Moodie DS. Association between primary pulmonary hypertension and portal hypertension: analysis of its pathophysiology and clinical, laboratory and hemodynamic manifestations. J Am Coll Cardiol 1991;17(2):492–8.

31. Benza RL, Miller DP, Gomberg-Maitland M, et al. Predicting survival in pulmonary arterial hypertension: insights from the Registry to Evaluate Early and Long-Term Pulmonary Arterial Hypertension Disease Management (REVEAL). Circulation 2010;122(2):164–72.

32. Safdar Z, Bartolome S, Sussman N. Portopulmonary hypertension: an update. Liver Transpl 2012; 18(8):881–91.

33. Edwards BS, Weir EK, Edwards WD, et al. Coexistent pulmonary and portal hypertension: morphologic and clinical features. J Am Coll Cardiol 1987;10(6):1233–8.

34. Naeye RL. "Primary" pulmonary hypertension with coexisting portal hypertension. A retrospective study of six cases. Circulation 1960;22:376–84.

35. Krowka MJ, Edwards WD. A spectrum of pulmonary vascular pathology in portopulmonary hypertension. Liver Transpl 2000;6(2):241–2.

36. Tuder RM, Cool CD, Geraci MW, et al. Prostacyclin synthase expression is decreased in lungs from patients with severe pulmonary hypertension. Am J Respir Crit Care Med 1999;159(6):1925–32.

37. Wagenvoort CA, Mulder PG. Thrombotic lesions in primary plexogenic arteriopathy. Similar pathogenesis or complication? Chest 1993;103(3):844–9.

38. Lee SD, Shroyer KR, Markham NE, et al. Monoclonal endothelial cell proliferation is present in primary but not secondary pulmonary hypertension. J Clin Invest 1998;101(5):927–34.

39. Morrell NW, Adnot S, Archer SL, et al. Cellular and molecular basis of pulmonary arterial hypertension. J Am Coll Cardiol 2009;54(Suppl 1):S20–31.

40. Iwakiri Y, Groszmann RJ. Vascular endothelial dysfunction in cirrhosis. J Hepatol 2007;46(5):927–34.

41. Groszmann RJ. Hyperdynamic state in chronic liver diseases. J Hepatol 1993;17(Suppl 2):S38–40.

42. Kowalski HJ, Abelmann WH. The cardiac output at rest in Laennec's cirrhosis. J Clin Invest 1953;32(10):1025–33.

43. Duncan BW, Desai S. Pulmonary arteriovenous malformations after cavopulmonary anastomosis. Ann Thorac Surg 2003;76(5):1759–66.

44. Freedom RM, Yoo SJ, Perrin D. The biological "scrabble" of pulmonary arteriovenous malformations: considerations in the setting of cavopulmonary surgery. Cardiol Young 2004;14(4):417–37.

45. Srivastava D, Preminger T, Lock JE, et al. Hepatic venous blood and the development of pulmonary arteriovenous malformations in congenital heart disease. Circulation 1995;92(5):1217–22.

46. Rossi SO, Gilbert-Barness E, Saari T, et al. Pulmonary hypertension with coexisting portal hypertension. Pediatr Pathol 1992;12(3):433–9.

47. Talwalkar JA, Swanson KL, Krowka MJ, et al. Prevalence of spontaneous portosystemic shunts in patients with portopulmonary hypertension and effect on treatment. Gastroenterology 2011;141(5):1673–9.

48. Geerts AM, De Vriese AS, Vanheule E, et al. Increased angiogenesis and permeability in the mesenteric microvasculature of rats with cirrhosis and portal hypertension: an in vivo study. Liver Int 2006;26(7):889–98.

49. Fernandez M, Mejias M, Angermayr B, et al. Inhibition of VEGF receptor-2 decreases the development of hyperdynamic splanchnic circulation and portal-systemic collateral vessels in portal hypertensive rats. J Hepatol 2005;43(1):98–103.

50. Fernandez M, Mejias M, Garcia-Pras E, et al. Reversal of portal hypertension and hyperdynamic splanchnic circulation by combined vascular endothelial growth factor and platelet-derived growth factor blockade in rats. Hepatology 2007;46(4):1208–17.

51. Van Steenkiste C, Geerts A, Vanheule E, et al. Role of placental growth factor in mesenteric neoangiogenesis in a mouse model of portal hypertension. Gastroenterology 2009;137(6):2112–24.e1–6.

52. Guevara M, Gines P, Jimenez W, et al. Increased adrenomedullin levels in cirrhosis: relationship with hemodynamic abnormalities and vasoconstrictor systems. Gastroenterology 1998;114(2):336–43.

53. Kakishita M, Nishikimi T, Okano Y, et al. Increased plasma levels of adrenomedullin in patients with pulmonary hypertension. Clin Sci (Lond) 1999;96(1):33–9.

54. Mok MY, Cheung BM, Lo Y, et al. Elevated plasma adrenomedullin and vascular manifestations in patients with systemic sclerosis. J Rheumatol 2007;34(11):2224–9.

55. Stewart DJ, Levy RD, Cernacek P, et al. Increased plasma endothelin-1 in pulmonary hypertension: marker or mediator of disease? Ann Intern Med 1991;114(6):464–9.

56. Beaudry P, Hadengue A, Callebert J, et al. Blood and plasma 5-hydroxytryptamine levels in patients with cirrhosis. Hepatology 1994;20(4 Pt 1):800–3.

57. Eddahibi S, Humbert M, Fadel E, et al. Serotonin transporter overexpression is responsible for pulmonary artery smooth muscle hyperplasia in primary pulmonary hypertension. J Clin Invest 2001;108(8):1141–50.

58. Martinet JP, Legault L, Cernacek P, et al. Changes in plasma endothelin-1 and Big endothelin-1 induced by transjugular intrahepatic portosystemic shunts in patients with cirrhosis and refractory ascites. J Hepatol 1996;25(5):700–6.

59. Pellicelli AM, Barbaro G, Puoti C, et al. Plasma cytokines and portopulmonary hypertension in patients with cirrhosis waiting for orthotopic liver transplantation. Angiology 2010;61(8):802–6.

60. El Chami H, Hassoun PM. Immune and inflammatory mechanisms in pulmonary arterial hypertension. Prog Cardiovasc Dis 2012;55(2):218–28.

61. Kherbeck N, Tamby MC, Bussone G, et al. The role of inflammation and autoimmunity in the pathophysiology of pulmonary arterial hypertension. Clin Rev Allergy Immunol 2013;44(1):31–8.

62. Savale L, Tu L, Rideau D, et al. Impact of interleukin-6 on hypoxia-induced pulmonary hypertension and lung inflammation in mice. Respir Res 2009;10:6.

63. Bhargava A, Kumar A, Yuan N, et al. Monocrotaline induces interleukin-6 mRNA expression in rat lungs. Heart Dis 1999;1(3):126–32.

64. Miyata M, Ito M, Sasajima T, et al. Effect of a serotonin receptor antagonist on interleukin-6-induced pulmonary hypertension in rats. Chest 2001; 119(2):554–61.

65. Soon E, Holmes AM, Treacy CM, et al. Elevated levels of inflammatory cytokines predict survival in idiopathic and familial pulmonary arterial hypertension. Circulation 2010;122(9):920–7.

66. Furuya Y, Satoh T, Kuwana M. Interleukin-6 as a potential therapeutic target for pulmonary arterial hypertension. Int J Rheumatol 2010;2010:720305.

67. Genesca J, Gonzalez A, Segura R, et al. Interleukin-6, nitric oxide, and the clinical and hemodynamic alterations of patients with liver cirrhosis. Am J Gastroenterol 1999;94(1):169–77.

68. Lee FY, Lu RH, Tsai YT, et al. Plasma interleukin-6 levels in patients with cirrhosis. Relationship to endotoxemia, tumor necrosis factor-alpha, and hyperdynamic circulation. Scand J Gastroenterol 1996;31(5):500–5.

69. Chang SW, Ohara N. Chronic biliary obstruction induces pulmonary intravascular phagocytosis and endotoxin sensitivity in rats. J Clin Invest 1994;94(5):2009–19.

70. Thenappan T, Goel A, Marsboom G, et al. A central role for CD68(+) macrophages in hepatopulmonary syndrome. Reversal by macrophage depletion. Am J Respir Crit Care Med 2011;183(8): 1080–91.

71. Roberts KE, Fallon MB, Krowka MJ, et al. Genetic risk factors for portopulmonary hypertension in patients with advanced liver disease. Am J Respir Crit Care Med 2009;179(9):835–42.

72. Roberts KE, Fallon MB, Krowka MJ, et al. Serotonin transporter polymorphisms in patients with portopulmonary hypertension. Chest 2009;135(6):1470–5.

73. Gaine S. Pulmonary hypertension. JAMA 2000; 284(24):3160–8.

74. Krowka MJ. Pulmonary hypertension: diagnostics and therapeutics. Mayo Clin Proc 2000;75(6): 625–30.

75. Benjaminov FS, Prentice M, Sniderman KW, et al. Portopulmonary hypertension in decompensated cirrhosis with refractory ascites. Gut 2003;52(9): 1355–62.

76. Sood G, Fallon MB, Niwas S. Utility of dyspnea-fatigue index for screening liver transplant candidates for hepatopulmonary syndrome. Hepatology 1998;28(Suppl):742A.

77. Fallon MB, Abrams GA. Pulmonary dysfunction in chronic liver disease. Hepatology 2000;32(4 Pt 1): 859–65.

78. Chan T, Palevsky HI, Miller WT. Pulmonary hypertension complicating portal hypertension: findings on chest radiographs. AJR Am J Roentgenol 1988;151(5):909–14.

79. Kuo PC, Plotkin JS, Johnson LB, et al. Distinctive clinical features of portopulmonary hypertension. Chest 1997;112(4):980–6.

80. Hourani JM, Bellamy PE, Tashkin DP, et al. Pulmonary dysfunction in advanced liver disease: frequent occurrence of an abnormal diffusing capacity. Am J Med 1991;90(6):693–700.

81. Swanson KL, Krowka MJ. Arterial oxygenation associated with portopulmonary hypertension. Chest 2002;121(6):1869–75.

82. Degano B, Mittaine M, Guenard H, et al. Nitric oxide and carbon monoxide lung transfer in patients with advanced liver cirrhosis. J Appl Physiol 2009;107(1):139–43.

83. Rodriguez-Roisin R, Krowka MJ. Hepatopulmonary syndrome–a liver-induced lung vascular disorder. N Engl J Med 2008;358(22):2378–87.

84. Forfia PR, Vachiery JL. Echocardiography in pulmonary arterial hypertension. Am J Cardiol 2012; 110(Suppl 6):16S–24S.

85. Hua R, Sun YW, Wu ZY, et al. Role of 2-dimensional Doppler echo-cardiography in screening portopulmonary hypertension in portal hypertension patients. Hepatobiliary Pancreat Dis Int 2009;8(2):157–61.

86. Cotton CL, Gandhi S, Vaitkus PT, et al. Role of echocardiography in detecting portopulmonary hypertension in liver transplant candidates. Liver Transpl 2002;8(11):1051–4.

87. Kim WR, Krowka MJ, Plevak DJ, et al. Accuracy of Doppler echocardiography in the assessment of pulmonary hypertension in liver transplant candidates. Liver Transpl 2000;6(4):453–8.

88. Raevens S, Colle I, Reyntjens K, et al. Echocardiography for the detection of portopulmonary hypertension in liver transplant candidates: an analysis of cutoff values. Liver Transpl 2013;19(6):602–10.

89. Forfia PR, Fisher MR, Mathai SC, et al. Tricuspid annular displacement predicts survival in pulmonary hypertension. Am J Respir Crit Care Med 2006;174(9):1034–41.

90. Brown SB, Raina A, Katz D, et al. Longitudinal shortening accounts for the majority of right ventricular contraction and improves after pulmonary vasodilator therapy in normal subjects and patients with pulmonary arterial hypertension. Chest 2011; 140(1):27–33.

91. Tei C, Dujardin KS, Hodge DO, et al. Doppler echocardiographic index for assessment of global right ventricular function. J Am Soc Echocardiogr 1996; 9(6):838–47.

92. Galie N, Hoeper MM, Humbert M, et al. Guidelines for the diagnosis and treatment of pulmonary hypertension. Eur Respir J 2009;34(6):1219–63.

93. Krowka MJ. Hepatopulmonary syndromes. Gut 2000;46(1):1–4.

94. Murray KF, Carithers RL Jr. AASLD practice guide-lines: evaluation of the patient for liver transplantation. Hepatology 2005;41(6):1407–32.

95. Torregrosa M, Genesca J, Gonzalez A, et al. Role of Doppler echocardiography in the assessment of portopulmonary hypertension in liver transplantation candidates. Transplantation 2001;71(4): 572–4.

96. Shub C, Tajik AJ, Seward JB, et al. Detecting intrapulmonary right-to-left shunt with contrast echocardiography. Observations in a patient with diffuse pulmonary arteriovenous fistulas. Mayo Clin Proc 1976;51(2):81–4.

97. Montani D, Savale L, Natali D, et al. Long-term response to calcium-channel blockers in non-idiopathic pulmonary arterial hypertension. Eur Heart J 2010;31(15):1898–907.

98. Sitbon O, Humbert M, Jais X, et al. Long-term response to calcium channel blockers in idiopathic pulmonary arterial hypertension. Circulation 2005; 111(23):3105–11.

99. Ricci GL, Melgosa MT, Burgos F, et al. Assessment of acute pulmonary vascular reactivity in portopulmonary hypertension. Liver Transpl 2007;13(11): 1506–14.

100. Golbin JM, Krowka MJ. Portopulmonary hypertension. Clin Chest Med 2007;28(1):203–18, ix.

101. Ota K, Shijo H, Kokawa H, et al. Effects of nifedipine on hepatic venous pressure gradient and portal vein blood flow in patients with cirrhosis. J Gastroenterol Hepatol 1995;10(2):198–204.

102. Provencher S, Herve P, Jais X, et al. Deleterious effects of beta-blockers on exercise capacity and hemodynamics in patients with portopulmonary hypertension. Gastroenterology 2006;130(1):120–6.

103. Van der Linden P, Le Moine O, Ghysels M, et al. Pulmonary hypertension after transjugular intrahepatic portosystemic shunt: effects on right ventricular function. Hepatology 1996;23(5):982–7.

104. Krowka MJ, Swanson KL. How should we treat portopulmonary hypertension? Eur Respir J 2006; 28(3):466–7.

105. Badesch DB, Abman SH, Ahearn GS, et al. Medical therapy for pulmonary arterial hypertension: ACCP evidence-based clinical practice guidelines. Chest 2004;126(Suppl 1):35S–62S.

106. Rubin LJ, Badesch DB, Barst RJ, et al. Bosentan therapy for pulmonary arterial hypertension. N Engl J Med 2002;346(12):896–903.

107. Barst RJ, Gibbs JSR, Ghofrani HA, et al. Updated Evidence-Based Algorithm in Pulmonary Arterial Hypertension. J Am Coll Cardiol 2009;54:S78–84.

108. Krowka MJ, Frantz RP, McGoon MD, et al. Improvement in pulmonary hemodynamics during intravenous epoprostenol (prostacyclin): a study of 15 patients with moderate to severe portopulmonary hypertension. Hepatology 1999;30(3):641–8.

109. Melgosa MT, Ricci GL, Garcia-Pagan JC, et al. Acute and long-term effects of inhaled iloprost in portopulmonary hypertension. Liver Transpl 2010; 16(3):348–56.

110. Hoeper MM, Seyfarth HJ, Hoeffken G, et al. Experience with inhaled iloprost and bosentan in portopulmonary hypertension. Eur Respir J 2007;30(6): 1096–102.

111. Findlay JY, Plevak DJ, Krowka MJ, et al. Progressive splenomegaly after epoprostenol therapy in portopulmonary hypertension. Liver Transpl Surg 1999;5(5):362–5.

112. Garcia-Pagan JC, Bosch J, Rodes J. The role of vasoactive mediators in portal hypertension. Semin Gastrointest Dis 1995;6(3):140–7.

113. Sitzmann JV, Bulkley GB, Mitchell MC, et al. Role of prostacyclin in the splanchnic hyperemia contributing to portal hypertension. Ann Surg 1989; 209(3):322–7.

114. Hoeper MM, Halank M, Marx C, et al. Bosentan therapy for portopulmonary hypertension. Eur Respir J 2005;25(3):502–8.

115. Savale L, Magnier R, Le Pavec J, et al. Efficacy, safety, and pharmacokinetics of bosentan in portopulmonary hypertension. Eur Respir J 2013;41(1): 96–103.

116. Halank M, Knudsen L, Seyfarth HJ, et al. Ambrisentan improves exercise capacity and symptoms in patients with portopulmonary hypertension. Z Gastroenterol 2011;49(9):1258–62.

117. Cartin-Ceba R, Swanson K, Iyer V, et al. Safety and efficacy of ambrisentan for the treatment of portopulmonary hypertension. Chest 2011;139(1):109–14.

118. Eriksson C, Gustavsson A, Kronvall T, et al. Hepatotoxicity by bosentan in a patient with portopulmonary hypertension: a case-report and review of the literature. J Gastrointestin Liver Dis 2011;20(1):77–80.

119. Gough MS, White RJ. Sildenafil therapy is associated with improved hemodynamics in liver transplantation candidates with pulmonary arterial hypertension. Liver Transpl 2009;15(1):30–6.

120. Hemnes AR, Robbins IM. Sildenafil monotherapy in portopulmonary hypertension can facilitate liver transplantation. Liver Transpl 2009;15(1):15–9.

121. Bremer HC, Kreisel W, Roecker K, et al. Phosphodiesterase 5 inhibitors lower both portal and pulmonary pressure in portopulmonary hypertension: a case report. J Med Case Rep 2007;1:46.

122. Deibert P, Bremer H, Roessle M, et al. PDE-5 inhibitors lower portal and pulmonary pressure in portopulmonary hypertension. Eur Respir J 2007;29(1): 220–1.

123. Wang YW, Lin HC, Yang YY, et al. Sildenafil decreased pulmonary arterial pressure but may have exacerbated portal hypertension in a patient with cirrhosis and portopulmonary hypertension. J Gastroenterol 2006;41(6):593–7.

124. Ghofrani HA, Rose F, Schermuly RT, et al. Oral sildenafil as long-term adjunct therapy to inhaled iloprost in severe pulmonary arterial hypertension. J Am Coll Cardiol 2003;42(1):158–64.

125. Ghofrani HA, Wiedemann R, Rose F, et al. Combination therapy with oral sildenafil and inhaled iloprost for severe pulmonary hypertension. Ann Intern Med 2002;136(7):515–22.

126. Hoeper MM, Faulenbach C, Golpon H, et al. Combination therapy with bosentan and sildenafil in idiopathic pulmonary arterial hypertension. Eur Respir J 2004;24(6):1007–10.

127. Humbert M, Barst RJ, Robbins IM, et al. Combination of bosentan with epoprostenol in pulmonary arterial hypertension: BREATHE-2. Eur Respir J 2004;24(3):353–9.

128. McLaughlin VV, Oudiz RJ, Frost A, et al. Randomized study of adding inhaled iloprost to existing bosentan in pulmonary arterial hypertension. Am J Respir Crit Care Med 2006;174(11):1257–63.

129. Wilkens H, Guth A, Konig J, et al. Effect of inhaled iloprost plus oral sildenafil in patients with primary pulmonary hypertension. Circulation 2001; 104(11):1218–22.

130. Austin MJ, McDougall NI, Wendon JA, et al. Safety and efficacy of combined use of sildenafil, bosentan, and iloprost before and after liver transplantation in severe portopulmonary hypertension. Liver Transpl 2008;14(3):287–91.

131. Reichenberger F, Voswinckel R, Steveling E, et al. Sildenafil treatment for portopulmonary hypertension. Eur Respir J 2006;28(3):563–7.

132. Fix OK, Bass NM, De Marco T, et al. Long-term follow-up of portopulmonary hypertension: effect of treatment with epoprostenol. Liver Transpl 2007;13(6):875–85.

133. Ghofrani HA, Seeger W, Grimminger F. Imatinib for the treatment of pulmonary arterial hypertension. N Engl J Med 2005;353(13):1412–3.

134. Zhou H, Liu H, Porvasnik SL, et al. Heme oxygenase-1 mediates the protective effects of rapamycin in monocrotaline-induced pulmonary hypertension. Lab Invest 2006;86(1):62–71.

135. Gerasimovskaya EV, Tucker DA, Stenmark KR. Activation of phosphatidylinositol 3-kinase, Akt, and mammalian target of rapamycin is necessary for hypoxia-induced pulmonary artery adventitial fibroblast proliferation. J Appl Physiol 2005;98(2): 722–31.

136. Gerasimovskaya EV, Tucker DA, Weiser-Evans M, et al. Extracellular ATP-induced proliferation of adventitial fibroblasts requires phosphoinositide 3-kinase, Akt, mammalian target of rapamycin, and p70 S6 kinase signaling pathways. J Biol Chem 2005;280(3):1838–48.

137. Tapper EB, Knowles D, Heffron T, et al. Portopulmonary hypertension: imatinib as a novel treatment

and the Emory experience with this condition. Transplant Proc 2009;41(5):1969–71.

138. Wessler JD, Steingart RM, Schwartz GK, et al. Dramatic improvement in pulmonary hypertension with rapamycin. Chest 2010;138(4):991–3.

139. Krowka MJ, Plevak DJ, Findlay JY, et al. Pulmonary hemodynamics and perioperative cardiopulmonary-related mortality in patients with portopulmonary hypertension undergoing liver transplantation. Liver Transpl 2000;6(4):443–50.

140. Krowka MJ, Mandell MS, Ramsay MA, et al. Hepatopulmonary syndrome and portopulmonary hypertension: a report of the multicenter liver transplant database. Liver Transpl 2004;10(2):174–82.

141. Ramsay MA, Simpson BR, Nguyen AT, et al. Severe pulmonary hypertension in liver transplant candidates. Liver Transpl Surg 1997;3(5):494–500.

142. McGlothlin D, Ivascu N, Heerdt PM. Anesthesia and pulmonary hypertension. Prog Cardiovasc Dis 2012;55(2):199–217.

143. Steadman RH. Anesthesia for liver transplant surgery. Anesthesiol Clin North America 2004;22(4): 687–711.

144. Cheng EY, Woehlck HJ. Pulmonary artery hypertension complicating anesthesia for liver transplantation. Anesthesiology 1992;77(2):389–92.

145. Estrin JA, Belani KG, Ascher NL, et al. Hemodynamic changes on clamping and unclamping of major vessels during liver transplantation. Transplant Proc 1989;21(3):3500–5.

146. Acosta F, Sansano T, Palenciano CG, et al. Portopulmonary hypertension and liver transplantation: hemodynamic consequences at reperfusion. Transplant Proc 2005;37(9):3865–6.

147. Aggarwal S, Kang Y, Freeman JA, et al. Postreperfusion syndrome: cardiovascular collapse following hepatic reperfusion during liver transplantation. Transplant Proc 1987;19(4 Suppl 3):54–5.

148. Bandara M, Gordon FD, Sarwar A, et al. Successful outcomes following living donor liver transplantation for portopulmonary hypertension. Liver Transpl 2010;16(8):983–9.

149. Ashfaq M, Chinnakotla S, Rogers L, et al. The impact of treatment of portopulmonary hypertension on survival following liver transplantation. Am J Transplant 2007;7(5):1258–64.

150. Martinez-Palli G, Taura P, Balust J, et al. Liver transplantation in high-risk patients: hepatopulmonary syndrome and portopulmonary hypertension. Transplant Proc 2005;37(9):3861–4.

151. Yoshida EM, Erb SR, Pflugfelder PW, et al. Single-lung versus liver transplantation for the treatment of portopulmonary hypertension–a comparison of two patients. Transplantation 1993;55(3):688–90.

152. Hollatz TJ, Musat A, Westphal S, et al. Treatment with sildenafil and treprostinil allows successful liver transplantation of patients with moderate to

severe portopulmonary hypertension. Liver Transpl 2012;18(6):686–95.

153. Aucejo F, Miller C, Vogt D, et al. Pulmonary hypertension after liver transplantation in patients with antecedent hepatopulmonary syndrome: a report of 2 cases and review of the literature. Liver Transpl 2006;12(8):1278–82.

154. Kaspar MD, Ramsay MA, Shuey CB Jr, et al. Severe pulmonary hypertension and amelioration of hepatopulmonary syndrome after liver transplantation. Liver Transpl Surg 1998;4(2):177–9.

155. Koneru B, Fisher A, Wilson DJ, et al. De novo diagnosis of portopulmonary hypertension following liver transplantation. Am J Transplant 2002;2(9): 883–6.

156. Mandell MS, Groves BM, Duke J. Progressive plexogenic pulmonary hypertension following liver transplantation. Transplantation 1995;59(10): 1488–90.

157. Martinez-Palli G, Barbera JA, Taura P, et al. Severe portopulmonary hypertension after liver transplantation in a patient with preexisting hepatopulmonary syndrome. J Hepatol 1999;31(6):1075–9.

158. Shirouzu Y, Kasahara M, Takada Y, et al. Development of pulmonary hypertension in 5 patients after pediatric living-donor liver transplantation: de novo or secondary? Liver Transpl 2006;12(5):870–5.

159. Koch DG, Caplan M, Reuben A. Pulmonary hypertension after liver transplantation: case presentation and review of the literature. Liver Transpl 2009;15(4):407–12.

160. Swanson KL, Wiesner RH, Nyberg SL, et al. Survival in portopulmonary hypertension: Mayo Clinic experience categorized by treatment subgroups. Am J Transplant 2008;8(11):2445–53.

161. Sussman N, Kaza V, Barshes N, et al. Successful liver transplantation following medical management of portopulmonary hypertension: a single-center series. Am J Transplant 2006;6(9):2177–82.

162. OPTN/UNOS Liver and Intestinal Organ Transplantation Committee. Report to the Board of Directors, November 16-17, 2009. Available at: http://optn. transplant.hrsa.gov/CommitteeReports/board_main_ Liver&IntestinalOrganTransplantationCommittee_11_ 20_2009_12_1.pdf. Accessed June 11, 2013.

163. Ogawa E, Hori T, Doi H, et al. Living-donor liver transplantation for moderate or severe porto-pulmonary hypertension accompanied by pulmonary arterial hypertension: a single-centre experience over 2 decades in Japan. J Hepatobiliary Pancreat Sci 2012; 19(6):638–49.

164. Sugimachi K, Soejima Y, Morita K, et al. Rapid normalization of portopulmonary hypertension after living donor liver transplantation. Transplant Proc 2009;41(5):1976–8.

165. Sulica R, Emre S, Poon M. Medical management of porto-pulmonary hypertension and right heart failure prior to living-related liver transplantation. Congest Heart Fail 2004;10(4):192–4.

166. Krowka MJ, Wiesner RH, Heimbach JK. Pulmonary contraindications, indications and MELD exceptions for liver transplantation: a contemporary view and look forward. J Hepatol 2013;59(2):367–74.

167. Grannas G, Neipp M, Hoeper MM, et al. Indications for and outcomes after combined lung and liver transplantation: a single-center experience on 13 consecutive cases. Transplantation 2008;85(4): 524–31.

168. Pirenne J, Verleden G, Nevens F, et al. Combined liver and (heart-)lung transplantation in liver transplant candidates with refractory portopulmonary hypertension. Transplantation 2002;73(1):140–2.

169. Raichlin E, Daly RC, Rosen CB, et al. Combined heart and liver transplantation: a single-center experience. Transplantation 2009;88(2):219–25.

170. Scouras NE, Matsusaki T, Boucek CD, et al. Portopulmonary hypertension as an indication for combined heart, lung, and liver or lung and liver transplantation: literature review and case presentation. Liver Transpl 2011;17(2):137–43.

171. Wallwork J, Williams R, Calne RY. Transplantation of liver, heart, and lungs for primary biliary cirrhosis and primary pulmonary hypertension. Lancet 1987;2(8552):182–5.

Pulmonary Hypertension Associated with Chronic Hemolytic Anemia and Other Blood Disorders

Roberto F. Machado, MD[a],*, Harrison W. Farber, MD[b]

KEYWORDS

- Pulmonary hypertension • Sickle cell disease • Thalassemia • Myeloproliferative disorders
- Splenectomy

KEY POINTS

- Pulmonary hypertension (PH) has emerged as a major complication of several hematologic disorders.
- With the exception of sickle cell disease, there are a limited number of studies evaluating the prevalence of PH using the gold standard right heart catheterization.
- The cause of the PH in patients with hematologic disorders is multifactorial.
- There are virtually no high-quality data on the safety and efficacy of PH-targeted therapy in this patient population.

INTRODUCTION

Pulmonary hypertension (PH) has emerged as a major complication of several hematologic disorders. Here the authors review the clinical manifestations, epidemiology, pathophysiology, and treatment of PH-complicating disorders of the hematologic system.

HEMOGLOBINOPATHIES

The oxygen-carrying capacity of erythrocytes relies, in part, on the presence of functional hemoglobin. The normal hemoglobin molecule, hemoglobin A (HbA), is typically comprised of 2 α-globin subunits and 2 β-globin subunits. Genetic defects may produce abnormal subunits/dysfunctional proteins or lower levels of normal hemoglobins. In addition to the specific defects associated with the different hemoglobinopathies, anemia should also be considered in the evaluation of PH in patients with these diseases. The signs and symptoms induced by anemia depend on the degree of anemia, the rate at which it evolves, the oxygen demands of patients, and the presence of chronic cardiopulmonary disease.[1–3] From the hemodynamic standpoint, as the hemoglobin level decreases (particularly with hemoglobin values less than 7 g/dL), blood viscosity

Disclosures: Institutional research (no salary) support from Actelion and United Therapeutics and honoraria for advisory board participation for Gilead Sciences and United Therapeutics (R.F. Machado). Speakers' bureau: Actelion, Gilead; consultant: Actelion, Gilead, United Therapeutics, Novartis, BMS, Ikaria, Bayer; research grants: United Therapeutics, Gilead (H.W. Farber).
Funding: National Heart, Lung, and Blood Institute of the National Institutes of Health (R01HL111656, K23HL098454 to R.F. Machado).
[a] Section of Pulmonary, Critical Care Medicine, Sleep and Allergy, Department of Medicine, Institute for Personalized Respiratory Medicine, University of Illinois at Chicago, 909 South Wolcott Avenue, M/C 719, Chicago, IL 60612, USA; [b] Pulmonary Center, Boston University School of Medicine, 72 East Concord Street, R-304, Boston, MA 02118, USA
* Corresponding author.
E-mail address: machador@uic.edu

decreases, cardiac output increases, filling pressures tend to decrease, and systemic and pulmonary vascular resistances decrease substantially. Such abnormalities are readily reversible with red blood cell transfusions.[2–4]

Sickle Cell Disease

Sickle cell disease (SCD) is one of the most common monogenetic diseases in the world. Sickle cell anemia, the most common and most severe form of SCD, occurs in individuals who are homozygous for a single nucleotide change from thymine to adenine, with the sixth amino acid in the β-globin chain becoming valine instead of glutamic acid, resulting in the production of hemoglobin S (HbS). Other types of SCD are the result of compound heterozygotes of one copy of HbS and one copy of another β-globin mutation, such as hemoglobin SC or hemoglobin S-beta-thalassemia.[5]

Approximately 250,000 children worldwide are born with homozygous sickle cell anemia every year[6]; 0.15% of African Americans are homozygous for SCD and 8% have sickle cell trait.[6] In sub-Saharan Africa, up to 40% of the population carry sickle cell trait and up to 1% of children are born with SCD.[7]

HbS is much less soluble than HbA when deoxygenated.[8,9] Deoxygenated HbS polymerizes and aggregates inside sickle erythrocytes and as they traverse the microcirculation these rigid, dense and sickled cells become entrapped in the microcirculation. This process is also enhanced by inflammation and integrin molecule expression, causing red cell and leukocyte adhesion to the endothelium. These episodes of microvascular occlusion result in an interruption in blood flow, ischemia, and reperfusion injury, with secondary inflammatory, thrombotic, and oxidant stress.[10–17] SCD is characterized by a chronic hemolytic anemia. Intravascular hemolysis releases cell-free hemoglobin into the plasma, which scavenges nitric oxide (NO), and releases red blood cell arginase-1 into the plasma, which catabolizes arginine, the substrate for NO synthesis,[18–20] and ultimately produces a state of endothelial dysfunction, vascular proliferation, and pro-oxidant and proinflammatory stress.[21–23]

Among the chronic cardiopulmonary complications of SCD, PH has emerged as a major cause of morbidity and mortality. A great deal of recent data has significantly added to the understanding of the prevalence, mechanisms, and clinical characterization of PH in patients with SCD. Retrospective and prospective cohort studies using Doppler echocardiography have reported that 20% to 30% of patients with SCD have an elevated estimated pulmonary artery systolic pressure that is 2 standard deviations more than the normal mean value (tricuspid regurgitant jet velocity [TRV] ≥2.5 m/s), whereas approximately 8% to 10% of patients have values 3 standard deviations more than the population normal mean (TRV ≥3.0 m/s).[21,24–27] Further, the measurement of N-terminal pro brain natriuretic peptide (NT-proBNP) in stored plasma samples showed that 30% of individuals enrolled in the Multicenter Study of Hydroxyurea in 1996 had elevated levels, suggesting the presence of elevated pulmonary pressures and strain in the right side of the heart.[28] Similarly, in the Cooperative Study of Sickle Cell Disease from 1978 and 1988, 27.6% of adults had elevated levels of NT-proBNP.[29] In both studies, elevated study entry levels of NT-proBNP were independently associated with a higher risk of death.

Three recent studies using the gold standard diagnostic test for the disease, right heart catheterization (RHC), have provided new insights into PH in SCD (Table 1). The National Institutes of Health (NIH) screening study has followed 533 patients for a median follow-up of 4.4 years.[31] Using preestablished inclusion criteria, 86 patients underwent RHC, of which 56 were diagnosed with PH (10.5% of the total study population). Similar findings were observed in a study of 80 patients with SCD in Brazil, which revealed a 10% prevalence of PH.[26] In a study of 398 patients with SCD in France, Parent and colleagues[27] observed a 6% prevalence of PH. Differences in the study design could explain discrepancies in the PH prevalence between the French study and both the US and Brazilian studies. Parent and colleagues[27] excluded approximately 10% of screened patients, including those with severe renal (creatinine clearance of less than 30 mL/min), liver (international normalized ratio >1.7), or lung disease (total lung capacity of less than 70% predicted).

The epidemiologic risk factors associated with an elevated TRV and PH documented by RHC include a history of renal or cardiovascular complications; increased systemic systolic blood pressure; abnormalities in markers of hemolytic anemia (anemia, reticulocytosis, increased lactate dehydrogenase, aspartate aminotransferase, and bilirubin); iron overload; cholestatic liver dysfunction (elevations in alkaline phosphatase); renal insufficiency; a history of cutaneous leg ulceration; and, in men, a history of priapism.[21,26,28,31–33] The development of and elevated TRV and PH was not associated with the number of vasoocclusive episodes or acute chest syndrome, markers of inflammation, fetal hemoglobin levels, or platelet counts.[21,26,28,31–33] These data provide support

Table 1
RHC-based PH screening studies in SCD

	Parent[27]	Fonseca[26]	Mehari[31,32]
Subjects screened (N)	398	80	531
Number of subjects with PH	24	8	55
Percent of screened population	6.0	10.0	10.5
mPAP, mm Hg	30 ± 6	33 ± 9	36 ± 9
CO, l/min	9 ± 2	5 ± 2[a]	9 ± 2
PVR, dyn×s/cm^5	138 ± 58	179 ± 120[b]	227 ± 149
6MWD, m	404 ± 94	460 ± 152	358 ± 115
Number of subjects with precapillary PH (% of screened population)	11 (2.7)	3 (3.75)	31 (6.0)
Number of subjects with postcapillary PH (% of screened population)	13 (3.3)	5 (6.25)	24 (4.5)
Mortality in PH/no PH group (%)	12.5/1.4	38.0/5.5	36.0/13.0

Abbreviations: 6MWD, 6-minute walk distance; CO, cardiac output; mPAP, mean pulmonary artery pressure; PVR, pulmonary vascular resistance.
[a] Cardiac index (l/min/m^2).
[b] Converted mean value: PVR measured in Wood units.

to the hypothesis that PH arises secondary to chronic hemolytic anemia and end-organ dysfunction (renal and liver disease) rather than secondary to episodes of acute chest syndrome and related pulmonary fibrosis.

An elevated estimated pulmonary artery systolic pressure by Doppler echocardiographic screening is a significant risk factor for death in patients with SCD. In the NIH study, compared with patients with TRV less than 2.5 m/s, the rate ratio for death for a TRV of 2.5 to 2.9 m/s and greater than 3.0 m/s was 4.4 (95% confidence interval [CI] 1.6–12.2) and 10.6 (95% CI 3.3–33.6), respectively.[21] De Castro and colleagues[25] also found that 6 of 42 patients (14%) with an elevated TRV and 2 of 83 patients (2%) with normal TRV died during a 2-year follow-up period.[25] Similarly, in the study by Ataga and colleagues,[24] 9 of 36 patients with an elevated TRV and 1 of 57 patients with normal TRV died during the 2.5-year follow-up period (relative risk 9.24 [95% CI 1.2–73.3]). In both the French and Brazilian screening studies, most of the deaths occurred in patients with TRV values greater than 2.5 m/s.

The presence of PH documented by RHC is a major risk factor for death in patients with SCD. Castro and colleagues[30] reported a 50% 2-year mortality rate in patients with SCD with PH, and each increase of 10 mm Hg in mean pulmonary artery pressure (PAP) was associated with a 1.7-fold increase in the rate of death (95% CI, 1.1–2.7). In the NIH study, the mortality rate was significantly higher in the PH group overall (20 deaths, 36%) than either the group without

PH by RHC (3 deaths, 10%) or the general sickle cell group with normal Doppler echocardiographic estimates of pulmonary artery systolic pressure (50 deaths, 13%).[31] In both the Brazilian[26] and French[27] cohorts, the mortality rate was significantly higher in the PH group (38% and 23%, respectively).

Mehari and colleagues[32] analyzed specific hemodynamic predictors of mortality in the NIH cohort. Hemodynamic variables independently associated with mortality included mean PAP (hazard ratio [HR] 1.61, 95% CI 1.05–2.45 per 10 mm Hg increase), diastolic PAP (HR 1.83, 95% CI 1.09–3.08 per 10 mm Hg increase), diastolic PAP–pulmonary capillary wedge pressure (HR 2.19, 95% CI 1.23–3.89 per 10 mm Hg increase), transpulmonary gradient (HR 1.78, 95% CI 1.14–2.79 per 10 mm Hg increase), and pulmonary vascular resistance (HR 1.44, 95% CI 1.09–1.89 per Wood unit increase). These data suggest that mortality in adults with SCD and PH is proportional to the severity of precapillary PH.

An association between the development of PH and the intensity of hemolytic anemia has been observed in prospective screening studies of patients with SCD.[21,24,25,27,33–38] Although this hypothesis has been challenged in editorials and commentaries,[39,40] there is strong clinical and experimental evidence suggesting that hemolysis is related mechanistically to PH. Hemolysis releases plasma-free hemoglobin that inactivates the intrinsic vasodilator NO[19,20] and arginase-1, which depletes L-arginine, the substrate for NO synthesis.[18] The result of these combined pathologic processes is a state of decreased NO bioavailability and resistance to NO-dependent vasodilation.[20]

There is a correlation between the rate of hemolysis and the levels of procoagulant factors in blood in patients with SCD[41–43] and hemolysis; decreased NO bioavailability induces platelet activation,[44] thrombin generation, and tissue factor activation.[45] Hemolysis is also associated with the formation of red blood cell microvesicles expressing phosphatidyl serine, which activate tissue factor.[43,46]

Splenectomy has been reported to be a risk factor for the development of PH,[47] particularly in patients with hemolytic disorders.[48–50] Thus, functional or surgical asplenia could also contribute to the development of PH in patients with SCD. Loss of splenic function may trigger platelet activation, promoting pulmonary microthrombosis and red cell adhesion to the endothelium.[51] In addition, patients with SCD have increased levels of cell-free hemoglobin and red cell prothrombotic microvesicles; following splenectomy, the rate of intravascular hemolysis increases.[43]

In patients with SCD, both at steady state and during vasoocclusive pain crises, plasma endothelin-1 levels are increased.[52] In vitro, sickle erythrocytes increase endothelin-1 production by cultured human endothelial cells. In addition, endothelin receptor A antagonism abolishes the vasoconstrictive effects of media from pulmonary endothelial cells exposed to sickled erythrocytes on aortic rings.[52] Finally, a high PAP could also result from the high-cardiac-output state associated with chronic anemia. It is possible that a high-cardiac-output state combined with hemolytic anemia and other risk factors, such as renal insufficiency and iron overload, act synergistically to cause pathologic pulmonary vascular remodeling.

The diagnostic evaluation of patients with SCD suspected of having PH should follow the same guidelines established for other causes of PH.[53,54] Given the high prevalence of PH in this population and the associated high mortality, the authors recommend noninvasive screening of all symptomatic adults with Doppler echocardiography and assessment of steady state plasma NT-proBNP levels and functional capacity. It is important that such screening be performed in the steady state because pulmonary pressures increase during vasoocclusive painful crisis and acute chest syndrome.[55,56] An elevated TRV cannot be used to diagnose PH. For example, only 25% of patients with a TRV of 2.5 m/s or more will actually have PH at RHC.[29] A TRV of 2.9 m/s or more has a higher positive predictive value of 64% but a very high false-negative rate of 42%.[27] The measurement of NT-proBNP levels

can be used to suggest PH or for risk stratification in patients with SCD[28] because plasma levels are higher in patients with sickle cell PH and correlate directly with the severity of the PH and the degree of functional impairment. An NT-proBNP level of 160 pg/mL or more is also an independent predictor of mortality (risk ratio 5.1, 95% CI 2.1–12.5). Combining a TRV of 2.5 m/s or more, a high NT-proBNP level (>164.5 pg/mL) and a low 6-minute walk distance of less than 333 m, the positive predictive value for PH was 62%, with a false-negative rate of 7%.[27] However, as in other diseases associated with PH, RHC is absolutely necessary to confirm the diagnosis and to determine its cause in these patients.

Most adult patients with SCD develop abnormal pulmonary function characterized by mild restrictive lung disease, abnormal diffusing capacity, and radiographic signs of mild pulmonary fibrosis[57–62]; the severity of these defects seems slightly greater in patients with PH.[63] In aggregate, however, the degree of pulmonary function abnormalities in these patients is rarely severe enough to be a major contributor to the cause of PH. Evidence suggestive of chronic thromboembolic pulmonary hypertension (CTEPH) occurs in approximately 5% of patients with SCD with PH[63]; this entity has been successfully treated surgically in at least 2 such patients.[64]

In studies of patients with SCD undergoing RHC, the mean cardiac output and pulmonary vascular resistance for patients without PH were 10 L/min and 59 dyn/s/cm[5], respectively.[3,30,63] It is within the context of these data that one must consider the impact of PH and an elevated pulmonary vascular resistance in patients who are chronically anemic with hemolytic disorders. In patients with SCD and PH, the degree of elevation in mean pulmonary pressures is mild to moderate (30–40 mm Hg), with mild elevations in pulmonary vascular resistance.[3,26,27,30,31,63] RHC data from these studies show that the hemodynamic cause of the PH in patients with SCD is multifactorial: precapillary PH (defined by a mean PAP ≥25 mm Hg and a wedge pressure ≤15 mm Hg) is present in 50% of catheterized patients, whereas pulmonary venous hypertension (postcapillary PH) secondary to left ventricular dysfunction (defined by a mean PAP ≥25 mm Hg, a wedge pressure >15 mm Hg) is present in 50%.[3,26,27,30,31,63] An echocardiographic study of a cohort of 141 patients with SCD found that 47% of them had a high TRV, diastolic dysfunction, or both (29% had a high TRV alone, 11% had diastolic dysfunction and a high TRV, and 7% had diastolic dysfunction alone). An elevated TRV and diastolic dysfunction were associated with a relative risk of death of 5.1 (95% CI

2.0–13.3) and 4.8 (95% CI 1.9–12.1), respectively, whereas the relative risk of death when both were present was 12.0 (95% CI 3.8–38.1).[65] In addition, in a series of 483 patients with homozygous SCD, markers of diastolic dysfunction were independently associated with a low 6-minute-walk distance.[33]

From a functional standpoint, patients with SCD are impaired by mild increases in PAP and pulmonary vascular resistance. When compared with age-, gender-, and hemoglobin-matched patients with SCD without PH, individuals with pulmonary hypertension exhibit lower 6-minute walk distance (435 ± 31 m vs 320 ± 20 m) and peak oxygen consumption (50% ± 3% vs 41% ± 2% of predicted) and higher ventilatory equivalent for carbon dioxide at the anaerobic threshold (31.6% ± 1.5% vs 39.2% ± 1.6%).[63] The 6-minute walk distance is inversely correlated with pulmonary vascular resistance and mean PAP and directly correlated with maximal oxygen consumption, supporting the contribution of increasing PAP to the loss of exercise capacity. PAP and pulmonary vascular resistance sharply increase with exercise, suggesting that pulmonary vascular disease contributes to functional limitation in these patients.[55] In addition, a lower exercise capacity (assessed by the 6-minute walk test) in patients with PH has also been demonstrated in larger cohorts of patients with SCD.[26,27,31,33]

There are very limited data on the specific management of patients with SCD and PH. Although this has not been tested in randomized trials of patients with SCD and PH, a reasonable approach should include maximization of SCD-specific therapy (ie, treatment of primary hemoglobinopathy with hydroxyurea or transfusion therapy according to published treatment guidelines[66,67]), treatment of hypoxia with chronic oxygen therapy, and treatment of associated cardiopulmonary conditions (such as iron overload, chronic liver disease, human immunodeficiency virus infection, nocturnal hypoxemia, thromboembolic disorders, and left ventricular disease). In patients with SCD with pulmonary arterial hypertension (PAH) (mean PAP ≥25 mm Hg and wedge pressures <15 mm Hg, with a relatively high pulmonary vascular resistance [eg, >160 dyn/cm⁵]), PAH-specific therapy can be considered. In addition, there are no randomized controlled trials (RCT) demonstrating the benefit of any PAH-specific therapy in SCD-associated PAH. Therapy should only be initiated and monitored by a team comprised of a PAH specialist and a hematologist specializing in SCD care.

In a series of 7 patients with either thalassemia or sickle thalassemia and PH treatment with sildenafil from 4 weeks to 48 months resulted in an improvement in TRV, New York Heart Association functional class, and 6-minute walk distance.[68] In another case series, 12 patients with SCD were treated with sildenafil for a mean of 6 months with improvements in estimated pulmonary artery systolic pressure, 6-minute walk distance, and NT-proBNP levels.[69] However, these preliminary data were not supported by the results of the Pulmonary Hypertension and Sickle Cell Disease with Sildenafil Therapy (Walk-PHaSST) study.[70] This 16-week, NIH-sponsored multicenter, double-blind, placebo-controlled trial of sildenafil in patients with SCD with increased TRV and a low exercise capacity was stopped early, before enrollment of the planned 132 patients, because of a higher incidence of serious adverse events in the sildenafil arm (45% of sildenafil, 22% placebo, $P = .022$). Hospitalization for vasoocclusive pain crisis was the predominant cause for this difference: 35% sildenafil versus 14% placebo ($P = .029$). Importantly, there was no signal of a treatment effect on the 6-minute walk distance or NT-proBNP in the 74 patients enrolled in the study at the time of suspension. Based on these findings, phosphodiesterase type 5 inhibitors should not be used as first-line agents in patients with SCD and PAH.

Minniti and colleagues[71] reported on the use of bosentan and ambrisentan (either as monotherapy or in combination with sildenafil) in a cohort of 14 patients with SCD and PH documented by RHC; with this treatment, there was a modest improvement in the 6-minute walk distance, NT-proBNP levels, and estimated pulmonary artery systolic pressure. The ASSET-1 (Assessment in Patients with Sickle Cell Disease of the Efficacy and Safety of Bosentan Therapy on Pulmonary Arterial Hypertension) and ASSET-2 studies enrolled patients with pulmonary arterial hypertension and pulmonary venous hypertension, respectively, who were randomized to bosentan or placebo. After the enrollment of 26 patients, the studies were terminated because of slow site activation and withdrawal of support by the sponsor. In this small number of patients, bosentan was well tolerated, with no significant differences in serious adverse events or laboratory tests between patients receiving the study drug; however, there was no evidence of a beneficial effect with treatment.[72] Acute administration of epoprostenol decreases PAP and pulmonary vascular resistance and increases cardiac output in patients with PH and SCD,[30] but chronic therapy with these agents has not been described in the literature.

β-Thalassemia

Thalassemia refers to a spectrum of diseases characterized by reduced or absent production of one or more α- or β-globin chains. β-thalassemia is caused by impaired production of β-globin chains, which leads to a relative excess of α-globin chains.[73] These excess α-globin chains are unstable, incapable of forming soluble tetramers on their own, and precipitate within the cell, leading to ineffective erythropoiesis and hemolytic anemia.[74] Thalassemia major (TM), or homozygous β-thalassemia, is a severe disorder caused by the inheritance of 2 β-thalassemia alleles. Patients with this disorder develop severe and lifelong transfusion-dependent anemia, hepatosplenomegaly, and skeletal deformities caused by bone marrow expansion; they are prone to infection and skeletal fractures. β-thalassemia intermedia (TI), an entity of intermediate severity, occurs in patients with heterozygotes of 2 thalassemic variants; these patients may have skeletal abnormalities and hepatosplenomegaly similar to those seen in TM, but they usually have milder anemia. The development of PH in patients with thalassemia is likely multifactorial, involving interactions among erythrocytes via intravascular hemolysis, platelets, the coagulation system, endothelial cells, and mediators of inflammation and vascular tone.

PH is a common finding in patients with β-thalassemia; the prevalence, however, is variable, depending on the method used for screening and the type of thalassemia (**Table 2**). In most studies, the prevalence has been determined by echocardiography; however, the accuracy of echocardiography in the evaluation of PH in this entity is currently unknown. In one report, 7 patients with TI and heart failure were found to have preserved left ventricular function and severe PH by RHC.[81] In a larger study of 110 patients with TI,[82] PH was suggested by echocardiography in 60% of cases. Among these patients, 6 with heart failure and preserved systolic function underwent RHC that confirmed PH.[82] A study comparing cardiovascular involvement in 205 patients with TI and TM, the most prevalent form of the disease, confirmed the aforementioned findings in TI[80]; in contrast, in TI, the main cardiac manifestation was left ventricular dysfunction.[76,77,80] In 2 small studies of patients with TM, the prevalence of PH suggested by echocardiography was 75% and 79%[75,76]; however, these patients were poorly managed by current standards and had a high prevalence of left ventricular systolic dysfunction. In summary, the true prevalence of PH in patients with thalassemia is unknown and should be determined.

Given the potential prevalence of PH, especially in TI, and the increased prevalence of left heart disease in thalassemia in general, it is reasonable to suggest that transthoracic Doppler echocardiography screening be performed in these patients; but, as in other diseases associated with PH, the diagnosis must be confirmed by RHC. Moreover, because there is an increased prevalence of left-sided cardiac disease in these patients, the cause of PH can only be conclusively differentiated by RHC.

Despite its potential complications, chronic transfusion therapy in severe thalassemia has changed the clinical course of the disease and is likely to have a favorable impact in individuals with PH. The management of those patients should focus on the disease-specific therapeutic targets that arise from the diverse pathogenetic mechanisms involved. Proper transfusion therapy restores tissue oxygen delivery and

Table 2
PH studies in thalassemia

Study	Number of Patients	Type of Thalassemia	Criteria for PH	Prevalence of PH (%)
Grisaru et al,[75] 1990	35	Major	ECHO: PAT/RVET	75
Du et al,[76] 1997	33	Major	ECHO: TPG+ RAP >30 mm Hg	79
Derchi et al,[77] 1999	130	Major	ECHO: TPG	10
Aessopos et al,[78] 2004	202	Major	ECHO: TPG >30	10
Hagar et al,[79] 2006	36	Major	ECHO: TRV >2.5 m/s	44
Aessopos et al,[80] 2005	36	Major	ECHO: TPG >30	10
Aessopos et al,[80] 2005	74	Intermedia	ECHO: TPG >30	60
Aessopos et al,[81] 1995	7	Intermedia	RHC	100
Aessopos et al,[82] 2001	110	Intermedia	ECHO: TPG >30 and RHC	59

Abbreviations: ECHO, echocardiography; PAT/RVET, ratio of pulmonary valve acceleration time to right ventricular ejection time; RAP, right atrial pressure; TPG, tricuspid systolic pressure gradient.

suppresses the synthesis of native defective erythrocytes, presumably ameliorating hemolysis, hypercoagulability, tissue hypoxia, and volume overload. In theory, this might obviate the development of PAH in these patients.[83,84] Combined with transfusions, iron chelation therapy prevents iron accumulation and the resulting oxidative tissue damage. This idea is supported by a report that, in well-transfused, iron-chelated patients with TM, PH was completely prevented.[78] Hydroxyurea modifies defective hemoglobin synthesis and reduces thrombocytosis, presumably decreasing hemolysis and hypercoagulability. In a recently published study of 584 patients with TI, the use of these modalities seemed protective against the development of PH.[85] However, the study was not randomized, was retrospective, and used echocardiography for the diagnosis of PH. Yet, other small studies and case reports in these patients have reported similar observations.[86,87] Prospective RCT of the adjuvant therapies noted earlier have not been performed and are an important area for future research.

The treatment of patients with thalassemia with confirmed PAH (group 1 PH) seems reasonable according to the current PAH guidelines, but that has never been tested in an RCT; moreover, they have been routinely excluded from the major RCT of approved pulmonary vasodilators. In a recent open-label study of 10 patients with β-thalassemia and an TRV greater than 2.5 m/s on Doppler echocardiography (none of the patients underwent confirmatory RHC), treatment with sildenafil resulted in a significant decrease in tricuspid regurgitant jet velocity and improved left ventricular end systolic/diastolic volume but did not change the 6-minute walk distance.[88] There are also case reports of favorable response to bosentan[89] and epoprostenol[90] in patients with RHC-confirmed precapillary PH. Given the lack of data, an RCT of pulmonary vasodilators in these patients should be considered. Because of the potential differences in PH causes in patients with TI and TM (eg, PAH in TI, left heart disease in TM), combining phenotypes in clinical trials is not ideal and should be avoided.

RED BLOOD CELL MEMBRANE DISORDERS
Paroxysmal Nocturnal Hemoglobinuria

Paroxysmal nocturnal hemoglobinuria (PNH) is a progressively debilitating and life-threatening hemolytic disease caused by an acquired clonal genetic deficiency of glycosylphosphatidylinositol-linked proteins on the surface of blood cells.[91] This deficiency results in complement-mediated chronic intravascular hemolysis and subsequent life-threatening thromboembolic disease and PH. Similarly to SCD, the mechanism by which PH evolves in these patients is thought to be caused by the vascular effect of intravascular hemolysis.

There are several case reports of patients with PNH who have developed PH.[92,93] Some of these patients have disease similar to PAH, whereas others have PH caused by thromboembolic disease (CTEPH). In the largest study,[94] 29 patients with PNH were evaluated for PH by echocardiography as well as for evidence of red cell hemolysis and NO resistance. The investigators found that 36% of the patients had elevated pulmonary artery systolic pressure (PASP), but no patient underwent confirmatory RHC. Patients with evidence of more severe hemolysis were more likely to have elevated PAP.

There are no studies of PH treatment in these patients. However, treatment with eculizumab does decrease intravascular hemolysis and might decrease the risk of the development of PH.[94–97]

Hereditary Spherocytosis

PH has been reported in patients with hereditary spherocytosis (HS), especially following splenectomy.[98–100] However, PH in these small studies or case reports has been only documented by echocardiography; confirmation with RHC is lacking. In the largest study, 36 patients with HS (78% with previous splenectomy) were evaluated for PH using echocardiography and NT-proBNP.[101] In this group of patients, the investigators observed no evidence of a significantly increased risk of developing PH and certainly not to the degree reported in either thalassemia or SCD.

These findings may have implications for the understanding of the cause of PH associated with hemoglobinopathies and other hemolytic disorders. Although this has been challenged in several forums,[39,40] there is strong evidence suggesting that hemolysis is critical for the development of vascular complications, especially PH, in these diseases with other factors, such as splenectomy being another potential contributor. As previously discussed, case reports of PH in patients with prior splenectomy and the observation that a substantial proportion of patients with thalassemia and SCD have had a prior splenectomy or have functional asplenia suggest that it is not solely the hemolysis that increases the risk of PH but that the absence of a spleen is also a contributor. However, in HS, because splenectomy effectively eliminates hemolysis, the aforementioned observations suggest it may be of greater importance in increasing the risk for the development of PH in these patients.

Hereditary Stomatocytosis

Hereditary stomatocytosis is a rare autosomal dominant red cell membrane protein disorder, characterized by plasma membrane leakage of sodium and potassium.[102] Because of this membrane instability, these red cells can exhibit abnormal responses to changes in temperature and are subject to intravascular hemolysis.[103]

Recent reports suggest that hereditary stomatocytosis carries a high risk of thrombotic complications, especially after splenectomy. In fact, all cases of PH reported in patients with hereditary stomatocytosis are seemingly related to thromboembolic disease,[104–107] including one in which the patient underwent pulmonary thromboendarterectomy[106] and another in which the patient underwent a heart-lung transplant.[107]

CHRONIC MYELOPROLIFERATIVE DISORDERS

Chronic myeloproliferative disorders (CMPD) include many hematopoietic disorders; some CMPD are well characterized, such as chronic myelogenous leukemia, chronic neutrophilic leukemia, chronic eosinophilic leukemia, polycythemia vera, idiopathic myelofibrosis, and essential thrombocytosis; others are rare or poorly characterized.[108] Each involves a multipotent hematopoietic progenitor cell with overproduction of one or more of the formed elements of the blood without significant dysplasia; there is also a predilection to extramedullary hematopoiesis, myelofibrosis, and transformation at varying rates to acute leukemia.

The possible association of PH with CMPD has been suggested by several case reports and small case series.[109–122] However, the exact incidence and prevalence is not currently known. On one hand, because clinical signs of PH appear at an advanced stage of disease and, in some cases, the diagnosis of CMPD is difficult to establish because of chronic hypoxemia, the prevalence of PH may be underestimated. On the other hand, the rate of PH may be overestimated because, in almost all cases, diagnosis has been made by echocardiography and not confirmed by RHC; thus, a secondary cause, such as left ventricular dysfunction or a high output state, has not been excluded.

Two distinct clinical forms of PH have been described in patients with CMPD: CTEPH and precapillary PH mimicking PAH (reviewed in Ref.[123]).

CTEPH: CMPD, especially polycythemia vera and essential thrombocytosis, is often characterized by a thrombophilic state, hyperviscosity, increased white blood cell count (WBC), all of which lead to microcirculatory disturbances and a very high rate of arterial and venous thromboses. In many cases, CTEPH has been the initial manifestation of CMPD. Also, in patients with CMPD, therapeutic splenectomy causes worsening of extramedullary hematopoiesis, increased platelet counts, and increased hematocrit, all of which may increase the risk of CTEPH.

The treatment of venous thromboses in patients with polycythemia vera and essential thrombocytosis does not differ from that of other patients. As in other cases of CTEPH, pulmonary endarterectomy (PTE) is the treatment of choice in these patients. In patients who are inoperable or have PH after PTE, medical therapy including diuretics, anticoagulants, and specific PAH therapy can be considered. However, no data on specific PAH therapy exist for patients with CTEPH associated with CMPD. In patients with a high thrombotic risk, therapy with hydroxyurea is recommended.[124]

Precapillary PH mimicking PAH[73,110,120,125–137]: Several factors have been suggested for the pathogenesis of PAH in patients with CMPD: (1) Portal hypertension, which is a cause of PAH and is a well-known complication of myeloid metaplasia with myelofibrosis.[138] (2) Chemotherapeutic agents or stem cell transplantation, both of which are treatment options for these conditions and have been associated with pulmonary venoocclusive disease.[125] (3) Tumor microembolism.[120,129] (4) Extramedullary hematopoiesis, although rare, is often associated with several of these syndromes. Pulmonary myeloid infiltration may be related to development of PH.[139] (5) Blood cell proliferation (platelets, WBC, or red blood cell count) in patients with CMPD may contribute to the development of PH.[73,122,136] (6) Enhanced angiogenesis in the peripheral blood and bone marrow might also be a possible link between CMPD and PH.[130,131] (7) Drug toxicity: There are recent reports of reversible PH in patients with chronic myelogenous leukemia (CML) treated with dasatinib.[137] This PH has improved or even resolved after discontinuation of dasatinib.[137]

Considering the many proposed possible links between CMPD and development of PH, many therapies have been suggested. However, there are no RCT of any of these interventions, such as cytoreductive therapy[124]; hematological control[124]; whole-lung, low-dose, external beam radiotherapy[133,134,139]; anticoagulation and antiplatelet agents[140]; and pulmonary-specific vasodilators.[109] All of these strategies should be studied further.

In summary, the incidence and prevalence of PH in patients with CMPD have not been defined in large prospective studies. Two distinct forms of PH have been described in patients with CMPD: CTEPH and precapillary PH mimicking PAH.

PAH-like PH is usually diagnosed late in the course of CMPD, whereas CTEPH is usually diagnosed earlier. Treatment of PH associated with CMPD has not been rigorously studied, and RCT have not been performed with any of the proposed therapies. PTE, however, is the treatment of choice in eligible patients with CTEPH.

SPLENECTOMY

Splenectomy has long been recognized as a risk factor for PH.[47,141] A recent study of 43 patients with various disorders and reasons for splenectomy found a higher occurrence of PH in these patients than in case controls; however, the diagnosis was made by echocardiography and not confirmed by RHC.[142]

The exact mechanism by which PH develops after splenectomy remains unclear.[143] In thalassemia and SCD, PH has been described following splenectomy, with some studies reporting the prevalence of PH as high as 75%. Asplenia has also been reported as an independent risk factor for PH following splenectomy for HS,[98–100] idiopathic thrombocytopenic purpura,[47] and other hemolytic disorders.[104,105,142] There is also evidence that splenectomy can increase the risk of PH in patients who do not have hemolytic disorders, such as trauma[47] and Gaucher disease.[144] These observations suggest that asplenia may be a risk factor for PH regardless of the underlying condition.

Several mechanisms have been postulated for PH following splenectomy: (1) platelet and/or endothelial activation by abnormal red cells and red cell fragments with subsequent deposition of platelet-rich microthrombi in the pulmonary vasculature; and (2) decreased NO bioavailability secondary to intravascular hemolysis resulting in endothelial dysfunction and/or platelet activation.[143] Although these mechanisms may contribute to PH in SCD and thalassemia (continued intravascular hemolysis following splenectomy), they do not explain conditions such as HS (splenectomy effectively eliminates hemolysis) or trauma (no significant hemolysis). Thus, it has been proposed that splenectomized individuals have increased levels of circulating prothrombotic microparticles, which have been associated with PH.[41]

SUMMARY

PH complicates several hematologic disorders. The cause of PH in patients with hematologic disorders is multifactorial, and a thorough diagnostic evaluation following established guidelines for PH is essential at the individual patient level and also in large studies designed to determine disease prevalence, mechanisms, and causes. There are virtually no high-quality data on the safety and efficacy of PH-targeted therapy in this patient population, and trials of therapies in these patients are needed.

REFERENCES

1. Weiskopf RB, Viele MK, Feiner J, et al. Human cardiovascular and metabolic response to acute, severe isovolemic anemia. JAMA 1998;279:217–21.
2. Brannon ES, Merrill AJ, Warren JV, et al. The cardiac output in patients with chronic anemia as measured by the technique of right atrial catheterization. J Clin Invest 1945;24:332–6.
3. Leight L, Snider TH, Clifford GO, et al. Hemodynamic studies in sickle cell anemia. Circulation 1954;10:653–62.
4. Roy SB, Bhatia ML, Mathur VS, et al. Hemodynamic effects of chronic severe anemia. Circulation 1963;28:346–56.
5. Ashley-Koch A, Yang Q, Olney RS. Sickle hemoglobin (HbS) allele and sickle cell disease: a HuGE review. Am J Epidemiol 2000;151:839–45.
6. Serjeant GR. Sickle-cell disease. Lancet 1997;350:725–30.
7. Aliyu ZY, Gordeuk V, Sachdev V, et al. Prevalence and risk factors for pulmonary artery systolic hypertension among sickle cell disease patients in Nigeria. Am J Hematol 2008;83:485–90.
8. Bunn HF. Pathogenesis and treatment of sickle cell disease. N Engl J Med 1997;337:762–9.
9. Noguchi CT, Schechter AN, Rodgers GP. Sickle cell disease pathophysiology. Baillieres Clin Haematol 1993;6:57–91.
10. Aslan M, Ryan TM, Adler B, et al. Oxygen radical inhibition of nitric oxide-dependent vascular function in sickle cell disease. Proc Natl Acad Sci U S A 2001;98:15215–20.
11. Belcher JD, Mahaseth H, Welch TE, et al. Critical role of endothelial cell activation in hypoxia-induced vasoocclusion in transgenic sickle mice. Am J Physiol Heart Circ Physiol 2005;288:H2715–25.
12. Belcher JD, Marker PH, Weber JP, et al. Activated monocytes in sickle cell disease: potential role in the activation of vascular endothelium and vasoocclusion. Blood 2000;96:2451–9.
13. Frenette PS. Sickle cell vaso-occlusion: multistep and multicellular paradigm. Curr Opin Hematol 2002;9:101–6.
14. Kaul DK, Hebbel RP. Hypoxia/reoxygenation causes inflammatory response in transgenic sickle mice but not in normal mice. J Clin Invest 2000;106:411–20.
15. Platt OS. Sickle cell anemia as an inflammatory disease. J Clin Invest 2000;106:337–8.

16. Wood KC, Hebbel RP, Granger DN. Endothelial cell NADPH oxidase mediates the cerebral microvascular dysfunction in sickle cell transgenic mice. FASEB J 2005;19:989–91.

17. Wood KC, Hebbel RP, Lefer DJ, et al. Critical role of endothelial cell-derived nitric oxide synthase in sickle cell disease-induced microvascular dysfunction. Free Radic Biol Med 2006;40:1443–53.

18. Morris CR, Kato GJ, Poljakovic M, et al. Dysregulated arginine metabolism, hemolysis-associated pulmonary hypertension, and mortality in sickle cell disease. JAMA 2005;294:81–90.

19. Reiter CD, Wang X, Tanus-Santos JE, et al. Cell-free hemoglobin limits nitric oxide bioavailability in sickle-cell disease. Nat Med 2002;8:1383–9.

20. Rother RP, Bell L, Hillmen P, et al. The clinical sequelae of intravascular hemolysis and extracellular plasma hemoglobin: a novel mechanism of human disease. JAMA 2005;293:1653–62.

21. Gladwin MT, Sachdev V, Jison ML, et al. Pulmonary hypertension as a risk factor for death in patients with sickle cell disease. N Engl J Med 2004;350:886–95.

22. Frei AC, Guo Y, Jones DW, et al. Vascular dysfunction in a murine model of severe hemolysis. Blood 2008;112:398–405.

23. Hsu L, McDermott T, Brown L, et al. Transgenic HbS mouse neutrophils in increased susceptibility to acute lung injury: implications for sickle acute chest syndrome. Chest 1999;116:92S.

24. Ataga KI, Moore CG, Jones S, et al. Pulmonary hypertension in patients with sickle cell disease: a longitudinal study. Br J Haematol 2006;134:109–15.

25. De Castro LM, Jonassaint JC, Graham FL, et al. Pulmonary hypertension associated with sickle cell disease: clinical and laboratory endpoints and disease outcomes. Am J Hematol 2008;83:19–25.

26. Fonseca GH, Souza R, Salemi VM, et al. Pulmonary hypertension diagnosed by right heart catheterisation in sickle cell disease. Eur Respir J 2012;39:112–8.

27. Parent F, Bachir D, Inamo J, et al. A hemodynamic study of pulmonary hypertension in sickle cell disease. N Engl J Med 2011;365:44–53.

28. Machado RF, Anthi A, Steinberg MH, et al. N-terminal pro-brain natriuretic peptide levels and risk of death in sickle cell disease. JAMA 2006;296:310–8.

29. Machado RF, Hildesheim M, Mendelsohn L, et al. NT-pro brain natriuretic peptide levels and the risk of death in the cooperative study of sickle cell disease. Br J Haematol 2011;154:512–20.

30. Castro O, Hoque M, Brown BD. Pulmonary hypertension in sickle cell disease: cardiac catheterization results and survival. Blood 2003;101:1257–61.

31. Mehari A, Gladwin MT, Tian X, et al. Mortality in adults with sickle cell disease and pulmonary hypertension. JAMA 2012;307:1254–6.

32. Mehari A, Alam S, Tan X, et al. Hemodynamic predictors of mortality in adults with sickle cell disease. Am J Respir Crit Care Med 2013;187(8):840–7.

33. Sachdev V, Kato GJ, Gibbs JS, et al. Echocardiographic markers of elevated pulmonary pressure and left ventricular diastolic dysfunction are associated with exercise intolerance in adults and adolescents with homozygous sickle cell anemia in the United States and United Kingdom. Circulation 2011;124:1452–60.

34. Ambrusko SJ, Gunawardena S, Sakara A, et al. Elevation of tricuspid regurgitant jet velocity, a marker for pulmonary hypertension in children with sickle cell disease. Pediatr Blood Cancer 2006;47:907–13.

35. Liem RI, Young LT, Thompson AA. Tricuspid regurgitant jet velocity is associated with hemolysis in children and young adults with sickle cell disease evaluated for pulmonary hypertension. Haematologica 2007;92:1549–52.

36. Kato GJ, Onyekwere OC, Gladwin MT. Pulmonary hypertension in sickle cell disease: relevance to children. Pediatr Hematol Oncol 2007;24:159–70.

37. Pashankar FD, Carbonella J, Bazzy-Asaad A, et al. Prevalence and risk factors of elevated pulmonary artery pressures in children with sickle cell disease. Pediatrics 2008;121:777–82.

38. Onyekwere OC, Campbell A, Teshome M, et al. Pulmonary hypertension in children and adolescents with sickle cell disease. Pediatr Cardiol 2008;29:309–12.

39. Bunn HF, Nathan DG, Dover GJ, et al. Pulmonary hypertension and nitric oxide depletion in sickle cell disease. Blood 2010;116:687–92.

40. Hebbel RP. Reconstructing sickle cell disease: a data-based analysis of the "hyperhemolysis paradigm" for pulmonary hypertension from the perspective of evidence-based medicine. Am J Hematol 2011;86:123–54.

41. Ataga KI, Moore CG, Hillery CA, et al. Coagulation activation and inflammation in sickle cell disease-associated pulmonary hypertension. Haematologica 2008;93:20–6.

42. van Beers EJ, Spronk HM, Ten Cate H, et al. No association of the hypercoagulable state with sickle cell disease related pulmonary hypertension. Haematologica 2008;93:e42–4.

43. Westerman M, Pizzey A, Hirschman J, et al. Microvesicles in haemoglobinopathies offer insights into mechanisms of hypercoagulability, haemolysis and the effects of therapy. Br J Haematol 2008;142:126–35.

44. Villagra J, Shiva S, Hunter LA, et al. Platelet activation in patients with sickle disease, hemolysis-associated pulmonary hypertension, and nitric oxide scavenging by cell-free hemoglobin. Blood 2007;110:2166–72.

45. Hagger D, Wolff S, Owen J, et al. Changes in coagulation and fibrinolysis in patients with sickle cell disease compared with healthy black controls. Blood Coagul Fibrinolysis 1995;6:93–9.

46. Setty BN, Rao AK, Stuart MJ. Thrombophilia in sickle cell disease: the red cell connection. Blood 2001;98:3228–33.

47. Hoeper MM, Niedermeyer J, Hoffmeyer F, et al. Pulmonary hypertension after splenectomy? Ann Intern Med 1999;130:506–9.

48. Atichartakarn V, Likittanasombat K, Chuncharunee S, et al. Pulmonary arterial hypertension in previously splenectomized patients with beta-thalassemic disorders. Int J Hematol 2003;78:139–45.

49. Chou R, DeLoughery TG. Recurrent thromboembolic disease following splenectomy for pyruvate kinase deficiency. Am J Hematol 2001;67:197–9.

50. Hayag-Barin JE, Smith RE, Tucker FC Jr. Hereditary spherocytosis, thrombocytosis, and chronic pulmonary emboli: a case report and review of the literature. Am J Hematol 1998;57:82–4.

51. Atichartakarn V, Angchaisuksiri P, Aryurachai K, et al. In vivo platelet activation and hyperaggregation in hemoglobin E/beta-thalassemia: a consequence of splenectomy. Int J Hematol 2003;77:299–303.

52. Ergul S, Brunson CY, Hutchinson J, et al. Vasoactive factors in sickle cell disease: in vitro evidence for endothelin-1-mediated vasoconstriction. Am J Hematol 2004;76:245–51.

53. Barst RJ, McGoon M, Torbicki A, et al. Diagnosis and differential assessment of pulmonary arterial hypertension. J Am Coll Cardiol 2004;43:40S–7S.

54. McGoon M, Gutterman D, Steen V, et al. Screening, early detection, and diagnosis of pulmonary arterial hypertension: ACCP evidence-based clinical practice guidelines. Chest 2004;126:14S–34S.

55. Machado RF, Kyle Mack A, Martyr S, et al. Severity of pulmonary hypertension during vaso-occlusive pain crisis and exercise in patients with sickle cell disease. Br J Haematol 2007;136:319–25.

56. Mekontso Dessap A, Leon R, Habibi A, et al. Pulmonary hypertension and cor pulmonale during severe acute chest syndrome in sickle cell disease. Am J Respir Crit Care Med 2008;177:646–53.

57. Koumbourlis AC, Hurlet-Jensen A, Bye MR. Lung function in infants with sickle cell disease. Pediatr Pulmonol 1997;24:277–81.

58. Koumbourlis AC, Zar HJ, Hurlet-Jensen A, et al. Prevalence and reversibility of lower airway obstruction in children with sickle cell disease. J Pediatr 2001;138:188–92.

59. Lonsdorfer J, Bogui P, Otayeck A, et al. Cardiorespiratory adjustments in chronic sickle cell anemia. Bull Eur Physiopathol Respir 1983;19:339–44.

60. Powars D, Weidman JA, Odom-Maryon T, et al. Sickle cell chronic lung disease: prior morbidity and the risk of pulmonary failure. Medicine 1988;67:66–76.

61. Santoli F, Zerah F, Vasile N, et al. Pulmonary function in sickle cell disease with or without acute chest syndrome. Eur Respir J 1998;12:1124–9.

62. Young RC Jr, Rachal RE, Reindorf CA, et al. Lung function in sickle cell hemoglobinopathy patients compared with healthy subjects. J Natl Med Assoc 1988;80:509–14.

63. Anthi A, Machado RF, Jison ML, et al. Hemodynamic and functional assessment of patients with sickle cell disease and pulmonary hypertension. Am J Respir Crit Care Med 2007;175:1272–9.

64. Yung GL, Channick RN, Fedullo PF, et al. Successful pulmonary thromboendarterectomy in two patients with sickle cell disease. Am J Respir Crit Care Med 1998;157:1690–3.

65. Sachdev V, Machado RF, Shizukuda Y, et al. Diastolic dysfunction is an independent risk factor for death in patients with sickle cell disease. J Am Coll Cardiol 2007;49:472–9.

66. Platt OS. Hydroxyurea for the treatment of sickle cell anemia. N Engl J Med 2008;358:1362–9.

67. Lanzkron S, Strouse JJ, Wilson R, et al. Systematic review: hydroxyurea for the treatment of adults with sickle cell disease. Ann Intern Med 2008;148:939–55.

68. Derchi G, Forni GL, Formisano F, et al. Efficacy and safety of sildenafil in the treatment of severe pulmonary hypertension in patients with hemoglobinopathies. Haematologica 2005;90:452–8.

69. Machado RF, Martyr S, Kato GJ, et al. Sildenafil therapy in patients with sickle disease and pulmonary hypertension. Br J Haematol 2005;130:445–53.

70. Machado RF, Barst RJ, Yovetich NA, et al. Hospitalization for pain in patients with sickle cell disease treated with sildenafil for elevated TRV and low exercise capacity. Blood 2011;118:855–64.

71. Minniti CP, Machado RF, Coles WA, et al. Endothelin receptor antagonists for pulmonary hypertension in adult patients with sickle cell disease. Br J Haematol 2009;147:737–43.

72. Barst RJ, Mubarak KK, Machado RF, et al. Exercise capacity and haemodynamics in patients with sickle cell disease with pulmonary hypertension treated with bosentan: results of the ASSET studies. Br J Haematol 2010;149:426–35.

73. Koch CA, Li CY, Mesa RA, et al. Nonhepatosplenic extramedullary hematopoiesis: associated diseases, pathology, clinical course, and treatment. Mayo Clin Proc 2003;78:1223–33.

74. Weatherall DJ. The thalassaemias. BMJ 1997;314: 1675–8.

75. Grisaru D, Rachmilewitz EA, Mosseri M, et al. Cardiopulmonary assessment in beta-thalassemia major. Chest 1990;98:1138–42.

76. Du ZD, Roguin N, Milgram E, et al. Pulmonary hypertension in patients with thalassemia major. Am Heart J 1997;134:532–7.

77. Derchi G, Fonti A, Forni GL, et al. Pulmonary hypertension in patients with thalassemia major. Am Heart J 1999;138:384.

78. Aessopos A, Farmakis D, Hatziliami A, et al. Cardiac status in well-treated patients with thalassemia major. Eur J Haematol 2004;73:359–66.

79. Hagar RW, Morris CR, Vichinsky EP. Pulmonary hypertension in thalassaemia major patients with normal left ventricular systolic function. Br J Haematol 2006;133:433–5.

80. Aessopos A, Farmakis D, Deftereos S, et al. Thalassemia heart disease: a comparative evaluation of thalassemia major and thalassemia intermedia. Chest 2005;127:1523–30.

81. Aessopos A, Stamatelos G, Skoumas V, et al. Pulmonary hypertension and right heart failure in patients with beta-thalassemia intermedia. Chest 1995;107:50–3.

82. Aessopos A, Farmakis D, Karagiorga M, et al. Cardiac involvement in thalassemia intermedia: a multicenter study. Blood 2001;97:3411–6.

83. Aessopos A, Farmakis D. Pulmonary hypertension in beta-thalassemia. Ann N Y Acad Sci 2005; 1054:342–9.

84. Aessopos A, Kati M, Meletis J. Thalassemia intermedia today: should patients regularly receive transfusions? Transfusion 2007;47:792–800.

85. Taher AT, Musallam KM, Karimi M, et al. Overview on practices in thalassemia intermedia management aiming for lowering complication rates across a region of endemicity: the OPTIMAL CARE study. Blood 2010;115:1886–92.

86. Atichartakarn V, Chuncharunee S, Chandanamattha P, et al. Correction of hypercoagulability and amelioration of pulmonary arterial hypertension by chronic blood transfusion in an asplenic hemoglobin E/beta-thalassemia patient. Blood 2004;103:2844–6.

87. Karimi M, Borzouee M, Mehrabani A, et al. Echocardiographic finding in beta-thalassemia intermedia and major: absence of pulmonary hypertension following hydroxyurea treatment in beta-thalassemia intermedia. Eur J Haematol 2009;82:213–8.

88. Morris CR, Kim HY, Wood JC, et al. Sildenafil therapy in thalassemia patients with Doppler-defined risk for pulmonary hypertension. Haematologica 2013;98:1359–67.

89. Anthi A, Tsangaris I, Hamodraka ES, et al. Treatment with bosentan in a patient with thalassemia intermedia and pulmonary arterial hypertension. Blood 2012;120:1531–2.

90. Tam DH, Farber HW. Pulmonary hypertension and beta-thalassemia major: report of a case, its treatment, and a review of the literature. Am J Hematol 2006;81:443–7.

91. Brodsky RA. Paroxysmal nocturnal hemoglobinuria. In: Hoffman R, Benz EJ, Shattil SJ, editors. Hematology: basic principles and practice. 4th edition. Philadelphia: Elsevier Churchill Livingstone; 2005. p. 419–27.

92. Heller PG, Grinberg AR, Lencioni M, et al. Pulmonary hypertension in paroxysmal nocturnal hemoglobinuria. Chest 1992;102:642–3.

93. Szer J, Hill A, Weitz IC. Clinical roundtable monograph: paroxysmal nocturnal hemoglobinuria: a case-based discussion. Clin Adv Hematol Oncol 2012;10:1–16.

94. Hill A, Sapsford RJ, Scally A, et al. Under-recognized complications in patients with paroxysmal nocturnal haemoglobinuria: raised pulmonary pressure and reduced right ventricular function. Br J Haematol 2012;158:409–14.

95. Hill A, Rother RP, Wang X, et al. Effect of eculizumab on haemolysis-associated nitric oxide depletion, dyspnoea, and measures of pulmonary hypertension in patients with paroxysmal nocturnal haemoglobinuria. Br J Haematol 2010;149:414–25.

96. Hillmen P, Hall C, Marsh JC, et al. Effect of eculizumab on hemolysis and transfusion requirements in patients with paroxysmal nocturnal hemoglobinuria. N Engl J Med 2004;350:552–9.

97. Hillmen P, Muus P, Duhrsen U, et al. Effect of the complement inhibitor eculizumab on thromboembolism in patients with paroxysmal nocturnal hemoglobinuria. Blood 2007;110:4123–8.

98. Schilling RF, Gangnon RE, Traver MI. Delayed adverse vascular events after splenectomy in hereditary spherocytosis. J Thromb Haemost 2008; 6:1289–95.

99. Jardine DL, Laing AD. Delayed pulmonary hypertension following splenectomy for congenital spherocytosis. Intern Med J 2004;34:214–6.

100. Smedema JP, Louw VJ. Pulmonary arterial hypertension after splenectomy for hereditary spherocytosis. Cardiovasc J Afr 2007;18:84–9.

101. Crary SE, Ramaciotti C, Buchanan GR. Prevalence of pulmonary hypertension in hereditary spherocytosis. Am J Hematol 2011;86:E73–6.

102. Chetty MC, Stewart GW. Pseudohyperkalaemia and pseudomacrocytosis caused by inherited red-cell disorders of the 'hereditary stomatocytosis' group. Br J Biomed Sci 2001;58:48–55.

103. Coles SE, Stewart GW. Temperature effects on cation transport in hereditary stomatocytosis and allied disorders. Int J Exp Pathol 1999;80: 251–8.

104. Yoshimoto A, Fujimura M, Nakao S. Pulmonary hypertension after splenectomy in hereditary stomatocytosis. Am J Med Sci 2005;330:195–7.

105. Stewart GW, Amess JA, Eber SW, et al. Thromboembolic disease after splenectomy for hereditary stomatocytosis. Br J Haematol 1996;93:303–10.

106. Murali B, Drain A, Seller D, et al. Pulmonary thromboendarterectomy in a case of hereditary stomatocytosis. Br J Anaesth 2003;91:739–41.

107. Jais X, Till SJ, Cynober T, et al. An extreme consequence of splenectomy in dehydrated hereditary stomatocytosis: gradual thrombo-embolic pulmonary hypertension and lung-heart transplantation. Hemoglobin 2003;27:139–47.

108. Swerdlow SH, Campo E, Harris NL. WHO classification of tumors of haematopoietic and lymphoid tissues. 4th edition. 2008.

109. Guilpain P, Montani D, Damaj G, et al. Pulmonary hypertension associated with myeloproliferative disorders: a retrospective study of ten cases. Respiration 2008;76:295–302.

110. Cortelezzi A, Gritti G, Del Papa N, et al. Pulmonary arterial hypertension in primary myelofibrosis is common and associated with an altered angiogenic status. Leukemia 2008;22:646–9.

111. Cortelezzi A, Colombo G, Pellegrini C, et al. Bone marrow glycophorin-positive erythroid cells of myelodysplastic patients responding to high-dose rHuEPO therapy have a different gene expression pattern from those of nonresponders. Am J Hematol 2008;83:531–9.

112. Altintas A, Karahan Z, Pasa S, et al. Pulmonary hypertension in patients with essential thrombocythemia and reactive thrombocytosis. Leuk Lymphoma 2007;48:1981–7.

113. Gupta R, Perumandla S, Patsiornik Y, et al. Incidence of pulmonary hypertension in patients with chronic myeloproliferative disorders. J Natl Med Assoc 2006;98:1779–82.

114. Di Stefano F. Pulmonary arterial hypertension and chronic myeloproliferative disorders. Am J Respir Crit Care Med 2006;174:616.

115. Ziakas PD, Voulgarelis M, Felekouras E, et al. Myelofibrosis-associated massive splenomegaly: a cause of increased intra-abdominal pressure, pulmonary hypertension, and positional dyspnea. Am J Hematol 2005;80:128–32.

116. Popat U, Frost A, Liu E, et al. New onset of myelofibrosis in association with pulmonary arterial hypertension. Ann Intern Med 2005;143:466–7.

117. Garypidou V, Vakalopoulou S, Dimitriadis D, et al. Incidence of pulmonary hypertension in patients with chronic myeloproliferative disorders. Haematologica 2004;89:245–6.

118. Dingli D, Utz JP, Krowka MJ, et al. Unexplained pulmonary hypertension in chronic myeloproliferative disorders. Chest 2001;120:801–8.

119. Garcia-Manero G, Schuster SJ, Patrick H, et al. Pulmonary hypertension in patients with myelofibrosis secondary to myeloproliferative diseases. Am J Hematol 1999;60:130–5.

120. Hill G, McClean D, Fraser R, et al. Pulmonary hypertension as a consequence of alveolar capillary plugging by malignant megakaryocytes in essential thrombocythaemia. Aust N Z J Med 1996;26:852–3.

121. Nand S, Orfei E. Pulmonary hypertension in polycythemia vera. Am J Hematol 1994;47:242–4.

122. Marvin KS, Spellberg RD. Pulmonary hypertension secondary to thrombocytosis in a patient with myeloid metaplasia. Chest 1993;103:642–4.

123. Adir Y, Humbert M. Pulmonary hypertension in patients with chronic myeloproliferative disorders. Eur Respir J 2010;35:1396–406.

124. Spivak JL. Polycythemia vera: myths, mechanisms, and management. Blood 2002;100:4272–90.

125. Willems E, Canivet JL, Ghaye B, et al. Pulmonary veno-occlusive disease in myeloproliferative disorders. Eur Respir J 2009;33:213–6.

126. Zetterberg E, Popat U, Hasselbalch H, et al. Angiogenesis in pulmonary hypertension with myelofibrosis. Haematologica 2008;93:945–6.

127. Landolfi R, Di Gennaro L, Falanga A. Thrombosis in myeloproliferative disorders: pathogenetic facts and speculation. Leukemia 2008;22:2020–8.

128. Gomez N, Sierra MV, Cortelezzi A, et al. Effects of discharges from the textile industry on the biotic integrity of benthic assemblages. Ecotoxicol Environ Saf 2008;69:472–9.

129. Dot JM, Sztrymf B, Yaici A, et al. Pulmonary arterial hypertension due to tumor emboli. Rev Mal Respir 2007;24:359–66.

130. Popat U, Frost A, Liu E, et al. High levels of circulating CD34 cells, dacrocytes, clonal hematopoiesis, and JAK2 mutation differentiate myelofibrosis with myeloid metaplasia from secondary myelofibrosis associated with pulmonary hypertension. Blood 2006;107:3486–8.

131. Fadini GP, Schiavon M, Cantini M, et al. Circulating CD34+ cells, pulmonary hypertension, and myelofibrosis. Blood 2006;108:1776–7 [author reply: 7].

132. Halank M, Marx C, Baretton G, et al. Severe pulmonary hypertension in chronic idiopathic myelofibrosis. Onkologie 2004;27:472–4.

133. Weinschenker P, Kutner JM, Salvajoli JV, et al. Whole-pulmonary low-dose radiation therapy in agnogenic myeloid metaplasia with diffuse lung involvement. Am J Hematol 2002;69:277–80.

134. Steensma DP, Hook CC, Stafford SL, et al. Low-dose, single-fraction, whole-lung radiotherapy for pulmonary hypertension associated with myelofibrosis with myeloid metaplasia. Br J Haematol 2002;118:813–6.

135. Haznedaroglu IC, Atalar E, Ozturk MA, et al. Thrombopoietin inside the pulmonary vessels in patients with and without pulmonary hypertension. Platelets 2002;13:395–9.
136. Hibbin JA, Njoku OS, Matutes E, et al. Myeloid progenitor cells in the circulation of patients with myelofibrosis and other myeloproliferative disorders. Br J Haematol 1984;57:495–503.
137. Montani D, Bergot E, Gunther S, et al. Pulmonary arterial hypertension in patients treated by dasatinib. Circulation 2012;125:2128–37.
138. Lee WC, Lin HC, Tsay SH, et al. Esophageal variceal ligation for esophageal variceal hemorrhage in a patient with portal and primary pulmonary hypertension complicating myelofibrosis. Dig Dis Sci 2001;46:915–9.
139. Trow TK, Argento AC, Rubinowitz AN, et al. 71-year-old woman with myelofibrosis, hypoxemia, and pulmonary hypertension. Chest 2010;138:1506–10.
140. Streiff MB, Smith B, Spivak JL. The diagnosis and management of polycythemia vera in the era since the Polycythemia Vera Study Group: a survey of American Society of Hematology members' practice patterns. Blood 2002;99:1144–9.
141. Simonneau G, Robbins IM, Beghetti M, et al. Updated clinical classification of pulmonary hypertension. J Am Coll Cardiol 2009;54:S43–54.
142. Meera V, Jijina F, Ghosh K. Pulmonary hypertension in patients with hematological disorders following splenectomy. Indian J Hematol Blood Transfus 2010;26:2–5.
143. Peacock AJ. Pulmonary hypertension after splenectomy: a consequence of loss of the splenic filter or is there something more? Thorax 2005;60:983–4.
144. Lo SM, Liu J, Chen F, et al. Pulmonary vascular disease in Gaucher disease: clinical spectrum, determinants of phenotype and long-term outcomes of therapy. J Inherit Metab Dis 2011;34:643–50.

World Health Organization Group 5 Pulmonary Hypertension

Tim Lahm, MD[a],*, Murali M. Chakinala, MD[b],*

KEYWORDS

- Sarcoidosis • Lymphangioleiomyomatosis • Pulmonary Langerhans cell histiocytosis • Renal failure
- Splenectomy • Fibrosing mediastinitis • Myeloproliferative disorders • Metabolic disorders

KEY POINTS

- World Health Organization group 5 PH entails PH caused by hematologic disorders, systemic diseases, metabolic disorders, and other entities (eg, chronic renal failure, pulmonary vascular obstruction).
- Although the prevalence of PH in group 5 conditions is variable, the presence of PH is frequently associated with worse outcomes.
- Major mechanisms for PH development in group 5 conditions include left heart disease, high-output heart failure, parenchymal lung disease, proinflammatory states, proliferative arteriopathy, chronic thromboemboli, pulmonary veno-occlusive disease, and obstruction or compression of the pulmonary vasculature.
- Pulmonary venous hypertension needs to be excluded as a cause of PH in group 5 conditions, because therapeutic approaches differ significantly from those for other causes of PH.
- Treatment of PH in group 5 conditions focuses on treatment of the underlying disorder.
- The role of pulmonary vasodilators, although conceptually appealing in certain conditions, is understudied in group 5 PH and needs further investigation.

INTRODUCTION

Pulmonary hypertension (PH) with unclear multifactorial mechanisms or group 5 PH is an important category in the Dana Point classification scheme (**Box 1**).[1] Although often overlooked, there are many interesting and challenging entities in this heterogeneous category. Because the diseases in this category do not share a common vascular pathobiology (as is the case in other Dana Point categories), group 5 was assembled because PH occurs for either unclear reasons or because of multiple mechanisms, some of which mirror the pathways of group 1 to 4 PH.

This article first discusses common pathogenic mechanisms leading to PH. The bulk of the article is devoted to specific disorders that can be complicated by PH, including various hematologic disorders, systemic disorders, and metabolic

Disclosures: T. Lahm, research support for investigator-initiated research from Pfizer and Gilead. M. M. Chakinala, consultant for Actelion, Gilead, United Therapeutics; speaker's bureau for Gilead and United Therapeutics; research support from Actelion, Gilead, United Therapeutics, Novartis, Medtronics, Bayer, Ikaria, Aires.
[a] Division of Pulmonary, Allergy, Critical Care, Occupational and Sleep Medicine, Department of Medicine, Richard L. Roudebush VA Medical Center, Center for Immunobiology, Indiana University School of Medicine, 980 West Walnut Street, Room C400, Indianapolis, IN 46202, USA; [b] Division of Pulmonary and Critical Care Medicine, Department of Medicine, Washington University School of Medicine, 660 South Euclid Avenue, Campus Box 8052, St Louis, MO 63110, USA
* Corresponding authors.
E-mail addresses: tlahm@iu.edu (T. Lahm); mchakina@dom.wustl.edu (M.M. Chakinala).

Clin Chest Med 34 (2013) 753–778
http://dx.doi.org/10.1016/j.ccm.2013.08.005

Box 1
Overview of World Health Organization (WHO)
PH groups with emphasis on WHO group 5

1. WHO group 1 PH: pulmonary arterial hypertension (PAH)

2. WHO group 2 PH: pulmonary hypertension caused by left heart disease

3. WHO group 3 PH: pulmonary hypertension caused by lung diseases and/or hypoxia

4. WHO group 4 PH: Chronic thromboembolic pulmonary hypertension (CTEPH)

5. WHO group 5 PH: Pulmonary hypertension with unclear multifactorial mechanisms

   5.1. Hematologic disorders: *myeloproliferative disorders, splenectomy,* hemoglobinopathies

   5.2. Systemic disorders: *sarcoidosis, pulmonary Langerhans cell histiocytosis, lymphangioleiomyomatosis, neurofibromatosis, vasculitis,* Whipple disease, POEMS (Polyneuropathy, Organomegaly, Endocrinopathy, Monoclonal protein, Skin changes) syndrome

   5.3. Metabolic disorders: *glycogen storage disorder, Gaucher disease, thyroid disorders,* Hurler syndrome/Hurler-Scheie syndrome

   5.4. Others: compression of pulmonary vessels (*fibrosing mediastinitis,* lymphadenopathy, tumor), obstruction of pulmonary vessels (endovascular tumor, *tumor emboli, pulmonary tumor thrombotic microangiopathy, pulmonary vein stenosis*), *chronic renal failure* on dialysis

Group 5 entities listed in italics are discussed in detail in this article.

disorders. Key aspects of PH in these various conditions, including epidemiology, pathogenesis, and disease-specific management, are emphasized. In addition, off-label use of vasomodulatory therapies, typically indicated for pulmonary arterial hypertension (PAH, group 1), in certain group 5 conditions is discussed. However, many of the group 5 disorders are either rare, or PH is an uncommon manifestation of the primary disorder, leading to an overall dearth of published experience, which primarily comprises small case series or individual case reports. Nevertheless, many of these conditions are frequently encountered in clinical practice, especially by pulmonologists and other specialists, and PH can have significant implications for overall management, thus warranting attention in this issue.

In order to understand the complex and variable pathophysiology of group 5 PH, it is vital to understand the various physiologic determinants of the pulmonary artery (PA) pressure (PAP), because derangements in any of these determinants can increase PAPs (**Fig. 1**). The pulmonary vascular resistance (PVR) is the ratio of pressure decline across the pulmonary circuit (ie, difference between precapillary pressure [mean PAP (mPAP)] and postcapillary pressure [pulmonary capillary wedge pressure (PCWP)], as an estimate of the left atrial pressure) and blood flow per minute through the circuit (ie, cardiac output [CO]). Rearranging this equation for PAP reveals that the pulmonary pressure is determined by postcapillary pressure (left atrial pressure), blood flow (CO), and the resistance to flow (PVR). Each of these three broad components (postcapillary pressures, blood flow, and vascular resistance) can be abnormal in group 5 and lead to PH (see **Fig. 1**).

PATHOGENESIS OF GROUP 5 PH

The mechanisms for development of group 5 PH are multiple and incompletely understood. The major recurring pathogenic mechanisms are summarized in **Fig. 1**. *Pulmonary vasoconstriction* may result from hypoxia in cases of chronic lung disease, from release of vasoactive cytokines in proinflammatory states, and from a vasoconstrictor/vasodilator imbalance similar to that observed in PAH.[2,3] *Compression of pulmonary vessels* may occur at a distal alveolar level caused by fibrotic lung disease or alveolar hyperinflation, or in a more proximal location caused by compression of central arteries or veins from fibrosing mediastinitis,[4,5] lymphadenopathy,[6] or tumor burden. *Destruction of alveolar vessels* can be seen as a consequence of structural distortion of the lung in conditions like sarcoidosis[6] or lymphangioleiomyomatosis (LAM).[7]

Pulmonary venous hypertension may occur as a consequence of central vein stenosis or left atrial stiffening after pulmonary vein isolation/ablation,[8,9] or may be caused by stiffness of left-sided cardiac chambers when systolic and/or diastolic left ventricular (LV) dysfunction complicates sarcoidosis,[10] sickle cell disease,[11,12] or chronic renal failure (CRF).[13] *Volume overload* contributes to pulmonary pressure increases in CRF-PH.[13] *Veno-occlusive changes* have been described in myeloproliferative disorders (MPDs), sarcoidosis, and pulmonary Langerhans cell histiocytosis (PLCH).[6,14–17]

PA occlusion can result as a consequence of tumor emboli, emboli with other material (eg, amniotic fluid, foreign material), or intravascular tumors

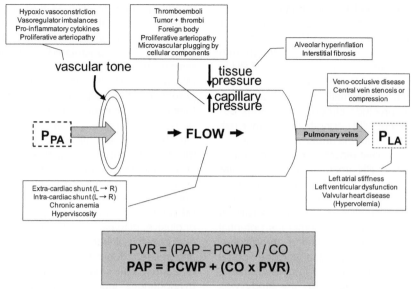

Fig. 1. Determinants of PAP and pathogenic mechanisms of group 5 PH. PAP is determined by PCWP, CO, and PVR. These variables are influenced by pulmonary blood flow, vascular tone, tissue pressure, capillary pressure, and resistance in the pulmonary venous system and left atrium. Each of these components can be altered in group 5 PH. CO, cardiac output; PCWP, pulmonary capillary wedge pressure; P_{LA}, left atrial pressure; P_{PA}, PA pressure; PVR, pulmonary vascular resistance. (*Courtesy of* John Newman, Vanderbilt University, with permission.)

(eg, PA sarcoma).[18–21] In MPDs, circulating megakaryocytes can also obstruct the pulmonary vasculature and secrete vasoactive cytokines.[22–24] MPDs and splenectomy are associated with *pulmonary vascular thrombosis* and subsequent development of *chronic thromboembolic PH* (CTEPH).[25]

A *proliferative arteriopathy* has been described in sarcoidosis, PLCH, and in glycogen storage disease (GSD), mediated at least in part by activation of proinflammatory cytokines and growth factors.[6,17,26–29] *Inflammation and growth factor activation* are also purported to be prominent contributors to PH pathogenesis in the context of other systemic disorders and MPDs.[30–32] For example, PH development in the latter condition has been associated with pulmonary myeloid infiltration,[33,34] and PH in PLCH, LAM, or CRF has been linked to direct actions of proinflammatory and proproliferative mediators on the pulmonary vasculature.[35–38]

A *high-output circulatory state* contributes to the pathogenesis of PH in patients with chronic hemolytic anemias,[11,12] hyperthyroidism,[39,40] or artificial shunts (eg, arteriovenous fistulas in CRF,[41,42] even though this association has recently been disputed[43]).

Drugs or procedures used to treat systemic disorders may also be implicated in development of group 5 PH. Examples include dasatinib, a tyrosine kinase inhibitor used to treat refractory chronic myelogenous leukemia,[44] or hemodialysis, which contributes to PH development via blood-membrane interactions and a subsequent proinflammatory state.[38,45]

In addition, *portal hypertension with portosystemic shunting*, which is encountered in systemic diseases as well as MPDs,[32,46] and *portocaval shunting* and/or *atrial septal defects*, as seen in metabolic disorders,[28,29] can lead to PH through a proliferative vasculopathy.

OVERVIEW OF DISEASE ENTITIES ASSOCIATED WITH GROUP 5 PH
Group 5.1: Hematologic Disorders

PH has been described in 3 broad categories of hematologic disorders: MPDs, postsplenectomy state, and chronic hemolytic anemia (or hemoglobinopathy); the first 2 categories are discussed in this article, while chronic hemolytic anemia is covered separately by Machado and Farber elsewhere in this issue.

PH in patients with myeloproliferative diseases (MPDs)

MPDs linked to PH (polycythemia vera [PV], essential thrombocythemia [ET], and primary myelofibrosis) comprise 1 subcategory of the World Health Organization (WHO) grouping of chronic myeloproliferative diseases, and associations with PH date back as far as the early 1990s. Several groups have described PH occurring in 30% to 50% of their cohorts of patients with MPDs, but based only on an echo-derived PA systolic pressure (PASP) greater than or equal to 35 mm Hg[31,47–49]; therefore, the true prevalence of PH in MPD is unknown (but likely less than these estimates suggest). The small numbers of cases in these series preclude strong associations between the different MPD conditions or other risk factors associated with the underlying disorder.

In one of the earliest reports, 26 patients developed unexplained PH (median right ventricular [RV] systolic pressure [RVSP] 71 mm Hg, range 32–105 mm Hg) at a median of 8 years after MPD had been established.[50] Characteristic of this subtype of group 5 PH, numerous potential causes for PH existed, including thrombosis, drug-induced mechanisms (eg, anagrelide), portal hypertension, splenectomy, high-output states, and postcapillary PH. However, the study was limited by incomplete work-up for CTEPH and a lack of lung histology. Serial assessments noted persistent PH in spite of controlling underlying MPD, and 80% of patients died at a median of only 18 months after PH was diagnosed. In contrast, Guilpain and colleagues[51] thoroughly evaluated 10 patients with MPD, including heart catheterization, and separated cases into 2 PH groups: CTEPH and PAH (later referred to as precapillary PH mimicking PAH by Adir and Humbert[32]).

Patients with MPDs, particularly those with PV and ET, are prone to thrombophilia with arterial and venous thromboses caused by a combination of increased cell counts, hyperviscosity, increased platelet activation, increased red cell aggregation, and polymorphonuclear cell (PMN) activation.[32] A JAK-2 gene mutation (V617F) that underlies nearly all cases of PV and roughly half of the cases of ET and myelofibrosis may provide the genetic underpinning to many of these prothrombotic mechanisms.[52–56] In addition, splenectomy, which is a therapy for certain forms of MPD, may further predispose individuals to CTEPH (discussed later). In Guilpain and colleagues'[51] series, CTEPH cases were detected at a much younger age than the precapillary PH cases, and at the same time that an underlying MPD was recognized.

The other form of PH in MPD (precapillary PH) involves the microcirculation and typically presents years after the diagnosis of MPD has been established; limited histologic examinations have revealed infiltration of the lung by hematopoietic cells, consistent with pulmonary myeloid metaplasia, or acute leukemic cells.[33,34,51,57] In addition, microcirculatory obstruction by circulating megakaryocytes and increased levels of

thrombopoietin, as well as thrombocytosis with increased platelet activation and secretion of platelet-derived growth factor (PDGF) or serotonin, have been postulated to induce vascular remodeling and PH.[22,23,58,59] Patients with MPDs with PH also have increased angiogenic potential with increased levels of vascular endothelial growth factor and increased microvessel density in the bone marrow; this may carry over into the pulmonary microcirculation.[30,31] Furthermore, portal hypertension is a known long-term consequence of the myeloid metaplasia that accompanies myelofibrosis, which makes portopulmonary hypertension a consideration in MPD.[50,51,60,61] In addition, pulmonary venoocclusive disease (PVOD) has been described and possibly linked to the cytoreductive agent, anagrelide.[15] More recently dasatinib, a multitargeted tyrosine kinase inhibitor used in chronic myelogenous leukemia, has been linked to a form of precapillary PH that is at least partially reversible soon after drug discontinuation.[44,62]

PH in patients after splenectomy

Asplenia increases the risk for PH after splenectomy for trauma, MPDs, or Gaucher disease (GD).[63–66] One of the first reports linking asplenia to PAH came from Hoeper and colleagues,[65] who estimated an 11.5% prevalence of splenectomy in patients with idiopathic PAH (IPAH), which is significantly higher than the splenectomy rate in the general population. Explants from 3 of the patients revealed a plexogenic arteriopathy with abundant thrombotic lesions.[65] In contrast, Jais and colleagues[63] determined a splenectomy frequency of 8.5% in a large cohort of patients with CTEPH but only a 2.5% rate in an IPAH group, which was still considerably higher than in a comparator group of other pulmonary disorders. It is unclear what accounted for the significant difference in splenectomy rates in the IPAH cohorts between the two studies; misclassification of IPAH and missed cases of CTEPH by Hoeper and colleagues[65] is unlikely because most of their IPAH cohort had negative pulmonary angiograms. Nevertheless, splenectomy has been accepted as a risk factor for developing CTEPH.[25] Length of time between splenectomy and PAH detection was long: 16 years[63] and 22 years.[65] The risk of CTEPH seems to be particularly high when splenectomy is performed for a hemolytic process,[66,67] suggesting a synergistic effect of the two conditions; however, patients with posttraumatic splenectomy are also susceptible to PAH.[63]

PH after splenectomy seems to be caused by a hypercoagulable state and subsequent in situ thrombosis as a consequence of megakaryocytes lodging in the pulmonary capillary bed and releasing platelets, inadequate removal of platelets, platelet activation by activated PMNs, and by inadequately cleared senescent and/or damaged red cells.[52,67–70] Excessive red cell thrombin generation further contributes to hypercoagulability.[67] Supportive evidence comes from an animal model of splenectomy in which intravenous injection of hemolysate induced platelet-rich thrombi in the pulmonary circulation.[71] In addition to activating platelets and generating thrombin, hemolyzed red cells may also contribute to postsplenectomy PH development via release of free hemoglobin and subsequent nitric oxide (NO) scavenging.[72,73]

In summary, asplenic patients are susceptible to PH after an extended period of time, regardless of the indication for splenectomy. Furthermore, in situ thrombosis seems to be an integral part of the disorder with a continuum of clinical presentations from surgically accessible proximal vessel involvement (ie, CTEPH) to medically managed distal thrombi as part of plexogenic arteriopathy (IPAH).

Patients with known or suspected MPD and/or asplenia require a comprehensive evaluation of PH when present.[74] Emphasis is placed on excluding thromboembolic disease, preferably with ventilation-perfusion scanning followed by pulmonary angiogram or computed tomography (CT) angiogram with experienced radiologic interpretation, especially in asplenic patients. Right heart catheterization (RHC) is paramount to exclude left-sided cardiac dysfunction and a high-output state. Given its rarity and limited published experience, management of PH in MPD is extrapolated from other PH populations, based on mechanistic similarities. Steps should be taken to control the underlying MPD with cytoreductive therapy and potentially plateletpheresis, if platelet counts are extremely high, based on isolated reports of improved hemodynamics with cell reduction.[75] Whole-lung low-dose radiation has been used in pulmonary myeloid metaplasia as a palliative intervention.[33,34] Antiplatelet therapy has not had an impact even though platelet dysfunction is speculated to be a key element in MPD.[50] CTEPH should be managed similar to any other case of CTEPH with anticoagulation, right heart failure management (ie, diuretics, oxygen), and thromboendarterectomy if the organized thrombus involves proximal pulmonary vessels.

Group 5.2: Systemic Disorders

Several systemic disorders have been shown to cause PH. These disorders include sarcoidosis,

PLCH, LAM, neurofibromatosis type 1 (NF1), and pulmonary vasculitides. These entities are discussed in detail in this chapter. A summary of the characteristics of PH in these settings is provided in **Table 1**. Other systemic disorders that may cause PH (eg, Whipple disease,[76] POEMS (Polyneuropathy, Organomegaly, Endocrinopathy, Monoclonal protein, Skin changes) syndrome[77]) are not reviewed because of space limitations.

Sarcoidosis-associated PH (SAPH)

Pulmonary involvement in sarcoidosis occurs in more than 90% of patients.[78] The overall prevalence of PH in sarcoidosis has been reported to be 5% to 15%[79,80]; however, prevalence increases to 50% to 60% in dyspneic patients,[81–83] and to 74% to 79% in patients listed for lung transplantation.[84,85] Even though these studies are confounded by the use of different methodologies for PH assessment (echocardiogram vs RHC): and because of inherent referral bias, these data indicate that sarcoidosis-associated PH (SAPH) is frequently associated with parenchymal lung disease.[86,87] SAPH most commonly occurs in the context of advanced stage IV disease; however, the severity of SAPH does not correlate with the severity of parenchymal lung disease or blood gas abnormalities, and SAPH may even be more severe in the setting of normal lung function and preserved parenchymal architecture.[6,82,84]

Even though SAPH is frequently mild to moderate in severity, mPAP greater than 40 mm Hg can be observed in more than a third of patients with advanced sarcoidosis and/or dyspnea despite immunosuppressive treatment.[10,86] The occurrence of PH in sarcoidosis is associated with impaired functional status and worse survival.[10,86,88]

Several potential causes of SAPH have been described (**Box 2**).[46,78,83] Although fibrotic lung disease with destruction and/or compression of alveolar vessels is a major contributor to SAPH development (seen in 68% of cases in the series by Nunes and colleagues[6]), the observation that SAPH can occur with normal lung function and preserved parenchymal architecture suggests that other factors play a significant role. These factors include a granulomatous pulmonary arteriopathy, PVOD, compression of pulmonary arteries caused by lymphadenoadenopathy or mediastinal fibrosis, LV systolic or diastolic dysfunction, pulmonary vasculitis, and portopulmonary hypertension.[46,78,83,89,90] In addition, obstructive sleep apnea is common in patients with sarcoidosis, and may also contribute to the development of PH.[91] These causes are reviewed in detail below.

Fibrocavitary disease may directly compress and/or destroy the pulmonary vasculature, or

Table 1
Differences and similarities between sarcoidosis-associated PH (SAPH), pulmonary Langerhans cell histiocytosis-PH (PLCH-PH), lymphangioleiomyomatosis-PH (LAM-PH), and neurofibromatosis type 1-PH (NF1-PH)

	PH Prevalence	Correlation with Structural Lung Disease	Severity of PH	Treatment Response
SAPH	Overall prevalence 5%–15% 50%–60% in patients with otherwise unexplained dyspnea 74%–79% in patients listed for lung transplants	Prevalence highest in stage IV disease PH severity not correlating with severity of parenchymal lung disease PH most severe in patients with preserved parenchymal architecture	Frequently mild to moderate mPAP >40 mm Hg in > one-third of patients with advanced sarcoidosis and/or dyspnea	PH in setting of fibrocavitary disease poorly responsive to therapy PH in absence of fibrotic disease fairly responsive to corticosteroid treatment ± pulmonary vasodilators
PLCH-PH	10.6% in unselected patients with PLCH 92%–100% in patients with advanced PLCH referred for lung transplantation	Predominantly seen in patients with significant parenchymal disease, but vascular changes frequently observed in regions not affected by PLCH lesions No significant correlation between lung function and hemodynamic parameters	Severe PH common Average mPAP in French PLCH registry 45 mm Hg; 66% of patients with mPAP $\geq$40 mm Hg	Use of PAH therapy associated with trend toward better survival rate in French registry
LAM-PH	7% in unselected patients with LAM 45% in patients with LAM referred for lung transplantation	Most common in patients with severe parenchymal disease No correlation between hemodynamic parameters and Pao_2	PH usually mild to moderate (mPAP 32 ± 6 mm Hg; PVR 376 ± 184 dyn·s·cm^{-5}) Significant impact of PH on oxygenation and functional capacity despite mild hemodynamic alterations	Significant hemodynamic improvements with PAH therapy in French registry Emerging role of sirolimus?
NF1-PH	Unknown	Concomitant lung disease (ILD, cysts, or bullae) described in 5 of 8 patients	Severe PH common Reported mean and median mPAPs 55 and 48 mm Hg RV failure and poor exercise capacity common	Poor outcomes despite treatment with PAH-specific drugs Early referral for lung transplantation recommended

Abbreviation: ILD, interstitial lung disease.

more indirectly lead to vessel tortuosity, turbulent pulmonary vascular flow, and shear stress, thus causing or exacerbating increases in PAP.[92] In addition, fibrosis and external compression may lead to vascular stiffness and decreased pulmonary vascular compliance.

Granulomatous involvement of the pulmonary arteries is common in SAPH. A series of 40

Box 2
Purported causes of SAPH

Fibrotic lung disease with destruction and/or compression of alveolar vessels

Granulomatous pulmonary arteriopathy

PVOD

Compression of pulmonary arteries by lymphadenopathy or fibrosing mediastinitis

LV systolic or diastolic dysfunction

Systemic vasculitis with pulmonary vascular involvement

Portopulmonary hypertension

autopsy cases reported these changes in 69% to 100% of patients with SAPH.[27] Sarcoid granulomas are predominantly located in the lymphatics adjacent to the pulmonary vasculature, and granulomatous involvement is observed at all levels from large elastic pulmonary arteries to venules.[27] Sarcoid granulomas tend to invade the vasculature and can be found throughout all layers of the pulmonary vascular wall. They are frequently accompanied by intimal fibrosis and medial proliferation, inflammatory changes, necrosis, and destruction of the architecture of small and medium-sized vessels, ultimately leading to an occlusive vasculopathy.[6,26,27] Vaso-occlusion may be caused directly by active granulomatous inflammation or may be an indirect consequence of the associated fibrosis and scarring. These changes are predominantly seen in small arterioles, as well as in pulmonary venules.[27] If the granulomatous inflammation predominantly involves the pulmonary venous system, a PVOD-like phenotype ensues.[6,16,93,94] Perivascular fibrosis, hemosiderosis, and iron deposits in elastic laminae have been described as well, whereas plexiform lesions seem to be absent or at least rare in SAPH.[6,95]

One of the hallmarks of SAPH is a heterogeneous involvement of the pulmonary vasculature. Although fibrocavitary disease usually favors central and upper lobe segments of the pulmonary vascular tree, granulomatous vascular involvement tends to occur in a patchy manner, thus differentiating SAPH from the more homogeneous vascular involvement seen in PAH.[6,46]

Although fibrocavitary disease usually affects small and intermediate-sized vessels, central blood vessels may be compressed by mediastinal or hilar lymph nodes or by mediastinal fibrosis.[46,78,89,90] An additional mechanical phenomenon contributing to SAPH development is pulmonary venous congestion from myocardial granulomatous inflammation and fibrosis with subsequent LV systolic or diastolic dysfunction[96] or mitral valve disease.[97] Approximately 15% of patients with persistent dyspnea despite immunosuppressive treatment may have PH caused by LV dysfunction; hemodynamic alterations in these cases are usually less severe, and overall survival is better than in SAPH with normal LV function.[10] For example, in one study, 5-year-survival with SAPH caused by LV dysfunction was 85% versus 40% with SAPH caused by other mechanisms.

In rare cases, a systemic vasculitis involving the pulmonary vasculature can complicate sarcoidosis. These patients have arteriographic evidence of large and small vessel vasculitis.[98] Many published cases involve children.[98] In addition, and also rare, portopulmonary hypertension from granulomatous infiltration of the liver or from Budd-Chiari syndrome can be seen.[99–101]

On a molecular level, hypoxic pulmonary vasoconstriction and vasoconstrictive effects of proinflammatory cytokines (eg, tumor necrosis factor alpha and endothelin-1 [ET-1]) on the pulmonary vasculature are potential contributors to SAPH development. For example, ET-1 has been shown to be significantly upregulated in sarcoidosis.[102] In contrast, vasodilators such as NO and prostacyclin are decreased. Some investigators have postulated that this vasoconstrictor/vasodilator imbalance may be caused by endothelial cell damage by infiltrating granulomas.[46] A strong vasoconstrictor component is supported by a small but prospective study of 8 patients with SAPH, 7 of whom showed a vasodilator response to inhaled NO despite significantly altered hemodynamics at baseline (mPAP, 55 mm Hg; mean PVR, 896 dyn·s·cm^{-5}).[103]

Symptoms of SAPH are nonspecific and often difficult to differentiate from underlying parenchymal lung disease or cardiac disease. However, SAPH should be suspected in patients with dyspnea that is disproportionate to pulmonary function or significant decreases in oxygenation or functional capacity. Severe exercise-induced desaturations, as well as the presence of signs of right heart failure, should raise suspicion for the presence of SAPH. In one series, the prevalence of right heart failure was 21%[82]; however, this is generally a late finding. In addition, decreases in lung diffusing capacity of carbon monoxide (DLCO) that are out of proportion to the decrease in lung volume may suggest SAPH. For example, in the series by Nunes and colleagues,[6] the patients with the most pronounced PH had a ratio of forced vital capacity (FVC; expressed as percentage of predicted) over DLCO (expressed as percentage of predicted) of 2.1, although this ratio was 1.3 in the patients with less pronounced PH. In the same series, 2 major groups of SAPH were identified: (1) PH in the setting of fibrocavitary disease (stage IV sarcoidosis), a scenario in which the hemodynamic alterations tend to be moderate in severity, and in which patients are primarily limited by ventilatory impairments; and (2) a more severe PH phenotype that occurs in the absence of significant fibrosis, characterized by the presence of ground-glass infiltrates on high-resolution CT, and an isolated reduction in diffusing capacity (and thus a higher FVC/DLCO ratio). Nunes and colleagues[6] reported this latter phenotype in 32% of patients. Because of lack of autopsy data, it is unclear whether the ground-glass opacities represent a PVOD-like component or active alveolitis. Despite having more pronounced hemodynamic alterations, the nonfibrotic

phenotype seemed to be more responsive to treatment with corticosteroids, suggesting that a more pronounced inflammatory reaction is present in these patients. In both phenotypes, mPAP was inversely correlated with DLCO. Examples of both phenotypes are shown in **Fig. 2**.

Diagnostic approaches for SAPH are similar to those of the other types of PH. Even though they are not uniform across studies, predictors of SAPH are supplemental oxygen use,[86] oxygen saturation less than 90% on 6-minute walk distance (6MWD) test,[80] decreased total lung capacity,[79] and DLCO less than 60% of predicted.[80] Because none of these abnormalities are specific for SAPH per se, such findings particularly indicate SAPH when accompanied by otherwise unexplained increases in B-natriuretic peptide (BNP) levels and/or by PH-related abnormalities on echocardiogram.[80] In contrast, the absence of

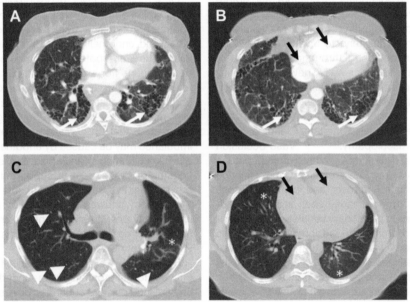

Fig. 2. Phenotypes of SAPH. (*A, B*) SAPH in the setting of fibrotic lung disease. Chest CT images from a 50-year-old woman with fibrocystic lung involvement (stage 4 sarcoidosis) that presented with dyspnea on exertion and fatigue. Note diffuse fibrotic and cystic changes (*white arrows*). Right atrial and RV enlargement is seen as well (*black arrows*). Pulmonary function testing showed a total lung capacity that was 65% of predicted. RHC revealed a mPAP of 66 mm Hg with a cardiac index of 1.6 L/min/m² and a PVR of 21.5 Wood units. The patient's symptoms and hemodynamics did not improve with corticosteroids, methotrexate, or pulmonary vasodilator therapy, and she developed intractable right heart failure. She eventually underwent successful heart and lung transplant. (*C, D*) SAPH in absence of fibrocystic lung disease. Chest CT images from a 40-year-old woman with sarcoidosis with mediastinal lymphadenopathy and ocular involvement that presented with a several-month history of exertional dyspnea, fatigue, and syncope. Symptoms did not improve after an increase prednisone dose. Chest CT revealed nodular opacities (*arrowheads*) in multiple lobes with mild ground-glass changes (*asterisk*), but no significant fibrosis. Right atrial and RV enlargement is suggested as well (*black arrows*), and was confirmed by echocardiogram; this also showed severe RV hypokinesis. Total lung capacity was 80% of predicted. RHC revealed an mPAP of 50 mm Hg with a cardiac index of 1.5 L/min/m² and a PVR of 17.1 Wood units. The patient was treated with treprostinil, ambrisentan, and tadalafil while being maintained on low-dose prednisone (5 mg/d). New York Heart Association (NYHA) functional class improved from IV to II. Six-minute walk distance increased from 229 m (750 feet) to 439 m (1440 feet), and PVR decreased to 12 Wood units.

hypoxemia at rest or exercise makes significant SAPH unlikely. Although pulmonary function tests tend to be more severely impaired in patients with SAPH,[79] they do not correlate well with increases in PAP.[6,83] Chest CT is particularly helpful in the work-up of suspected SAPH, because it may help detect fibrocavitary disease, compression of pulmonary vessels by lymphadenopathy or fibrosis, or pulmonary venous involvement with a PVOD-like phenotype as causes of PH.

Because of the high reported rate of pulmonary vasoreactivity,[103–105] a vasodilator challenge during RHC should be considered. However, the role of calcium channel blockers in SAPH has not been tested. The high incidence of pulmonary venous involvement should be kept in mind, and signs and symptoms suggesting PVOD should be aggressively looked for. Because of its therapeutic implications, left heart disease also needs to be ruled out as a cause of SAPH.

PH in pulmonary Langerhans cell histiocytosis (PLCH)

PLCH is a rare lung disease that almost exclusively affects current or prior cigarette smokers. The disease is characterized by the emergence of cystic lesions and nodules in the lung parenchyma.[106–108] Disease activity generally tracks with smoking status, and end-stage lung disease is predominantly seen in patients with ongoing tobacco use; however, rarely, disease progression occurs despite smoking cessation.[109,110]

PH seems to be frequent in PLCH. Using a PH definition of SPAP greater than 35 mm Hg on echocardiogram, one retrospective cohort analysis of 123 unselected patients with PLCH reported a prevalence of 10.6%.[111] However, echocardiography was only performed in symptomatic patients (n = 17), thus potentially underestimating the true prevalence of PLCH-PH. In studies of patients with advanced PLCH referred for lung transplantation, RHC-confirmed PH was present in 92% to 100% of patients.[17,112] Hemodynamic alterations were pronounced in both studies, with 73% of patients having an mPAP greater than 35 mm Hg in one study,[112] and with mPAP being 59 ± 4 mm Hg in the other.[17] In a more recent study of 29 patients from the French PLCH registry, average mPAP was 45 mm Hg, and 19 patients had an mPAP greater than or equal to 40 mm Hg, consistent with severe PH.[35] These studies indicate that PH is not only common in PLCH but may also be severe. Studies also found hemodynamic alterations in PLCH to be more pronounced than in the setting of idiopathic pulmonary fibrosis (IPF)[17,113] or chronic obstructive pulmonary disease.[17] These observations corroborate earlier studies showing that exercise capacity in patients with PLCH generally is limited by pulmonary vascular disease rather than ventilatory limitations.[114,115]

Survival data in PLCH-PH are sparse, but a recent study from the French registry reported 1-year, 3-year, and 5-year overall survival of 96%, 92%, and 73%, respectively.[35] In the same study, WHO functional class was the only variable significantly associated with death from PLCH-PH.[35]

The pathogenesis of PLCH-PH is not well understood. Infiltration of the walls of small and medium-sized pulmonary arteries with Langerhans cell granuloma has been described in lung regions with prominent parenchymal PLCH nodules, suggesting that a specific pulmonary vasculopathy may contribute to PLCH-PH development.[35,116] However, this finding was rare in another study.[17] Plexogenic lesions are not typically seen in PLCH-PH, but have been described in 1 case report.[117] A more consistent finding is diffuse medial hypertrophy with intimal fibrosis and/or proliferation.[17,35,116] These changes are frequently found even in regions not involved with PLCH nodules.[17] Furthermore, proliferative involvement of pulmonary veins has been described as well, and aspects of PVOD-like disease were detected in one-third of investigated specimens of patients in the series by Fartoukh and colleagues.[17] Even though prominent vascular changes frequently occur in regions not affected by parenchymal PLCH lesions, PH seems to develop predominantly in patients with significant parenchymal disease. One potential explanation for this phenomenon is the induction of diffuse pulmonary vascular remodeling as a consequence of the release of proinflammatory cytokines and growth factors by PLCH granuloma. In fact, PLCH granulomas have been shown to produce interleukin (IL)-1 and IL-6, transforming growth factor beta, and PDGF,[118–120] all of which have been implicated in PAH pathogenesis.[2] No significant correlations exist between lung function parameters and hemodynamic end points, suggesting that PH development in PLCH is unlikely to be related to pulmonary mechanics or hypoxemia.[17] In contrast, cigarette smoke is a known inducer of pulmonary vascular remodeling,[121] and may contribute to increases in PAP in PLCH.

In the French registry,[35] most of the patients were diagnosed with PH at an average of 11 years after PLCH diagnosis, which is similar to the report by Fartoukh and colleagues.[17] In both studies, patients were young (mean ages 39 and 45 years, respectively), and had an obstructive physiology with moderate to severe airflow obstruction (forced expiratory volume in 1 second [FEV_1], 46% and

52% of predicted), air trapping, and maintained total lung capacity. DLCO was significantly decreased at 27% and 28% of predicted. Mean 6MWD was 355 m. Mean PVR was 6.9 Wood units (WU), cardiac index (CI) was maintained at 3.2 L/min/m^2, and 38% of patients were using supplemental oxygen. Almost 50% of patients were on PAH-specific therapy, suggesting that baseline hemodynamics and functional parameters may be more severe in treatment-naive patients; this is also suggested by the more profound alteration of these parameters in the study by Fartoukh and colleagues[17] (CI, 2.6 L/min/m^2; PVR index, 25 WU/m^2). Despite severely altered hemodynamics, a positive vasodilator response may be seen in up to one-third of patients,[17] but the clinical significance of this finding is unknown. The presence of pulmonary venous involvement may predispose patients to pulmonary edema with pulmonary vasodilators,[35,122,123] as seen in 2 patients in the series by Fartoukh and colleagues.[17]

Predictors of PH development in PLCH have not yet been described, as no formal comparisons exist between patients with PLCH with and without PH. As in other diseases, disproportionate decreases in DLCO, poor exercise capacity, and exertional decreases in oxygen saturations may indicate the presence of PH.[17,35,114,115]

PH in lymphangioleiomyomatosis (LAM)

LAM is a disease characterized by proliferation of abnormal smooth muscle–like cells in the lymphatic system of the lungs and abdomen that primarily affects young or middle-aged women and that is characterized by diffuse pulmonary thin-walled cysts.[124–128]

Three studies have evaluated the prevalence of PH in LAM. An echocardiographic study of 95 patients with LAM estimated PH (estimated PASP>35 mm Hg) to be 7%.[129] A similar prevalence was found in a recent study from the French LAM registry, in which RHC-confirmed PH was seen in 7.4% of patients, after an average of 9.2 years following LAM diagnosis.[7] In contrast, an RHC study of 20 patients with LAM evaluated for lung transplantation documented PH in 45% of patients.[130] As in other lung diseases, the prevalence of PH in LAM seems to increase with worsening severity of lung disease.

The presence of PH in patients with LAM has significant clinical implications. In a study by Taveira-DaSilva and colleagues,[129] PAP during peak exercise correlated negatively with oxygen saturation, and increases in PAP were noted even during low-level exercise such as performing activities of daily living. A large number of patients

with LAM-PH (6/20) died or underwent lung transplantation within 2 years of PH diagnosis in the recent series by Cottin and colleagues,[7] with transplant-free probability of survival being 87% at 1 year, 78% at 2 years, and 56% at 3 years.

Mechanisms of LAM-PH are not well defined, but likely include vascular rarefaction from parenchymal lung destruction and vascular compression from obstructive lung disease and hyperinflation. The role of hypoxia in LAM-PH development is questionable, as no correlation was found between hemodynamic parameters and partial pressure of arterial oxygen (Pao$_2$). Involvement of the PA wall by characteristic human melanoma black 45–positive LAM cells (referred to as perivascular epithelioid cells) may contribute to PH pathogenesis as well,[7,131,132] potentially via activation of mammalian target of rapamycin (mTOR) signaling.[133] LAM cells are also found in the pulmonary venous compartment,[7] but PVOD in the setting of LAM has not been described.

In the Cottin and colleagues[7] series, there was no difference between patients with LAM with or without PH with regard to age, menopause, smoking history, imaging patterns, occurrence of renal angiomyolipomas, pneumothoraces, chylothoraces, chylous ascites, or association with tuberous sclerosis complex. However, patients with LAM-PH had more dyspnea, and more functional limitations (with most patients being in New York Heart Association [NYHA] functional class 3 or 4). Patients with LAM-PH were characterized by more pronounced airway obstruction (FEV$_1$, 42% ± 24% vs 63% ± 25% of predicted), lower DLCO (29% ± 13% vs 50% ± 25% of predicted), worse oxygenation, and a lower 6MWD (340 ± 84 vs 474 ± 144 m) with more pronounced exercise-induced desaturations (81% ± 9% vs 88% ± 8%). mPAP was 32 ± 6 mm Hg, with PVR being 376 ± 184 dyn·s·cm^{-5}. PH was seen despite preserved lung volumes, suggesting that LAM-PH may progress independently of parenchymal lung disease. CO and saturation of venous oxygen (Svo$_2$) were preserved at 5.4 ± 1.9 L/min and 69% ± 7%, respectively, and 0 of 8 patients were reactive to inhaled NO. Severe PH or right heart failure was generally absent. Therefore, even though LAM-PH seems to be only mild to moderate in severity, its impact on oxygenation and functional capacity seems to be substantial.

PH in neurofibromatosis type 1 (NF1)

NF1, or von Recklinghausen disease, is multisystem genetic disease characterized by café-au-lait spots, axillary or groin freckling, and neurofibromas.[134] Interstitial lung disease (ILD) with cystic and bullous changes or vascular involvement may be seen.[134,135] The prevalence of PH in NF1 is not known. Outcomes of patients with NF1-PH reported in case series were uniformly poor. Despite treatment with PAH-specific drugs, most patients with NF1-PH died of progressive respiratory failure and/or cor pulmonale within less than 6 years of diagnosis.[136–138]

The pathogenesis of NF1-PH is not known. Intimal thickening and fibrosis, hyperplasia of pericytes and smooth muscle cells, as well as a plexiform arteriopathy similar to the one observed in PAH have been described,[136,137,139] but histologic examinations of the pulmonary vasculature in NF1-PH are limited to case reports. PH may also occur as a consequence of ILD. NF1 is a tumor suppressor gene, and a direct contribution of the NF1 gene mutation to pulmonary vascular remodeling via PDGF, Ras, mTOR, and extracellular signal-related kinase activation with subsequent proproliferative signaling and misguided angiogenesis has been postulated.[136,140–142] NF1-PH seems to predominantly affect women[136–138]; however, whether this is caused by estrogens or altered estrogen signaling has not yet been determined.

PH seems to develop late in the course of NF1, and most reported patients are more than 50 years of age.[136–139] For example, in the series by Montani and colleagues,[136] the median delay between PH and NF1 diagnosis was 44 years. In 2 separate series, patients tended to have significantly altered hemodynamics with severe increases of mPAP, mildly reduced CI, high PVR, and lack of acute vasodilator responsiveness.[136,137] As a result, in the series by Montani and colleagues,[136] most patients had NYHA class 3 symptoms, signs of RV failure, and severely decreased 6MWD (median 180 m). Concomitant lung disease (ILD, cysts, or bullae) was described in 5 of 8 patients. A mosaic pattern of lung attenuation on high-resolution CT was frequently noted in the series by Stewart and colleagues.[137] Patients may have normal, restrictive, or obstructive respiratory physiology, but DLCO seems to be decreased out of proportion in most patients.[136,137]

PH in pulmonary vasculitis

PH can be seen in the setting of various vasculitides, such as Takayasu arteritis, giant-cell arteritis (GCA), Behçet disease, and vasculitis associated with rheumatoid arthritis, systemic lupus erythematosus, or other connective tissue diseases. The incidence of PA involvement in Takayasu arteritis seems to be between 50% and 80%, often as a late manifestation of the disease.[143] Typical findings are stenosis or occlusion, mostly involving the segmental and subsegmental arteries and less commonly lobar or main PAs.[144] In contrast, pulmonary vascular involvement is rare in GCA, and its exact prevalence is unknown.[143] Pulmonary involvement in Behçet disease ranges from 1% to 7.7%[145]; however, PA aneurysms rather than PH are the predominant finding. PH is a rare occurrence in the necrotizing antinuclear cytoplasm antibody–associated vasculitides (granulomatosis with polyangiitis, Churg-Strauss, microscopic polyangiitis), but isolated reports exist.[146] In children, PH may be seen in the context of PA stenoses from Moyamoya.[147,148]

Group 5.3: Metabolic Disorders

Metabolic diseases linked to PH are GSDs, lysosomal storage disorders, and thyroid disorders. Mucopolysaccharidoses known to cause PH (eg, Hurler syndrome or Hurler-Scheie syndrome[149]) are not reviewed because of space limitations.

PH in glycogen storage disease (GSD)

GSDs are a group of genetic disorders that are typically diagnosed in the first few months to years of life. They are characterized by abnormal glycogen deposition in muscles, liver, and other cell types that result from enzyme deficiencies in the synthesis or breakdown of glycogen.[150] Based on the underlying enzyme deficiency, 11 different types of GSDs have been described; hypoglycemia, hyperlipidemia, hepatomegaly, myopathy, and growth retardation are the most common findings.

Although recent publications reported PH in 2 patients with GSD type III (Cori disease or Fabry disease),[151] and PVOD in a patient with type II GSD (Pompe disease),[152] PH has primarily been described in GSD type I (von Gierke disease).[28,29,153,154] Information on the prevalence of PH in GSD is limited; in the report by Humbert and colleagues,[28,29] 30 patients with type Ia GSD were regularly followed over 3 years, and only 1 had GSD-PH. However, when present, PH seems to have a significant and negative impact on outcomes.[151,153,155]

The pathogenesis of GSD-PH remains unknown. Histologic evaluations of lungs from patients with type I GSD show pathologic changes similar to those in idiopathic PAH.[28,29,153,156] Because only a minority of patients with GSD develop PH, genetic or environmental modifiers may be needed for PH to develop. As such, abnormalities in serotonin metabolism with increased levels caused by liver dysfunction or creation of portocaval shunts have been postulated to contribute.[28,29,153] Other purported mechanisms include glycogen accumulation in the pulmonary vasculature, as well as pulmonary accumulation of a mitogenic and vasoconstrictive humoral mediator other than serotonin.[151,153] A case of PVOD in late-onset type II GSD has recently been reported.[152] Cardiac involvement may occur in GSDs and can thus lead to pulmonary venous hypertension.[157]

There seems to be a long latency between GSD diagnosis and PH diagnosis, and reported patients with GSD-PH are predominantly women in their second or third decade (**Table 2**).[28,29,151,153,154] GSD-PH may thus be a consequence of long-term metabolic abnormalities. Hemodynamic alterations in GSD-PH are severe, and several reported patients died within a few months of PH diagnosis.[28,29,151,153,155] Whether GSD-PH improves with enzyme replacement therapy (ERT) has not been adequately defined, but it is notable that severe PH seems to develop despite use of ERT.

PH in Gaucher disease (GD)

GD is a lysosomal storage disorder caused by decreased activity of the lysosomal enzyme acid-beta-glucosidase. This disorder leads to accumulation of glucosylceramide, predominantly in cells of macrophage lineage (known as Gaucher cells) and their subsequent organ infiltration.[158] Three major subtypes of GD have been described. Type 1 GD is associated with ILD and PH; the latter (diagnosed by echocardiography) occurring in up to 30% of untreated patients and in 7% of patients treated with ERT.[64,159] Risk factors for developing significant PH in GD include mutations other than the most common mutation (N370S), a family history of GD-PH, polymorphisms in the angiotensin-converting enzyme I gene, lack of ERT, splenectomy, and female sex.[159] Although

GD-PH is usually mild to moderate in severity, severe, life-threatening PH occurs in approximately 1% of patients with GD.[160] Before the ERT era, PH was one of the major causes of premature death in GD.[160]

GD-PH seems to be caused at least in part by pulmonary capillary infiltration and plugging by glycolipid-laden macrophages, resulting in a classic plexogenic vasculopathy.[161–164] Obstruction of pulmonary capillaries from bone marrow emboli has been described as well.[162] GD-PH can also occur in the setting of alveolar, interstitial, or myocardial infiltration with Gaucher cells.[162,165] Additional purported mechanisms of PH development in GD include asplenia, alterations in pulmonary vascular cell cycle and apoptosis pathways, and a systemic proinflammatory state with increased plasma levels of proinflammatory cytokines (eg, IL-1β, IL-6).[158–160,166,167] In particular, it has been postulated that splenectomy, in addition to creating a hypercoagulable state with increased platelet counts and accumulation of megakaryocytes, allows reduced clearance and increased deposition of macrophages in the pulmonary vasculature.[159] An association with ERT in the setting of hepatopulmonary syndrome (HPS) has been described as well,[160,168] suggesting that improvement in HPS after ERT initiation may unmask concomitant PH.

Based on the small series by Lo and colleagues[160] (n = 14 patients), patients with GD-PH are female predominant, have a history of splenectomy, and are diagnosed with PH several decades after GD (see **Table 2**). In general, PH severity does not correlate well with GD severity, suggesting a potential impact of a hitherto unidentified genetic or environmental modifier. In the largest series, mean RVSP was 30 ± 10 mm Hg

Table 2
Differences and similarities between PH in glycogen storage disease (GSD-PH) and PH in Gaucher disease (GD-PH)

	Age at Onset	Gender Predominance	Severity of PH	Treatment of PH
GSD-PH	Second or third decade of life	Female	Usually severe	Concomitant treatment of GSD and PH usually required (but limited experience)
GD-PH	Third, fourth, or fifth decade of life	Female	Usually mild; severe only in a subtype of patients	Mild GD-PH may improve with ERT alone; pulmonary vasodilators used in moderate to severe cases

Abbreviation: ERT, enzyme replacement therapy.

in untreated patients, and only 23 ± 8 mm Hg in patients on ERT.[159] Only 1 of 134 patients had an RVSP greater than 50 mm Hg, and many patients were asymptomatic. The only study that included patients with RHC data (n = 7) reported a wide range of mPAPs (32–57 mm Hg) and PVRs (2.8–19.2 WU).[160] However, a subgroup of patients had more pronounced PH and were younger, more likely to be female, more likely to have undergone splenectomy, had mutations other than the N370S mutation, had a sibling with GD-PH, and had a lack of or poor adherence to ERT.[159] Patients with GD characterized by these features are considered an at-risk population that warrants close observation and more aggressive treatment. C-reactive protein (CRP) and N-terminal pro-BNP levels have been identified as surrogate markers of GD-PH.[169] In selected patients characterized by severe GD, PH may be preceded by or occur simultaneously with HPS.[160]

GD-PH usually improves with ERT,[159] and treatment with high-dose imiglucerase remains the cornerstone of therapy. ERT alone may be sufficient to significantly improve mild PH; however, in patients with more severe hemodynamic alterations, combination with pulmonary vasodilators and anticoagulants may be required[159] (see "PAH-specific therapy" section later in this chapter).

PH associated with thyroid disorders

An association between PH and hypothyroidism was described in 1993,[170] and subsequently confirmed by other reports.[171–175] The exact prevalence of PH in the setting of hypothyroidism is unknown, and most existing reports focus on the prevalence of thyroid abnormalities in cohorts with preexisting PAH. These studies have reported a 3-fold to 6-fold increase in prevalence of thyroid disease in patients with PAH.[171,174,176] For example, in a recent survey of female patients with PAH, the prevalence of self-reported thyroid disease was 41%,[171] a rate 6 times that of large population-based estimates of thyroid disease.[176] Other studies reported hypothyroidism rates of 20.1% to 22.5% in patients with PAH.[172,173] In particular, a connection seems to exist between autoimmune thyroiditis and PAH, as evidenced by a study that reported autoimmune thyroid disease in 49% of patients with PAH.[175] However, these studies, although showing associations between thyroid disease and PAH, do not allow definite conclusions regarding cause and effect.

Associations also exist between PAH and hyperthyroid conditions. Even though hyperthyroidism seems to be less commonly found in PAH cohorts than hypothyroidism,[174] series of patients with Graves disease or multinodular goiter reported a 34% to 65% prevalence of patients with echocardiographic evidence of PH.[40,177–181]

In addition, reports exist of the development of hyperthyroid disease in patients with idiopathic PAH after treatment initiation with intravenous prostacyclins.[182,183] For example, one study noted a prevalence of 6.7% of thyroid-stimulating immunoglobulin-negative thyrotoxicosis in adults with preexisting PAH being treated with epoprostenol.[183]

Given that thyroid dysfunction is frequently of autoimmune cause,[184] and given the known association between autoimmunity and PAH, a common autoimmune pathogenesis has been postulated as the cause for the association between PH and thyroid disorders.[170] Antithyroglobulin and antithyroperoxidase antibodies are frequently found in patients with PAH.[175,185] In addition, thyroid abnormalities are common in systemic autoimmune diseases known to cause PAH, such as scleroderma or systemic lupus erythematosus.[186,187] LV systolic or diastolic dysfunction can be seen in the setting of hypothyroidism or hyperthyroidism and may contribute to PH development in these settings. In addition, thyroid hormones may have direct effects on the pulmonary vasculature, as shown by reports of hypothyroidism-associated Raynaud phenomenon improving with thyroid hormone replacement.[188,189] Because Raynaud phenomenon is associated with increased PA pressures,[190] thyroid hormone may thus attenuate PA vasoconstriction. However, animal studies suggest that the proproliferative and angiogenic effects of thyroid hormones may worsen pulmonary vascular remodeling in the setting of PAH.[191] Such a mechanism, as well as a hyperdynamic, high cardiac output state may contribute to PH pathogenesis in patients with hyperthyroidism.[40,191] Hyperthyroidism-induced increases in metabolism of pulmonary vasodilators, decreases in cholinergic output, and increases in blood volume have been postulated as well.[192–194] The underlying mechanisms of epoprostenol-induced hyperthyroidism have not yet been elucidated. Stimulatory effects on thyroid tissue with subsequent goiter formation have been proposed.[183]

The currently available studies and reports describe associations between PAH and clinical (autoimmune thyroiditis, Graves disease, multinodular goiter) or subclinical (abnormal thyroid-stimulating hormone [TSH] levels, increased antithyroglobulin antibody titers) thyroid abnormalities. Such associations are not limited to idiopathic PAH, but are also seen with PAH associated with connective tissue disease, human immunodeficiency virus (HIV), drugs, or liver cirrhosis.[175] Hypothyroidism seems to be more commonly associated with PAH than hyperthyroidism, but TSH levels are usually only mildly increased (5–10 mIU/L).[174] Thyroid abnormalities seem to be more common in female patients with PAH.[174]

The observation that both hypothyroidism as well as hyperthyroidism are associated with PAH suggests that increased PA pressures do not derive from a particular direction of disturbance in thyroid hormone levels. Other than the described thyroid abnormalities, no specific phenotype of PAH in the setting of thyroid disease has been described, and currently described patient cohorts show similar epidemiologic features to PAH cohorts without thyroid abnormalities. The same study that documented a high prevalence of autoimmune thyroid disease in PAH also reported a strong first-degree family history of autoimmune thyroiditis (seen in 25% of patients).[175] Because most studies used an echocardiography-based definition of PH, no detailed descriptions of the hemodynamic alterations in thyroid disease–associated PAH are currently available. One study of hypothyroid patients with PAH that included RHC data reported an mPAP of 58.7 ± 14.8 mm Hg.[172] Echocardiography studies of hyperthyroid patients predominantly documented mildly to moderately increased estimated PASPs.[40,177–182] Hyperthyroid patients with PH typically have features of a hyperdynamic state, such as high CO and a low peripheral resistance.[40] Most of the published literature suggests that treatment of thyroid dysfunction improves the PH, particularly in cases of PH with accompanying thyrotoxicosis. One study suggested that PA pressures decrease faster with methimazole than with surgical therapy.[177]

Group 5.4: Other Disorders

There is a heterogeneous list of diseases associated with PH development. PH caused by CRF, fibrosing mediastinitis, and tumor emboli are reviewed. Other entities categorized in this group (eg, PA occlusion by endovascular tumors such as sarcomas,[195,196] PA compression from massive lymphadenopathy, pulmonary vein stenosis after catheter ablation for atrial fibrillation[197]) are not reviewed because of space limitations.

PH in patients with chronic renal failure (CRF) on dialysis

Patients with CRF maintained on dialysis are susceptible to PH through a myriad of mechanisms. The prevalence of PH in the CRF population is controversial as studies have primarily relied on echocardiography without confirmatory

catheterization, and used only a PASP greater than 35 mm Hg to define PH.[198] Mindful of these shortcomings, multiple studies primarily of cross-sectional design report a prevalence of 30% to 60% in patients undergoing dialysis. Also, prevalence seems to increase after initiating dialysis, is greater with hemodialysis (vs peritoneal dialysis), and is often associated with left heart dysfunction (ie, suggestive of group 2 PH).[199–203]

Patients with CRF may develop PH for multiple reasons, including increased flow, increased postcapillary or left atrial pressures, and increased PVR (see **Fig. 1**).[204] Most often, mild PH (PASP<50 mm Hg or mPAP<30 mm Hg) is linked to left-sided heart disease with increased PCWP stemming from valvular heart disease, systolic heart failure, or heart failure with preserved ejection fraction (caused by diastolic dysfunction).[200,204,205] The recent PEPPER study (prevalence of precapillary pulmonary arterial hypertension in patients with end-stage renal disease) confirmed through RHC in 62 dyspneic patients with CRF on hemodialysis or advanced chronic kidney disease (CKD) that postcapillary (postpulmonary) hypertension (group 2 PH) was overwhelmingly the most common type.[13] In addition, PAPs declined by an average of 6 mm Hg when measured after dialysis, indicating hypervolemia as an important driving factor. Given that hypervolemia is a frequent precipitant of PH in LV disease and that myocardial dysfunction is commonly associated with CKD, patients with CRF are particularly susceptible to group 2 PH. An additional contributing factor is the arteriovenous fistula (AVF), a surgically created left-to-right shunt that increases cardiac preload to the heart. Once thought to be a significant factor in the pathogenesis of PH in the CRF population, more recent studies have been conflicting about the causal role of AVF.[43,206–209] Given that PH is more common after AVF placement, associated with higher CO, and that PA pressures may decline with transient occlusion of an AVF, a reasonable explanation is that shunt flow can contribute to PH in patients with underlying cardiac dysfunction who cannot cope with the increased preload without increasing left-sided pressures.[206,207,210] In some, high shunt flow rates caused by an overgrown AVF may have a more prominent role; Basile and colleagues[209] determined (by receiver operating characteristic curves) that shunt flow greater than 2.0 L/min or shunt flow/CO greater than 20% strongly predict high-output failure.

Chronic anemia leading to increased CO, chronic thromboembolic disease emanating from recurrent graft/fistula thrombosis, and hypoxic lung diseases (ie, chronic obstructive pulmonary disease and obstructive sleep apnea) may also cause PH in patients with renal failure.[204] Patients with CRF can, rarely, develop PAH from a proliferative vasculopathy if the cause of CRF overlaps with the underlying cause of group 1 conditions: connective tissue disorders (eg, scleroderma or systemic lupus erythematosus), HIV, or cirrhosis; in distinction from most patients with CRF, mPAP and PVR are much higher and the transpulmonary gradient is abnormal (ie, >12–15) in these situations, signifying a precapillary component.

In the PEPPER study, 10% of dyspneic patients with CRF with invasively documented PH had no significant cardiac disease, pulmonary disease, or anemia, and constituted a CRF subgroup with unexplained PH.[13] Unique attributes of CRF that are linked to systemic vascular disorders (uremia-induced endothelial dysfunction, extraosseous vascular calcifications caused by derangement of the calcium/phosphorus–parathyroid hormone–vitamin D axis, and inflammation from repeated exposure to dialysis membranes) are speculated to also affect the pulmonary circulation.[204]

Chronic uremia is characterized by systemic imbalances in vasoconstrictors (increased endothelin-1, thromboxane) and vasodilators (reduced NO).[205,211] In particular, the NO pathway is underexpressed from a combination of reduced NO production, increased levels of its inhibitor, asymmetric dimethylarginine, and decreased responsiveness of the endothelium to NO.[42,212,213] These derangements, which are integral to the pathogenesis of PAH, cumulatively promote vasoconstriction and cellular proliferation and may be the genesis for unexplained PH in CRF.[42,205]

The occurrence of PH in CRF seems to confer greater risk of death and worse outcomes for patients undergoing kidney transplantation.[199,200,214] Stallworthy and colleagues[215] recently showed that PH and/or RV dysfunction (as a marker of PH) along with advanced age and echo-derived measures of LV dysfunction independently predict mortality in patients with CRF. However, because of the retrospective nature of most studies, a dearth of pulmonary vascular histology, and the strong association with left-sided cardiac disease, a direct causal link between PH and these important clinical outcomes cannot be made. The rarity of severe RV failure and the milder degree of hemodynamic derangements, in contrast with patients with PAH (group 1), makes it more likely that PH is a marker of more advanced left-sided heart disease in most patients with CRF.

The extent to which PH should be evaluated in the context of CRF is contingent on the potential cause of the PH, attributable symptoms, and clinical circumstances. Patients with more than mild

PH (ie, PASP>50 mm Hg), notable RV dysfunction, hemodynamic intolerance to hemodialysis, or patients who are being considered for kidney transplantation warrant a more thorough diagnostic evaluation. Echocardiography should search for LV (systolic or diastolic) dysfunction, valvular dysfunction, and a high-output state. In these situations, it is imperative to invasively determine the PCWP, CO, and PVR, preferably after dialysis while patients are at their dry weight, in order to isolate the origin(s) of PH and guide management. If a high-output state exists in the presence of an AVF, temporary occlusion of the AVF with a sphygmomanometer has been described as a useful diagnostic tool for measuring the impact of the left-to-right shunt.[206,209]

Management should focus on optimizing the various factors leading to the development of PH: controlling LV failure through control of systemic blood pressures and achieving dry weight, adequate iron and erythropoietin supplementation to avoid anemia, and lowering the calcium-phosphate product to acceptable levels. If an overgrown AVF is causing a high-output state, downsizing or even ligation of the AVF may be necessary.

PH in fibrosing mediastinitis (mediastinal fibrosis)

Extensive fibrosis in the mediastinum occurs rarely after exposure to certain infectious organisms, most notably *Histoplasma capsulatum*.[216] An aberrant host response in the form of dense fibrosis and mild mononuclear inflammation develops in areas surrounding central lymph nodes of the chest, which consequently can narrow or obliterate vital mediastinal structures, including central pulmonary arteries and/or veins. PH can ensue if enough central veins and/or arteries are affected by the underlying fibroproliferative process; histopathology reveals thickening of the intima, medial, and adventitial layers of the pulmonary veins and arteries.[217] Clinical presentation includes dyspnea, either from cardiovascular limitations and/or increased dead space as a consequence of segmental or lobar perfusion defects, as well as hemoptysis from erosive broncholiths, pulmonary venous edema, or aberrant systemic-to-pulmonary collaterals of bronchial submucosa.

Imaging is crucial in displaying the extent of mediastinal involvement and determining the best course of action. Chest CT angiography should focus on the pulmonary veins, as they are particularly vulnerable. Ground-glass infiltrates in a patchy but central distribution in the region of the lung affiliated with the compromised vein represents venous edema. Some other potential CT findings include densely calcified lymph nodes, which if present support the diagnosis of *Histoplasma*; as well as pulmonary infarction, pleural thickening, bronchiectasis, pericardial effusion, pleural effusion, and abnormal venovenous communications across fissures. The ventilation-perfusion scan provides complementary information by showing physiologic consequences of vascular occlusion and quantifying regional ventilation and perfusion.

In general, vascular treatment indications in fibrosing mediastinitis include severe dyspnea, presence of moderate-severe PH, or recurrent significant hemoptysis. Patients without additional lung disorders tolerate the physiologic loss of a single lung and probably do not need an intervention. In contrast, the presence of significant bilateral disease usually warrants intervention. Surgical experience has been disappointing because of the challenges of surgical exposure and the limited durable options for overcoming large vessel disease.[218,219] Isolated case reports of improvement with corticosteroids likely represents a different mediastinal disease, distinct from the more common fibrotic and calcified form encountered after remote granulomatous infections.[220,221]

Success with congenital pulmonary vein stenosis has led to percutaneous stenting of fibrosing mediastinitis–related pulmonary veins and/or arteries (**Fig. 3**).[5,222–224] However, stenting is challenging and should be performed by centers equipped to comprehensively evaluate the condition and perform complex and risky percutaneous procedures that may include transatrial septal puncture.[222] Selection of the patient and the vascular territory for intervention is paramount, as corresponding ventilation should be preserved and the end-result should be an intact arterial-venous relationship to a region of the lung. The choice of stents continues to evolve with technological advances and is beyond the scope of this article. PH can improve considerably, especially when proximal PAs are involved, and symptoms lessen dramatically.[222] However, durability of pulmonary venous stents is suboptimal because stents are susceptible to early and late restenosis and often require reintervention within 1 to 2 years.[5,223] In addition, lung transplantation may be an option in carefully selected individuals with predominantly distal disease who have identifiable surgical planes for explantation and anastomoses of the allograft (personal observation, MMC).

PH from tumor emboli

Certain tumors can invade systemic veins and release tumor fragments, which can evade

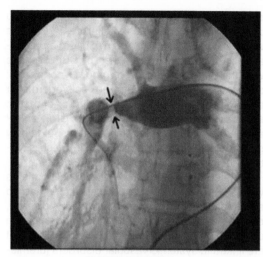

RLLPA stenosis

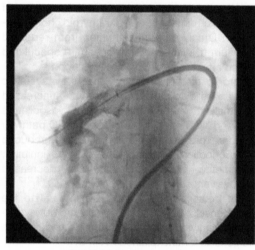

RLLPA following stenting

Fig. 3. Percutaneous vascular stenting of central PA in fibrosing mediastinitis. An 18-year-old woman with exertional dyspnea, orthopnea, episodes of massive hemoptysis, and moderate PH (mPAP, 40 mm Hg). There was severe stenosis of the right lower lobe PA (*arrows, top panel*) and significant improvement in blood flow after stent placement (*bottom panel*) with resolution in orthopnea, reduced dyspnea, and resolution of hemoptysis.

peripheral destruction and ultimately be trapped by the pulmonary microcirculation. One autopsy series showed that 25% of patients with cancer dying from pulmonary embolism had tumor emboli.[225] This phenomenon has most often been seen with primary gastric, breast, ovary, lung, kidney, and colon malignancies, but the list of culpable cancers is long.[226] In some of these instances, embolization of tumorlets leads to the more profound process of pulmonary tumor thrombotic microangiopathy (PTTM), which involves significant activation of coagulation and inflammatory cascades. Proliferative cellular changes eventually occur within the intima, notable for fibromuscular/fibrocellular remodeling of pulmonary arteries and arterioles.[227,228]

However, cases of PTTM are rarely suspected before a fatal event because presenting symptoms are nonspecific (primarily dyspnea and cough).[225] The unique aspect to these cases is the significant and progressive PH and right-sided heart failure that accompanies the diffuse histopathology of PTTM, and the lack of evidence for pulmonary thromboemboli. Ventilation-perfusion scans may have small, peripheral, subsegmental perfusion defects that could suggest PTTM; whereas thin-cut CT images could spotlight RV or PA enlargement, and small centrilobular nodules that may appear in a tree-in-bud pattern and could also be seen in PVOD.[229,230] A conclusive diagnosis of PTTM can only made by showing vascular occlusion by tumor cells through surgical lung biopsy, which can be risky because these individuals are typically compromised by their underlying malignancy and/or severe PH.[231] Another novel way to confirm the diagnosis of PTTM is to show tumor cells through cytologic analysis of blood aspirated from a PA catheter in its wedged position. Even with proper collection (ie, slow aspiration of blood, wasting the initial 10 to 15 mL of aspirated blood, and placing in a heparinized tube for cytologic evaluation), false-negatives occur and a negative sample should not exclude PTTM.[232]

Prognosis with PTTM is poor, given the distribution of the primary tumor and the rapidly progressive PH and right-sided heart failure. Treatment should focus on the primary malignancy, and a chemotherapy-responsive tumor can regress within the pulmonary vasculature.[233]

PAH-SPECIFIC PULMONARY VASODILATOR THERAPY FOR GROUP 5 PH
PH in Patients with Hematologic Disorders

In general, treatment of PH associated with hematologic disorders is directed toward the underlying disease, and improvements in hemodynamics with such interventions have been reported.[33,34,75] External beam radiation against pulmonary myeloid metaplasia may regress PH, as shown in one case report.[234] Meanwhile, experience with pulmonary vasodilators has not been reported in cases of precapillary PH, despite this group's dismal prognosis and thus needs investigation. Caution must be exercised for unmasking a PVOD phenotype with pulmonary vasodilators. Because plexogenic arteriopathy has been showed in the postsplenectomy population, PAH-specific therapies are reasonable

to consider, if surgically accessible thromboembolic disease is excluded.

PH in Patients with Systemic Disorders

Similar to group 5.1 PH, the first line of treatment in PH from systemic disorders is directed toward the underlying disease. However, in sarcoid, treatment with corticosteroids alone seems to have only a modest and inconsistent impact on PH. For example, in the series by Gluskowski and colleagues,[87] only 50% of patients showed improved hemodynamics. Nunes and colleagues[6] suggested that patients with nonfibrotic sarcoidosis and underlying sarcoid vasculopathy may respond to corticosteroid treatment, whereas in patients with fibrotic disease, corticosteroids seem to be inactive. These latter patients should be referred for lung transplantation sooner than would be considered solely from lung function.

Sarcoid vasculitis is usually treated with corticosteroids and cytotoxic therapy. Even though clinical response is common, relapses and morbidity from disease and/or treatment are frequent.[98] Other vasculitides leading to PH development are also usually treated with corticosteroids and cytotoxic therapy.[146]

Several PAH-specific therapies have been studied in PH associated with systemic disorders, but at this point no randomized, controlled trials and no survival data exist. In small series of patients with SAPH, prostacyclin analogues, endothelin receptor antagonists, and phosphodiesterase type 5 inhibitors have been shown to improve hemodynamics, functional status, and/or outcomes.[83,85,105,235,236] Similar to what is reported for corticosteroids, patients with a higher FVC seem to respond better to treatment than patients with more fibrotic disease.[236]

Studies investigating the treatment of PH in systemic disorders other than sarcoidosis are rare and involve a limited number of patients. In PLCH-PH, PAH therapies improved hemodynamics without worsening oxygenation or causing pulmonary edema, and the use of PAH therapy was associated with a trend toward a better survival rate.[35] In addition, the successful use of sildenafil in PLCH-PH was documented in a case report.[237] In 6 patients with LAM-PH, PAH therapy similarly led to significant hemodynamic improvements.[7] The mTOR inhibitor rapamycin (sirolimus) attenuates PH in animal models,[238,239] and improves lung volumes and quality of life in patients with LAM[240]; however, its specific use for LAM-PH, although theoretically appealing, has not yet been investigated. Specific PH therapies seem to have only a modest effect in patients with

NF1.[136,137] Because of poor outcomes and limited impact of specific PH therapy, eligible patients with NF1 and PH are therefore recommended to undergo early referral for lung transplantation.[136]

The potential for pulmonary edema development in cases of PVOD (as in sarcoidosis or PLCH), as well as the potential for worsening ventilation/perfusion mismatch in the setting of parenchymal lung disease, needs to be kept in mind when treating patients with systemic disorders with pulmonary vasodilators.

PH in Patients with Metabolic Disorders

Data on the treatment of PH associated with metabolic disorders are limited to case reports or small case series. GD-PH usually improves with ERT,[159] and high doses of ERT are recommended.[160] Although mild GD-PH may respond to treatment with imiglucerase alone, patients with more severe hemodynamic alterations usually require a combination of ERT with pulmonary vasodilators and anticoagulants.[159] Epoprostenol has been most commonly used,[159,241,242] but experience with sildenafil or bosentan is evolving.[160,243]

In contrast, GSD-PH seems to develop despite ongoing ERT, suggesting that ERT alone may be less efficacious for PH in this setting. Data for GSD-PH treatment are even more limited than they are for GD-PH. The severity of histologic changes and hemodynamic alterations in GSD-PH provide a rationale for prostacyclins, but at this point only the successful use of sildenafil has been reported.[151,154]

Most of the published literature suggests that treatment of thyroid dysfunction improves cardiopulmonary hemodynamics, particularly in cases of PH with accompanying thyrotoxicosis.[40,177–182] Pulmonary vasodilators are indicated if a PAH phenotype persists despite normalization of thyroid function. Whether epoprostenol-induced hyperthyroidism improves after dose adjustment is unknown, but a decrease in dose is recommended.[183]

PH in Patients with Other Disorders

Data on the use of PAH-specific therapies in this category are sparse. In CRF-PH, aggressive volume management and treatment of comorbidities are paramount. For the minority of patients with CRF with otherwise unexplained PH, PAH-specific therapies could be considered, similar to patients without CRF. However, tadalafil has a prolonged half-life in CRF and should not be used in patients with a creatinine clearance less than 30 mL/min.[204] There are no data for the use of PAH-specific therapy for fibrosing mediastinitis, tumor emboli, PTTM, or tumor obstruction.

SUMMARY

Group 5 is a fascinating and complex group of disorders that manifest PH by several mechanisms, such as a proliferative pulmonary arteriopathy, pulmonary vascular obliteration, asplenia, high-output failure, or PVOD. The presence of PH affects most patients and often alters their prognosis. Similar to PAH, a diagnosis of group 5 PH can only be made after thorough evaluations to exclude other relevant cardiopulmonary issues that could affect overall management. However, because of the rarity of these heterogeneous conditions, much is unknown about mechanisms of disease and treatment. PAH-specific vasodilators should be used cautiously in this population, and only by providers experienced with the medications and the underlying disease process. Eligible patients should be referred for lung transplantation expediently when severe group 5 PH is documented. Until larger cohorts of group 5 patients can be assembled into observation registries and clinical trials, especially with the more common disorders (eg, SAPH and PH associated with CRF), it will be difficult to further the understanding of this important group of patients with PH.

REFERENCES

1. Simonneau G, Robbins IM, Beghetti M, et al. Updated clinical classification of pulmonary hypertension. J Am Coll Cardiol 2009;54:S43–54.
2. Hassoun PM, Mouthon L, Barbera JA, et al. Inflammation, growth factors, and pulmonary vascular remodeling. J Am Coll Cardiol 2009;54:S10–9.
3. Hoeper MM, Barbera JA, Channick RN, et al. Diagnosis, assessment, and treatment of nonpulmonary arterial hypertension pulmonary hypertension. J Am Coll Cardiol 2009;54:S85–96.
4. Berry DF, Buccigrossi D, Peabody J, et al. Pulmonary vascular occlusion and fibrosing mediastinitis. Chest 1986;89:296–301.
5. Ferguson ME, Cabalka AK, Cetta F, et al. Results of intravascular stent placement for fibrosing mediastinitis. Congenit Heart Dis 2010;5:124–33.
6. Nunes H, Humbert M, Capron F, et al. Pulmonary hypertension associated with sarcoidosis: mechanisms, haemodynamics and prognosis. Thorax 2006;61:68–74.
7. Cottin V, Harari S, Humbert M, et al. Pulmonary hypertension in lymphangioleiomyomatosis: characteristics in 20 patients. Eur Respir J 2012;40:630–40.
8. Gibson DN, Di Biase L, Mohanty P, et al. Stiff left atrial syndrome after catheter ablation for atrial

fibrillation: clinical characterization, prevalence, and predictors. Heart Rhythm 2011;8:1364–71.

9. Shoemaker MB, Hemnes AR, Robbins IM, et al. Left atrial hypertension after repeated catheter ablations for atrial fibrillation. J Am Coll Cardiol 2011; 57:1918–9.

10. Baughman RP, Engel PJ, Taylor L, et al. Survival in sarcoidosis-associated pulmonary hypertension: the importance of hemodynamic evaluation. Chest 2010;138:1078–85.

11. Parent F, Bachir D, Inamo J, et al. A hemodynamic study of pulmonary hypertension in sickle cell disease. N Engl J Med 2011;365:44–53.

12. Fonseca GH, Souza R, Salemi VM, et al. Pulmonary hypertension diagnosed by right heart catheterisation in sickle cell disease. Eur Respir J 2012;39: 112–8.

13. Pabst S, Hammerstingl C, Hundt F, et al. Pulmonary hypertension in patients with chronic kidney disease on dialysis and without dialysis: results of the pepper-study. PLoS One 2012;7:e35310.

14. Montani D, Price LC, Dorfmuller P, et al. Pulmonary veno-occlusive disease. Eur Respir J 2009; 33:189–200.

15. Willems E, Canivet JL, Ghaye B, et al. Pulmonary veno-occlusive disease in myeloproliferative disorder. Eur Respir J 2009;33:213–6.

16. Jones RM, Dawson A, Jenkins GH, et al. Sarcoidosis-related pulmonary veno-occlusive disease presenting with recurrent haemoptysis. Eur Respir J 2009;34:517–20.

17. Fartoukh M, Humbert M, Capron F, et al. Severe pulmonary hypertension in histiocytosis X. Am J Respir Crit Care Med 2000;161:216–23.

18. Roberts KE, Hamele-Bena D, Saqi A, et al. Pulmonary tumor embolism: a review of the literature. Am J Med 2003;115:228–32.

19. Conde-Agudelo A, Romero R. Amniotic fluid embolism: an evidence-based review. Am J Obstet Gynecol 2009;201:445.e1–13.

20. Wang LJ, Yang HL, Shi YX, et al. Pulmonary cement embolism associated with percutaneous vertebroplasty or kyphoplasty: a systematic review. Orthop Surg 2012;4:182–9.

21. Yi ES. Tumors of the pulmonary vasculature. Cardiol Clin 2004;22:431–40, vi–vii.

22. Hill G, McClean D, Fraser R, et al. Pulmonary hypertension as a consequence of alveolar capillary plugging by malignant megakaryocytes in essential thrombocythaemia. Aust N Z J Med 1996;26:852–3.

23. Hibbin JA, Njoku OS, Matutes E, et al. Myeloid progenitor cells in the circulation of patients with myelofibrosis and other myeloproliferative disorders. Br J Haematol 1984;57:495–503.

24. Halank M, Marx C, Baretton G, et al. Severe pulmonary hypertension in chronic idiopathic myelofibrosis. Onkologie 2004;27:472–4.

25. Bonderman D, Jakowitsch J, Adlbrecht C, et al. Medical conditions increasing the risk of chronic thromboembolic pulmonary hypertension. Thromb Haemost 2005;93:512–6.

26. Corte TJ, Wells AU, Nicholson AG, et al. Pulmonary hypertension in sarcoidosis: a review. Respirology 2011;16:69–77.

27. Takemura T, Matsui Y, Saiki S, et al. Pulmonary vascular involvement in sarcoidosis: a report of 40 autopsy cases. Hum Pathol 1992;23:1216–23.

28. Humbert M, Labrune P, Simonneau G. Severe pulmonary arterial hypertension in type 1 glycogen storage disease. Eur J Pediatr 2002;161(Suppl 1): S93–6.

29. Humbert M, Labrune P, Sitbon O, et al. Pulmonary arterial hypertension and type-I glycogen-storage disease: the serotonin hypothesis. Eur Respir J 2002;20:59–65.

30. Zetterberg E, Popat U, Hasselbalch H, et al. Angiogenesis in pulmonary hypertension with myelofibrosis. Haematologica 2008;93:945–6.

31. Cortelezzi A, Gritti G, Del Papa N, et al. Pulmonary arterial hypertension in primary myelofibrosis is common and associated with an altered angiogenic status. Leukemia 2008;22:646–9.

32. Adir Y, Humbert M. Pulmonary hypertension in patients with chronic myeloproliferative disorders. Eur Respir J 2010;35:1396–406.

33. Weinschenker P, Kutner JM, Salvajoli JV, et al. Whole-pulmonary low-dose radiation therapy in agnogenic myeloid metaplasia with diffuse lung involvement. Am J Hematol 2002;69:277–80.

34. Steensma DP, Hook CC, Stafford SL, et al. Low-dose, single-fraction, whole-lung radiotherapy for pulmonary hypertension associated with myelofibrosis with myeloid metaplasia. Br J Haematol 2002;118:813–6.

35. Le Pavec J, Lorillon G, Jais X, et al. Pulmonary Langerhans cell histiocytosis-associated pulmonary hypertension: clinical characteristics and impact of pulmonary arterial hypertension therapies. Chest 2012;142:1150–7.

36. Goncharova EA, Goncharov DA, Eszterhas A, et al. Tuberin regulates p70 S6 kinase activation and ribosomal protein S6 phosphorylation. A role for the TSC2 tumor suppressor gene in pulmonary lymphangioleiomyomatosis (LAM). J Biol Chem 2002;277:30958–67.

37. Kosmadakis G, Aguilera D, Carceles O, et al. Pulmonary hypertension in dialysis patients. Ren Fail 2013;35(4):514–20.

38. Craddock PR, Fehr J, Brigham KL, et al. Complement and leukocyte-mediated pulmonary dysfunction in hemodialysis. N Engl J Med 1977;296:769–74.

39. Vallabhajosula S, Radhi S, Cevik C, et al. Hyperthyroidism and pulmonary hypertension: an important association. Am J Med Sci 2011;342:507–12.

40. Siu CW, Zhang XH, Yung C, et al. Hemodynamic changes in hyperthyroidism-related pulmonary hypertension: a prospective echocardiographic study. J Clin Endocrinol Metab 2007;92:1736–42.

41. Beigi AA, Sadeghi AM, Khosravi AR, et al. Effects of the arteriovenous fistula on pulmonary artery pressure and cardiac output in patients with chronic renal failure. J Vasc Access 2009;10:160–6.

42. Nakhoul F, Yigla M, Gilman R, et al. The pathogenesis of pulmonary hypertension in haemodialysis patients via arterio-venous access. Nephrol Dial Transplant 2005;20:1686–92.

43. Unal A, Tasdemir K, Oymak S, et al. The long-term effects of arteriovenous fistula creation on the development of pulmonary hypertension in hemodialysis patients. Hemodial Int 2010;14:398–402.

44. Montani D, Bergot E, Gunther S, et al. Pulmonary arterial hypertension in patients treated by dasatinib. Circulation 2012;125:2128–37.

45. Kiykim AA, Horoz M, Ozcan T, et al. Pulmonary hypertension in hemodialysis patients without arteriovenous fistula: the effect of dialyzer composition. Ren Fail 2010;32:1148–52.

46. Shlobin OA, Nathan SD. Management of end-stage sarcoidosis: pulmonary hypertension and lung transplantation. Eur Respir J 2012;39:1520–33.

47. Garypidou V, Vakalopoulou S, Dimitriadis D, et al. Incidence of pulmonary hypertension in patients with chronic myeloproliferative disorders. Haematologica 2004;89:245–6.

48. Altintas A, Karahan Z, Pasa S, et al. Pulmonary hypertension in patients with essential thrombocythemia and reactive thrombocytosis. Leuk Lymphoma 2007;48:1981–7.

49. Gupta R, Perumandla S, Patsiornik Y, et al. Incidence of pulmonary hypertension in patients with chronic myeloproliferative disorders. J Natl Med Assoc 2006;98:1779–82.

50. Dingli D, Utz JP, Krowka MJ, et al. Unexplained pulmonary hypertension in chronic myeloproliferative disorders. Chest 2001;120:801–8.

51. Guilpain P, Montani D, Damaj G, et al. Pulmonary hypertension associated with myeloproliferative disorders: a retrospective study of ten cases. Respiration 2008;76:295–302.

52. Carobbio A, Finazzi G, Guerini V, et al. Leukocytosis is a risk factor for thrombosis in essential thrombocythemia: interaction with treatment, standard risk factors, and JAK2 mutation status. Blood 2007;109:2310–3.

53. Baxter EJ, Scott LM, Campbell PJ, et al. Acquired mutation of the tyrosine kinase JAK2 in human myeloproliferative disorders. Lancet 2005;365: 1054–61.

54. Campbell PJ, Scott LM, Buck G, et al. Definition of subtypes of essential thrombocythaemia and relation to polycythaemia vera based on JAK2 V617F mutation status: a prospective study. Lancet 2005;366:1945–53.

55. Arellano-Rodrigo E, Alvarez-Larran A, Reverter JC, et al. Increased platelet and leukocyte activation as contributing mechanisms for thrombosis in essential thrombocythemia and correlation with the JAK2 mutational status. Haematologica 2006;91:169–75.

56. Falanga A, Marchetti M, Vignoli A, et al. V617F JAK-2 mutation in patients with essential thrombocythemia: relation to platelet, granulocyte, and plasma hemostatic and inflammatory molecules. Exp Hematol 2007;35:702–11.

57. Garcia-Manero G, Schuster SJ, Patrick H, et al. Pulmonary hypertension in patients with myelofibrosis secondary to myeloproliferative diseases. Am J Hematol 1999;60:130–5.

58. Haznedaroglu IC, Atalar E, Ozturk MA, et al. Thrombopoietin inside the pulmonary vessels in patients with and without pulmonary hypertension. Platelets 2002;13:395–9.

59. Perros F, Montani D, Dorfmuller P, et al. Platelet-derived growth factor expression and function in idiopathic pulmonary arterial hypertension. Am J Respir Crit Care Med 2008;178:81–8.

60. Ito H, Adachi Y, Arimura Y, et al. A 25-year clinical history of portopulmonary hypertension associated with latent myeloproliferative disorder. J Gastroenterol 2003;38:488–92.

61. Perrone C, Cartolari R, Lupi B, et al. Pulmonary hypertension diagnosed by echocardiography during idiopathic myelofibrosis. A case report and a brief review of the literature. Multidiscip Respir Med 2010;5:267–70.

62. Hennigs JK, Keller G, Baumann HJ, et al. Multi tyrosine kinase inhibitor dasatinib as novel cause of severe pre-capillary pulmonary hypertension? BMC Pulm Med 2011;11:30.

63. Jais X, Ioos V, Jardim C, et al. Splenectomy and chronic thromboembolic pulmonary hypertension. Thorax 2005;60:1031–4.

64. Elstein D, Klutstein MW, Lahad A, et al. Echocardiographic assessment of pulmonary hypertension in Gaucher's disease. Lancet 1998;351:1544–6.

65. Hoeper MM, Niedermeyer J, Hoffmeyer F, et al. Pulmonary hypertension after splenectomy? Ann Intern Med 1999;130:506–9.

66. Aessopos A, Farmakis D, Karagiorga M, et al. Cardiac involvement in thalassemia intermedia: a multicenter study. Blood 2001;97:3411–6.

67. Cappellini MD, Robbiolo L, Bottasso BM, et al. Venous thromboembolism and hypercoagulability in splenectomized patients with thalassaemia intermedia. Br J Haematol 2000;111:467–73.

68. Peacock AJ. Pulmonary hypertension after splenectomy: a consequence of loss of the splenic filter or is there something more? Thorax 2005;60: 983–4.

69. Landolfi R, Di Gennaro L, Falanga A. Thrombosis in myeloproliferative disorders: pathogenetic facts and speculation. Leukemia 2008;22:2020–8.

70. Thachil J. The enigma of pulmonary hypertension after splenectomy–does the megakaryocyte provide a clue? QJM 2009;102:743–5.

71. Kisanuki A, Kietthubthew S, Asada Y, et al. Intravenous injection of sonicated blood induces pulmonary microthromboembolism in rabbits with ligation of the splenic artery. Thromb Res 1997; 85:95–103.

72. Reiter CD, Wang X, Tanus-Santos JE, et al. Cell-free hemoglobin limits nitric oxide bioavailability in sickle-cell disease. Nat Med 2002;8:1383–9.

73. Gladwin MT, Vichinsky E. Pulmonary complications of sickle cell disease. N Engl J Med 2008;359: 2254–65.

74. Badesch DB, Champion HC, Sanchez MA, et al. Diagnosis and assessment of pulmonary arterial hypertension. J Am Coll Cardiol 2009;54:S55–66.

75. Marvin KS, Spellberg RD. Pulmonary hypertension secondary to thrombocytosis in a patient with myeloid metaplasia. Chest 1993;103:642–4.

76. Najm S, Hajjar J, Nelson RP Jr, et al. Whipple's disease-associated pulmonary hypertension with positive vasodilator response despite severe hemodynamic derangements. Can Respir J 2011; 18:e70–2.

77. Allam JS, Kennedy CC, Aksamit TR, et al. Pulmonary manifestations in patients with POEMS syndrome: a retrospective review of 137 patients. Chest 2008;133:969–74.

78. Baughman RP, Culver DA, Judson MA. A concise review of pulmonary sarcoidosis. Am J Respir Crit Care Med 2011;183:573–81.

79. Handa T, Nagai S, Miki S, et al. Incidence of pulmonary hypertension and its clinical relevance in patients with sarcoidosis. Chest 2006;129: 1246–52.

80. Bourbonnais JM, Samavati L. Clinical predictors of pulmonary hypertension in sarcoidosis. Eur Respir J 2008;32:296–302.

81. Rizzato G, Pezzano A, Sala G, et al. Right heart impairment in sarcoidosis: haemodynamic and echocardiographic study. Eur J Respir Dis 1983; 64:121–8.

82. Sulica R, Teirstein AS, Kakarla S, et al. Distinctive clinical, radiographic, and functional characteristics of patients with sarcoidosis-related pulmonary hypertension. Chest 2005;128:1483–9.

83. Baughman RP, Engel PJ, Meyer CA, et al. Pulmonary hypertension in sarcoidosis. Sarcoidosis Vasc Diffuse Lung Dis 2006;23:108–16.

84. Shorr AF, Helman DL, Davies DB, et al. Pulmonary hypertension in advanced sarcoidosis: epidemiology and clinical characteristics. Eur Respir J 2005;25:783–8.

85. Milman N, Burton CM, Iversen M, et al. Pulmonary hypertension in end-stage pulmonary sarcoidosis: therapeutic effect of sildenafil? J Heart Lung Transplant 2008;27:329–34.

86. Shorr AF, Davies DB, Nathan SD. Predicting mortality in patients with sarcoidosis awaiting lung transplantation. Chest 2003;124:922–8.

87. Gluskowski J, Hawrylkiewicz I, Zych D, et al. Effects of corticosteroid treatment on pulmonary haemodynamics in patients with sarcoidosis. Eur Respir J 1990;3:403–7.

88. Arcasoy SM, Christie JD, Pochettino A, et al. Characteristics and outcomes of patients with sarcoidosis listed for lung transplantation. Chest 2001; 120:873–80.

89. Toonkel RL, Borczuk AC, Pearson GD, et al. Sarcoidosis-associated fibrosing mediastinitis with resultant pulmonary hypertension: a case report and review of the literature. Respiration 2010;79:341–5.

90. Hamilton-Craig CR, Slaughter R, McNeil K, et al. Improvement after angioplasty and stenting of pulmonary arteries due to sarcoid mediastinal fibrosis. Heart Lung Circ 2009;18:222–5.

91. Turner GA, Lower EE, Corser BC, et al. Sleep apnea in sarcoidosis. Sarcoidosis Vasc Diffuse Lung Dis 1997;14:61–4.

92. Thannickal VJ, Toews GB, White ES, et al. Mechanisms of pulmonary fibrosis. Annu Rev Med 2004; 55:395–417.

93. Portier F, Lerebours-Pigeonniere G, Thiberville L, et al. Sarcoidosis simulating a pulmonary veno-occlusive disease. Rev Mal Respir 1991;8:101–2.

94. Hoffstein V, Ranganathan N, Mullen JB. Sarcoidosis simulating pulmonary veno-occlusive disease. Am Rev Respir Dis 1986;134:809–11.

95. Diaz-Guzman E, Farver C, Parambil J, et al. Pulmonary hypertension caused by sarcoidosis. Clin Chest Med 2008;29:549–63, x.

96. Nunes H, Freynet O, Naggara N, et al. Cardiac sarcoidosis. Semin Respir Crit Care Med 2010;31: 428–41.

97. Cross B, Nicolarsen J, Bullock J, et al. Cardiac sarcoidosis presenting as mitral regurgitation. J Am Soc Echocardiogr 2007;20:906.e9–13.

98. Fernandes SR, Singsen BH, Hoffman GS. Sarcoidosis and systemic vasculitis. Semin Arthritis Rheum 2000;30:33–46.

99. Efe C, Shorbagi A, Ozseker B, et al. Budd-Chiari syndrome as a rare complication of sarcoidosis. Rheumatol Int 2012;32:3319–20.

100. Delfosse V, de Leval L, De Roover A, et al. Budd-Chiari syndrome complicating hepatic sarcoidosis: definitive treatment by liver transplantation: a case report. Transplant Proc 2009;41:3432–4.

101. Salazar A, Mana J, Sala J, et al. Combined portal and pulmonary hypertension in sarcoidosis. Respiration 1994;61:117–9.

102. Terashita K, Kato S, Sata M, et al. Increased endothelin-1 levels of BAL fluid in patients with pulmonary sarcoidosis. Respirology 2006;11:145–51.

103. Preston IR, Klinger JR, Landzberg MJ, et al. Vasoresponsiveness of sarcoidosis-associated pulmonary hypertension. Chest 2001;120:866–72.

104. Jones K, Higenbottam T, Wallwork J. Pulmonary vasodilation with prostacyclin in primary and secondary pulmonary hypertension. Chest 1989;96: 784–9.

105. Fisher KA, Serlin DM, Wilson KC, et al. Sarcoidosis-associated pulmonary hypertension: outcome with long-term epoprostenol treatment. Chest 2006; 130:1481–8.

106. Sundar KM, Gosselin MV, Chung HL, et al. Pulmonary Langerhans cell histiocytosis: emerging concepts in pathobiology, radiology, and clinical evolution of disease. Chest 2003;123:1673–83.

107. Tazi A. Adult pulmonary Langerhans' cell histiocytosis. Eur Respir J 2006;27:1272–85.

108. Vassallo R, Ryu JH, Colby TV, et al. Pulmonary Langerhans'-cell histiocytosis. N Engl J Med 2000;342:1969–78.

109. Delobbe A, Durieu J, Duhamel A, et al. Determinants of survival in pulmonary Langerhans' cell granulomatosis (histiocytosis X). Groupe d'etude en pathologie interstitielle de la societe de pathologie thoracique du nord. Eur Respir J 1996;9: 2002–6.

110. Vassallo R, Ryu JH, Schroeder DR, et al. Clinical outcomes of pulmonary Langerhans'-cell histiocytosis in adults. N Engl J Med 2002;346:484–90.

111. Chaowalit N, Pellikka PA, Decker PA, et al. Echocardiographic and clinical characteristics of pulmonary hypertension complicating pulmonary Langerhans cell histiocytosis. Mayo Clin Proc 2004;79:1269–75.

112. Dauriat G, Mal H, Thabut G, et al. Lung transplantation for pulmonary Langerhans' cell histiocytosis: a multicenter analysis. Transplantation 2006;81: 746–50.

113. Harari S, Simonneau G, De Juli E, et al. Prognostic value of pulmonary hypertension in patients with chronic interstitial lung disease referred for lung or heart-lung transplantation. J Heart Lung Transplant 1997;16:460–3.

114. Keogh BA, Lakatos E, Price D, et al. Importance of the lower respiratory tract in oxygen transfer. Exercise testing in patients with interstitial and destructive lung disease. Am Rev Respir Dis 1984;129: S76–80.

115. Crausman RS, Jennings CA, Tuder RM, et al. Pulmonary histiocytosis X: pulmonary function and exercise pathophysiology. Am J Respir Crit Care Med 1996;153:426–35.

116. Travis WD, Borok Z, Roum JH, et al. Pulmonary Langerhans cell granulomatosis (histiocytosis X). A clinicopathologic study of 48 cases. Am J Surg Pathol 1993;17:971–86.

117. Sumino KC, Chakinala MM. A 45-year-old female with a history of dyspnea. Breathe 2006;2:11–4.

118. Tazi A, Bonay M, Grandsaigne M, et al. Surface phenotype of Langerhans cells and lymphocytes in granulomatous lesions from patients with pulmonary histiocytosis X. Am Rev Respir Dis 1993;147: 1531–6.

119. Asakura S, Colby TV, Limper AH. Tissue localization of transforming growth factor-beta1 in pulmonary eosinophilic granuloma. Am J Respir Crit Care Med 1996;154:1525–30.

120. Sauder DN, Dinarello CA, Morhenn VB. Langerhans cell production of interleukin-1. J Invest Dermatol 1984;82:605–7.

121. Barbera JA. Mechanisms of development of chronic obstructive pulmonary disease-associated pulmonary hypertension. Pulm Circ 2013;3: 160–4.

122. Hamada K, Teramoto S, Narita N, et al. Pulmonary veno-occlusive disease in pulmonary Langerhans' cell granulomatosis. Eur Respir J 2000; 15:421–3.

123. Harari S, Brenot F, Barberis M, et al. Advanced pulmonary histiocytosis X is associated with severe pulmonary hypertension. Chest 1997;111: 1142–4.

124. Johnson SR. Lymphangioleiomyomatosis. Eur Respir J 2006;27:1056–65.

125. McCormack FX. Lymphangioleiomyomatosis: a clinical update. Chest 2008;133:507–16.

126. Cottin V, Archer F, Leroux C, et al. Milestones in lymphangioleiomyomatosis research. Eur Respir Rev 2011;20:3–6.

127. Harari S, Torre O, Moss J. Lymphangioleiomyomatosis: what do we know and what are we looking for? Eur Respir Rev 2011;20:34–44.

128. Johnson SR, Cordier JF, Lazor R, et al. European Respiratory Society guidelines for the diagnosis and management of lymphangioleiomyomatosis. Eur Respir J 2010;35:14–26.

129. Taveira-DaSilva AM, Hathaway OM, Sachdev V, et al. Pulmonary artery pressure in lymphangioleiomyomatosis: an echocardiographic study. Chest 2007;132:1573–8.

130. Reynaud-Gaubert M, Mornex JF, Mal H, et al. Lung transplantation for lymphangioleiomyomatosis: the French experience. Transplantation 2008; 86:515–20.

131. Corrin B, Liebow AA, Friedman PJ. Pulmonary lymphangiomyomatosis. A review. Am J Pathol 1975; 79:348–82.

132. Carrington CB, Cugell DW, Gaensler EA, et al. Lymphangioleiomyomatosis. Physiologic-pathologic-radiologic correlations. Am Rev Respir Dis 1977; 116:977–95.

133. Krymskaya VP, Snow J, Cesarone G, et al. mTOR is required for pulmonary arterial vascular smooth muscle cell proliferation under chronic hypoxia. FASEB J 2011;25:1922–33.

134. Reynolds RM, Browning GG, Nawroz I, et al. Von Recklinghausen's neurofibromatosis: neurofibromatosis type 1. Lancet 2003;361:1552–4.

135. Zamora AC, Collard HR, Wolters PJ, et al. Neurofibromatosis-associated lung disease: a case series and literature review. Eur Respir J 2007;29:210–4.

136. Montani D, Coulet F, Girerd B, et al. Pulmonary hypertension in patients with neurofibromatosis type I. Medicine (Baltimore) 2011;90:201–11.

137. Stewart DR, Cogan JD, Kramer MR, et al. Is pulmonary arterial hypertension in neurofibromatosis type 1 secondary to a plexogenic arteriopathy? Chest 2007;132:798–808.

138. Aoki Y, Kodama M, Mezaki T, et al. Von Recklinghausen disease complicated by pulmonary hypertension. Chest 2001;119:1606–8.

139. Samuels N, Berkman N, Milgalter E, et al. Pulmonary hypertension secondary to neurofibromatosis: intimal fibrosis versus thromboembolism. Thorax 1999;54:858–9.

140. Munchhof AM, Li F, White HA, et al. Neurofibroma-associated growth factors activate a distinct signaling network to alter the function of neurofibromin-deficient endothelial cells. Hum Mol Genet 2006;15:1858–69.

141. Xu J, Ismat FA, Wang T, et al. NF1 regulates a ras-dependent vascular smooth muscle proliferative injury response. Circulation 2007;116:2148–56.

142. Li F, Munchhof AM, White HA, et al. Neurofibromin is a novel regulator of ras-induced signals in primary vascular smooth muscle cells. Hum Mol Genet 2006;15:1921–30.

143. McCann C, Gopalan D, Sheares K, et al. Imaging in pulmonary hypertension, part 2: large vessel diseases. Postgrad Med J 2012;88:317–25.

144. Matsunaga N, Hayashi K, Sakamoto I, et al. Takayasu arteritis: protean radiologic manifestations and diagnosis. Radiographics 1997;17:579–94.

145. Erkan F, Gul A, Tasali E. Pulmonary manifestations of Behcet's disease. Thorax 2001;56:572–8.

146. Guillevin L. Vasculopathy and pulmonary arterial hypertension. Rheumatology (Oxford) 2009;48(Suppl 3):iii54–7.

147. Kapusta L, Daniels O, Renier WO. Moya-moya syndrome and primary pulmonary hypertension in childhood. Neuropediatrics 1990;21:162–3.

148. Ou P, Dupont P, Bonnet D. Fibromuscular dysplasia as the substrate for systemic and pulmonary hypertension in the setting of Moya-moya disease. Cardiol Young 2006;16:495–7.

149. Valayannopoulos V, de Blic J, Mahlaoui N, et al. Laronidase for cardiopulmonary disease in Hurler syndrome 12 years after bone marrow transplantation. Pediatrics 2010;126:e1242–7.

150. Hicks J, Wartchow E, Mierau G. Glycogen storage diseases: a brief review and update on clinical features, genetic abnormalities, pathologic features, and treatment. Ultrastruct Pathol 2011;35:183–96.

151. Lee TM, Berman-Rosenzweig ES, Slonim AE, et al. Two cases of pulmonary hypertension associated with type III glycogen storage disease. JIMD Rep 2011;1:79–82.

152. Kobayashi H, Shimada Y, Ikegami M, et al. Prognostic factors for the late onset Pompe disease with enzyme replacement therapy: from our experience of 4 cases including an autopsy case. Mol Genet Metab 2010;100:14–9.

153. Pizzo CJ. Type I glycogen storage disease with focal nodular hyperplasia of the liver and vasoconstrictive pulmonary hypertension. Pediatrics 1980;65:341–3.

154. Ueno M, Murakami T, Takeda A, et al. Efficacy of oral sildenafil in a beraprost-treated patient with severe pulmonary hypertension secondary to type I glycogen storage disease. Circ J 2009;73:1965–8.

155. Furukawa N, Kinugasa A, Inoue F, et al. Type I glycogen storage disease with vasoconstrictive pulmonary hypertension. J Inherit Metab Dis 1990;13:102–7.

156. Hamaoka K, Nakagawa M, Furukawa N, et al. Pulmonary hypertension in type I glycogen storage disease. Pediatr Cardiol 1990;11:54–6.

157. Kishnani PS, Austin SL, Arn P, et al. Glycogen storage disease type III diagnosis and management guidelines. Genet Med 2010;12:446–63.

158. Jmoudiak M, Futerman AH. Gaucher disease: pathological mechanisms and modern management. Br J Haematol 2005;129:178–88.

159. Mistry PK, Sirrs S, Chan A, et al. Pulmonary hypertension in type 1 Gaucher's disease: genetic and epigenetic determinants of phenotype and response to therapy. Mol Genet Metab 2002;77:91–8.

160. Lo SM, Liu J, Chen F, et al. Pulmonary vascular disease in Gaucher disease: clinical spectrum, determinants of phenotype and long-term outcomes of therapy. J Inherit Metab Dis 2011;34:643–50.

161. Roberts WC, Fredrickson DS. Gaucher's disease of the lung causing severe pulmonary hypertension with associated acute recurrent pericarditis. Circulation 1967;35:783–9.

162. Smith RL, Hutchins GM, Sack GH Jr, et al. Unusual cardiac, renal and pulmonary involvement in Gaucher's disease: Interstitial glucocerebroside accumulation, pulmonary hypertension and fatal bone marrow embolization. Am J Med 1978;65:352–60.

163. Ross DJ, Spira S, Buchbinder NA. Gaucher cells in pulmonary-capillary blood in association with

pulmonary hypertension. N Engl J Med 1997;336: 379–81.

164. Amir G, Ron N. Pulmonary pathology in Gaucher's disease. Hum Pathol 1999;30:666–70.

165. Schneider EL, Epstein CJ, Kaback MJ, et al. Severe pulmonary involvement in adult Gaucher's disease. Report of three cases and review of the literature. Am J Med 1977;63:475–80.

166. Bouguila J, Rouatbi H, Tej A, et al. Hepatopulmonary syndrome: a complication of type 1 Gaucher disease. Rev Pneumol Clin 2012;68:58–62.

167. Mistry PK, Liu J, Yang M, et al. Glucocerebrosidase gene-deficient mouse recapitulates Gaucher disease displaying cellular and molecular dysregulation beyond the macrophage. Proc Natl Acad Sci U S A 2010;107:19473–8.

168. Dawson A, Elias DJ, Rubenson D, et al. Pulmonary hypertension developing after alglucerase therapy in two patients with type 1 Gaucher disease complicated by the hepatopulmonary syndrome. Ann Intern Med 1996;125:901–4.

169. Elstein D, Nir A, Klutstein M, et al. C-reactive protein and NT-proBNP as surrogate markers for pulmonary hypertension in Gaucher disease. Blood Cells Mol Dis 2005;34:201–5.

170. Badesch DB, Wynne KM, Bonvallet S, et al. Hypothyroidism and primary pulmonary hypertension: an autoimmune pathogenetic link? Ann Intern Med 1993;119:44–6.

171. Sweeney L, Voelkel NF. Estrogen exposure, obesity and thyroid disease in women with severe pulmonary hypertension. Eur J Med Res 2009;14:433–42.

172. Curnock AL, Dweik RA, Higgins BH, et al. High prevalence of hypothyroidism in patients with primary pulmonary hypertension. Am J Med Sci 1999;318:289–92.

173. Ghamra ZW, Dweik RA, Arroliga AC. Hypothyroidism and pulmonary arterial hypertension. Am J Med 2004;116:354–5.

174. Li JH, Safford RE, Aduen JF, et al. Pulmonary hypertension and thyroid disease. Chest 2007;132: 793–7.

175. Chu JW, Kao PN, Faul JL, et al. High prevalence of autoimmune thyroid disease in pulmonary arterial hypertension. Chest 2002;122:1668–73.

176. Aoki Y, Belin RM, Clickner R, et al. Serum TSH and total T4 in the United States population and their association with participant characteristics: National Health And Nutrition Examination Survey (NHANES 1999-2002). Thyroid 2007;17: 1211–23.

177. Marvisi M, Zambrelli P, Brianti M, et al. Pulmonary hypertension is frequent in hyperthyroidism and normalizes after therapy. Eur J Intern Med 2006; 17:267–71.

178. Guntekin U, Gunes Y, Tuncer M, et al. QTc dispersion in hyperthyroidism and its association with

pulmonary hypertension. Pacing Clin Electrophysiol 2009;32:494–9.

179. Merce J, Ferras S, Oltra C, et al. Cardiovascular abnormalities in hyperthyroidism: a prospective Doppler echocardiographic study. Am J Med 2005;118:126–31.

180. Yazar A, Doven O, Atis S, et al. Systolic pulmonary artery pressure and serum uric acid levels in patients with hyperthyroidism. Arch Med Res 2003; 34:35–40.

181. Armigliato M, Paolini R, Aggio S, et al. Hyperthyroidism as a cause of pulmonary arterial hypertension: a prospective study. Angiology 2006;57:600–6.

182. Ferris A, Jacobs T, Widlitz A, et al. Pulmonary arterial hypertension and thyroid disease. Chest 2001; 119:1980–1.

183. Chadha C, Pritzker M, Mariash CN. Effect of epoprostenol on the thyroid gland: enlargement and secretion of thyroid hormone. Endocr Pract 2009; 15:116–21.

184. Singer PA, Cooper DS, Levy EG, et al. Treatment guidelines for patients with hyperthyroidism and hypothyroidism. Standards of Care Committee, American Thyroid Association. JAMA 1995;273: 808–12.

185. Yanai-Landau H, Amital H, Bar-Dayan Y, et al. Autoimmune aspects of primary pulmonary hypertension. Pathobiology 1995;63:71–5.

186. Miller FW, Moore GF, Weintraub BD, et al. Prevalence of thyroid disease and abnormal thyroid function test results in patients with systemic lupus erythematosus. Arthritis Rheum 1987;30:1124–31.

187. Akikusa B, Kondo Y, Iemoto Y, et al. Hashimoto's thyroiditis and membranous nephropathy developed in progressive systemic sclerosis (PSS). Am J Clin Pathol 1984;81:260–3.

188. Lateiwish AM, Feher J, Baraczka K, et al. Remission of Raynaud's phenomenon after l-thyroxine therapy in a patient with hypothyroidism. J Endocrinol Invest 1992;15:49–51.

189. Shagan BP, Friedman SA. Raynaud's phenomenon and thyroid deficiency. Arch Intern Med 1980;140: 832–3.

190. Ohar JM, Robichaud AM, Fowler AA, et al. Increased pulmonary artery pressure in association with Raynaud's phenomenon. Am J Med 1986;81:361–2.

191. Al Husseini A, Bagnato G, Farkas L, et al. Thyroid hormone is highly permissive in angioproliferative pulmonary hypertension in rats. Eur Respir J 2013;41:104–14.

192. Klein I. Thyroid hormone and the cardiovascular system. Am J Med 1990;88:631–7.

193. Nakchbandi IA, Wirth JA, Inzucchi SE. Pulmonary hypertension caused by Graves' thyrotoxicosis: normal pulmonary hemodynamics restored by (131)I treatment. Chest 1999;116:1483–5.

194. Arroliga AC, Dweik RA, Rafanan AL. Primary pulmonary hypertension and thyroid disease. Chest 2000;118:1224–5.

195. Mayer E, Kriegsmann J, Gaumann A, et al. Surgical treatment of pulmonary artery sarcoma. J Thorac Cardiovasc Surg 2001;121:77–82.

196. Anderson MB, Kriett JM, Kapelanski DP, et al. Primary pulmonary artery sarcoma: a report of six cases. Ann Thorac Surg 1995;59:1487–90.

197. Robbins IM, Colvin EV, Doyle TP, et al. Pulmonary vein stenosis after catheter ablation of atrial fibrillation. Circulation 1998;98:1769–75.

198. Kawar B, Ellam T, Jackson C, et al. Pulmonary hypertension in renal disease: epidemiology, potential mechanisms and implications. Am J Nephrol 2013;37:281–90.

199. Yigla M, Fruchter O, Aharonson D, et al. Pulmonary hypertension is an independent predictor of mortality in hemodialysis patients. Kidney Int 2009;75:969–75.

200. Agarwal R. Prevalence, determinants and prognosis of pulmonary hypertension among hemodialysis patients. Nephrol Dial Transplant 2012;27:3908–14.

201. Fabbian F, Cantelli S, Molino C, et al. Pulmonary hypertension in dialysis patients: a cross-sectional Italian study. Int J Nephrol 2011;2011:283475.

202. Kumbar L, Fein PA, Rafiq MA, et al. Pulmonary hypertension in peritoneal dialysis patients. Adv Perit Dial 2007;23:127–31.

203. Unal A, Sipahioglu MH, Kavuncuoglu F, et al. A rare cause of peritoneal dialysis-related peritonitis: *Gemella haemolysans*. Perit Dial Int 2009;29:482.

204. Sise ME, Courtwright AM, Channick RN. Pulmonary hypertension in patients with chronic and end-stage kidney disease. Kidney Int 2013. [Epub ahead of print].

205. Abdelwhab S, Elshinnawy S. Pulmonary hypertension in chronic renal failure patients. Am J Nephrol 2008;28:990–7.

206. Yigla M, Nakhoul F, Sabag A, et al. Pulmonary hypertension in patients with end-stage renal disease. Chest 2003;123:1577–82.

207. Havlucu Y, Kursat S, Ekmekci C, et al. Pulmonary hypertension in patients with chronic renal failure. Respiration 2007;74:503–10.

208. Acarturk G, Albayrak R, Melek M, et al. The relationship between arteriovenous fistula blood flow rate and pulmonary artery pressure in hemodialysis patients. Int Urol Nephrol 2008;40:509–13.

209. Basile C, Lomonte C, Vernaglione L, et al. The relationship between the flow of arteriovenous fistula and cardiac output in haemodialysis patients. Nephrol Dial Transplant 2008;23:282–7.

210. Yigla M, Banderski R, Azzam ZS, et al. Arteriovenous access in end-stage renal disease patients and pulmonary hypertension. Ther Adv Respir Dis 2008;2:49–53.

211. Dhaun N, Goddard J, Webb DJ. The endothelin system and its antagonism in chronic kidney disease. J Am Soc Nephrol 2006;17:943–55.

212. Schmidt RJ, Baylis C. Total nitric oxide production is low in patients with chronic renal disease. Kidney Int 2000;58:1261–6.

213. Vallance P, Leone A, Calver A, et al. Accumulation of an endogenous inhibitor of nitric oxide synthesis in chronic renal failure. Lancet 1992;339:572–5.

214. Issa N, Krowka MJ, Griffin MD, et al. Pulmonary hypertension is associated with reduced patient survival after kidney transplantation. Transplantation 2008;86:1384–8.

215. Stallworthy EJ, Pilmore HL, Webster MW, et al. Do echocardiographic parameters predict mortality in patients with end-stage renal disease? Transplantation 2013;95:1225–32.

216. Loyd JE, Tillman BF, Atkinson JB, et al. Mediastinal fibrosis complicating histoplasmosis. Medicine (Baltimore) 1988;67:295–310.

217. Chazova I, Robbins I, Loyd J, et al. Venous and arterial changes in pulmonary veno-occlusive disease, mitral stenosis and fibrosing mediastinitis. Eur Respir J 2000;15:116–22.

218. Mitchell IM, Saunders NR, Maher O, et al. Surgical treatment of idiopathic mediastinal fibrosis: report of five cases. Thorax 1986;41:210–4.

219. Garrett HE Jr, Roper CL. Surgical intervention in histoplasmosis. Ann Thorac Surg 1986;42:711–22.

220. Davis AM, Pierson RN, Loyd JE. Mediastinal fibrosis. Semin Respir Infect 2001;16:119–30.

221. Cordasco EM Jr, Ahmad M, Mehta A, et al. The effects of steroid therapy on pulmonary hypertension secondary to fibrosing mediastinitis. Cleve Clin J Med 1990;57:647–52.

222. Doyle TP, Loyd JE, Robbins IM. Percutaneous pulmonary artery and vein stenting: a novel treatment for mediastinal fibrosis. Am J Respir Crit Care Med 2001;164:657–60.

223. Fontaine AB, Borsa JJ, Hoffer EK, et al. Stent placement in the treatment of pulmonary artery stenosis secondary to fibrosing mediastinitis. J Vasc Interv Radiol 2001;12:1107–11.

224. Smith JS, Kadiev S, Diaz P, et al. Pulmonary artery stenosis secondary to fibrosing mediastinitis: management with cutting balloon angioplasty and endovascular stenting. Vasc Endovascular Surg 2011;45:170–3.

225. Goldhaber SZ, Dricker E, Buring JE, et al. Clinical suspicion of autopsy-proven thrombotic and tumor pulmonary embolism in cancer patients. Am Heart J 1987;114:1432–5.

226. von Herbay A, Illes A, Waldherr R, et al. Pulmonary tumor thrombotic microangiopathy with pulmonary hypertension. Cancer 1990;66:587–92.

227. Chinen K, Tokuda Y, Fujiwara M, et al. Pulmonary tumor thrombotic microangiopathy in patients with gastric carcinoma: an analysis of 6 autopsy cases and review of the literature. Pathol Res Pract 2010; 206:682–9.

228. Patrignani A, Purcaro A, Calcagnoli F, et al. Pulmonary tumor thrombotic microangiopathy: the challenge of the antemortem diagnosis. J Cardiovasc Med (Hagerstown) 2013. [Epub ahead of print].

229. Crane R, Rudd TG, Dail D. Tumor microembolism: pulmonary perfusion pattern. J Nucl Med 1984; 25:877–80.

230. Franquet T, Gimenez A, Prats R, et al. Thrombotic microangiopathy of pulmonary tumors: a vascular cause of tree-in-bud pattern on CT. AJR Am J Roentgenol 2002;179:897–9.

231. Seki Y, Gotou M, Yasuda A, et al. Secondary pulmonary hypertension due to pulmonary tumor thrombotic microangiopathy diagnosed by open lung biopsy. Kyobu Geka 2011;64:916–9.

232. Masson RG, Ruggieri J. Pulmonary microvascular cytology. A new diagnostic application of the pulmonary artery catheter. Chest 1985;88:908–14.

233. Ishiguro T, Takayanagi N, Ando M, et al. Pulmonary tumor thrombotic microangiopathy responding to chemotherapy. Nihon Kokyuki Gakkai Zasshi 2011;49:681–7.

234. Trow TK, Argento AC, Rubinowitz AN, et al. A 71-year-old woman with myelofibrosis, hypoxemia, and pulmonary hypertension. Chest 2010;138: 1506–10.

235. Baughman RP, Judson MA, Lower EE, et al. Inhaled iloprost for sarcoidosis associated pulmonary hypertension. Sarcoidosis Vasc Diffuse Lung Dis 2009;26:110–20.

236. Barnett CF, Bonura EJ, Nathan SD, et al. Treatment of sarcoidosis-associated pulmonary hypertension. A two-center experience. Chest 2009;135:1455–61.

237. Held M, Schnabel P, Warth A, et al. Pulmonary hypertension in pulmonary Langerhans cell granulomatosis. Case Rep Med 2012;2012:378467.

238. Houssaini A, Abid S, Mouraret N, et al. Rapamycin reverses pulmonary artery smooth muscle cell proliferation in pulmonary hypertension. Am J Respir Cell Mol Biol 2013;48:568–77.

239. Nishimura T, Faul JL, Berry GJ, et al. 40-O-(2-hydroxyethyl)-rapamycin attenuates pulmonary arterial hypertension and neointimal formation in rats. Am J Respir Crit Care Med 2001;163:498–502.

240. McCormack FX, Inoue Y, Moss J, et al. Efficacy and safety of sirolimus in lymphangioleiomyomatosis. N Engl J Med 2011;364:1595–606.

241. Elstein D, Zimran A. IV epoprostenol in Gaucher's disease. Chest 2000;117:1821.

242. Bakst AE, Gaine SP, Rubin LJ. Continuous intravenous epoprostenol therapy for pulmonary hypertension in Gaucher's disease. Chest 1999;116: 1127–9.

243. Fernandes CJ, Jardim C, Carvalho LA, et al. Clinical response to sildenafil in pulmonary hypertension associated with Gaucher disease. J Inherit Metab Dis 2005;28:603–5.

Chronic Thromboembolic Pulmonary Hypertension

Peter S. Marshall, MD, MPH[a],*, Kim M. Kerr, MD[b],
William R. Auger, MD[b]

KEYWORDS

- Chronic thromboembolic pulmonary hypertension • Pulmonary hypertension • Pulmonary embolus
- Pulmonary thromboendarterectomy • Epidemiology • Diagnosis • Therapy
- Percutaneous pulmonary angioplasty

KEY POINTS

- Chronic thromboembolic pulmonary hypertension (CTEPH) is an uncommon, but serious, complication of acute pulmonary embolus.
- Several risk factors for the development of CTEPH have been identified and many are not directly associated with thrombophilia.
- More research into the mechanisms whereby acute thrombus fails to resolve and results in increased pulmonary artery pressures is needed.
- Presenting signs and symptoms of CTEPH are nonspecific.
- The diagnostic evaluation confirms the diagnosis of CTEPH, helps determine the appropriateness for pulmonary thromboendarterectomy (also referred to as pulmonary endarterectomy), assesses for comorbidities, and determines prognosis.
- Use of pulmonary arterial hypertension-modifying agents may improve hemodynamics and functional capacity but their role in CTEPH is yet to be determined.
- Percutaneous pulmonary angioplasty may improve hemodynamics and functional capacity in patients who are not surgical candidates, but has significant procedural risk.
- Pulmonary thromboendarterectomy is the treatment of choice in appropriate patients.

INTRODUCTION AND DEFINITION

Chronic thromboembolic pulmonary hypertension (CTEPH) or World Health Organization (WHO) class IV pulmonary hypertension is defined by a mean pulmonary artery pressure (mPAP) greater than 25 mm Hg in the presence of organized, nonacute thrombus within the pulmonary vascular bed. The syndrome of chronic thromboembolic disease includes not only patients with overt thromboembolic pulmonary hypertension and right heart dysfunction, but those nonpulmonary hypertensive patients symptomatic because of dead space ventilation, referred to as thromboembolic-related respiratory insufficiency (TERRI).[1,2]

CTEPH arises from an initial thromboembolism or multiple events. However, 1 year after a thromboembolic event, patients are usually left with more than 90% of their pulmonary vascular bed unaffected.[1] Some individuals do not completely resolve clot and experience a series of pathobiological changes that lead to chronic large vessel narrowing and distal small vessel vasculopathy causing increased pulmonary artery pressures. It is unclear whether these pathophysiologic changes have a genetic basis, are related to the anatomy involved, or involve alterations in fibrinolysis. The reasons for the failure to handle the clot burden and elucidation of the pathobiology are the subject of much research.

a Yale University School of Medicine, Section of Pulmonary, Critical Care & Sleep Medicine, 15 York Street, LCI 101, New Haven, CT 06510, USA; b Division of Pulmonary & Critical Care Medicine, University of California, San Diego Health Care System, 9300 Campus Point Drive, La Jolla, CA 92037, USA
* Corresponding author.
E-mail address: peter.marshall@yale.edu

Clin Chest Med 34 (2013) 779–797
http://dx.doi.org/10.1016/j.ccm.2013.08.012
0272-5231/13/$ – see front matter © 2013 Elsevier Inc. All rights reserved.

EPIDEMIOLOGY

Approximately 600,000 acute pulmonary emboli (PEs) occur yearly in the United States, resulting in 200,000 to 300,000 deaths.[3] Only 150,000 of all patients with PE are diagnosed, indicating that thousands of PEs are undetected.[4] Some patients with acute PE, whether diagnosed or undiagnosed, develop chronically increased pulmonary artery pressures. Registry data suggest that the incidence of CTEPH is between 3 and 30 per 1 million in the general population.[5] There are an estimated 500 to 2500 new cases of CTEPH in the United States each year and only 60% to 74.8% of patients diagnosed with CTEPH have a history of documented acute PE, reinforcing the concept that acute PE may go undiagnosed.[6–9] The lack of documented PE in some patients has prompted some investigators to suggest that thromboembolism may not always be the inciting event in CTEPH.[10]

The percentage of patients with acute PE who develop CTEPH is unknown but ranges from 0.6% to 8.8%.[11–14] A prospective study identified 223 eligible patients with acute PE and followed patients for up to 10 years.[14] Patients with conditions that predisposed them to nonthromboembolic pulmonary hypertension were not included in the analysis (N = 81). The cumulative incidence of CTEPH at 6 months was 1% (95% confidence interval [CI], 0.0–2.4), at 1 year 3.1% (95% CI, 0.7–5.5), and at 2 years 3.8% (95% CI, 1.1–6.5). Predictors for the development of CTEPH included multiple episodes of PE, larger perfusion defect, and younger age. No new cases of CTEPH were identified after 2 years of follow-up.

A screening program for CTEPH was devised for 866 unselected patients with acute PE. The overall incidence of CTEPH was 0.57% (95% CI, 0.02–1.2).[15] In patients with provoked PE the incidence of CTEPH was 0, and in patients with unprovoked PE it was 1.5% (95% CI, 0.08–3.1). Only 68% of the original cohort completed the study. CTEPH could not be definitively excluded in the deceased or those not reporting for follow-up and this may have underestimated the incidence of CTEPH. In addition, the inclusion of patients with conditions predisposing them to pulmonary hypertension in the screening program may have resulted in an underestimation of the incidence of CTEPH compared with the results of other studies.[12,13] Studies offering higher estimates of the incidence of CTEPH used only echocardiography to detect CTEPH in symptomatic (and asymptomatic) patients, which may account for the higher estimates, whereas all cases in the screening program cohort were confirmed by right heart catheterization.[13,15]

The incidence of CTEPH after acute PE is probably 0.5% to 3.8%, with few cases identified more than 2 years after acute PE. The relationship between prior thromboembolism and CTEPH is stronger in patients with a prior episode of deep vein thrombosis (DVT), whose incidence of CTEPH is 5.2%, and in patients with a prior episode of PE, whose incidence is 33%.[14]

It is widely accepted that incompletely resolved PE is a risk factor for the development of CTEPH after acute PE, and that larger perfusion defects are correlated with the development of CTEPH.[11,14,16,17] The development of CTEPH after acute PE may also be related to the degree of increase in pulmonary pressures at diagnosis of acute PE. A cohort of 78 patients was followed for 5 years and those who had persistent increases in pulmonary artery pressures after 1 year had significantly higher pulmonary pressures at the time of diagnosis.[17] In other studies, patients with a right ventricular systolic pressure (RVSP) greater than 50 mm Hg at PE diagnosis had a 3-fold to 5-fold greater increase in persistent pulmonary hypertension by transthoracic echocardiography (TTE).[17,18] Reidel and colleagues[19] noted that a mPAP greater than 30 mm Hg at PE diagnosis was associated with further increases in pulmonary artery pressure during long-term follow-up. Although data are limited, there is some evidence that use of lytic therapy in those PE patients with significant pulmonary hypertension at presentation may reduce the occurrence of sustained increases in pulmonary artery pressures, although this remains controversial.[18,20]

Factors other than thromboembolic disease have been identified for the development of CTEPH.[7,21] A cohort of patients with CTEPH was compared with a cohort of patients with precapillary nonthrombotic pulmonary arterial hypertension (PAH).[7] In addition to prior venous thromboembolism and recurrent venous thromboembolism, multivariate analysis revealed that independent risk factors for the development of CTEPH included thyroid replacement (odds ratio [OR], 6.10; 95% CI, 2.73–15.05), a history of malignancy (OR, 3.76; 95% CI, 1.47–10.43), ventriculoatrial shunt (for hydrocephalus) and infected pacemaker (OR, 76.40; 95% CI, 7.67–10351), and a history of splenectomy (OR, 17.87; 95% CI, 1.56–2438). These risk factors are relevant to those without PE or DVT because only 40% of the patients in this cohort had a history of prior thromboembolic disease. Other risk factors include the presence of antiphospholipid antibodies/lupus anticoagulant, inflammatory bowel disease, chronic osteomyelitis, infected tunneled catheter systems, fibrinogen variants resistant to lysis, histocompatibility locus antigen (HLA) polymorphisms, and non-O blood groups.[7,22–25]

The concept that prothrombotic states may predispose patients to the development of CTEPH is supported by several observations. First, prior venous thromboembolism is clearly associated with the development of CTEPH (OR, 4.5; 95% CI, 2.4–9.1), as is recurrent venous thromboembolism (OR, 15; CI, 95% 5.4–43).[7,22] Increased levels of factor VIII have been identified in a greater proportion of individuals with CTEPH (41%) than patients with nonthromboembolic pulmonary hypertension (22%; $P = .022$) and healthy controls (5%; $P<.0001$).[26] After successful pulmonary endarterectomy (PEA), increased levels of factor VIII remain, whereas successful treatment of PAH with prostanoids results in a decrease in the levels of factor VIII.[27] Inborn thrombotic disorders such as factor V Leiden, protein C and S deficiency, and antithrombin III are not consistently associated with the development of CTEPH, however.[21,28]

A diagnosis of CTEPH with mean pulmonary artery pressure greater than 50 mm Hg before the advent of PEA implied a 2-year mortality of greater than 80%.[19] Despite anticoagulation, the 3-year mortality for patients with a mPAP greater than 30 mm Hg is estimated at 90%.[29] Given the overall incidence of CTEPH after acute PE of approximately 0.5% to 3.8%, the incidence of 33% after multiple episodes of PE, and the existence of effective treatment, consideration should be given to screening symptomatic and asymptomatic patients with acute PE with TTE, looking for the presence of increased pulmonary artery pressures, which may signal the development of CTEPH.[30] Many would limit screening to certain groups, such as those with thrombus in central vessels, those with significant hemodynamic changes (or evidence of right ventricle [RV] dysfunction), and those with documented thrombophilia.[31] The interval for scheduling serial TTE is unknown. Following patients for as much as 2 years after the acute event is reasonable given that cases of CTEPH after acute PE have not been discovered after greater than 2 years of follow-up.[14] Patients who have persistently increased or increasing pulmonary artery pressures should be considered for right heart catheterization and treatment.

PATHOBIOLOGY OF CTEPH

In most instances the inciting event for CTEPH is an acute thrombotic event. This event may be symptomatic or silent.[7–9,31] A subset of patients with acute PE fail to resolve thrombus. The resultant pulmonary vascular changes can be described as taking place in dual compartments:

the large vessel compartment and small vessel compartment (pulmonary arteriopathy).[1] The larger vessels in CTEPH are affected to a greater extent than in PAH and undergo remodeling as a result of thrombus that is slow to resolve.[32] The failure to resolve thrombus may be caused by the presence of thrombotic, genetic, or medical risk factors (**Fig. 1**).[21,22,33] The changes observed in the small vessel compartment are similar to those observed in PAH.[5,32]

The pathophysiologic alterations by which an acute thrombus evolves to a chronic vascular lesion continue to be the focus of several investigative efforts. Under normal circumstances the endothelium of vessels affected by thrombus are activated and penetrate thrombus.[34] Areas of endothelial lined spaces are created and eventually form vascular channels. It is thought that the formation of these channels is mediated by vascular endothelial growth factor and basic fibroblastic growth factor.[35] In patients with CTEPH, collagen-secreting cells cause dysfunction of the endothelial cells, causing ineffective angiogenesis.[36] Inflammatory changes may also contribute to the failure to resolve thrombus normally.[5] Levels of the proinflammatory cytokine macrophage chemoattractant protein-1 have been shown to be increased in patients with CTEPH.[37]

The presence of abnormal fibrinogen types and failure to cleave fibrinogen by plasminogen is another possible explanation for incomplete clot resolution.[24,38,39] The (Fg)-Aa Thr312Ala fibrinogen genotype has been identified in greater frequency in patients with CTEPH and is associated with increased risk of VTE.[40,41]

Fibrotic changes in pulmonary arteries can also contribute to vascular narrowing and occlusion. The abnormal migration and proliferation of fibroblasts and myofibroblasts causes vascular wall thickening and loss of vascular reactivity.[5] Vessel wall thickening is produced by the formation of fibrous and atherosclerotic plaques.[42]

The development of a small vessel arteriopathy has been shown to be a feature of those patients with CTEPH,[43] and may be a response to larger vessel narrowing and shear stress (see **Fig. 1**). It is characterized by extension of muscularization into distal vessels, concentric intimal fibroelastosis, intimal fibrosis, medial hypertrophy, and plexiform lesions.[5,43] In CTEPH, arteriopathy is thought to be caused by abnormal endothelial function, abnormal proliferation and migration of smooth muscle cells, abnormal fibroblast migration, inhibition of apoptosis in vascular smooth muscle cells, and in situ thrombosis.[41,43] The importance of pulmonary arteriolar remodeling is supported by several observations: (1) there is often a lack of

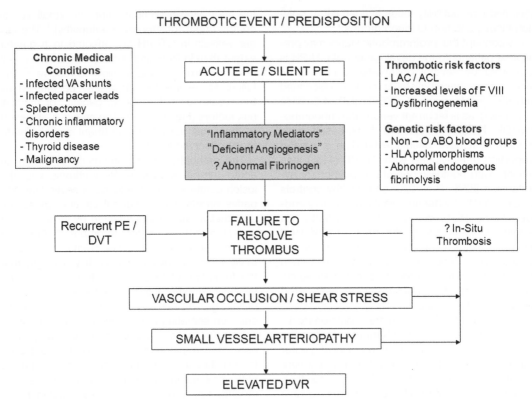

Fig. 1. Proposed pathobiology in the development of CTEPH. ACL, anti-cardiolipin; LAC, lupus anti-coagulant; PVR, pulmonary vascular resistance.

correlation between pulmonary artery pressures and the degree of angiographic pulmonary vascular obstruction, (2) pulmonary hypertension can progress in the absence of recurrent thromboembolism, and (3) the total pulmonary vascular resistance (PVR) is significantly higher in patients with CTEPH than in patients with acute PE and a similar degree of proximal vessel occlusion.[30]

The presence of small vessel disease may be associated with some of the medical conditions cited as risk factors for CTEPH: VA shunts, inflammatory bowel disease, splenectomy, malignancy, and thyroid replacement may correlate with small vessel disease.[24] In addition, in vivo data and animal data suggest that infection with *Staphylococcus* contributes to delayed thrombus resolution (and progression to arteriopathy) and *Staphylococcus* species are often the infectious agent in device-related infections.[33]

Persistent vasoconstriction may also play a role in the pathophysiology of CTEPH.[30] Plasma levels of endothelin-1 are increased in patients with this form of pulmonary hypertension in addition to increased expression of type B endothelin receptors.[44,45] Changes in the endothelin signaling cascade promote chronic vasoconstriction. Similar observations have been made in PAH.

The end result of these changes is the development of increased pulmonary artery pressures. The pulmonary vascular bed is narrowed by an initial occlusion with thrombus and remodeling of adjacent vessels, ultimately resulting in proximal obstruction and secondary distal vasculopathy.[30] With the RV working against the high resistance of a compromised pulmonary vascular bed, progressive RV dilatation and dysfunction ensues, and, if left untreated, patients succumb to progressive RV failure.

CLINICAL PRESENTATION

Patients with CTEPH typically present with progressive dyspnea and a decrease in exercise tolerance. Because these symptoms are nonspecific they are typically attributed to more common diseases such as obstructive lung disease, cardiac abnormalities, obesity, and deconditioning.[1] The symptoms arise from limitations in cardiac output caused by an increased PVR as well as increased minute ventilation requirements secondary to increased dead space ventilation.[46–48] As previously noted, although most patients with CTEPH have a history of at least one previous acute thromboembolic event, approximately 30% to

40% have no such history, thereby making the diagnosis of CTEPH more challenging.[7,8] Early in the course of the disease, physical examination findings may be normal or limited to a subtle accentuation of the pulmonic component of the second heart sound, which can be easily missed. Approximately 30% of patients have a pulmonary flow murmur, a bruit caused by turbulent blood flow through pulmonary arteries partially obstructed by chronic thrombus.[49] Pulmonary flow murmurs do not occur in small vessel PAH and should alert the clinician to search for other causes of pulmonary hypertension when present. As the disease progresses, patients develop exertional syncope and signs and symptoms of RV failure. Findings on physical examination to support the diagnosis of RV failure include jugular venous distension, RV lift, fixed splitting of the second heart sound, RV gallop, a murmur of tricuspid regurgitation, hepatomegaly, ascites, and edema. Cyanosis may be a sign of right-to-left shunting through a patent foramen ovale (PFO).[1]

EVALUATION OF CHRONIC THROMBOEMBOLIC DISEASE

The diagnostic evaluation of CTEPH serves 4 purposes: (1) to confirm obstructing chronic thromboembolic disease as the cause of pulmonary hypertension and quantify its hemodynamic impact, (2) to determine the surgical accessibility of the disease, (3) to estimate the likelihood of symptomatic and hemodynamic benefit from surgical resection, and (4) to assess comorbidities that may affect perioperative short-term and long-term outcomes of PEA surgery.

Any patient with unexplained pulmonary hypertension should be evaluated for the presence of CTEPH because the optimal treatment option for CTEPH is surgical rather than the medical therapy used in other forms of pulmonary hypertension. In addition, survivors of acute PE should be followed after the acute event to detect signs and symptoms of CTEPH. Patients with acute PE with evidence of pulmonary hypertension or RV dysfunction at any time during the acute event should receive a follow-up echocardiogram. Although recommendations for the ideal timing of this evaluation may vary (to be conducted after 6 vs 12 weeks of anticoagulation), a delay in time to echocardiography after the acute PE is meant to determine whether or not pulmonary hypertension and right ventricular strain have resolved.[30,50]

Patients diagnosed with CTEPH are often initially referred to physicians for dyspnea. The evaluation typically begins with chest radiography, echocardiography, and pulmonary function tests.

Once pulmonary vascular disease is suspected, the evaluation becomes more focused.

Routine hematologic and biochemical analyses are usually normal, but may show abnormalities reflecting hepatic congestion and reduced renal perfusion caused by right heart failure. Because it may affect decision making with regard to the intensity of long-term anticoagulation, an assessment for thrombophilic states should be performed. Although the prevalence of hereditary thrombophilic states (deficiencies of antithrombin III, protein C, protein S, as well as factor II [also known as prothrombin 20210A] and factor V Leiden mutations) is similar to that in normal control subjects or in patients with PAH, antiphospholipid antibodies (lupus anticoagulant, anticardiolipin antibodies) may be found in up to 21% of patient with CTEPHs.[21] As previously noted, higher levels of factor VIII have been found in patients with CTEPH compared with patients with PAH or healthy controls.[26]

General Diagnostics

Chest radiography

Findings on the chest radiograph in the early stages of disease may be normal, but as disease progresses RV enlargement may be observed with obliteration of the retrosternal airspace and prominence of the right heart border. Central pulmonary artery enlargement often occurs with more advanced disease; the vessels may be irregular and asymmetric in appearance.[51] The lung fields may be clear, have areas of hypoperfusion (Westermark sign), or have evidence of previous infarction (Hampton hump).

Pulmonary function tests

Pulmonary function testing is commonly performed in the assessment of dyspnea. Although there are no specific findings that suggest CTEPH, pulmonary function testing is helpful in excluding significant coexistent airway or parenchymal lung disease. In the absence of other lung disease, patients with CTEPH typically have normal spirometry and lung volumes. Up to 20% may show a mild restrictive defect related to parenchymal scarring from previous lung infarction.[52] The diffusing capacity of carbon monoxide (DL_{CO}) may be may be normal, mildly reduced, or moderately reduced.[53,54] However, severe reductions in DL_{CO} should prompt consideration of underlying parenchymal abnormalities such as emphysema or interstitial lung disease. Patients with CTEPH may have a normal resting partial pressure of arterial oxygen (Pao_2), but may desaturate with exercise. Hypoxemia is caused by ventilation-perfusion mismatching and is exacerbated by a reduced mixed venous partial pressure of oxygen.[46] Right-to-left shunting through a PFO may also contribute to hypoxemia. When dead space is measured, it is frequently increased and can result in inefficient ventilation, particularly during exercise. This condition has been shown to contribute to the sensation of dyspnea with exertion.[47,48]

Transthoracic echocardiogram

Transthoracic echocardiography (TTE) is a valuable, noninvasive tool for evaluating the patient with unexplained dyspnea. Pulmonary artery systolic pressure can be estimated using Doppler analysis of the tricuspid regurgitant envelope, cardiac output (CO) can be estimated, and right-sided chamber size and systolic function can be assessed. The interventricular septum may show paradoxic motion or bowing in the setting of right ventricular volume overload.[55] Echocardiography is also useful for excluding left ventricular dysfunction, valvular heart disease, and congenital heart disease as causes of pulmonary hypertension. Quality of imaging can be limited by obesity and operator skill. In addition, although Doppler-derived pressure estimations in general correlate with invasive measurements of right ventricular pressures, they may be inaccurate in an individual patient. Pulmonary artery systolic pressure may be underestimated in severe tricuspid regurgitation and overestimations by greater than 10 mm Hg for pulmonary artery systolic pressure may also occur.[56] Right heart catheterization is required to confirm the diagnosis and to define the hemodynamic profile in greater detail and accuracy.[57]

Lung ventilation-perfusion scan

All patients diagnosed with pulmonary hypertension should undergo radioisotope ventilation/perfusion (V/Q) scanning, which plays an essential role in distinguishing patients with CTEPH from patients with small vessel pulmonary hypertension.[50,56,57] Patients with CTEPH show one or more segmental or larger unmatched perfusion defects (**Fig. 2**). In contrast, patients with pulmonary hypertension caused by small vessel disease such as PAH have normal or mottled perfusion scans with subsegmental perfusion defects.[58,59] A normal perfusion pattern on V/Q scan excludes the diagnosis of surgically accessible chronic thromboembolic disease.[60] A large, retrospective study of 227 patients with CTEPH found that V/Q scanning had a greater sensitivity than CT pulmonary angiography (CTPA) in detecting chronic thromboembolic disease (97.4% vs 51%).[61] In a smaller study of 12 patients with documented CTEPH, single-photon emission computed

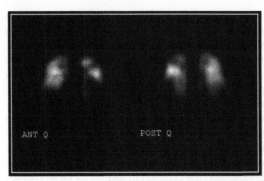

Fig. 2. Perfusion scan of patient with CTEPH with large perfusion defects in the right and left lower lobes and areas of decreased perfusion (*graying*) in both upper lobes.

tomography (CT) perfusion scintigraphy was also more sensitive than CTPA in detecting obstructed vascular segments documented by surgery.[62]

The magnitude of perfusion defects often underestimates the degree of vascular obstruction in CTEPH. This is caused by organization and recanalization of clot resulting in partial rather than complete obstruction of pulmonary arteries that allows limited passage of radiolabeled aggregated albumin, resulting in gray zones in areas of hypoperfused lung on the perfusion scan.[63] Because of this, further evaluation for chronic thromboembolic disease should be conducted even when the V/Q scan shows a limited number of mismatched perfusion defects.

Imaging of Pulmonary Vasculature

In patients with CTEPH, the aim of preoperative imaging is to assess the extent of accessible disease. The quality of the imaging must be adequate to detect chronic thromboembolic disease from the central pulmonary arteries down to the segmental level vessels. Imaging of the pulmonary vasculature can be done with CT, magnetic resonance imaging (MRI), or pulmonary angiography, depending on the pulmonary hypertension center's preference and expertise.

CT pulmonary angiography

CT pulmonary angiography (CTPA) is a commonly used method in the diagnosis of acute PE, but the sensitivity of CTPA to detect CTEPH has been considered lower than that of conventional angiography. However, with technological advances and increased experience, the accuracy of CTPA in detection of chronic thromboembolic disease has improved.[64,65] CTPA provides the benefit of additional imaging of the lung parenchyma, airways, mediastinum, pleura, and chest wall. Findings characteristic of chronic thromboembolic disease are different from those of acute PE and may be misinterpreted by physicians lacking experience in the imaging of CTEPH. Chronic thromboemboli may appear as complete vascular obstruction or partial vascular obstruction, with organized lining thrombus mimicking thickening of the vascular wall, eccentric filling defects, intraluminal webs or bands, or abrupt vessel narrowing (**Fig. 3**A).[66,67] Other findings suggesting CTEPH include enlarged bronchial arteries and collateral arteries from the systemic circulation to the lung. These dilated bronchial arteries are seen in roughly half of patients with CTEPH and are helpful in distinguishing CTEPH from patients with acute PE or PAH, in which dilated bronchial arteries are rarely present.[68,69] Lymph node enlargement was seen in 36% percent of patients in one study specifically analyzing adenopathy in patients with CTEPH. The subcarinal space was the most frequent location for enlarged lymph nodes, followed by the anterior mediastinum and left hilum. Pleural and pericardial effusion were more common in those with lymph node enlargement and it is postulated that the enlarged lymph nodes are caused by slowing of lymph flow because of increased central venous pressure.[70] Lung parenchymal changes include mosaic attenuation caused by areas of relative hypoperfusion or hyperperfusion (see **Fig. 3**B) and peripheral irregular, wedge-shaped, or linear opacities caused by pulmonary infarction.[66,67] CT imaging also allows the surgeon to assess the topographic relationship of the sternum to the medistinal structures before sternotomy.[64] This assessment can sometimes be important in patients with previous mediastinal surgery or massive right heart chamber enlargement. CT scanning also plays a valuable role in assessing the patient for the presence and location of underlying parenchymal disease such as emphysema or fibrotic lung disease.[60]

Chronic thromboembolic disease is bilateral in most patients, with unilateral disease seen in only 3% of 410 patients in one study. If unilateral hypoperfusion of 1 lung is identified with scintigraphy, this should prompt further investigation (CT or MRI) to search for other diseases that may lead to central pulmonary artery occlusion such as pulmonary artery sarcoma, large vessel arteritis, or extrinsic compression of the pulmonary artery from fibrosing mediastinitis or malignancy.[71,72]

Although CTPA can play a valuable role in the evaluation of patients with CTEPH, 2 caveats must be kept in mind: (1) CTPA alone is not sensitive enough to rule out chronic thromboembolic disease, and (2) the presence of chronic clots on CT does not confirm the diagnosis of CTEPH. A study comparing V/Q scanning with CTPA found that perfusion scanning was more sensitive (96%–97.4%) than CT angiography (51%) in detecting CTEPH.[61] In addition, chronic lining thrombus identical to that seen in CTEPH can also be seen in Eisenmenger syndrome, other causes of PAH, and chronic obstructive pulmonary disease (COPD).[73,74] These clots seem to be nonobstructive in situ thrombosis that develops in the central pulmonary arteries. Surgically removing these clots does not result in hemodynamic improvement and poses considerable risk to such patients. Hence, distinguishing in situ thrombosis from CTEPH is critical in the evaluation process and can be accomplished by V/Q scanning. Patients with in situ thrombosis do not show the segmental or larger unmatched perfusion defects that are seen in CTEPH.

MRI of the pulmonary vessels

There is increasing interest in the role of MRI not only in the detection of chronic thromboembolic disease but also in the assessment of right ventricular function and its response to therapy. With

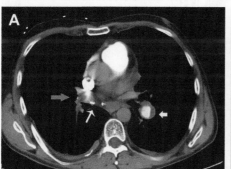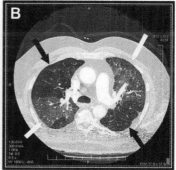

Fig. 3. (*A*) CT angiogram of patient with CTEPH. Note the lining thrombus in the left descending pulmonary artery (*white block arrow*) with occlusion of the right interlobar artery (*gray arrow*) and mediastinal collateral vessels (*white line arrow*). (*B*) Chest CT of patient with CTEPH showing mosaicism reflecting areas of hyperperfusion (*white arrows*) and hypoperfusion (*black arrows*).

experienced clinicians, magnetic resonance (MR) angiography has been shown to accurately show findings of CTEPH (intraluminal webs/bands, vessel cutoffs, and organized central thromboemboli) up to the segmental level.[75,76] In addition, three-dimensional contrast-enhanced lung perfusion MRI tracks the dynamic passage of a contrast bolus, allowing imaging of regional pulmonary perfusion. A recent study investigated 132 patients with pulmonary hypertension, all of whom underwent perfusion scintigraphy, lung perfusion MRI, CTPA, and right heart catheterization at a large pulmonary hypertension referral center. Seventy-eight patients were confirmed to have CTEPH. Sensitivity in the diagnosis of CTEPH was 96% for perfusion scintigraphy, 97% for MR perfusion, and 94% for CTPA.[77] Cardiac MR has been proved useful in the evaluation of right heart function and detection of anatomic abnormalities, and can be used to assess right ventricular volumes, left ventricular septal bowing, muscle mass, and calculation of stroke volume. MRI is particularly advantageous in patients with suboptimal echocardiographic imaging and also allows pulmonary angiographic imaging without exposure to radiation or iodinated contrast.[75,78] Disadvantages include the usual contraindications to MRI such as claustrophobia, pacemakers, and foreign metallic objects.

Conventional pulmonary angiography

Pulmonary angiography (either conventional or digital subtraction) remains the gold standard in the evaluation of CTEPH and can be performed safely by experienced individuals, even in patients with severe hemodynamic impairment.[79] The angiographic appearance of chronic thromboembolic disease is different from that of acute PE because of the organization and recanalization that takes place during partial embolic resolution. Characteristic angiographic findings in CTEPH include vascular webs or bandlike narrowings, intimal irregularities, pouch defects, abrupt narrowing of vessels, and proximal obstruction of pulmonary arteries (**Figs. 4** and **5**).[80] Biplane imaging is optimal because lateral images provide better detail of lobar and segmental vessels that overlap on anterior-posterior images.[1]

Cardiac Catheterization

Cardiac catheterization may be performed at the time of pulmonary angiography.[81] Right heart catheterization defines the severity of the pulmonary hypertension and degree of cardiac dysfunction, which are helpful in assessing the risk of surgical intervention. For symptomatic patients without significant pulmonary hypertension at rest, and who show angiographic evidence of chronic thromboembolic disease, exercise hemodynamic measurements can be obtained. A significant increase in pulmonary artery pressures as CO is augmented is an abnormal physiologic response to exercise, and, with enough chronic thromboembolic involvement of the pulmonary vessels, the normal compensatory mechanism of vessel recruitment and dilation with exertion can be overcome. This information provides objective evidence for a patient's symptoms during exertion, and likely reflects a clinically relevant stage in the evolution of CTEPH.

TREATMENT
Surgical Approach to Chronic Thromboembolic Disease

Preoperative assessment

With the diagnosis confirmed or suspected, assessment of surgical candidacy for PTE should

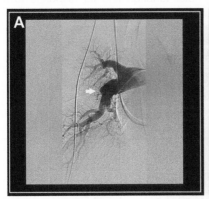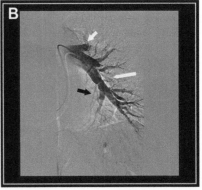

Fig. 4. Right (*A*) and left (*B*) pulmonary digital subtraction angiography. Pouch deformities with lobar occlusions are noted in the proximal right middle lobe and left upper lobes (*white block arrows*). A prominent band is seen at the origin of the left lower lobe (*long white arrow*) and abrupt vessel narrowing can be seen in the antero-medial segment of the left lower lobe (*black arrow*). All are findings of chronic thromboembolic disease.

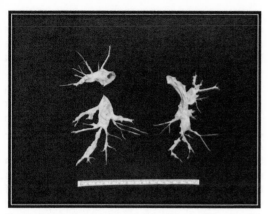

Fig. 5. Surgical specimen from patient in **Figs. 2** and **4**.

be performed at centers with expertise in the management of CTEPH.[50] To be considered surgical candidates, patients must have surgically accessible chronic thromboembolic disease. The definition of surgically accessible varies depending on the experience and skill of the surgeon. In addition to the location of chronic thrombi, the extent of vessel obstruction and its correlation with hemodynamic compromise are important in determining candidacy for surgery. Interpreting radiologic imaging and estimating postoperative hemodynamic outcome is largely subjective and requires extensive clinical experience. Proximal organized thrombi represent the ideal surgical circumstance, but patients with more distal obstruction (isolated segmental disease) often also derive hemodynamic benefit.[82] Because the increase in PVR arises not only from central surgically accessible lesions but also from distal, small vessel arteriopathy, patients with a significant component of small vessel arteriopathy may not experience a significant decrease in PVR following PTE, leaving them at increased risk of short-term and long-term adverse consequences. Determining the presence and extent of small vessel arteriopathy before surgery remains challenging, and is the subject of several recent investigative reports.[83–85]

Most patients who undergo PTE typically have PVRs greater than 300 dyn/s/cm^{-5} with most in the range of 700 to 1100 dyn/s/cm^{-5}. Surgery may be considered for patients with normal resting hemodynamics if they have significant obstruction of 1 main pulmonary artery, those who exhibit significant pulmonary hypertension with exercise, and those who are symptomatic from increased dead space ventilation.[47] Patients with preoperative PVRs greater than 1000 dyn/s/cm^{-5} have been shown to have a higher operative mortality,[82,86,87] but a markedly increased preoperative PVR does not exclude the patient from being a surgical candidate.[82,88]

Comorbid diseases must also be assessed as part of the preoperative evaluation. Coronary artery disease and valvular heart disease can be corrected at the time of PTE.[89] Severe underlying parenchymal disease, particularly involving regions of the lung anticipated to be reperfused with an endarterectomy, is a contraindication to surgery, which has the potential to increase V/Q mismatch and worsen hypoxemia. The postoperative course in these patients is frequently complicated by prolonged mechanical ventilation and they may experience minimal improvement in symptoms following surgery.[90] Hepatic and renal insufficiency may complicate the perioperative period, but may improve with correction of pulmonary hypertension and right ventricular failure. Advanced age increases perioperative risks, but is not an absolute contraindication to surgery.[91]

Pulmonary thromboendarterectomy

Pulmonary thromboendarterectomy (PTE; also referred to as PEA) is the surgical intervention to remove obstructive, adherent chronic thromboembolic lesions from within the pulmonary vascular bed and is considered the treatment of best option for those patients with CTEPH.[92] During the 3 decades following the first attempts in the early 1960s to surgically treat CTEPH, there were several essential surgical modifications that have led to the current success of this procedure.[93–95] Performance of a median sternotomy provides access to the central pulmonary vessels of both lungs, thereby avoiding the disruption of the extensive bronchial artery collateral circulation and pleural adhesions that may develop following long-standing pulmonary arterial obstruction. The use of cardiopulmonary bypass with periods of hypothermic circulatory arrest is the crucial element of the surgical procedure. Deep hypothermia provides for tissue protection, whereas intermittent circulatory arrest periods avoid back-bleeding from bronchial artery to pulmonary artery anastomoses and provides the necessary bloodless field to allow the optimal dissection of chronic thromboembolic material from the pulmonary vessels. The importance of this phase of the operation has grown as dissection from the segmental arteries has become technically feasible, making adequate visualization of these more distal vessels imperative.[82] Modifications of this technique have been used with the intent of minimizing neurologic risks of deep hypothermia and circulatory arrest periods. Those described include the use of moderate hypothermia (23–32°C), aortic bronchial artery occlusion with a balloon catheter, shortening circulatory arrest periods (20 minute to 7 minutes) with more frequent reperfusion periods, antegrade cerebral artery perfusion with and without total circulatory arrest, and application of negative pressure in the left ventricle.[96–100] Data are lacking as to whether any of these technical modifications has substantively affected postoperative outcomes following this surgical procedure.[101]

Most patients undergoing PTE surgery experience both short-term and long-term pulmonary hemodynamic improvement. Immediately following surgery, a reduction in mPAP with augmentation in CO has been a consistent observation, although results vary between experienced centers.[8,82,102–105] In a recent report of the surgical outcomes in a series of 500 patients undergoing PTE between 2006 and 2010, Madani and colleagues[82] showed a reduction in PVR from a preoperative mean value of 719.0 ± 383.2 dyn/s/cm^{-5} to 253.4 ± 148.6 dyn/s/cm^{-5} after surgery. This reduction was the result of a decline in mPAP of 45.5 ± 11.6 mm Hg to 26.0 ± 8.4 mm Hg, and an improvement in CO from 4.3 ± 1.4 L/min to 5.6 ± 1.4 L/min after surgery. As longer term data have become available, the hemodynamic and resultant functional status improvements are sustained in most patients, with a favorable impact on long-term survivorship.[106–111]

There are patients who do not achieve normal pulmonary pressures and right heart function following PTE surgery, although the definition of residual pulmonary hypertension varies between reporting centers. Occurrence estimates vary between 5% and 35% of operated patients, although long-term information as to what level of residual pulmonary hypertension negatively affects functional status and survivorship is lacking.[25,88,106,109,112,113] Possible explanations for this postoperative outcome include chronic thromboembolic disease that could not be surgically resected, or a significant amount of coexisting distal vasculopathy.

Mortalities reported from centers performing PTE surgery have steadily declined over the years, currently in the range of 2.2% to 11.4%,[82,102–105] with the lower perioperative mortality figures at centers with more extensive experience. For low-risk patients based on a preoperative PVR of less than 1000 dyn/s/cm^{-5}, postoperative mortalities have been reported to be as low as 1.6%.[82] However, the presence of residual pulmonary hypertension after endarterectomy represented a considerable risk factor for doing poorly in the postoperative period. Madani and colleagues[82] reported a mortality of 10.3% for those individuals left with a PVR greater than 500 dyn/s/cm^{-5} following surgery, compared with 0.9% when the postoperative PVR was less than this value. As has been the experience for CTEPH centers

worldwide, the overall decline in mortalities is likely a result of expanding surgical capabilities, better understanding of the natural history of the disease leading to earlier and more selective surgical referral, and better coordinated postoperative care.

Nonsurgical Approach to Chronic Thromboembolic Disease

Medical therapy

Several PAH-specific medical therapies have been developed over the past few decades, and have proved to be effective in the treatment of various types of small vessel pulmonary arterial disease. These therapies include several prostanoid derivatives, endothelin receptor antagonists, phophodiesterase-5 inhibitors, and, most recently, stimulators of soluble guanylate cyclase. With the heterogeneity in pulmonary vascular lesions known to exist in CTEPH,[43,114] and especially given the similarities in small vessel disorders shared with idiopathic PAH, efficacy studies have been pursued in several subgroups of patients with chronic thromboembolic disease.[115] The most targeted subgroup in which medical therapy has been tested are those patients deemed to have inoperable CTEPH. Other patient groups in which PAH-specific medical therapy might prove to be of benefit are in patients after PTE showing residual pulmonary hypertension and as a therapeutic bridge in those patients with operable chronic thromboembolic disease with severe pulmonary hypertension and right heart dysfunction. At present, there are only limited data examining disease-modifying therapies for each of these indications.

Most of the published information examining medical therapy for inoperable CTEPH comes from trials with the dual endothelin receptor antagonist, bosentan. In a meta-analysis involving 11 studies comprising 269 patients (39 patients with persistent pulmonary hypertension following endarterectomy), treatment with bosentan was associated with an improvement in 6-minute walk distance (6MWD) of 35.9 m after 3 to 6 months of therapy. Approximately 25% of patients experienced an improvement in New York Heart Association (NYHA) functional class during this same follow-up period. An additional gain of 21 m at 1 year was achieved for patients receiving drug for a more extended period. Hemodynamic data available from 7 studies (185 patients) revealed a weighted improvement in cardiac index (0.23 L/min/m^2), reduction in mPAP (2.62 mm Hg), and, in 5 studies (164 patients), a reported weighted mean reduction in PVR of 159.7 dyne/s/cm^{-5} (20% of baseline).[116]

The only randomized controlled trial examining the efficacy of bosentan in inoperable CTEPH was reported in 2008. Jais and colleagues[117] enrolled 157 patients (bosentan use in 77 patients) with approximately 28% having previously undergone PTE surgery. Compared with baseline, 16-week treatment with bosentan resulted in an improvement in pulmonary hemodynamic parameters: a 24.1% reduction in PVR, a decline in total pulmonary resistance (treatment effect, -193 dyne/s/cm^{-5}) with an increase in cardiac index (treatment effect, 0.3 L/min/m^2). There was also a decrease in N-terminal probrain natriuretic peptide (NT-proBNP) levels (-622 ng/L) in the bosentan-treated patients relative to those receiving placebo. However, at 16 weeks, there was no definable improvement in exercise capacity (6MWD) and no statistically significant treatment effect of bosentan on WHO functional class.

Available studies examining the efficacy of other classes of PAH-specific medical therapy for patients with inoperable CTEPH are more limited. In a double-blind, placebo-controlled, 12-week pilot study, Suntharalingham and colleagues[118] enrolled 19 patients with inoperable CTEPH, assessing the benefit of sildenafil (9 patients receiving drug) in this group. There was no significant difference detected in 6MWD (primary end point). However, an improvement in WHO functional class and PVR were noted. Control subjects were then transitioned to open-label sildenafil use and reassessed at 12 months. Significant improvement in 6-minute walk distance, activity, and symptom scores (as measured on the Cambridge pulmonary hypertension outcome review [CAMPHOR] Quality of Life questionnaire), cardiac index, PVR, and NT-proBNP values (1000–811 pg/mL) were noted. In a larger patient group, Reichenberger and colleagues[119] conducted an open-label study of sildenafil (50 mg 3 times a day) in 104 patients with inoperable CTEPH. After 3 months of therapy, there was a modest decrease in PVR (863 ± 38 dyn/s/cm^{-5} to 759 ± 62 dyn/s/cm^{-5}), with an increase in 6MWD from 310 ± 11 m to 361 ± 15 m; this distance further improved to 366 ± 18 m after 12 months of sildenafil.

The use of intravenous epoprostenol, a prostacyclin derivative, in patients with inoperable CTEPH has also been examined.[120,121] In a recent study specifically addressing this issue, Cabrol and colleagues[121] retrospectively analyzed 27 patients with inoperable CTEPH who were treated with epoprostenol. After 3 months of therapy, there was a decrease in mean pulmonary artery pressure (56 ± 9 mm Hg to 51 ± 8 mm Hg), total pulmonary resistance (29.3 ± 7.0 U/m^2 to 23.0 ± 5.0 U/m^2), and an increase in 6MWD of 66 m.

NYHA functional class improved by 1 tier in 11 of 23 patients. In a single-center uncontrolled observational study, 28 patients with severe inoperable CTEPH were treated with subcutaneous treprostinil (a prostacyclin analogue). Right heart catheterization was repeated in 19 patients after 19 ± 6.3 months of treatment. Treprostinil therapy was associated not only with a significant reduction in PVR but also an improvement 6MWD, WHO functional class, brain natriuretic peptide (BNP) levels, and CO. Five-year survival rate was 53% compared with 16% in untreated historical controls.[122] Although the long-term benefit of inhaled iloprost (an aerosolized prostacyclin analogue) in patients with inoperable CTEPH has not been established, an acute pulmonary hemodynamic benefit has been observed with its use in this patient subgroup. With the administration of 5 μg of inhaled iloprost to 20 patients with CTEPH (12 with distal chronic thromboembolic lesions), Krug and colleagues[123] showed a decline in PVR from 1057 ± 404.3 dyn/s/cm^{-5} to 821.3 ± 294.3 dyn/s/cm^{-5}, and a reduction in mPAP from 50.55 + 8.43 mm Hg to 45.75 ± 8.09 mm Hg accompanied by an increase in CO from 3.66 ± 1.05 L/min to 4.05 ± 0.91 L/min. Acknowledging that 16 of the 20 patients were already receiving one or more PAH-specific medical therapies at the time, the investigators' observation of an acute hemodynamic response to inhaled iloprost suggested there might be a component of vasoconstriction in this subgroup of patients with CTEPH. This finding supports a similar observation made by Ulrich and colleagues[124] in which acute vasoreactivity to 10 μg of inhaled iloprost was shown in 22 patients with CTEPH.

Riociguat, a soluble guanylate cyclase stimulator, has been trialed in patients with pulmonary hypertension and inoperable CTEPH. In a multicenter, open-label, uncontrolled phase II trial, 41 patients with inoperable CTEPH (4 patients also receiving bosentan) were treated with riociguat for 12 weeks. An improvement in 6MWD of 55 m (17.0–105.0 m) from a baseline of 390.0 m (330.0–441.0 m) was observed. In a subgroup of 30 patients undergoing follow-up right heart catheterization, there was a significant decline in mPAP (median improvement of -4.5 mm Hg from a baseline of 42.5 mm Hg), accompanied by a significant decrease in PVR and systemic vascular resistance, along with an increase in cardiac index.[125] Results from a double-blind, placebo-controlled study examining the efficacy of riociguat in the treatment of inoperable CTEPH is awaiting publication.

The use of PAH-specific medical therapy in patients with residual pulmonary hypertension following PTE surgery can be extracted from studies involving patients with inoperable disease. Condliffe and colleagues[106] performed a retrospective observational study analyzing patients with inoperable CTEPH as well as those with persistent post-PTE pulmonary hypertension. Seventy of the 198 patients who survived PTE surgery (35%) showed persistent pulmonary hypertension, which was defined as a mPAP greater than or equal to 25 mm Hg and PVR of 240 mm Hg dyne/s/cm^{-5} or greater. Using treatment criteria of a mPAP of 30 mm Hg or greater and/or WHO functional class III or worse, 8% of survivors were receiving disease-modifying therapy at 3 months, with an increase to 18% at 2 years following surgery. An intention-to-treat analysis of patients with a baseline 6MWD test showed that the average improvement in distance walked was 97.0 ± 14.6 m at 3 months and 103.1 ± 22.7 m at 12 months. One-year and 3-year survival for those with post-PTE pulmonary hypertension was 99% and 94%, which was nearly identical for those patients without residual pulmonary hypertension. In the BENEFiT (Bosentan Effects in iNopErable Forms of chronic Thromboembolic pulmonary hypertension) study, as noted earlier, bosentan had a significantly positive effect on pulmonary hemodynamics but not on exercise capacity, both in patients with inoperable CTEPH and those with persistent pulmonary hypertension after PTE.[117]

Medical therapy has also been used as a therapeutic bridge in patients with CTEPH before thromboendarterectomy, the presumption being that, if pulmonary hypertension and right heart function can be improved in high-risk patients, a reduction in postoperative mortality might be realized. Nagaya and colleagues[126] administered intravenous prostacyclin at a mean dose of 6 ± 1 ng/kg/min for a duration of 46 ± 12 days before PTE surgery in 12 patients with operable CTEPH, each with a PVR greater than 1200 dyn/s/cm^{-5}. This treatment resulted in a significant preoperative reduction in PVR (1510 ± 53 to 1088 ± 58 dyn/s/cm^{-5}) and a decline in plasma BNP levels. After surgery, 1 patient in the treatment group died (8.3%) during the first 30 days, compared with none in the group of 21 patients with a preoperative PVR less than 1200 dyn/s/cm^{-5}. Most notable in study was the observation that the pulmonary hemodynamic outcomes in both patient groups were comparable.

More recently, Reesink and colleagues[127] conducted a randomized, controlled, single-blind study using bosentan as a bridge to PEA surgery. Twenty-five patients with operable CTEPH were enrolled, 13 receiving bosentan, for 16 weeks. Comparative differences from baseline between the groups, with therapeutic benefit achieved in those patients receiving bosentan, showed a change in total pulmonary resistance of 299 dyn/s/cm^{-5}, mPAP 11 mm Hg, cardiac index of 0.3 L/min/m^2, and 6MWD of 33 m. However, postoperative pulmonary hemodynamic outcomes were similar between the patient groups (although postoperative mPAP and total pulmonary resistance were lower in the bosentan group, this did not achieve statistical significance). Three patients died in the no-bosentan group after surgery, compared with no deaths in the bosentan-treated patients. Otherwise, for those who survived surgery, the short-term postoperative clinical courses between groups were comparable (intensive care unit days, ventilator days, occurrence of lung injury).

Further evaluation of the role of PAH-specific medical therapies in patients with CTEPH is required. A recent longer term observational study (32 patients over a mean follow-up of 3.4 years) revealed that, even with advancement of medical therapies, the 1-year and 3-year rates of freedom from clinical worsening were 74% and 60%, respectively. Mortality during this time period was 34% (11 of 32 patients).[128] These figures further emphasize the importance of ensuring that the chronic thromboembolic lesions in any patient with CTEPH are beyond surgical resection given the superior hemodynamic outcomes achieved with thromboendarterectomy surgery.

Disease-modifying therapy might also provide benefit for those patients with residual pulmonary hypertension following thromboendarterectomy surgery. The level of pulmonary hypertension that is clinically important, and the appropriate time to initiate therapy following surgery, require further clarification.

In addition, existing data have not justified the routine use of PAH-specific medical therapy in patients with operable CTEPH, although there may be clinical benefit achieved in a subgroup of these patients with severe pulmonary hypertension and right heart dysfunction. Jensen and colleagues,[129] in a retrospective analysis of patients referred for PTE surgery between 2005 and 2007, suggested that use of PAH-specific medical therapy in patients with surgical CTEPH (19.9% of patients in 2005, 37.0% in 2007) was associated with a significant delay in time to referral, without having a discernible benefit on postoperative hemodynamic outcomes.

Percutaneous pulmonary angioplasty

Published in 2001, Feinstein and colleagues[130] described balloon pulmonary angioplasty as an alternative approach to PTE surgery in selected patients with CTEPH with surgically inaccessible disease, or in those patients whose comorbidities precluded surgical consideration. Performed in 18 patients, averaging 2.6 procedures and 6 balloon dilations per patient, there was an overall decrease in mPAP (42 ± 12 to 33 ± 10 mm Hg), and improvement in functional status and 6MWD in those patients (17 of 18) followed at an average of 35.9 months after the initial catheterization. Only 1 patient died on postcatheterization day 7 (of right ventricular failure). However, the overall postprocedure cardiac index was not significantly improved, the hemodynamic improvement was not comparable with those obtained in patients undergoing endarterectomy, and the development of reperfusion lung injury after the procedure was considerable. Those patients with a mPAP greater than 35 mm Hg were at greatest risk (incidence of 61%; 3 patients requiring mechanical ventilation). In addition, comparisons with the use of PAH-specific medical therapies in this patient population were not available at the time these study results were reported.

With the publication of several recent studies, there has been a renewed interest in pulmonary angioplasty for patients with inoperable CTEPH. In a prospective study of 12 patients deemed to have nonsurgical CTEPH and stabilized with pulmonary vasodilators (including 2 patients with residual pulmonary hypertension after PTE), Sugimura and colleagues[131] performed multiple angioplasty sessions until the mPAP was less than 30 mm Hg. Not only did this approach result in an overall improvement in pulmonary hemodynamics and functional status but, compared with historical controls, an improvement in survivorship was shown. Mild to moderate hemoptysis was observed in 50% of patients following this procedure.

In a larger group of 68 patients, Mizoguchi and colleagues[132] reported a refinement of the angioplasty procedure with the selection of appropriate balloon size using intravascular ultrasound, asserting that this might reduce the incidence of postprocedure reperfusion lung injury. Although 60% of patients still developed a degree of reperfusion injury (including the development of hemosputum), an improvement in mPAP (45.4 ± 9.6 mm Hg to 24.0 ± 6.4 mm Hg) and functional status was reported. One patient died of right heart failure 28 days following the procedure. Results of right heart catheterization were available in 57 patients at an average of 1.0 ± 0.9 years after the final angioplasty procedure (0.3–7.0 years). The initial hemodynamic benefit was shown to be sustained; the mPAP in this group was 24.0 ± 5.8 mm Hg.

A more recent report from Kataoka and colleagues[133] included 29 patients with CTEPH undergoing pulmonary angioplasty. This patient group showed no immediate hemodynamic improvement (28 of 29 patients, 1 patient dying 2 days after angioplasty from wire perforation), although, in follow-up at 6.0 ± 6.9 months, functional status, plasma B-type natriuretic levels, and pulmonary hemodynamics (mPAP, 45 ± 9.9 mm Hg to 31.8 ± 10.0 mm Hg; CO, 3.6 ± 1.2 L/min to 4.6 ± 1.7 L/min) improved. Reperfusion lung injury complicated 27 of 51 (53%) procedures.

There is as yet limited information on the role of balloon pulmonary angioplasty in the treatment of patients with CTEPH. Further information about the long-term benefit of this procedure is warranted, especially compared with PTE of patients with more distal chronic thromboembolic disease. Studies comparing the efficacy of PAH-specific medical therapy versus angioplasty in patients with inoperable CTEPH also need to be conducted.

SUMMARY

CTEPH is a disease with significant morbidity and mortality. Diagnosis is often delayed because of the nonspecific signs and symptoms. The lack of a prior diagnosed pulmonary embolus in a significant number of patients diagnosed with CTEPH also contributes to the delay in diagnosis. As more is understood about the epidemiology and pathobiology of the disease, clinicians will improve their ability to detect this form of pulmonary hypertension.

The mainstay of therapy is surgery, namely PTE. Surgery results in improved hemodynamics, improved functional status, and improved survival compared with nonsurgical management. Over the years the mortality related to PTE has declined and this is likely related to better understanding of the natural history of CTEPH and early referral to selected surgical centers. Preoperative indicators of poor surgical results include markedly increased PVR (>1000 dyn/s/cm^{-5}), major comorbid conditions, and significant lung disease in areas of lung reperfused by PTE. Advanced age is also a predictor of poor outcome but not a contraindication to PTE.

Mortality after PTE is high among those with residual increase in PVR (>500 dyn/s/cm^{-5}). Before surgery, an attempt should be made to determine the extent of distal disease versus more proximal disease or upstream disease because patients with more distal disease often have residual increase in PVR after PTE.

The role of nonsurgical therapy in CTEPH has yet to be defined. Use of PAH disease-modifying agents in patients ineligible for PTE may be indicated, but mortality remains high despite modest short-term gains in functional status and hemodynamics. Medical therapies may be of use in patients with residual increased PVR after PTE but specific indications for their use in this population have yet to be clarified. Use of medical therapies as a bridge to PTE may improve preoperative hemodynamics but does not enhance postsurgical hemodynamics. Preoperative use may result in inadvisable delay of PTE in those patients suitable for surgery. Use of percutaneous pulmonary angioplasty in patients not eligible for PTE may result in sustained hemodynamic and symptomatic improvement. The procedure has a high incidence of postprocedure reperfusion lung injury but, in patients who cannot undergo PTE, may provide an alternative to medical therapy. Given the current understanding of CTEPH, referring suitable surgical candidates for PTE offers the best possible outcomes.

REFERENCES

1. Fedullo PF, Kerr KM, Kim NH, et al. Chronic thromboembolic pulmonary hypertension. Am J Respir Crit Care Med 2011;183:1605–13.
2. Auger WR, Fedullo PF. Chronic thromboembolic pulmonary hypertension. In: Klinger JR, Frantz RP, editors. Diagnosis and management of pulmonary hypertension. Springer, in press.
3. Fedullo P, Tapson V. Clinical practice. The evaluation of suspected pulmonary embolism. N Engl J Med 2003;349(13):1247–56.
4. Kucher N, Goldhaber S. Management of massive pulmonary embolism. Circulation 2005; 112(2):28–32.
5. Lang IM, Pasevento R, Bonderman D, et al. Risk factors and basic mechanisms of chronic thromboembolic pulmonary hypertension: a current understanding. Eur Respir J 2013;41:462–8.
6. Tapson VF, Humbert M. Incidence and prevalence of chronic thromboembolic pulmonary hypertension: from acute to chronic pulmonary embolism. Proc Am Thorac Soc 2006;3(7):564–7.
7. Bonderman D, Wilkens H, Wakaounig S, et al. Risk factors for chronic thromboembolic pulmonary hypertension. Eur Respir J 2009;33:325–31.
8. Pepke-Zaba J, Delcroix M, Lang I, et al. Chronic thromboembolic pulmonary hypertension (CTEPH): results from an international prospective registry. Circulation 2011;124:1973–81.
9. Meignan M, Rosso J, Gauthier H, et al. Systematic lung scans reveal a high frequency of silent pulmonary embolism in patients with proximal deep venous thrombosis. Arch Intern Med 2000;160: 159–64.
10. Egermayer P, Peacock AJ. Is pulmonary embolism a common cause of chronic pulmonary hypertension? Limitations of the embolic hypothesis. Eur Respir J 2000;15:440–8.
11. Miniati M, Monti S, Bottai M, et al. Survival and restoration of pulmonary perfusion in a long-term follow-up of patients after acute pulmonary embolism. Medicine 2006;85(5):253–62.
12. Beccatini C, Agnelli G, Pesaveno R, et al. Incidence of chronic thromboembolic pulmonary hypertension after first episode of pulmonary embolism. Chest 2006;130(1):172–5.
13. Dentali F, Donadini M, Gianni M, et al. Incidence of pulmonary hypertension in patients with previous pulmonary embolism. Thromb Res 2009;124(3): 256–8.
14. Pengo V, Lensing A, Prins M, et al. Incidence of chronic thromboembolic pulmonary hypertension after pulmonary embolism. N Engl J Med 2004; 350(22):2257–64.
15. Klok F, van Kralingen K, van Dijk AP, et al. Prospective cardiopulmonary screening program to detect chronic thromboembolic pulmonary hypertension in patients after acute pulmonary embolism. Haematologica 2010;95(6):970–5.
16. Golpe R, Pérez-de-Llano LA, Castro-Añón O, et al. Right ventricle dysfunction and pulmonary hypertension in hemodynamically stable pulmonary embolism. Respir Med 2010;104(9):1370–6.
17. Ribeiro A, Lindmarker P, Johnsson H, et al. Pulmonary embolism. One-year follow-up with echocardiography, Doppler and five-year survival analysis. Circulation 1999;99(10):1325–30.
18. Thomas D, Limbrey R. P145 Thrombolysis of acute PE patients reduces development of subsequent CTEPH. Thorax 2012;67:A125.
19. Riedel M, Stanek V, Widimsky J, et al. Longterm follow-up of patients with pulmonary thromboembolism. Late prognosis and evolution of hemodynamic and respiratory data. Chest 1982;81:151–8.
20. Kline J, Steuerwald M, Marchick M, et al. Prospective evaluation of right ventricular function and functional status 6 months after acute submassive pulmonary embolism: frequency of persistent or subsequent elevation in estimated pulmonary artery pressure. Chest 2009;136(5):1202–10.
21. Wolf M, Boyer-Neumann C, Parent F, et al. Thrombotic risk factors in pulmonary hypertension. Eur Respir J 2000;15:395–9.
22. Bonderman D, Jakowitsch J, Adlbrecht C, et al. Medical conditions increasing the risk of chronic thromboembolic pulmonary hypertension. Thromb Haemost 2005;93:512–6.
23. Natali D, Jais X, Abraham M, et al. Chronic thromboembolic pulmonary hypertension associated with indwelling Port-A-Cath® central venous access systems. Am J Respir Crit Care Med 2011;183:A2409.

24. Morris TA, Marsh JJ, Chiles PG, et al. High prevalence of dyfibrinogenemia in patients with CTEPH. Blood 2009;114:1929–36.

25. Bonderman D, Skoro-Sajer N, Jakowitsch J, et al. Predictors of outcome in chronic thromboembolic pulmonary hypertension. Circulation 2007;115:2153–8.

26. Bonderman D, Turecek PL, Jakowitsche J, et al. High prevalence of elevated clotting factor VIII in chronic thromboembolic pulmonary hypertension. Thromb Haemost 2003;90:372–6.

27. Friedman R, Mears J, Barst R. Continuous infusion of prostacyclin normalizes plasma markers of endothelial cell injury and platelet aggregation in primary pulmonary hypertension. Circulation 1997;96:2782–5.

28. Wong CL, Szydlo R, Gibbs S, et al. Hereditary and acquired thrombotic risk factors for chronic thromboembolic pulmonary hypertension. Blood Coagul Fibrinolysis 2010;21:201–6.

29. Lewczuk J, Piszko P, Jagas J, et al. Prognostic factors in medically treated patients with chronic pulmonary embolism. Chest 2001;119:818–23.

30. Jaff M, McMurty S, Archer S, et al. Management of massive and submassive pulmonary embolism, iliofemoral deep vein thrombosis and chronic thromboembolic pulmonary hypertension: a scientific statement from the American Heart Association. Circulation 2011;123:1788–830.

31. McNeil K, Dunning J. Chronic thromboembolic pulmonary hypertension (CTEPH). Heart 2007;93:1152–8.

32. Humbert M. Pulmonary arterial hypertension and chronic thromboembolic pulmonary hypertension: pathophysiology. Eur Respir Rev 2010;19:59–63.

33. Bonderman D, Jakowitsch J, Redwan B, et al. Role for staphylococci in misguided thrombus resolution of chronic thromboembolic pulmonary hypertension. Arterioscler Thromb Vasc Biol 2008;28:678–84.

34. Distler JH, Hirth A, Kurowska-Stolarska M, et al. Angiogenic and angiostatic factors in the molecular control of angiogenesis. Q J Nucl Med 2003;47:149–61.

35. Waltham M, Burnand KG, Collins M, et al. Vascular endothelial growth factor and basic fibroblast growth factor are found in resolving venous thrombi. J Vasc Surg 2000;32:988–96.

36. Sakao S, Hao H, Tanabe N, et al. Endothelial-like cells in chronic thromboembolic pulmonary hypertension: crosstalk with myofibroblast-like cells. Respir Res 2011;12:109.

37. Kimura H, Okada O, Tanabe N, et al. Plasma monocyte chemoattractant protein-1 and pulmonary vascular resistance in chronic thromboembolic pulmonary hypertension. Am J Respir Crit Care Med 2001;164:319–24.

38. Miniati M, Fiorillo C, Becatti M, et al. Fibrin resistance to lysis in patients with pulmonary hypertension other than thromboembolic. Am J Respir Crit Care Med 2010;181:992–6.

39. Morris TA, Marsh JJ, Chiles PG, et al. Fibrin derived from patients with chronic thromboembolic pulmonary hypertension is resistant to lysis. Am J Respir Crit Care Med 2006;173:1270–5.

40. Le Gal G, Delahousse B, Lacut K, et al. Fibrinogen Aa-Thr312Ala and factor XIII-A Val34Leu polymorphisms in idiopathic venous thromboembolism. Thromb Res 2007;121:333–8.

41. Lang IM, Marsh JJ, Konopka RG, et al. Factors contributing to increased vascular fibrinolytic activity in mongrel dogs. Circulation 1993;87:1990–2000.

42. Arbustini E, Morbini P, D'Armini AM, et al. Plaque composition in plexogenic and thromboembolic pulmonary hypertension: the critical role of thrombotic material in pultaceous core formation. Heart 2002;88:177–82.

43. Moser KM, Bloor CM. Pulmonary vascular lesions occurring in patients with chronic major vessel thromboembolic pulmonary hypertension. Chest 1993;103(3):685–92.

44. Lang IM, Marsh JJ, Olman MA, et al. Parallel analysis of tissue-type plasminogen activator and type 1 plasminogen activator inhibitor in plasma and endothelial cells derived from patients with chronic pulmonary thromboemboli. Circulation 1994;90:706–12.

45. Bauer M, Wilkens H, Langer F, et al. Selective upregulation of endothelin B receptor gene expression in severe pulmonary hypertension. Circulation 2002;105:1034–6.

46. Kapitan KS, Buchbinder M, Wagner PD, et al. Mechanisms of hypoxemia in chronic thromboembolic pulmonary hypertension. Am Rev Respir Dis 1989;139:1149–54.

47. van der Plas MN, Reesink HJ, Roos CM, et al. Pulmonary endarterectomy improves dyspnea by the relief of dead space ventilation. Ann Thorac Surg 2010;89:347–52.

48. Zhai Z, Murphy K, Tighe H, et al. Differences in ventilatory inefficiency between pulmonary arterial hypertension and chronic thromboembolic pulmonary hypertension. Chest 2011;140:1284–91.

49. Auger WR, Moser KM. Pulmonary flow murmurs; a distinctive physical sign found in chronic thromboembolic disease. Clin Res 1989;37:145A.

50. Wilkens H, Lang I, Behr J, et al. Chronic thromboembolic pulmonary hypertension (CTEPH): updated recommendations of the Cologne Consensus Conference 2011. Int J Cardiol 2011;154(Suppl 1):S54–60.

51. Woodruff WW III, Hoeck BE, Chitwood WR, et al. Radiographic findings in pulmonary hypertension

from unresolved embolism. AJR Am J Roentgenol 1985;144:681–6.

52. Morris TA, Auger WR, Ysreal MZ, et al. Parenchymal scarring is associated with restrictive spirometric defects in patients with chronic thromboembolic pulmonary hypertension. Chest 1996; 110:399–403.

53. Bernstein RJ, Ford RL, Clausen JL, et al. Membrane diffusion and capillary blood volume in chronic thromboembolic pulmonary hypertension. Chest 1996;110:1430–6.

54. Steenhuis LH, Groen HJ, Koeter GH, et al. Diffusion capacity and haemodynamics in primary and chronic thromboembolic pulmonary hypertension. Eur Respir J 2000;16:276–81.

55. Dittrich HC, McCann HA, Blanchard DG. Cardiac structure and function in chronic thromboembolic pulmonary hypertension. Am J Card Imaging 1994;8:18–27.

56. Galie N, Hoeper MM, Humbert M, et al. Guidelines for the diagnosis and treatment pulmonary hypertension; the task force for the diagnosis and treatment of pulmonary hypertension of the European Society of Cardiology (ESC) and the European Respiratory Society (ERS), endorsed by the International Society of Heart and Lung Transplantation (ISHLT). Eur Heart J 2009;30:2493–537.

57. McLaughlin VV, Archer SL, Badesch DB, et al. ACCF/AHA 2009 expert consensus document on pulmonary hypertension: a report of the American College of Cardiology Foundation Task Force on Expert Consensus Documents and the American Heart Association developed in collaboration with the American College of Chest Physicians; American Thoracic Society, Inc and the Pulmonary Hypertension Association. Circulation 2009;119:2250–94.

58. Lisbona R, Kreisman H, Novales-Diaz J, et al. Perfusion lung scanning differentiation of primary from thromboembolic pulmonary hypertension. AJR Am J Roentgenol 1985;144:27–30.

59. Powe JE, Palevsky HI, McCarthey KE, et al. Pulmonary arterial hypertension: value of perfusion scintigraphy. Radiology 1987;164:727–30.

60. Auger WR, Kerr KM, Kim NH, et al. Evaluation of patients with chronic thromboembolic pulmonary hypertension for pulmonary endarterectomy. Pulm Circ 2012;2:155–61.

61. Tunariu N, Gibbs SJ, Win Z, et al. Ventilation-perfusion scintigraphy is more sensitive than multidetector CTPA in detecting chronic thromboembolic disease as a treatable cause of pulmonary hypertension. J Nucl Med 2007;48:680–4.

62. Soler X, Kerr KM, Marsh JJ, et al. Pilot study comparing SPECT perfusion scintigraphy with CT pulmonary angiography in chronic thromboembolic pulmonary hypertension. Respirology 2012;17:180–4.

63. Ryan KL, Fedullo PF, Davis GB, et al. Perfusion scan findings understate the severity of angiographic and hemodynamic compromise in chronic thromboembolic pulmonary hypertension. Chest 1988;93:1180–5.

64. Reichelt A, Hoeper MM, Galanski M, et al. Chronic thromboembolic pulmonary hypertension: evaluation with 64-detector row CT versus digital subtraction angiography. Eur J Radiol 2009;71:49–54.

65. Sugiura T, Tanabe N, Matsuura Y, et al. Role of 320-slice CT imaging in the diagnostic workup of patients with chronic thromboembolic pulmonary hypertension. Chest 2013;143:1070–7.

66. Bergin CJ, Sirlin CB, Hauschildt JP, et al. Chronic thromboembolism; diagnosis with helical CT and MR imaging with angiographic and surgical correlation. Radiology 1997;204:695–702.

67. Willemink MJ, van Es HW, Koobs L, et al. CT evaluation of chronic thromboembolic pulmonary hypertension. Clin Radiol 2012;67:277–85.

68. Heinrich M, Uder M, Tscholl D, et al. CT scan findings in chronic thromboembolic pulmonary hypertension. Chest 2005;127:1606–13.

69. Remy-Jardin M, Bouaziz N, Dumont P, et al. Comparison of systemic collateral supply in patients with chronic thromboembolic pulmonary hypertension; noninvasive assessment with multislice spiral CT angiography. Eur Radiol 2004;14(Suppl):163.

70. Bergin CJ, Park KJ. Lymph node enlargement in pulmonary arterial hypertension due to chronic thromboembolism. J Med Imaging Radiat Oncol 2008;52:18–23.

71. Bergin CJ, Hauschildt JP, Brown MA, et al. Identifying the cause of hypoperfusion in patients suspected to have chronic pulmonary thromboembolism: diagnostic accuracy of helical CT and conventional angiography. Radiology 1999;213:743–9.

72. Wijesuriya S, Chandratreya L, Medford AR. Chronic pulmonary emboli and radiologic mimics on CT pulmonary angiography. A diagnostic challenge. Chest 2013;143(5):1460–71.

73. Moser KM, Fedullo PF, Finkbeiner WE, et al. Do patients with primary pulmonary hypertension develop extensive central thrombi? Circulation 1995;91:741–5.

74. Russo A, De Luca M, Vigna C, et al. Central pulmonary artery lesions in chronic obstructive pulmonary disease. A transesophageal echocardiographic study. Circulation 1999;100:1808–15.

75. Kovacs G, Reiter G, Reiter U, et al. The emerging role of magnetic resonance imaging in the diagnosis and management of pulmonary hypertension. Respiration 2008;76:458–70.

76. Kreitner KF, Ley S, Kauczor HU, et al. Chronic thromboembolic pulmonary hypertension: pre- and postoperative assessment with breath-hold MR imaging techniques. Radiology 2004;232: 535–43.

77. Rajaram S, Swift AJ, Telfer A, et al. 3D contrast-enhanced lung perfusion MRI is an effective screening tool for chronic thromboembolic pulmonary hypertension: results from the ASPIRE registry. Thorax 2013;68(7):677–8.

78. Swift AJ, Rajaram S, Condliffe R, et al. Diagnostic accuracy of cardiovascular magnetic resonance imaging of right ventricular morphology and function in the assessment of suspected pulmonary hypertension results from the ASPIRE registry. J Cardiovasc Magn Reson 2012;14:40.

79. Pitton MB, Duber C, Mayer E, et al. Hemodynamic effects of nonionic contrast bolus injection and oxygen inhalation during pulmonary angiography in patients with chronic major-vessel thromboembolic pulmonary hypertension. Circulation 1996; 94:2485–91.

80. Auger WR, Fedullo PF, Moser KM, et al. Chronic major-vessel thromboembolic pulmonary artery obstruction: appearance at angiography. Radiology 1992;182:393–8.

81. Hoeper MM, Lee SH, Voswinckel R, et al. Complications of right heart catheterization procedures in patients with pulmonary hypertension in experienced centers. J Am Coll Cardiol 2006;48: 2546–52.

82. Madani MM, Auger WR, Pretorius V, et al. Pulmonary endarterectomy: recent changes in a single institution's experience of more than 2,700 patient. Ann Thorac Surg 2012;94:97–103.

83. Kim NH, Fessler P, Channick RN, et al. Preoperative partitioning of pulmonary vascular resistance correlates with early outcome after thromboendarterectomy for chronic thromboembolic pulmonary hypertension. Circulation 2004;109:18–22.

84. Hardziyenka M, Reesink HJ, Bouma BJ, et al. A novel echocardiographic predictor of in-hospital mortality and mid-term haemodynamic improvement after pulmonary endarterectomy for chronic thromboembolic pulmonary hypertension. Eur Heart J 2007;28:842–9.

85. Toshner M, Suntharalingam J, Fesler P, et al. Occlusion pressure analysis role in partitioning of pulmonary vascular resistance in CTEPH. Eur Respir J 2012;40:612–7.

86. Hartz RS, Byme JG, Levitsky S, et al. Predictors of mortality in pulmonary thromboendarterectomy. Ann Thorac Surg 1996;62:1255–60.

87. Darteville P, Fadel E, Mussot S, et al. Chronic thromboembolic pulmonary hypertension. Eur Respir J 2004;23:637–48.

88. Thistlethwaite PA, Kemp A, Du L, et al. Outcomes of pulmonary endarterectomy for treatment of extreme thromboembolic pulmonary hypertension. J Thorac Cardiovasc Surg 2006; 131:307–13.

89. Thistlethwaite PA, Auger WR, Madani MM, et al. Pulmonary thromboendarterectomy combined with other cardiac operations: indications, surgical approach, and outcome. Ann Thorac Surg 2001; 72:13–9.

90. Kunihara T, Gerdts J, Groesdonk H, et al. Predictors of postoperative outcome after pulmonary endarterectomy from a 14-year experience with 279 patients. Eur J Cardiothorac Surg 2011;40: 154–61.

91. Berman M, Hardman G, Sharples L, et al. Pulmonary endarterectomy: outcomes in patients >70. Eur J Cardiothorac Surg 2012;41:e154–60.

92. Jenkins DP, Madani M, Mayer E, et al. Surgical treatment of chronic thromboembolic pulmonary hypertension. Eur Respir J 2013;41:735–42.

93. Daily PO, Auger WR. Historical perspective: surgery for chronic thromboembolic disease. Semin Thorac Cardiovasc Surg 1999;11:143–51.

94. Winkler MH, Rohrer CH, Ratty SC, et al. Techniques of profound hypothermia and circulatory arrest for pulmonary thromboendarterectomy. J Extra Corp Tech 1990;22:57–60.

95. Madani MM, Jamieson SW. Technical advances of pulmonary endarterectomy for chronic thromboembolic disease. Semin Thorac Cardiovasc Surg 2006;18:243–9.

96. Hagl C, Khaladj N, Peters T, et al. Technical advances of pulmonary thromboendarterectomy for chronic thromboembolic pulmonary hypertension. Eur J Cardiothorac Surg 2003;23:776–81.

97. Thompson B, Tsui SS, Dunning J, et al. Pulmonary endarterectomy is possible and effective without the use of complete circulatory arrest–the UK experience in over 150 patients. Eur J Cardiothorac Surg 2008;33:157–63.

98. Mikus PM, Mikus E, Martin-Suarez S, et al. Pulmonary endarterectomy: an alternative to circulatory arrest and deep hypothermia: mid-term results. Eur J Cardiothorac Surg 2008; 34:159–63.

99. Lafci G, Tasoglu I, Ulas MM, et al. Pulmonary endarterectomy with use of moderate hypothermia and antegrade cerebral perfusion without circulatory arrest. Tex Heart Inst J 2012;39:65–7.

100. Morsolini M, Nicolardi S, Milanesi E, et al. Evolving surgical techniques for pulmonary endarterectomy according to the changing features of chronic thromboembolic pulmonary hypertension patients during 17-year single-center experience. J Thorac Cardiovasc Surg 2012;144:100–7.

101. Vuylsteke A, Sharples L, Charman G, et al. Circulatory arrest versus cerebral perfusion during pulmonary endarterectomy surgery (PEACOG): a randomized controlled trial. Lancet 2011;378:1379–87.

102. Mayer E, Jenkins D, Lindner J, et al. Surgical management and outcome of patients with chronic thromboembolic pulmonary hypertension: results from an international prospective registry. J Thorac Cardiovasc Surg 2011;141:702–10.

103. Ogino H, Ando M, Matsuda H, et al. Japanese single-center experience of surgery for chronic thromboembolic pulmonary hypertension. Ann Thorac Surg 2006;82:630–6.

104. de Perrot M, McRae K, Shargall Y, et al. Pulmonary thromboendarterectomy for chronic thromboembolic pulmonary hypertension: the Toronto experience. Can J Cardiol 2011;27:692–7.

105. Maliyasena VA, Hopkins PM, Thomson BM, et al. An Australian tertiary referral center experience of the management of chronic thromboembolic pulmonary hypertension. Pulm Circ 2012;2:359–64.

106. Condliffe R, Kiely DG, Gibbs JS, et al. Improved outcomes in medically and surgically treated chronic thromboembolic pulmonary hypertension. Am J Respir Crit Care Med 2008;177:1122–7.

107. Saouti N, Morshuis WJ, Heijmen RH, et al. Long-term outcome after pulmonary endarterectomy for chronic thromboembolic pulmonary hypertension: a single institution experience. Eur J Cardiothorac Surg 2009;35:947–52.

108. Freed DH, Thomson BM, Tsui SS, et al. Functional and haemodynamic outcome 1 year after pulmonary thromboendarterectomy. Eur J Cardiothorac Surg 2008;34:525–30.

109. Corsico AG, D'Armini AM, Cerveri I, et al. Long term outcome after pulmonary thromboendarterectomy. Am J Respir Crit Care Med 2008;178:419–24.

110. Ishida K, Masuda M, Tanabe N, et al. Long-term outcome after pulmonary endarterectomy for chronic thromboembolic pulmonary hypertension. J Thorac Cardiovasc Surg 2012;144:321–6.

111. Oh SJ, Bok JS, Hwang HY, et al. Clinical outcomes of thromboendarterectomy for chronic thromboembolic pulmonary hypertension: 12-year experience. Korean J Thorac Cardiovasc Surg 2013;46:41–8.

112. Freed DH, Thomson BM, Berman M, et al. Survival after pulmonary thromboendarterectomy: effect of residual pulmonary hypertension. J Thorac Cardiovasc Surg 2011;141:383–7.

113. Kepez A, Sunbul M, Kivrak T, et al. Evaluation of improvement in exercise capacity after pulmonary endarterectomy in patients with chronic thromboembolic pulmonary hypertension: correlation with echocardiographic parameters. Thorac Cardiovasc Surg 2013. [Epub ahead of print].

114. Yi ES, Kim H, Ahn H, et al. Distribution of obstructive intimal lesions and their cellular phenotypes in chronic pulmonary hypertension. A morphometric and immunohistochemical study. Am J Respir Crit Care Med 2000;162:1577–86.

115. Bresser P, Pepke-Zaba J, Jais X, et al. Medical therapies for chronic thromboembolic pulmonary hypertension. An evolving treatment paradigm. Proc Am Thorac Soc 2006;3:594–600.

116. Becattini C, Manina G, Busti C, et al. Bosentan for chronic thromboembolic pulmonary hypertension: findings from a systemic review and a meta-analysis. Thromb Res 2010;126:e51–6.

117. Jais X, D'Armini A, Jansa P, et al. Bosentan for treatment of inoperable chronic thromboembolic pulmonary hypertension: BENEFiT (Bosentan effects in iNopErable Forms of chronIc Thromboembolic pulmonary hypertension), a randomized, placebo-controlled trial. J Am Coll Cardiol 2008;52:2127–34.

118. Suntharalingham J, Treacy CM, Doughty NJ, et al. Long-term use of sildenafil in inoperable chronic thromboembolic pulmonary hypertension. Chest 2008;134:229–36.

119. Reichenberger F, Voswinckel R, Enke B, et al. Long-term treatment with sildenafil in chronic thromboembolic pulmonary hypertension. Eur Respir J 2007;30:922–7.

120. Scelsi L, Ghio S, Campana C, et al. Epoprostenol in chronic thromboembolic pulmonary hypertension with distal lesions. Ital Heart J 2004;5:618–23.

121. Cabrol S, Souza R, Jais X, et al. Intravenous epoprostenol in inoperable chronic thromboembolic pulmonary hypertension. J Heart Lung Transplant 2007;26:357–62.

122. Skoro-Sajer N, Bonderman D, Wiesbauer F, et al. Treprostinil for severe inoperable chronic thromboembolic pulmonary hypertension. J Thromb Haemost 2007;5:483–9.

123. Krug S, Hammerschmidt S, Pankau H, et al. Acute improved hemodynamics following inhaled iloprost in chronic thromboembolic pulmonary hypertension. Respiration 2008;76:154–9.

124. Ulrich S, Fischler M, Speich R, et al. Chronic thromboembolic and pulmonary arterial hypertension share acute vasoreactivity properties. Chest 2006;130:841–6.

125. Ghofrani HA, Hoeper MM, Halank M, et al. Riociguat for chronic thromboembolic pulmonary hypertension and pulmonary arterial hypertension: a phase II study. Eur Respir J 2010;36:792–9.

126. Nagaya N, Sasaki N, Ando M, et al. Prostacyclin therapy before pulmonary thromboendarterectomy in patients with chronic thromboembolic pulmonary hypertension. Chest 2003;123:338–43.

127. Reesink HJ, Surie S, Kloek JJ, et al. Bosentan as a bridge to pulmonary endarterectomy for chronic

thromboembolic pulmonary hypertension. J Thorac Cardiovasc Surg 2010;139:85–91.

128. Scholzel B, Post MC, Thijs Plokker HW, et al. Clinical worsening during long-term follow-up in inoperable chronic thromboembolic pulmonary hypertension. Lung 2012;190:161–7.

129. Jensen KW, Kerr KM, Fedullo PF, et al. Pulmonary hypertensive medical therapy in chronic thromboembolic pulmonary hypertension before pulmonary thromboendarterectomy. Circulation 2009;120: 1248–54.

130. Feinstein JA, Goldhaber SZ, Lock JE, et al. Balloon angioplasty for treatment of chronic thromboembolic pulmonary hypertension. Circulation 2001; 103:10–3.

131. Sugimura K, Fukumoto Y, Satoh K, et al. Percutaneous transluminal pulmonary angioplasty markedly improves pulmonary hemodynamics and long-term prognosis in patients with chronic thromboembolic pulmonary hypertension. Circ J 2012;76:485–8.

132. Mizoguchi H, Ogawa A, Munemasa M, et al. Refined balloon pulmonary angioplasty for inoperable patients with chronic thromboembolic pulmonary hypertension. Circ Cardiovasc Interv 2012;5: 748–55.

133. Katoaka M, Inami T, Hayashida K, et al. Percutaneous transluminal pulmonary angioplasty for the treatment of chronic thromboembolic pulmonary hypertension. Circ Cardiovasc Interv 2012;5: 756–62.

Standard Nonspecific Therapies in the Management of Pulmonary Arterial Hypertension

Maor Sauler, MD[a], Wassim H. Fares, MD, MSc[b],
Terence K. Trow, MD[c],*

KEYWORDS

- Pulmonary hypertension • Pulmonary arterial hypertension • Adjunct therapies • Oxygen therapy
- Diuretics • Anticoagulation • Digoxin • Calcium channel blockers

KEY POINTS

- Adjunct therapies in pulmonary arterial hypertension (PAH), including oxygen, diuretics, digoxin, and anticoagulation, are still relevant treatment options in PAH despite the lack of robust clinical data.
- Oxygen therapy is a low-risk intervention that has the physiologic benefit of improving hypoxemia and decreasing pulmonary vasoconstriction. Its use has been shown to be efficacious in chronic obstructive pulmonary disease and may be of benefit in PAH.
- Diuresis can improve right ventricular (RV) functioning if PAH results in RV pressure and volume overload.
- The use of digoxin is extrapolated from its use in left-sided systolic heart failure and may have a theoretic beneficial role in PAH.
- Because idiopathic pulmonary arterial hypertension is associated with hypercoagulability, anticoagulation may improve long-term outcomes in some patients, although its use should be weighed against the risk of bleeding.
- Acute vasoreactivity testing defines a small subset of patients with PAH in whom high-dose calcium channel blocker monotherapy can be effective.

INTRODUCTION

Recent advances in pulmonary arterial hypertension (PAH) research over the past 20 years have created a new era of PAH-specific therapies.[1–4] Although the advent of these therapeutics has revolutionized PAH therapy, their innovation was predated by supportive but nonspecific medical therapies that were adapted from their use in other more common cardiopulmonary diseases. Still in use today, these therapies include oxygen therapy, diuretics, digoxin, anticoagulation, and high-dose calcium channel blockers (CCBs).[1,2] Although never validated in robust, prospective, placebo-controlled trials to show a significant mortality difference in patients with PAH, expert

[a] Section of Pulmonary, Critical Care, & Sleep Medicine, Department of Internal Medicine, Yale University School of Medicine, 333 Cedar Street, PO Box 208057, New Haven, CT 06520-8057, USA; [b] Yale Pulmonary Vascular Disease Program, Section of Pulmonary, Critical Care, & Sleep Medicine, Department of Internal Medicine, Yale University School of Medicine, 333 Cedar Street, LLCI 105 C, New Haven, CT 06520-8057, USA; [c] Yale Pulmonary Vascular Disease Program, Department of Internal Medicine, Yale University School of Medicine, 333 Cedar Street, LLCI 105 D, New Haven, CT 06520-8057, USA
* Corresponding author.
E-mail address: terence.trow@yale.edu

Clin Chest Med 34 (2013) 799–810
http://dx.doi.org/10.1016/j.ccm.2013.08.013
0272-5231/13/$ – see front matter © 2013 Elsevier Inc. All rights reserved.

opinion continues to support the use of adjunct therapies based on the current pathologic understandings of PAH combined with some evidence extrapolated from small studies. This article discusses why these therapies continue to play an important role in the treatment of patients with PAH.[2–4]

OXYGEN THERAPY

The use of supplemental oxygen therapy in PAH is based on the understanding that hypoxemia is a strong stimulus for pulmonary vasoconstriction as the lung vasculature tries to match lung perfusion with ventilation. The mechanism underlying this process is not completely understood but research has suggested that decreased oxygen availability for respiration results in changes in reactive oxygen species production, which signals calcium influx leading to vasoconstriction.[5]

The role of oxygen therapy has not been specifically studied in PAH, but has been extrapolated from data in hypoxemic patients with chronic obstructive pulmonary disease (COPD). In particular, 2 landmark trials in the early 1980s showed a survival benefit if patients were treated with at least 15 hours/d of supplemental oxygen.[6,7] However, this improvement in mortality did not seem to occur as a result of decreasing hypoxic vasoconstriction. Oxygen therapy does not correct, or even nearly correct, pulmonary hypertension (PH) in patients with COPD. Although some reduction in pulmonary vascular resistance (PVR) can occur, improved survival in patients with COPD treated with oxygen is not thought to be caused by the modest reduction in pulmonary artery pressure (PAP).[8] Furthermore, a post hoc analysis from the Nocturnal Oxygen Therapy in Hypoxemic Chronic Obstructive Lung Disease Trial (NOTT) showed the greatest mortality benefit in patients with low baseline PVRs and patients with the greatest improvements in PVR paradoxically had the highest mortality.[6]

Similar to those with COPD-related hypoxemia, supplemental oxygen therapy is recommended in patients with PAH who have shown hypoxemia. At present, it is recommended that patients with PAH whose partial pressure of arterial oxygen (Pao$_2$) is consistently less than or equal to 55 mm Hg or whose oxyhemoglobin saturation is less than or equal to 88% at rest, during sleep, or with ambulation receive oxygen therapy.[2–4]

In addition, patients with evidence of chronic hypoxemia such as polycythemia (hematocrit >55%), signs of cor pulmonale, or suggestion of right heart failure (RHF) on an electrocardiogram (ECG) or echocardiography should receive oxygen therapy if the oxyhemoglobin saturation is less than or equal to 89% or if the Pao$_2$ is less than 60 mm Hg.[4,9,10] All patients with a moderate to severe impairment of diffusion of carbon monoxide (DLCO) warrant testing of oxyhemoglobin desaturation.[10,11] Hypoxemia at rest or intermittently with sleep or exercise is common in patients with PAH.[12] Intermittent worsening of oxygen saturation during exercise is occasionally a consequence of increased right-to-left shunting through a patent foramen ovale. In addition, if there is no evidence of hypoxemia during rest or exertion shown in the office, the clinician needs to be aware that nocturnal hypoxemia, even without evidence of sleep apnea, may occur in up to 60% of patients with PAH.[12]

The role of oxygen therapy in congenital heart disease (CHD)–associated PAH (CHD-APAH) is controversial. Nocturnal administration of oxygen in children with CHD-APAH has been shown to slow the rate of progression of polycythemia and to improve symptoms.[13,14] Whether or not oxygen therapy improves survival is not clear. One study of 15 nonrandomly assigned patients with CHD-APAH studied 15 hours/d or longer of oxygen supplementation more than 5 years. Nine patients received oxygen therapy and 6 did not. A mortality benefit was seen with 9 of the 9 alive in the oxygen therapy group and 1 of the 6 alive in the untreated group at the 5-year time point.[13] However, a recent well-designed, prospective, randomized, controlled study of 23 adult patients with CHD-APAH and Eisenmenger syndrome showed no survival benefit with nocturnal oxygen administration.[15] In addition, no improvement in 6-minute walk distances, hematocrit levels, or quality of life were seen in the oxygen-treated group.[15]

Patients with obstructive sleep apnea (OSA) generally have mild to moderate PH.[16–18] Moderate to severe PH should not be attributed to sleep disordered breathing in these patients and other causes such as pulmonary venous hypertension related to diastolic dysfunction from obesity cardiomyopathy or concurrent COPD should be looked for. In OSA-related PH, continuous positive airway pressure (CPAP) combined with oxygen therapy (when needed) result in a more pronounced decrease in mean PAP and PVR than that seen in patients treated with oxygen alone. Although resolution of mild PH may be reversible with early treatment, full resolution of more severe PH is not expected with even the most compliant use of CPAP.[19–21] However, patients with the obesity hypoventilation syndrome can develop severe PH and treatment requires noninvasive positive-pressure ventilation, which can reverse hypercapnea and signs of RHF within months.[22–24]

In patients who cannot tolerate such therapy, tracheostomy with chronic outpatient mechanical ventilation at night may be offered and has the potential to be lifesaving.[4,25,26]

Oxygen therapy carries with it several logistic and social stigma issues that need to be addressed with its recipients. The inconvenience of ambulatory systems, limitations of time that portable systems allow, danger of falls over long cords and tubing, risk as a fire hazard, and the stigma some patients feel when seen in public may all negatively affect patients' self-esteem. These issues need to be discussed frankly with patients before oxygen therapy is prescribed.

DIURETICS

Patients with PAH can show significant symptomatic relief from diuretic therapy.[2–4,27] As a consequence of increased pulmonary vasculature resistance, patients with PAH have increased right ventricular (RV) wall stress. If severe, this can result in paradoxic septal bowing, which leads to encroachment on the left ventricle as a result of right ventricle–left ventricle interdependence.[28–30] Diuretics can reduce RV filling pressures and therefore can be beneficial in patients with signs of volume overload as shown by peripheral edema, systemic venous congestion, severe tricuspid regurgitation, and/or RV failure.[2–4] Although never systematically studied, longstanding observations of the efficacy of diuretic therapy combined with sound physiologic evidence make it unlikely that this therapy will ever be studied in a randomized, double-blinded, placebo-controlled fashion. Loop diuretics are often the first-line therapy. Studies from patients with left ventricular (LV) systolic disease have shown a benefit from the use of aldosterone inhibitors in patients with New York Heart Association (NYHA) class III or IV functional status.[31] The addition of spironolactone to an angiotensin-converting enzyme (ACE) inhibitor and furosemide decreased 2-year mortality and need for subsequent hospitalization. Although never studied in patients with PAH and RHF, similarities in LV and RV failure on the renin-angiotensin-aldosterone system suggest that, in patients with class III or IV NYHA disease, the use of aldosterone may be a reasonable therapeutic option. However, the use of aldosterone antagonists should be used with caution in patients with renal failure, diabetes, or in those at risk for hyperkalemia or on medications with the potential for concomitant nephrotoxicity including ACE inhibitors and nonsteroidal antiinflammatory agents.[4,27] Amelioride, a potassium sparing diuretic, has been shown to reduce pulmonary arterial smooth muscle cell (PASMC) proliferation and significantly reduce PAP and total pulmonary resistance (TPR) compared with controls in a hypoxia-induced rat model of PH.[32] However, there are no clinical trial data to determine whether these experimental animal data are clinically relevant in humans.

The use of diuretics in patients with PAH requires careful monitoring. Rapid, large-volume diuresis should be avoided except when frank cardiogenic pulmonary edema and/or worsening hypoxemia are present because the preload-dependent right ventricle may react to underfilling with hypotension.[4] Any evidence of orthostatic hypotension as manifested by dizziness or near-syncope should also be addressed with dose adjustments accordingly to avoid hypotension. However, in general, systemic hypotension should not be considered an absolute contraindication to the use of diuretics, because the causative factor for decreased cardiac output in patients with PAH is typically increased PVR and not decreased circulating volume. Underdosing in the setting of the low blood pressure that these patients often have can result in overall clinical worsening, worsening hepatic congestion, or bowel wall edema with symptoms of early satiety.[4,33] The optimal volume status for patients with PAH often occurs within a narrow window and therefore diuretic therapy use requires frequent evaluations by health care providers. Patients with RHF often require salt and fluid restriction, leg elevation when not ambulating, and compressive stockings to control their edema in conjunction with judicious diuretic use. Electrolytes should be closely monitored because these patients are frequently on digoxin and are prone to arrhythmias.

DIGOXIN THERAPY

The use of cardiac glycosides dates back to Sir William Withering's 1785 description of the use of foxglove in the management of dropsy and other diseases.[34] Although its role in the management of many cardiac conditions has been supplanted by newer medications, it is still a useful adjunct in cardiac disease and has a role in the management of PAH.[35,36]

Digoxin and other cardiac glycosides can exert pleiotropic effects on cardiac function. Digoxin binds and inhibits the alpha subunit of the sodium-potassium ATPase pump. This binding promotes sodium-calcium exchange that results in an increase in intracellular calcium and a subsequent increase in cardiac contractility.[35–37] In healthy individuals, this increase in contractility does not result in an increase in cardiac output.[35,38–40] However, it does cause a significant improvement in LV ejection fraction in those with LV systolic heart failure.[39–43] Digoxin also exerts its cardioprotective effect via its modulation of neurohormonal activity, which occurs through increased baroreceptor sensitivity and vagal tone, and to a lesser extent decreased sympathetic nerve discharge and serum norepinephrine and plasma renin activity. Digoxin results in a parasympathomimetic effect that is advantageous in the treatment of both heart failure and atrial fibrillation.[44–48]

Digoxin has been studied in multiple double-blinded studies showing efficacy in the treatment of left heart failure.[41,46,49–52] Digoxin reduced the incidence of hospitalizations and the number of emergency room visits for left heart failure in the Captopril-Digoxin Multicenter Trial of 300 patients with mild to moderate heart failure.[41] Digoxin also increased the exercise time and reduced both plasma norepinephrine concentrations and renin activity at 6 months of therapy in the Dutch Ibopamine Multicenter Trial.[46] In addition, withdrawal of digoxin has been shown to result in an increase in heart failure–related hospitalizations.[49,51] In the Digitalis Investigation Group (DIG) trial, the largest trial of digoxin to date, there was no demonstrable improvement in mortality. However, there was a 25% reduction in the number of hospitalizations for worsening heart failure and a 65% reduction in total hospitalizations in the digoxin-treated group.[53] A subgroup analysis of patients with heart failure with preserved ejection fraction from this study showed a similar trend of reduction in heart failure symptoms and hospitalization without a change in mortality.[53]

As with other treatments, the abundance of data supporting digoxin use for patients with left heart failure resulted in extrapolation to patients with PAH and RHF. Rich and colleagues[54] gave 1 dose of intravenous (IV) digoxin to 17 consecutive patients with severe PAH and RHF with normal LV function. After 2 hours, cardiac output increased from 3.49 ± 1.2 L/min to 3.81 ± 1.2 L/min ($P = .028$), suggesting modest inotropic effect. Neurohormonal samples in this study also revealed a significant decrease in norepinephrine levels (680 ± 89 pg/mL to 580 ± 85 pg/mL; $P = .013$) and significant and unexpected increases in atrial natriuretic peptide (311 ± 44 pg/mL to 421 ± 9 pg/mL; $P = .010$) following digoxin administration. There was no significant difference in plasma renin activity or changes in PAPs.

Others have suggested a role for digoxin in those with COPD and associated PH (World Health Organization class 3 PH). In a chronic hypoxia murine model of PH, digoxin attenuated RV hypertrophy, pulmonary vascular remodeling, and RV pressure. When digoxin was given after the development of PH, RV pressures and proliferative changes in pulmonary artery smooth muscle cells were decreased.[55] In a study of 15 patients with COPD and RHF, Mathur and colleagues[56] showed that after 8 weeks of digoxin therapy RV ejection fraction, as measured by radionuclide angiography, improved in the 4 patients who had reduced LV ejection fractions (LVEFs) at the study outset but did not change in the remaining 11 patients who had normal LVEFs to begin with.

Because of limited human data, the use of digoxin in patients with PAH remains controversial and, if used, the clinician must be mindful of the potential for toxicity.[4,57–59] Because many of these patients are on diuretic therapy, it is of the utmost importance to monitor serum electrolytes because hypomagnesemia and hypokalemia can augment sodium-potassium pump inhibition by digoxin with resulting arrhythmogenic effects.[4,35–37,60] Because digoxin is renally cleared, it should be used with caution in patients with impaired renal function.[4,61,62]

A study of digoxin levels revealed that an increased mortality existed for those patients with higher serum digoxin levels, with optimum outcomes seen in those with serum digoxin levels of 0.5–0.8 ng/mL.[59] This is important because many laboratories still report the normal digoxin range to be 0.5 to 2.0 ng/mL. Mortality risk also seems increased in those with active myocardial ischemia and digoxin should not be used in this setting.[4,35,58] In addition, digoxin interacts with many agents such as macrolides, cyclosporine, amiodarone, and itraconazole, which can increase digoxin levels, increasing the potential for toxicity.[4,61,62]

ANTICOAGULATION

Patients with PAH are at an increased risk for the development of intrapulmonary thrombosis and thromboembolism. There are many factors that increase the tendency for patients with PAH to form clots. As right atrial pressures increase, patients with PAH develop increasing venous engorgement and stasis. Stasis also occurs as a result of decreased flow through the pulmonary circulation as a result of a failing RV.[4] As dyspnea and peripheral myopathy worsen, many patients with PAH develop an increasingly sedentary lifestyle, increasing the risk for venous thrombosis. Patients with PAH also develop endovascular remodeling that disrupts the homeostatic interactions between platelets and the pulmonary arterial endothelium, which increases the risk for in situ thrombus formation.[63–67]

Several studies have shown that idiopathic pulmonary arterial hypertension (IPAH) is a prothrombotic state.[68–84] This is not a result of inherited thrombophilias,[85–87] but a result of a dysregulated thrombin formation that is caused by endothelial cell dysfunction, platelet activation, and a disrupted balance of the proteins involved in clot formation and fibrinolysis (Table 1).[64,65,68–70,73,76,79–82,86] It remains unclear whether thrombotic arteriopathy contributes to the pathogenesis of PAH or occurs as a consequence of stasis and decreased flow,[84,88] although some coagulopathic abnormalities are reversed with the use of PAH-specific therapy.[89–92] Irrespective, thrombotic arteriopathy may alter the disease course and prognosis in IPAH and APAH. Anticoagulation is an irrefutable part of the treatment of chronic thromboembolic PH (CTEPH).

Four observational studies suggested a survival advantage for patients with IPAH treated with anticoagulation.[33,93–95] Three of these were retrospective and 1 was a nonblinded, uncontrolled prospective study. Fuster and colleagues[93] evaluated the course of 120 patients with IPAH at a single center and determined that only pulmonary arterial oxygen saturation and the use of anticoagulation were prognosticators of survival. Of 56 patients who underwent autopsy, 18 had plexogenic arteriopathy, whereas 32 had chronic thrombus as the major histologic feature. To further investigate the role of anticoagulation, 78 additional patients treated with anticoagulation were compared with 37 receiving no anticoagulation. This analysis showed a more favorable survivorship in the warfarin-treated group.[93] From a study design standpoint, the numbers were too small to reach statistical significance. In addition,

Table 1
Prothrombotic abnormalities in PAH

Abnormalities	Subjects	Reference
Platelet Aggregation Related		
Increased urinary thromboxane metabolite (11-dehydrothromboxane B2)	IPAH	68
Decreased urinary PGI2 metabolite	IPAH	68
Decreased nitric oxide (exhaled or urinary excretion)	IPAH, APAH	84
Increased circulating platelet aggregates	APAH	72
Increased thromboxane A2	IPAH	68
Decreased prostacyclin	IPAH	68
Increased circulating platelet aggregates	APAH	72
Increased plasma serotonin and decreased platelet serotonin	IPAH	79,80
Increased plasma P-selectin	IPAH	92
Decreased thrombomodulin	IPAH	69,76,92
Endothelial Function Related		
Decreased NO synthase	IPAH	83
Decreased prostacyclin synthase expression	IPAH	63
Decreased PGI2 metabolite	IPAH	68
Increased urinary thromboxane metabolite (11-dehydrothromboxane B2)	IPAH	68
Decreased thrombomodulin	IPAH	69,76,92
Increased von Willebrand factor	IPAH, APAH	69,70
Increased fibrinogen inhibitor plasminogen activator 1	IPAH	59,69
Coagulation and Fibrinolytic Related		
Increased prevalence of antiphospholipid Ab/lupus anticoagulant	IPAH, CTEPH	58
Increased von Willebrand factor antigen level	IPAH	69,70
Increased fibrinogen inhibitor plasminogen activator 1	IPAH	69,85
Increased euglobulin lysis time	IPAH	69
Increased fibrinogen level	APAH	69

Abbreviation: CTEPH, chronic thromboembolic PH.
Adapted from Alam S, Palevesky HI. Standard therapies for pulmonary arterial hypertension. Clin Chest Med 2007;28:91–115; with permission.

the criteria used to decide when not to antico-agulate were not clearly stated, leaving the potential for selection bias. A more contemporary retrospective study during the early era of PAH-specific therapy by Kawut and colleagues[33] reviewed 84 patients with newly diagnosed PAH that was idiopathic, heritable, or associated with anorexigen use. The use of warfarin was associated with a decrease in the combined end point of death or lung transplantation. However, the study failed to show an improvement in outcomes for PAH-specific therapy and also failed to provide criteria for deciding who not to anticoagulate, again raising concern over selection bias.[33] A third study by Frank and colleagues[94] retrospectively examined 173 patients with PAH, of whom 104 had taken the anorexigen aminorex, whereas the remaining 69 had IPAH. Fifty-six of the 104 aminorex-induced PAH and 24 of the 69 patients with IPAH received warfarin therapy. Patients with aminorex APAH fared better than those with IPAH (7.5 years vs 3.9 years median survival; $P \leq .001$) and, regardless of cause, anticoagulation showed an improvement in survival (7.2 years vs 4.9 years; $P < .05$) In addition, those receiving anticoagulation therapy early after onset of symptoms had a better prognosis than those commencing anticoagulation therapy 2 years or longer after symptomatic presentation.[94]

There has been 1 prospective observational trial of warfarin therapy in IPAH, but this single-center study used a historical control group form the National Institute of Health Primary Pulmonary Hypertension Registry. This study evaluated 64 patients for response to high-dose CCB administration (defined at the time as a $\geq 20\%$ decrease in mean PAP or a $\geq 20\%$ decrease in PVR). The decision to put patients on warfarin therapy was based on the finding of nonuniform perfusion on a nuclear lung scan. Warfarin therapy was associated with increased survival in the group as a whole, and showed a particular benefit in patients who were nonresponders to high-dose CCB administration.[95]

Although this literature suggests some evidence for the use of anticoagulation therapy, the decision to use warfarin therapy needs to be balanced against the risk for potential bleeding complications.[96,97] This need is especially applicable to patients with systemic sclerosis (SSc) in whom there is a high risk of gastrointestinal bleeding.[98] A recent retrospective study of 275 patients with SSc-APAH and 155 patients with IPAH used a Bayesian propensity score to adjust for baseline differences in PAH severity and medication, in patients exposed and not exposed to warfarin. This analysis suggested that there was a 70%

probability that warfarin provided no significant benefit or was harmful.[99] The investigators concluded that SSc-APAH should not receive warfarin therapy.

The current expert opinion is to treat patients with IPAH with warfarin anticoagulation in those without contraindications and to consider warfarin therapy in patients with APAH with advanced disease, such as those receiving continuous IV therapy.[2,3] This should be done in the absence of absolute contraindications and should be weighed against the risk of complications in patients with other forms of associated PAH. In addition, consideration of the other medications being used may influence the decision to anticoagulate, because concerning drug-drug interactions can occur.[100] In portopulmonary APAH, expert consensus advises against using anticoagulation because of the risk of bleeding.[2,3] The recommended anticoagulation dose of warfarin is the dose that achieves an international normalized ratio (INR) of 1.5 to 2.0 for those with IPAH, although some European experts recommend achieving INRs between 2.0 and 3.0.[2,3] In patients with CTEPH, anticoagulation is indicated, although a higher INRs goal of between 2.5 and 3.5 is usually advised.[101]

Although warfarin therapy is the recommended form of anticoagulation, other forms of anticoagulation have been considered. In a murine model of PH induced by chronic hypoxia, high-dose heparin therapy partially but significantly reduced RV systolic pressures and remodeling of distal small pulmonary arteries.[102] A similar finding has been reported in a guinea pig chronic hypoxia model in which PH and TPR were partially reversed with the continuous infusion of heparin.[103] When heparin and warfarin treatment were compared in the same guinea pig model, only heparin showed partial reversal of PH once established.[104] It is unclear why heparin seemed to have a more beneficial effect than warfarin. The mechanism for this effect of heparin is unclear but inhibition of platelet-derived growth factor and inhibition of smooth muscle growth in the pulmonary artery, perhaps by alterations in the regulation of cyclin-dependent kinase, and/or inhibition of the Rho GTPase pathway have all been suggested.[102,105] The direct factor Xa inhibitor rivaroxaban was recently compared with warfarin and enoxaparin in a monocrotaline rat model of PAH.[106] Rivoroxaban reduced systolic and end-diastolic RV pressure increases and RV hypertrophy, whereas warfarin reduced RV pressure increases only. Enoxaparin had no effect on either RV pressure or RV hypertrophy. Heparin, low-molecular-weight heparin, and direct factor Xa inhibitors have not been studied in humans with PAH.

CCBS

Early in the understanding of PAH, it was thought that the increased PAPs in patients with PAH were primarily caused by aberrant vasoconstriction and treatment was initially implemented using therapies used to treat systemic hypertension.[32,107–109] As understanding of the pathogenesis of PAH evolved, it became clear that vasoconstriction is only part of a broader and more complex disease that includes dysregulated endothelial cell function, PASMC proliferation, vascular inflammation, and in situ thrombosis.[63,65,66,110–112] The first landmark study, by Rich and colleagues,[95] showed that patients who responded to acute vasodilator therapy (PAP mean or PVR decrease by $\geq$20%) in the form of intravenous CCB administration had a 94% survival at 5 years compared with 55% in those who did not. This vasoresponsive group represented 26% of all patients with IPAH. However, as experience with the use of high-dose CCB increased it became clear that only a minority of patients with IPAH with this definition of vasoresponsiveness maintained a sustained response to CCB therapy after 1 year.[113] This finding led to a more stringent definition of vasoresponsiveness as recommended by the American College of Chest Physicians (ACCP). Current guidelines suggest that high-dose CCB should be used in patients in whom there is a reduction in PAP mean by 10 mm Hg or more to an absolute value of 40 mm Hg or less without a decrease in cardiac output or systemic blood pressure when challenged with inhaled nitric oxide, IV adenosine, or IV epoprostenol during right heart catheterization.[113] Using this definition, only 6.8% of patients with IPAH in a large cohort of patients with IPAH in France were deemed vasoresponders.[113] Acute vasoresponsiveness in APAH occurs even less often.[114,115] The role of acute vasoreactivity testing in APAH and the role of high-dose CCB therapy in these patients are not known, although the report of the French experience by Montani and colleagues[114] suggests they do not have a role in human immunodeficiency virus–APAH, connective-tissue disease APAH, or CHD-APAH, whereas there may be a role for high-dose CCB in anorexigen-APAH. Acute vasoreactivity testing is still routinely done, pragmatically, in many forms of APAH to show that cheaper CCB therapy is not appropriate in these patients.

The agent of choice for acute vasodilator testing has evolved over time. During testing, there is always a concern that vasodilation may lead to systemic hypotension or worsening hypoxemia.[112] Therefore, titration of IV CCB agents should no longer be used for acute vasodilator testing because these agents are longer acting than current alternatives and can cause side effects that are less readily reversed. Inhaled nitric oxide (iNO), IV prostacyclin (epoprostenol), or IV adenosine are all acceptable agents for acute testing.[116] There are few studies comparing these agents, but, in a recent study, 6 of 39 (15%) with IPAH were found to be responders by the current ACCP criteria to iNO, whereas none of these patients showed a vasodilator response to adenosine, perhaps because of side effect limitations in reaching the maximal adenosine dose.[117] Regardless of the agent selected, caution must be used in certain situations. Vasodilator testing should not be done in patients with severely depressed cardiac function (eg, cardiac index <2.0) because undesirable reductions in systemic blood pressure may occur. It should also be done with extreme caution in patients with pulmonary artery wedge pressures greater than 15 mm Hg and should be immediately aborted if patients develop any signs of worsening hypoxemia. Reports of acute pulmonary edema during acute vasodilator testing exist and death during vasodilator challenge has occurred.[118–121] Failure to respond acutely to vasodilator testing does not exclude improvement with long-term use of prostacyclin or other PAH-specific therapies.[122–124]

Patients who meet the ACCP criteria for vasoresponsiveness should be treated with high-dose CCB therapy.[2–4] Nifedipine is often initiated in those with heart rates less than 100 beats/min, whereas diltiazem is often initiated for those with heart rates of more than 100 beats/min.[4,95,112] Amlodipine is also an acceptable agent in vasoresponsive patients. Empiric CCB use is never indicated and may be fatal. Therapy can either be initiated as an inpatient with an RHC in place or through gradual up-titration of oral therapy as an outpatient. Close follow-up is essential because nearly half of all patients meeting acute vasodilator criteria do not have durable response and may require other PAH-specific therapies. A small observational study of 7 patients initially shown to be nonresponders seemed to develop a vasodilator response several months after treatment with epoprostenol.[125] The clinical significance of this and its implication for CCB use in this subgroup of patients is unknown.

SUMMARY

In the era preceding the development of PAH-specific therapies, the use of digoxin, anticoagulation, oxygen, and diuretics was advised in patients with IPAH from retrospective, uncontrolled studies or on assumptions from data in similar diseases.[2,3] Although PAH-specific therapies have changed the mainstay of treatment, the adjunct therapies still have an important role in the treatment of PAH. The use of oxygen, diuretics, and digoxin has been adopted from more common medical conditions and use of these agents is often advocated from sound physiologic reasoning. Because IPAH is associated with hypercoagulability, anticoagulation may improve long-term outcomes in some patients, although the clinician has to weigh the benefit of anticoagulation against the risk of bleeding, which can be significant, especially in SSc-APAH. A small subset of patients with IPAH who are vasoresponsive can be effectively managed with high-dose CCB monotherapy. These patients generally have a better prognosis and greater survival times but still require close monitoring for durability of response because many ultimately require the addition of other PAH-specific therapies.

REFERENCES

1. D'Alonzo GE, Barst RJ, Ayres SM, et al. Survival in patients with primary pulmonary hypertension. Results from a national prospective registry. Ann Intern Med 1991;115(5):343–9.
2. Badesch DB, Abman SH, Simonneau G, et al. Medical therapy for pulmonary arterial hypertension: updated ACCP evidence-based clinical practice guidelines. Chest 2007;131(6): 1917–28.
3. McLaughlin VV, Archer SL, Badesch DB, et al. ACCF/AHA 2009 expert consensus document on pulmonary hypertension a report of the American College of Cardiology Foundation Task Force on Expert Consensus Documents and the American Heart Association developed in collaboration with the American College of Chest Physicians; American Thoracic Society, Inc; and the Pulmonary Hypertension Association. J Am Coll Cardiol 2009; 53(17):1573–619.
4. Alam S, Palevsky HI. Standard therapies for pulmonary arterial hypertension. Clin Chest Med 2007; 28(1):91–115, viii.
5. Weissmann N, Tadic A, Hanze J, et al. Hypoxic vasoconstriction in intact lungs: a role for NADPH oxidase-derived H_2O_2? Am J Physiol Lung Cell Mol Physiol 2000;279(4):L683–90.
6. Continuous or nocturnal oxygen therapy in hypoxemic chronic obstructive lung disease: a clinical trial. Nocturnal Oxygen Therapy Trial Group. Ann Intern Med 1980;93(3):391–8.
7. Long term domiciliary oxygen therapy in chronic hypoxic cor pulmonale complicating chronic bronchitis and emphysema. Report of the Medical Research Council Working Party. Lancet 1981; 1(8222):681–6.
8. Timms RM, Khaja FU, Williams GW. Hemodynamic response to oxygen therapy in chronic obstructive pulmonary disease. Ann Intern Med 1985;102(1): 29–36.
9. Pauwels RA, Buist AS, Ma P, et al. Global strategy for the diagnosis, management, and prevention of chronic obstructive pulmonary disease: National Heart, Lung, and Blood Institute and World Health Organization Global Initiative for Chronic Obstructive Lung Disease (GOLD): executive summary. Respir Care 2001;46(8):798–825.
10. Owens GR, Rogers RM, Pennock BE, et al. The diffusing capacity as a predictor of arterial oxygen desaturation during exercise in patients with chronic obstructive pulmonary disease. N Engl J Med 1984;310(19):1218–21.
11. Kelley MA, Panettieri RA Jr, Krupinski AV. Resting single-breath diffusing capacity as a screening test for exercise-induced hypoxemia. Am J Med 1986;80(5):807–12.
12. Minai OA, Pandya CM, Golish JA, et al. Predictors of nocturnal oxygen desaturation in pulmonary arterial hypertension. Chest 2007;131(1):109–17.
13. Bowyer JJ, Busst CM, Denison DM, et al. Effect of long term oxygen treatment at home in children with pulmonary vascular disease. Br Heart J 1986;55(4):385–90.
14. Widlitz A, Barst RJ. Pulmonary arterial hypertension in children. Eur Respir J 2003;21(1):155–76.
15. Sandoval J, Aguirre JS, Pulido T, et al. Nocturnal oxygen therapy in patients with the Eisenmenger syndrome. Am J Respir Crit Care Med 2001; 164(9):1682–7.
16. Atwood CW Jr, McCrory D, Garcia JG, et al. Pulmonary artery hypertension and sleep-disordered breathing: ACCP evidence-based clinical practice guidelines. Chest 2004;126(Suppl 1):72S–7S.
17. Koo KW, Sax DS, Snider GL. Arterial blood gases and pH during sleep in chronic obstructive pulmonary disease. Am J Med 1975;58(5):663–70.
18. Podszus T, Bauer W, Mayer J, et al. Sleep apnea and pulmonary hypertension. Klin Wochenschr 1986;64(3):131–4.
19. Alchanatis M, Tourkohoriti G, Kakouros S, et al. Daytime pulmonary hypertension in patients with obstructive sleep apnea: the effect of continuous positive airway pressure on pulmonary hemodynamics. Respiration 2001;68(6):566–72.
20. Sajkov D, Wang T, Saunders NA, et al. Continuous positive airway pressure treatment improves pulmonary hemodynamics in patients with obstructive sleep apnea. Am J Respir Crit Care Med 2002; 165(2):152–8.
21. Arias MA, Garcia-Rio F, Alonso-Fernandez A, et al. Pulmonary hypertension in obstructive sleep

apnoea: effects of continuous positive airway pressure: a randomized, controlled cross-over study. Eur Heart J 2006;27(9):1106–13.

22. Kessler R, Chaouat A, Schinkewitch P, et al. The obesity-hypoventilation syndrome revisited: a prospective study of 34 consecutive cases. Chest 2001;120(2):369–76.

23. Littleton SW, Mokhlesi B. The pickwickian syndrome-obesity hypoventilation syndrome. Clin Chest Med 2009;30(3):467–78, vii–viii.

24. Masa JF, Celli BR, Riesco JA, et al. The obesity hypoventilation syndrome can be treated with noninvasive mechanical ventilation. Chest 2001; 119(4):1102–7.

25. Nowbar S, Burkart KM, Gonzales R, et al. Obesity-associated hypoventilation in hospitalized patients: prevalence, effects, and outcome. Am J Med 2004; 116(1):1–7.

26. Budweiser S, Riedl SG, Jorres RA, et al. Mortality and prognostic factors in patients with obesity-hypoventilation syndrome undergoing noninvasive ventilation. J Intern Med 2007;261(4): 375–83.

27. Chronic Heart Failure: National Clinical Guideline for Diagnosis and Management in Primary and Secondary Care: Partial Update. London 2010.

28. Dittrich HC, Chow LC, Nicod PH. Early improvement in left ventricular diastolic function after relief of chronic right ventricular pressure overload. Circulation 1989;80(4):823–30.

29. Gan C, Lankhaar JW, Marcus JT, et al. Impaired left ventricular filling due to right-to-left ventricular interaction in patients with pulmonary arterial hypertension. Am J Physiol Heart Circ Physiol 2006;290(4): H1528–33.

30. Krayenbuehl HP, Turina J, Hess O. Left ventricular function in chronic pulmonary hypertension. Am J Cardiol 1978;41(7):1150–8.

31. Pitt B, Zannad F, Remme WJ, et al. The effect of spironolactone on morbidity and mortality in patients with severe heart failure. Randomized Aldactone Evaluation Study Investigators. N Engl J Med 1999;341(10):709–17.

32. Quinn DA, Du HK, Thompson BT, et al. Amiloride analogs inhibit chronic hypoxic pulmonary hypertension. Am J Respir Crit Care Med 1998;157(4 Pt 1):1263–8.

33. Kawut SM, Horn EM, Berekashvili KK, et al. New predictors of outcome in idiopathic pulmonary arterial hypertension. Am J Cardiol 2005;95(2): 199–203.

34. Krishnamachari KA, Satyanarayana K. Resurgence of epidemic dropsy in India. Lancet 1972;2(7772): 339.

35. Eichhorn EJ, Gheorghiade M. Digoxin. Prog Cardiovasc Dis 2002;44(4):251–66.

36. Dec GW. Digoxin remains useful in the management of chronic heart failure. Med Clin North Am 2003;87(2):317–37.

37. Little WC, Rassi A Jr, Freeman GL. Comparison of effects of dobutamine and ouabain on left ventricular contraction and relaxation in closed-chest dogs. J Clin Invest 1987;80(3):613–20.

38. Hasenfuss G, Mulieri LA, Allen PD, et al. Influence of isoproterenol and ouabain on excitation-contraction coupling, cross-bridge function, and energetics in failing human myocardium. Circulation 1996;94(12):3155–60.

39. Braunwald E. Effects of digitalis on the normal and the failing heart. J Am Coll Cardiol 1985; 5(5 Suppl A):51A–9A.

40. Mason DT, Braunwald E. Studies on digitalis. IX. Effects of ouabain on the nonfailing human heart. J Clin Invest 1963;42(7):1105–11.

41. Comparative effects of therapy with captopril and digoxin in patients with mild to moderate heart failure. The Captopril-Digoxin Multicenter Research Group. JAMA 1988;259(4):539–44.

42. Gheorghiade M, Hall V, Lakier JB, et al. Comparative hemodynamic and neurohormonal effects of intravenous captopril and digoxin and their combinations in patients with severe heart failure. J Am Coll Cardiol 1989;13(1): 134–42.

43. Davies RF, Beanlands DS, Nadeau C, et al. Enalapril versus digoxin in patients with congestive heart failure: a multicenter study. Canadian Enalapril Versus Digoxin Study Group. J Am Coll Cardiol 1991;18(7):1602–9.

44. Ferguson DW, Berg WJ, Sanders JS, et al. Sympathoinhibitory responses to digitalis glycosides in heart failure patients. Direct evidence from sympathetic neural recordings. Circulation 1989;80(1): 65–77.

45. Newton GE, Tong JH, Schofield AM, et al. Digoxin reduces cardiac sympathetic activity in severe congestive heart failure. J Am Coll Cardiol 1996; 28(1):155–61.

46. van Veldhuisen DJ, Man in 't Veld AJ, Dunselman PH, et al. Double-blind placebo-controlled study of ibopamine and digoxin in patients with mild to moderate heart failure: results of the Dutch Ibopamine Multicenter Trial (DIMT). J Am Coll Cardiol 1993;22(6):1564–73.

47. Gheorghiade M, Ferguson D. Digoxin. A neurohormonal modulator in heart failure? Circulation 1991; 84(5):2181–6.

48. Krum H, Bigger JT Jr, Goldsmith RL, et al. Effect of long-term digoxin therapy on autonomic function in patients with chronic heart failure. J Am Coll Cardiol 1995;25(2):289–94.

49. Packer M, Gheorghiade M, Young JB, et al. Withdrawal of digoxin from patients with chronic

heart failure treated with angiotensin-converting-enzyme inhibitors. RADIANCE Study. N Engl J Med 1993;329(1):1–7.

50. DiBianco R, Shabetai R, Kostuk W, et al. A comparison of oral milrinone, digoxin, and their combination in the treatment of patients with chronic heart failure. N Engl J Med 1989;320(11): 677–83.

51. Uretsky BF, Young JB, Shahidi FE, et al. Randomized study assessing the effect of digoxin withdrawal in patients with mild to moderate chronic congestive heart failure: results of the PROVED trial. PROVED Investigative Group. J Am Coll Cardiol 1993;22(4):955–62.

52. Gheorghiade M, Zarowitz BJ. Review of randomized trials of digoxin therapy in patients with chronic heart failure. Am J Cardiol 1992;69(18): 48G–62G [discussion: 62G–3G].

53. The effect of digoxin on mortality and morbidity in patients with heart failure. The Digitalis Investigation Group. N Engl J Med 1997;336(8):525–33.

54. Rich S, Seidlitz M, Dodin E, et al. The short-term effects of digoxin in patients with right ventricular dysfunction from pulmonary hypertension. Chest 1998;114(3):787–92.

55. Abud EM, Maylor J, Undem C, et al. Digoxin inhibits development of hypoxic pulmonary hypertension in mice. Proc Natl Acad Sci U S A 2012; 109(4):1239–44.

56. Mathur PN, Powles P, Pugsley SO, et al. Effect of digoxin on right ventricular function in severe chronic airflow obstruction. A controlled clinical trial. Ann Intern Med 1981;95(3):283–8.

57. Marik PE, Fromm L. A case series of hospitalized patients with elevated digoxin levels. Am J Med 1998;105(2):110–5.

58. Leor J, Goldbourt U, Rabinowitz B, et al. Digoxin and increased mortality among patients recovering from acute myocardial infarction: importance of digoxin dose. The SPRINT Study Group. Cardiovasc Drugs Ther 1995;9(5):723–9.

59. Rathore SS, Curtis JP, Wang Y, et al. Association of serum digoxin concentration and outcomes in patients with heart failure. JAMA 2003;289(7):871–8.

60. Smith TW, Antman EM, Friedman PL, et al. Digitalis glycosides: mechanisms and manifestations of toxicity. Part I. Prog Cardiovasc Dis 1984;26(5): 413–58.

61. Jelliffe RW, Brooker G. A nomogram for digoxin therapy. Am J Med 1974;57(1):63–8.

62. Juurlink DN, Mamdani M, Kopp A, et al. Drug-drug interactions among elderly patients hospitalized for drug toxicity. JAMA 2003;289(13):1652–8.

63. Humbert M, Morrell NW, Archer SL, et al. Cellular and molecular pathobiology of pulmonary arterial hypertension. J Am Coll Cardiol 2004;43(12 Suppl S): 13S–24S.

64. Johnson SR, Granton JT, Mehta S. Thrombotic arteriopathy and anticoagulation in pulmonary hypertension. Chest 2006;130(2):545–52.

65. Wagenvoort CA. Lung biopsy specimens in the evaluation of pulmonary vascular disease. Chest 1980;77(5):614–25.

66. Bjornsson J, Edwards WD. Primary pulmonary hypertension: a histopathologic study of 80 cases. Mayo Clin Proc 1985;60(1):16–25.

67. Pietra GG, Edwards WD, Kay JM, et al. Histopathology of primary pulmonary hypertension. A qualitative and quantitative study of pulmonary blood vessels from 58 patients in the National Heart, Lung, and Blood Institute, Primary Pulmonary Hypertension Registry. Circulation 1989;80(5): 1198–206.

68. Christman BW, McPherson CD, Newman JH, et al. An imbalance between the excretion of thromboxane and prostacyclin metabolites in pulmonary hypertension. N Engl J Med 1992;327(2):70–5.

69. Welsh CH, Hassell KL, Badesch DB, et al. Coagulation and fibrinolytic profiles in patients with severe pulmonary hypertension. Chest 1996; 110(3):710–7.

70. Collados MT, Sandoval J, Lopez S, et al. Characterization of von Willebrand factor in primary pulmonary hypertension. Heart Vessels 1999;14(5): 246–52.

71. Lopes AA, Maeda NY. Circulating von Willebrand factor antigen as a predictor of short-term prognosis in pulmonary hypertension. Chest 1998; 114(5):1276–82.

72. Lopes AA, Maeda NY, Almeida A, et al. Circulating platelet aggregates indicative of in vivo platelet activation in pulmonary hypertension. Angiology 1993;44(9):701–6.

73. Geggel RL, Carvalho AC, Hoyer LW, et al. von Willebrand factor abnormalities in primary pulmonary hypertension. Am Rev Respir Dis 1987;135(2): 294–9.

74. Huber K, Beckmann R, Frank H, et al. Fibrinogen, t-PA, and PAI-1 plasma levels in patients with pulmonary hypertension. Am J Respir Crit Care Med 1994;150(4):929–33.

75. Lopes AA, Maeda NY, Aiello VD, et al. Abnormal multimeric and oligomeric composition is associated with enhanced endothelial expression of von Willebrand factor in pulmonary hypertension. Chest 1993;104(5):1455–60.

76. Cacoub P, Karmochkine M, Dorent R, et al. Plasma levels of thrombomodulin in pulmonary hypertension. Am J Med 1996;101(2):160–4.

77. Eisenberg PR, Lucore C, Kaufman L, et al. Fibrinopeptide A levels indicative of pulmonary vascular thrombosis in patients with primary pulmonary hypertension. Circulation 1990;82(3): 841–7.

78. Can MM, Tanboga IH, Demircan HC, et al. Enhanced hemostatic indices in patients with pulmonary arterial hypertension: an observational study. Thromb Res 2010;126(4):280–2.

79. Herve P, Drouet L, Dosquet C, et al. Primary pulmonary hypertension in a patient with a familial platelet storage pool disease: role of serotonin. Am J Med 1990;89(1):117–20.

80. Herve P, Launay JM, Scrobohaci ML, et al. Increased plasma serotonin in primary pulmonary hypertension. Am J Med 1995;99(3):249–54.

81. Kereveur A, Callebert J, Humbert M, et al. High plasma serotonin levels in primary pulmonary hypertension. Effect of long-term epoprostenol (prostacyclin) therapy. Arterioscler Thromb Vasc Biol 2000;20(10):2233–9.

82. Langleben D, Moroz LA, McGregor M, et al. Decreased half-life of fibrinogen in primary pulmonary hypertension. Thromb Res 1985;40(4):577–80.

83. Giaid A, Saleh D. Reduced expression of endothelial nitric oxide synthase in the lungs of patients with pulmonary hypertension. N Engl J Med 1995;333(4):214–21.

84. Archer SL, Djaballah K, Humbert M, et al. Nitric oxide deficiency in fenfluramine- and dexfenfluramine-induced pulmonary hypertension. Am J Respir Crit Care Med 1998;158(4):1061–7.

85. Hoeper MM, Sosada M, Fabel H. Plasma coagulation profiles in patients with severe primary pulmonary hypertension. Eur Respir J 1998;12(6):1446–9.

86. Wolf M, Boyer-Neumann C, Parent F, et al. Thrombotic risk factors in pulmonary hypertension. Eur Respir J 2000;15(2):395–9.

87. Lang CC, Choy AM, Pringle TH, et al. Renal, hemodynamic and neurohormonal effects of atrial natriuretic factor in cardiac allograft recipients treated with cyclosporin A. Am J Cardiol 1993;72(14):1083–4.

88. Chaouat A, Weitzenblum E, Higenbottam T. The role of thrombosis in severe pulmonary hypertension. Eur Respir J 1996;9(2):356–63.

89. Boyer-Neumann C, Brenot F, Wolf M, et al. Continuous infusion of prostacyclin decreases plasma levels of t-PA and PAI-1 in primary pulmonary hypertension. Thromb Haemost 1995;73(4):735–6.

90. Veyradier A, Nishikubo T, Humbert M, et al. Improvement of von Willebrand factor proteolysis after prostacyclin infusion in severe pulmonary arterial hypertension. Circulation 2000;102(20):2460–2.

91. Girgis RE, Champion HC, Diette GB, et al. Decreased exhaled nitric oxide in pulmonary arterial hypertension: response to bosentan therapy. Am J Respir Crit Care Med 2005;172(3):352–7.

92. Sakamaki F, Kyotani S, Nagaya N, et al. Increased plasma P-selectin and decreased thrombomodulin in pulmonary arterial hypertension were improved by continuous prostacyclin therapy. Circulation 2000;102(22):2720–5.

93. Fuster V, Steele PM, Edwards WD, et al. Primary pulmonary hypertension: natural history and the importance of thrombosis. Circulation 1984;70(4):580–7.

94. Frank H, Mlczoch J, Huber K, et al. The effect of anticoagulant therapy in primary and anorectic drug-induced pulmonary hypertension. Chest 1997;112(3):714–21.

95. Rich S, Kaufmann E, Levy PS. The effect of high doses of calcium-channel blockers on survival in primary pulmonary hypertension. N Engl J Med 1992;327(2):76–81.

96. Levine MN, Raskob G, Beyth RJ, et al. Hemorrhagic complications of anticoagulant treatment: the Seventh ACCP Conference on Antithrombotic and Thrombolytic Therapy. Chest 2004;126(Suppl 3):287S–310S.

97. Opitz CF, Kirch W, Mueller EA, et al. Bleeding events in pulmonary arterial hypertension. Eur J Clin Invest 2009;39(Suppl 2):68–73.

98. Duchini A, Sessoms SL. Gastrointestinal hemorrhage in patients with systemic sclerosis and CREST syndrome. Am J Gastroenterol 1998;93(9):1453–6.

99. Johnson SR, Granton JT, Tomlinson GA, et al. Warfarin in systemic sclerosis-associated and idiopathic pulmonary arterial hypertension. A Bayesian approach to evaluating treatment for uncommon disease. J Rheumatol 2012;39(2):276–85.

100. Spangler ML, Saxena S. Warfarin and bosentan interaction in a patient with pulmonary hypertension secondary to bilateral pulmonary emboli. Clin Ther 2010;32(1):53–6.

101. Poli D, Miniati M. The incidence of recurrent venous thromboembolism and chronic thromboembolic pulmonary hypertension following a first episode of pulmonary embolism. Curr Opin Pulm Med 2011;17(5):392–7.

102. Hales CA, Kradin RL, Brandstetter RD, et al. Impairment of hypoxic pulmonary artery remodeling by heparin in mice. Am Rev Respir Dis 1983;128(4):747–51.

103. Hassoun PM, Thompson BT, Hales CA. Partial reversal of hypoxic pulmonary hypertension by heparin. Am Rev Respir Dis 1992;145(1):193–6.

104. Hassoun PM, Thompson BT, Steigman D, et al. Effect of heparin and warfarin on chronic hypoxic pulmonary hypertension and vascular remodeling in the guinea pig. Am Rev Respir Dis 1989;139(3):763–8.

105. Yu L, Quinn DA, Garg HG, et al. Gene expression of cyclin-dependent kinase inhibitors and effect of

heparin on their expression in mice with hypoxia-induced pulmonary hypertension. Biochem Biophys Res Commun 2006;345(4):1565–72.

106. Delbeck M, Nickel KF, Perzborn E, et al. A role for coagulation factor Xa in experimental pulmonary arterial hypertension. Cardiovasc Res 2011;92(1): 159–68.

107. Rubin LJ, Peter RH. Oral hydralazine therapy for primary pulmonary hypertension. N Engl J Med 1980;302(2):69–73.

108. Camerini F, Alberti E, Klugmann S, et al. Primary pulmonary hypertension: effects of nifedipine. Br Heart J 1980;44(3):352–6.

109. Packer M, Greenberg B, Massie B, et al. Deleterious effects of hydralazine in patients with pulmonary hypertension. N Engl J Med 1982;306(22): 1326–31.

110. McLaughlin VV, McGoon MD. Pulmonary arterial hypertension. Circulation 2006;114(13):1417–31.

111. Newman JH, Phillips JA 3rd, Loyd JE. Narrative review: the enigma of pulmonary arterial hypertension: new insights from genetic studies. Ann Intern Med 2008;148(4):278–83.

112. Rich S, Kaufmann E. High dose titration of calcium channel blocking agents for primary pulmonary hypertension: guidelines for short-term drug testing. J Am Coll Cardiol 1991;18(5):1323–7.

113. Sitbon O, Humbert M, Jais X, et al. Long-term response to calcium channel blockers in idiopathic pulmonary arterial hypertension. Circulation 2005; 111(23):3105–11.

114. Montani D, Savale L, Natali D, et al. Long-term response to calcium-channel blockers in non-idiopathic pulmonary arterial hypertension. Eur Heart J 2010;31(15):1898–907.

115. Humbert M, Sitbon O, Chaouat A, et al. Pulmonary arterial hypertension in France: results from a national registry. Am J Respir Crit Care Med 2006; 173(9):1023–30.

116. Galie N, Torbicki A, Barst R, et al. Guidelines on diagnosis and treatment of pulmonary arterial hypertension. The Task Force on Diagnosis and Treatment of Pulmonary Arterial Hypertension of the European Society of Cardiology. Eur Heart J 2004;25(24):2243–78.

117. Oliveira EC, Ribeiro AL, Amaral CF. Adenosine for vasoreactivity testing in pulmonary hypertension: a head-to-head comparison with inhaled nitric oxide. Respir Med 2010;104(4):606–11.

118. Preston IR, Klinger JR, Houtchens J, et al. Pulmonary edema caused by inhaled nitric oxide therapy in two patients with pulmonary hypertension associated with the CREST syndrome. Chest 2002; 121(2):656–9.

119. Farber HW, Graven KK, Kokolski G, et al. Pulmonary edema during acute infusion of epoprostenol in a patient with pulmonary hypertension and limited scleroderma. J Rheumatol 1999;26(5): 1195–6.

120. Strange C, Bolster M, Mazur J, et al. Hemodynamic effects of epoprostenol in patients with systemic sclerosis and pulmonary hypertension. Chest 2000;118(4):1077–82.

121. Rubin LJ, Mendoza J, Hood M, et al. Treatment of primary pulmonary hypertension with continuous intravenous prostacyclin (epoprostenol). Results of a randomized trial. Ann Intern Med 1990; 112(7):485–91.

122. Barst RJ, Rubin LJ, McGoon MD, et al. Survival in primary pulmonary hypertension with long-term continuous intravenous prostacyclin. Ann Intern Med 1994;121(6):409–15.

123. Barst RJ, Rubin LJ, Long WA, et al. A comparison of continuous intravenous epoprostenol (prostacyclin) with conventional therapy for primary pulmonary hypertension. N Engl J Med 1996;334(5): 296–301.

124. Rich S, Brundage BH. High-dose calcium channel-blocking therapy for primary pulmonary hypertension: evidence for long-term reduction in pulmonary arterial pressure and regression of right ventricular hypertrophy. Circulation 1987;76(1):135–41.

125. Ziesche R, Petkov V, Wittmann K, et al. Treatment with epoprostenol reverts nitric oxide non-responsiveness in patients with primary pulmonary hypertension. Heart 2000;83(4):406–9.

Oral Therapies for Pulmonary Arterial Hypertension
Endothelin Receptor Antagonists and Phosphodiesterase-5 Inhibitors

Richard Channick, MD[a],*, Iona Preston, MD[b],
James R. Klinger, MD[c]

KEYWORDS

- Pulmonary arterial hypertension • Oral therapy • Endothelin receptor antagonists
- Phosphodiesterase-5 inhibitors

KEY POINTS

- The development of oral therapies for pulmonary arterial hypertension (PAH) has been a breakthrough in management for this life-threatening condition.
- Diagnosis and institution of treatment at earlier stages of disease has likely improved outcomes.
- Although data are limited because of the rare nature of PAH and lack of head-to-head comparisons between the various oral therapies, long-term data and clinical experience unequivocally support their critical role and clear clinical benefits.
- Novel oral agents are being developed that may further advance the field.

INTRODUCTION

The approval of oral therapies for pulmonary arterial hypertension (PAH) represented a breakthrough. Before approval of the first oral therapy, bosentan, in 2001, continuous intravenous epoprostenol was the only approved treatment. Although extremely effective, epoprostenol therapy requires significant time and resource commitment and is associated with a variety of side effects and challenges. Thus, availability of oral agents offers benefit to many patients with PAH. With the growing understanding of the importance of the endothelin and nitric oxide (NO) signaling pathways in the pathogenesis of PAH, the development of oral therapies targeted at these pathways ensued and led to the first randomized, placebo-controlled trials in PAH. This article reviews the profile, safety, and efficacy of the 4 available oral agents and discusses the overall approach to the use of these therapies.

ENDOTHELIN RECEPTOR ANTAGONISTS

The endothelins are a family of 21-amino-acid peptides that play a key role in the regulation

---

Disclosures: Klinger: Grant Support: Actelion, Bayer, Gilead, Ikaria, United Therapeutics. Consultant: Bayer, United Therapeutics. Steering Committee: Bayer; Channick: Grant Support: Actelion, Bayer, United Therapeutics. Consultant: Actelion, Bayer, United Therapeutics. Steering Committee: Bayer, Actelion; Preston: Grant Support: Actelion, Aires, GeNO, Gilead, United Therapeutics. Consultant: Actelion, Bayer, Gilead, United Therapeutics.

[a] Division of Pulmonary and Critical Care Medicine, Massachusetts General Hospital, Harvard Medical School, Boston, MA, USA; [b] Division of Pulmonary and Critical Care Medicine, New England Medical Center, Tufts University, Boston, MA, USA; [c] Division of Pulmonary, Sleep and Critical Care Medicine, Rhode Island Hospital, Alpert Medical School of Brown University, Providence, RI, USA
* Corresponding author.
E-mail address: rchannick@partners.org

Clin Chest Med 34 (2013) 811–824
http://dx.doi.org/10.1016/j.ccm.2013.09.005
0272-5231/13/$ – see front matter © 2013 Elsevier Inc. All rights reserved.

of vascular tone. The first member of this family identified was endothelin-1 (ET-1), a 2492-Da peptide with potent vasoconstrictor properties, isolated in 1988 by Yanagisawa and colleagues[1] (http://www.sciencedirect.com/science/article/pii/S0024320512003955 - bb0300 #bb0300). Two additional endothelin isopeptides, endothelin-2 (ET-2) and endothelin-3 (ET-3), were subsequently discovered.[2]

Vascular endothelial cells are the major source of endothelin production in humans. However, in addition, endothelin is produced in a wide range of additional cell types including bronchial epithelium, macrophages, cardiac myocytes, glomerular mesangium, and glial cells.[3–6]

Discovery of ET-1 derived from pulmonary artery endothelial cells and its receptors, expressed on pulmonary artery smooth muscle cells, led to the synthesis of endothelin receptor antagonists.

ET-1 Production

The human ET-1 gene is located on the telomeric region of chromosome 6p.[7] The ET-1 gene includes 5 exons that encode messenger ribonucleic acid (mRNA) for a large precursor protein, preproendothelin-1 (PPET-1), which is converted to ET-1 by endothelin-converting enzyme (**Fig. 1**). It seems that vascular endothelial cells are able to rapidly increase or inhibit ET-1 production to regulate vascular tone.[2]

Most of the ET-1 secreted from cultured endothelial cells is secreted from the abluminal side of the cells toward the adjacent vascular smooth muscle cells, which contain specific endothelin receptors.[8] This paracrine effect of ET-1 suggests that circulating levels of the peptide do not necessarily reflect local activity within the pulmonary vasculature.

Endothelin Receptors

There are 2 distinct receptors for the endothelin family of peptides: endothelin receptor A (ETA) and endothelin receptor B (ETB). The endothelin receptors belong to the family of receptors connected to guanine nucleotide-binding (G) proteins.[9] ETA receptors are expressed on pulmonary vascular smooth muscle cells, whereas ETB receptors are located on both pulmonary vascular endothelial cells and smooth muscle cells. When activated, the ETA receptor mediates vasoconstriction. The mechanism is thought to occur via G protein–induced phospholipase C activation; 1,4,5-inositol triphosphate (IP3) formation; and the consequent release of Ca^{2+} from intracellular stores.[9] In addition to mediating vasoconstriction, ET-1 is a potent mitogen, with the ability to produce proliferation in several cell types, including vascular smooth muscle cells.[10] The mitogenic actions of ET-1 are mediated by both the ETA and ETB receptors.[11] ETB receptors on endothelial cells mediate vasodilation via increased production of NO and prostacyclin.[12] In addition to potentially mediating pulmonary vasodilation, there are data suggesting that the ETB receptor may mediate a vasoconstrictive effect through a population of ETB receptors located on vascular smooth muscle cells.[13] The vasoconstrictive actions of ETB receptors may become more pronounced in the pathologic setting of pulmonary hypertension than in the normal pulmonary vasculature.[14]

In humans with pulmonary hypertension, the role of abnormal endothelin production and receptor-mediated effects have been well shown. Patients with idiopathic PAH (IPAH) have higher serum levels of ET-1 than control subjects. Lung specimens from patients with IPAH, compared with those from patients without pulmonary hypertension, show increased ET-1 staining of the muscular pulmonary arteries and increased expression of PPET-1 in the endothelial cells of the same vessels.[15] Increased ET-1 levels have similarly been seen in patients with PAH associated with congenital heart disease[16] and chronic thromboembolic pulmonary hypertension.[17,18]

The development of each of the 2 currently approved endothelin receptor antagonists, bosentan and ambrisentan, followed a similar path, with earlier phase studies showing hemodynamic benefits leading to larger trials in which placebo-corrected change in exercise capacity was the primary end point.

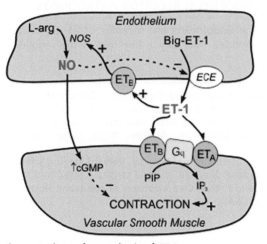

Fig. 1. Pathway for synthesis of ET-1.

CLINICAL DATA
Ambrisentan

Ambrisentan is a specific ETA receptor antagonist approved for PAH functional classes II and III at dosages of 5 mg or 10 mg once daily. Following a phase 2 dosing study showing improvement in pulmonary hemodynamics,[19] 2 randomized controlled trials, ARIES-1 and ARIES-2 (ARIES-1, 5 mg, 10 mg, placebo; ARIES-2, 2.5 mg, 5 mg, placebo) were conducted, enrolling a total of 394 patients.[20] Both trials showed improvement in the primary end point of placebo-corrected 6-minute walk distance (6MWD) (Fig. 2). In ARIES-2, there was a significant improvement in time to clinical worsening in the treatment group compared with placebo. There was a trend toward improvement in time to clinical worsening in the ARIES-1 study, but this was not statistically significant ($P = .307$). World Health Organization (WHO) functional class improvement was significant in ARIES-1 and there was a trend toward improvement in ARIES-2, but this did not reach statistical significance ($P = .117$). Two-hundred and ninety-eight patients were enrolled and followed in a long-term extension study over 48 weeks. Eighteen patients required additional therapies (prostanoids or phosphodiesterase type-5 [PDE-5] inhibitors). Of the 280 patients continued on ambrisentan monotherapy, the improvement in 6MWD at 12 weeks was 40 m and maintained at 39 m. Although there were no patients with increases in serum aminotransferases of more than 3 times the upper limit of normal while on ambrisentan, in the trials, long-term follow-up has revealed cases of transaminase increases that resolve on discontinuation of ambrisentan.

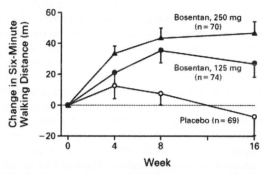

Fig. 2. Bosentan improved 6MWD compared with placebo, from Ref.[22] Although 250 mg twice a day led to a greater effect, the incidence of liver toxicity was significantly greater than in the group receiving 125 mg twice a day The US Food and Drug Administration (FDA)–approved dose is 125 mg twice a day.

Bosentan

Bosentan is a dual endothelin A and B receptor antagonist. Bosentan received US Food and Drug Administration (FDA) approval in November 2001 for patients with WHO functional class III or IV PAH. The first double-blind, placebo-controlled trial randomized 32 patients with IPAH (84%) or PAH associated with scleroderma, functional class III, to bosentan or placebo for 12 weeks.[21] The primary end point was the placebo-corrected change in 6MWD, with secondary end points including change in pulmonary hemodynamics, WHO functional class, Borg dyspnea index, and clinical worsening. The placebo-corrected improvement in 6MWD was 76 m in favor of the bosentan group. In addition, cardiac index (CI) and pulmonary vascular resistance (PVR) were significantly improved with bosentan. There were asymptomatic increases in liver aminotransferases in 2 patients on bosentan, but these returned to baseline without discontinuing or changing the dosage.

The subsequent BREATHE-1 (Bosentan Randomized Trial of Endothelin Antagonist Therapy) trial randomized 213 patients with IPAH (70%) and pulmonary hypertension associated with connective tissue disease who were WHO functional classes III and IV to placebo or bosentan at a dosage of 125 mg or 250 mg twice daily. At 16 weeks, the bosentan group had a placebo-corrected 6MWD improvement of 44 m ($P<.001$) (Fig. 3).[22] In addition, there were improvements in the Borg dyspnea score and time to clinical worsening in both bosentan groups. Increases in liver aminotransferases greater than 8 times the upper limit of normal was again noted in the bosentan group and was dosage-dependent with 2 patients in the 125-mg group and 5 patients in the 250-mg group.

In addition to the registration trials of bosentan discussed earlier, a randomized controlled trial of bosentan in less functionally impaired patients with PAH (WHO class II), the EARLY (Endothelin Antagonist Trial in Mildly Symptomatic Pulmonary Arterial Hypertension Patients) trial, showed a benefit in reducing PVR and preventing clinical worsening at 6 months. No statistically significant effect on 6MWD was seen, although baseline walk distance was greater than 400 m, confirming that this cohort had better baseline exercise capacity.[23]

Bosentan has also been studied in a randomized controlled trial in patients with congenital heart disease.[24] The BREATHE-5 study showed that, in a group of patients with either atrial or ventricular septal defects, compared with placebo, bosentan improved 6MWD without worsening hypoxemia.

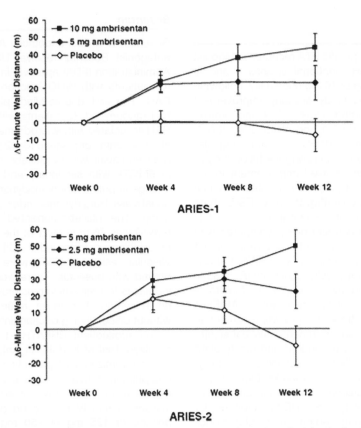

Fig. 3. Effects of ambrisentan on the primary end point, 6MWD in the 2 pivotal trials. Similar improvements were seen, although in ARIES 2, lower doses seemed to give similar effects compared with ARIES 1. The approved dose of ambrisentan is 5 mg or 10 mg once daily.

Long-term survival data in patients on bosentan, although uncontrolled, have been published. Of the 169 patients with IPAH enrolled in the 2 pivotal trials of bosentan, estimated survival at 1 and 2 years was 96% and 89% respectively, compared with the predicted survival of 69% and 57%[25] (based on a validated National Institutes of Health equation calculating predicted survival from baseline hemodynamics). However, there are no prospective controlled survival data with the newer agents, given obvious ethical concerns about such trials in the era of existing effective therapy.

SAFETY CONSIDERATIONS IN ENDOTHELIN RECEPTOR ANTAGONIST THERAPY

ET-1 antagonists are considered teratogenic, and therefore women of child-bearing potential require monthly pregnancy testing and the use of 2 reliable forms of birth control during therapy. Increases in liver aminotransferases, in some cases to greater than 5 times the upper limits of normal, were also noted with bosentan therapy during randomized controlled clinical trials, and, as a result, all patients receiving bosentan are required to undergo monthly liver function testing. The rate of liver function test abnormalities during ambrisentan administration has been found to be similar to that of the general population, and monthly testing is no longer required, although periodic testing at the discretion of the prescriber is recommended. In patients in whom liver function tests do become abnormal during therapy with either drug, namely aspartate transaminase (AST) or alanine transaminase (ALT) increases of more than 5-fold the upper limit of normal or total bilirubin levels greater than or equal to 2-fold the upper limit of normal require drug discontinuation. In addition, for bosentan, AST or ALT increases between 3 and 5 times the upper limit of normal require either a dosage reduction or drug cessation. Hemoglobin levels should also be monitored periodically, because anemia has been reported during therapy with ET-1 antagonists. ET-1 antagonists are well tolerated by most patients, but significant peripheral edema occurred during the clinical trials, particularly in older patients. Close monitoring of volume status is therefore indicated during drug initiation and up-titration. Nasal congestion has also been reported.[20–23]

Several significant drug interactions exist. For bosentan, both glyburide and cyclosporine are contraindicated, and strong p450 inhibitors (eg, rifampin) should be used only with caution. For ambrisentan, the only clinically relevant interaction that has been identified is an increase in ambrisentan levels with cyclosporine; as a result, the ambrisentan dosage should be limited to 5 mg daily when taken with cyclosporine (see package inserts for additional details on pregnancy prevention, drug interactions, and laboratory monitoring).

Phosphodiesterase Inhibitors

Phosphodiesterase inhibitors (PDEIs) work by inhibiting phosphodiesterase type-5 (PDE5), the primary metabolic enzyme of intracellular cyclic guanosine monophosphate (cGMP) in the pulmonary vasculature. Intracellular cGMP is the second messenger for NO and natriuretic peptide (NP) signaling and mediates most of the vasodilator effects of these agents on the pulmonary circulation. The discoveries of NP and NO toward the end of the last century ushered in a new age in pulmonary vascular research that has led to the discovery of myriad effects of intracellular cGMP, including inhibition of smooth muscle cell proliferation and platelet aggregation. cGMP also plays an important role in vascular endothelial cell and cardiomyocyte function.

An extensive body of literature has investigated the role of the NPs and NO in modulating systemic and pulmonary vascular tone.[26] Both NP and NO act as vasodilators on preconstricted pulmonary vessels and in lungs exposed to acute hypoxia,[27–29] and disrupted NP or NO signaling exaggerate pulmonary hypertensive responses.[30,31] More importantly, patients with PAH seem to have impairments in NP and NO signaling that may result in decreased intracellular cGMP availability.[32–34] These findings have led to the development of PDE5 inhibitors to ameliorate the increase in pulmonary vascular tone and remodeling that are characteristic of PAH.

cGMP is synthesized from its precursor, guanosine triphosphate (GTP), by a family of enzymes termed guanylate cyclases (GCs). The particulate GCs are membrane-bound receptors with high binding affinity for the NPs that have an intracellular GC domain. Binding of atrial natriuretic peptide (ANP) or brain natriuretic peptide (BNP) to the natriuretic peptide receptor A (NPR-A) results in activation of GC domain and an increase in intracellular cGMP levels (**Fig. 4**). A similar receptor, NPR-B, produces cGMP in response to C-type natriuretic peptide (CNP). In contrast, soluble GC (sGC) is an intracellular GC with a heme moiety that has high binding affinity for NO. Increase of intracellular cGMP by NO occurs via activation of sGC following synthesis of NO, primarily by endothelial cells, and diffusion into adjacent pulmonary vascular smooth muscle cGMP (see **Fig. 4**).

Most of the functional effects of cGMP occur via activation of cGMP-dependent protein kinase, or protein kinase G (PKG), which phosphorylates specific target molecules that decrease intracellular calcium concentration via activation of

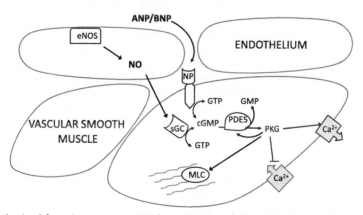

Fig. 4. cGMP is synthesized from its precursor, GTP by activation of the particulate GC NPR-A and NPR-B or activation of soluble guanylate cyclase (sGC) by NO. ANP and BNP are synthesized and released by atrial and ventricular cardiac myocytes and released into the circulation. NO is produced in endothelial cells and diffuses into adjacent pulmonary vascular smooth muscle. cGMP activates cGMP-dependent protein kinase (PKG) which phosphorylates specific target molecules that decrease intracellular calcium concentration via activation of calcium ion pumps and inhibition of transmembrane calcium channels. Decreased intracellular calcium concentration impedes myosin light chain phosphorylation leading to smooth muscle cell relaxation. PKG also increases the activity of PDE-5 and thereby increases metabolism of cGMP. See text for further explanation.

calcium ion pumps to remove intracellular calcium and by inhibition of transmembrane voltage-gated calcium channels that prevent calcium entry (see **Fig. 4**). In addition, PKG-dependent phosphorylation of the receptor for IP3 decreases calcium release from the sarcoplasmic reticulum.[35] In vascular smooth muscle, the decrease in intracellular calcium impedes myosin light chain phosphorylation and leads to smooth muscle relaxation. PKG may also relax vascular smooth muscle by phosphorylating myosin-binding proteins[36] and seems to mediate cGMP-induced inhibition of pulmonary vascular smooth muscle proliferation.[35] In addition, PKG has been shown to activate the PDEs that metabolize cGMP, providing a negative feedback loop that helps stabilize intracellular levels.[37]

The PDEs are a large family of enzymes that hydrolyze the 3′,5′-cyclic nucleotide monophosphates to their respective 5′- monophosphates.[38,39] More than a dozen PDE5 isoforms have been identified with different degrees of specificity for cAMP and cGMP. PDE-4, PDE-7, and PDE-8 hydrolyze cAMP, primarily, whereas PDE-5, PDE-6, and PDE-9 are selective for cGMP. The rest of the isozymes have substantial activity for both nucleotides. However, each cyclic nucleotide can act, to some degree, as a substrate for the other's PDE and each is capable of activating the other's downstream protein kinase, resulting in considerable crosstalk between pathways.[35,40]

Although the lung has the highest tissue concentration of PDE5,[41] the enzyme is found throughout the circulation including the corpus cavernosum where it plays a major role in modulating penile erection and is the primary target of PDE5 inhibitors used for the treatment of erectile dysfunction (ED). Several studies suggest that PDE5 activity in the lung is increased in pulmonary hypertensive diseases, thereby increasing cGMP metabolism and impairing cGMP-mediated pulmonary vasodilation.[42,43] Selective inhibition of PDE5 results in greater pulmonary than systemic vasodilation because of either greater concentration or activity of PDE5 in pulmonary than in systemic vasculature under these conditions.[44–46] Selective inhibitors of PDE5 have been shown to reverse acute pulmonary vasoconstriction and blunt the development of experimental pulmonary hypertension in animals.[45,47] These agents also blunt acute pulmonary vasoconstriction in man and have been shown to mitigate the development of high-altitude pulmonary edema.[48,49] These observations provided the rationale to target PDE5 for the treatment of pulmonary vascular disease and led to the clinical development of PDE5 inhibitors to treat PAH.

Sildenafil in PAH

After the approval of sildenafil for ED in 1998, there has been increasing interest in its effects on the pulmonary vasculature.

Experimental pulmonary hypertension More than 60 studies, many of which used sildenafil consistently, show that PDE5 inhibition alone or in combination with PDE3 inhibitors attenuate or reverse acute PAH.[46,50–52] This held true when PDE5 inhibition was achieved via intravenous, oral, or inhaled administration. Furthermore, augmentation of cGMP by a combination of inhaled NO and inhaled sildenafil,[53] or intravenous ANP and oral sildenafil,[54] produced more pulmonary vasodilation than sildenafil alone. Sildenafil has also been extensively tested in various in vivo models of pulmonary hypertension. In the chronic hypoxia model in rats, sildenafil reduced the right ventricular pressures and the proportion of muscularized distal pulmonary arteries. In monocrotaline-induced pulmonary hypertensive rats, sildenafil administered in drinking water for 6 weeks increased cGMP and reduced pulmonary hypertension, muscularization of the peripheral pulmonary arteries, and right ventricular hypertrophy without affecting gas exchange or systemic arterial pressure and, more importantly, also improved survival.[55] In addition, combination of sildenafil and beraprost (a prostacyclin analogue that stimulates cAMP production) limited progression of pulmonary hypertension and improved survival in the monocrotaline rat model.[56]

The complete vasodilator effect of PDE5 inhibition seems to depend on a preserved NO/NP-cGMP pathway. Sildenafil reduced pulmonary artery pressure in chronically hypoxic mice with targeted disruption of the gene encoding endothelial NO synthase less than in wild-type controls and failed to decrease right ventricular hypertrophy or pulmonary muscularization. In concordance with these observations, in chronically hypoxic mice lacking the GC-linked NPR-A, PDE5 inhibition blunted the increase in pulmonary artery pressures, right ventricular hypertrophy, and pulmonary vascular remodeling, but the effect was less than in wild-type mice.[57] These findings suggest that natriuretic peptides and NO contribute to the vasodilator response to sildenafil.

Acute effects of sildenafil on human PAH Several studies showed that sildenafil is a potent acute pulmonary vasodilator in patients with PAH. Oral sildenafil, inhaled NO, and aerosolized iloprost significantly improved pulmonary hemodynamics in 10 consecutive patients with idiopathic PAH.[58] In 13 patients with PAH, all but 1 in New York

Heart Association (NYHA) class III or IV, sildenafil reduced mean pulmonary artery pressure (mPAP) and PVR, and increased CI without affecting pulmonary artery wedge pressure. Sildenafil potentiated and prolonged the effects of inhaled NO and, when combined, the two agents reduced PVR and increased CI more than either agent alone.[45] In another cohort of 20 patients with different forms of PAH, sildenafil proved to be a potent acute pulmonary vasodilator, the effect potentiated by inhaled NO.[59] Sildenafil improved acutely pulmonary hemodynamics in 5 patients with idiopathic PAH and the inhaled prostacyclin analogue, iloprost, had additive effects with sildenafil.[60]

Chronic effects of sildenafil on human PAH Early nonrandomized, single-center studies of patients with PAH treated with long-term sildenafil (25–100 mg orally 3 times daily for 5–20 months) found significant improvements in functional class and 6MWD as well as a decrease in pulmonary artery systolic pressure on echocardiography compared with baseline. Two placebo-controlled crossover trials showed functional benefit, one with 2 weeks of therapy[61] and the other 6 weeks.[62] In the longer trial, 22 patients with PAH received placebo or sildenafil (25–100 mg 3 times daily). Exercise tolerance, CI, and the dyspnea and fatigue components of the quality-of-life score significantly improved with sildenafil, but there was no significant change in systolic pulmonary artery pressure estimated by echocardiography.

Based on this experimental data and early human studies, the pivotal randomized, placebo-controlled trial of sildenafil was conducted in idiopathic, connective tissue disease–associated and congenital heart disease–associated PAH (SUPER trial).[63] The trial enrolled patients in functional class II to IV whose 6MWDs were between 100 and 450 m at baseline. Two-hundred and seventy-eight patients were randomized to 3 treatment groups (20, 40, and 80 mg orally 3 times a day) or placebo for 12 weeks. The main outcome variable (6MWD) increased significantly (45, 46, and 50 m for the 3 dosages, respectively) compared with the placebo arm, but no dosage-response relationship was seen. Pulmonary hemodynamics also improved significantly, but time to clinical worsening was not significantly prolonged compared with controls. Among the 222 patients completing 1 year of sildenafil (most of whom had been on 80 mg 3 times a day), the average improvement from baseline in 6MWD was 51 m. The drug was well tolerated, with headache and epistaxis occurring significantly more often than in controls. Combination therapies of sildenafil and other compounds such as endothelin receptor antagonists and prostacyclins have been conducted or are underway and are discussed elsewhere.

PDE5 inhibition with sildenafil in other forms of pulmonary hypertension Given the successful results in improving human PAH, as well as the favorable safety profile, sildenafil has been also tested in forms of pulmonary hypertension other than PAH. For example, treatment with sildenafil improved pulmonary hemodynamics and exercise capacity in healthy subjects with both acute hypoxic PAH at rest[48] and with exercise,[64] as well as in chronic high-altitude PAH.[65] Sildenafil has also been tested as a therapy for chronic thromboembolic pulmonary hypertension in patients who are not candidates for thromboendarterectomy.[66] Administered at a daily dosage of 50 mg 3 times over approximately 6 months, sildenafil reduced average mPAPs and PVR by 15% and 30%, respectively, and increased CI and 6MWD by 17% and 54 m, respectively. Sildenafil caused acute pulmonary vasodilation and improved gas exchange in 16 patients with pulmonary hypertension secondary to severe lung fibrosis (WHO group 3).[67] In addition, sildenafil was tested in patients with pulmonary hypertension secondary to left heart disease (WHO group 2). In a small group of patients with pulmonary hypertension secondary to left ventricular systolic dysfunction caused by coronary artery disease or idiopathic dilated cardiomyopathy, PDE5 inhibition with sildenafil improved cardiac output and decreased pulmonary artery wedge pressure, while augmenting and prolonging the hemodynamic effects of inhaled NO.[68] Despite these preliminary positive data, there is no convincing evidence yet to warrant the use of sildenafil in pulmonary hypertension caused by left heart disease.

Tadalafil Tadalafil is a beta-carboline–based PDE5 inhibitor that was designed to inhibit PDE activity and to have high specificity for PDE5. The selectivity of tadalafil for PDE5 is reported to be 9000-fold to 10,000-fold greater than for PDE1 to PDE4 and PDE7 to PDE10[69 and package insert] and to be nearly 800-fold greater for PDE5 than for PDE6.[69] The clinical efficacy of tadalafil as a PDE5 inhibitor has been well shown in studies of ED and seems to be at least as effective as other PDE5 inhibitors.[70] Following successful reports of sildenafil for the treatment of PAH, several preliminary studies reported similar efficacy for this indication with tadalafil. The longer half-life of tadalafil, which allowed once-daily dosing, also made it an attractive alternative to sildenafil for the long-term treatment of PAH.

In 2004, Ghofrani and colleagues[71] compared the acute vasodilator effects of 3 PDE5 inhibitors in 60 consecutive patients as part of their initial evaluation of pulmonary hypertension. Compared with sildenafil and vardenafil, tadalafil produced similar decreases in mPAP and PVR and increases in CI. The peak vasodilator effect occurred after approximately 45 minutes for vardenafil (10 or 20 mg), 60 minutes for sildenafil (50 mg), and 75 to 90 minutes for tadalafil (20–60 mg). In the same year, the first of a few small open-label trials and case reports described the clinical benefits of extended treatment with tadalafil in PAH.[72,73] In 2007, 2 small open-label trials in India reported improvement in symptoms and pulmonary hemodynamics in patients with PAH treated with tadalafil.[74,75] A large, multicenter, randomized controlled trial of tadalafil called the PHIRST (Pulmonary Arterial Hypertension and Response to Tadalafil) study began to enrolled patients with idiopathic or associated PAH in 2005.[76] This pivotal trial randomized 405 patients to placebo, 2.5, 10, 20, or 40 mg of tadalafil once daily. Most patients had idiopathic or heritable PAH. Approximately one-quarter had PAH associated with connective tissue disease, and slightly more than half the patients were taking bosentan at the time of enrollment. Randomization was stratified for baseline 6MWD, type of PAH, and background treatment with bosentan. The primary end point was change from baseline to 16 weeks in 6MWD and was significantly greater for the 10-mg, 20-mg, and 40-mg tadalafil groups than for placebo (P = .047, P = .028, and P<.001), but the prespecified significance level of P<.01 was reached only

in the group that received 40 mg of tadalafil (**Fig. 5**). Time to clinical worsening defined as death, heart or lung transplantation, atrial septostomy, hospitalization for worsening PAH, initiation of a new therapy for PAH, or increase in WHO functional class was longer and the incidence of clinical worsening was less in patient who received 40 mg of tadalafil versus placebo. In a subgroup of 93 patients who underwent right heart catheterization at baseline and after 16 weeks of study drug, mPAP and PVR decreased significantly in patients who received 20 mg (n = 17) or 40 mg (n = 18) of tadalafil. CI was also significantly increased in the group treated with 40 mg of tadalafil. The improvement in 6MWD was sustained for 10 months in a subgroup of patients who were enrolled in a long-term extension study of 20 or 40 mg of tadalafil. Of the 213 patients who had completed at least 10 months of tadalafil therapy at the time of publication, the mean change in 6MWD was 37 m at 16 weeks and 38 m after 44 weeks.

Based on the results of this pivotal clinical trial, tadalafil was approved by the FDA in May, 2009, at a dosage of 40 mg once daily for the treatment of WHO group 1 PAH. Additional data from the long-term extension study were published separately in 2012. There were 357 patients who were enrolled in the double-blind, uncontrolled extension study (PHIRST-2) and 293 patients completed the 52-week trial. The 6MWD in the group assigned to 20 mg of tadalafil in the long-term extension trial was 406 ± 67 m achieved after 16 weeks of therapy and 415 ± 80 m after 52 weeks. The 6MWD in the

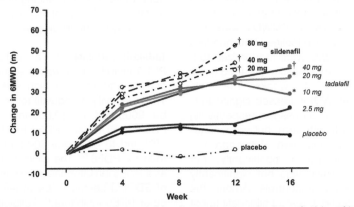

Fig. 5. Comparison of the primary outcome variables from the pivotal trials of sildenafil and tadalafil. Both studies examined the effect of various doses of drug compared with placebo. Change from baseline in 6MWD was measured after 12 weeks of treatment in the sildenafil trial (SUPER) and after 16 weeks of treatment in the PHIRST study. All 3 doses of sildenafil resulted in a significant increase in walk distance compared with placebo in the SUPER trial. Only the highest dose of tadalafil achieved the prespecified significance level of P<.01 in the PHIRST study. All patients in SUPER were treatment naive, whereas half the study population in PHIRST had been taking an endothelin receptor antagonist for at least 3 months at study entry.

group assigned to 40 mg of tadalafil was 413 ± 81 m after 16 weeks of therapy and 410 ± 78 m after 52 weeks. Deterioration in WHO functional class occurred in 9% of patients in the 20-mg group and 6% of patients taking 40 mg of tadalafil.

Few studies have examined the use of tadalafil to treat PAH in children, although patients as young as 12 and 13 years of age have been included in published trials of tadalafil in PAH.

In general, tadalafil has been well tolerated in patients with PAH. The most common adverse effects are headache, flushing, and myalgias including back pain. Serious adverse events were reported in 13% of patients in the PHIRST trial, but were judged by the investigators to be drug related in only 3.0%.

In a post hoc analysis of elderly patients who were treated with 40 mg of tadalafil[77] the incidence of adverse events was no different in patients greater than 65 years of age compared with those who were less than 65 years old.

Rare cases of vascular thrombosis have been reported following the use of PDE5 inhibitors, including a case of acute pulmonary embolism associated with tadalafil use in a patient with protein C deficiency.[78] Of particular concern is the possible relationship between PDE5 inhibitors and nonarteritic ischemic optic neuropathy (NAION). Although the number of cases has been too low to directly link the use of PDE5 inhibitors with NAION, several reports have raised the possibility of this association with sildenafil[37,38] and with tadalafil[79–82] when taken for ED.

Tadalafil is absorbed rapidly, reaching peak plasma concentrations approximately 2 hours after ingestion and is metabolized primarily in the liver via cytochrome P450 (CYP) 3A4 to an inactive catechol metabolite. Following extensive methylation and glucuronidation, the catechol metabolites are excreted primarily in the feces and urine (61% and 36%, respectively). Plasma elimination has a mean half-life of 17.5 hours in healthy volunteers, but may be greater than 30 hours in patients with PAH. Because of the hepatic and renal routes of elimination of catechol metabolites, it is advisable to start tadalafil at no more than 20 mg a day in patients with mild to moderate hepatic or renal disease and increase to 40 mg daily based on individual tolerance. Tadalafil should be avoided in patients with more severe liver or renal impairment. Like all PDE5 inhibitors, tadalafil should not be used with nitrates because of the potential for hypotension and coronary ischemia. Potent inhibitors of CYP3A such as itraconazole or ketoconazole should be avoided because they may prolong the metabolism of tadalafil.

Overview of Available Oral Therapies: Comparisons

At least 4 orally active medications are available for the treatment of PAH (**Table 1**) and it is anticipated that several more may be available within the next few years. Studies adequately powered to detect differences in clinical efficacy between sildenafil and tadalafil or between bosentan and ambrisentan have not been done. No study has yet to adequately address the relative efficacy of ERAs versus PDE5 inhibitors. However, results from the major pivotal studies of sildenafil, tadalafil, bosentan, and ambrisentan have been similar (**Table 2**). In general, study subjects enrolled in these trials were treatment naive and had IPAH or PAH associated with connective tissue disease. Most patients were WHO functional class III at baseline and the effect of therapy on 6MWD, pulmonary hemodynamics, and improvement in functional class were not appreciably different between medications or between the two classes of drug. In the lone study that attempted to compare differences in efficacy between an ERA

Table 1
Dose and monitoring of the 4 FDA approved oral therapies for PAH

	Approved Dose (mg)	Frequency	Suggest Laboratory Monitoring	Common Side Effects
Bosentan	62.5 or 125	bid	LFTs monthly CBC quarterly Urine pregnancy test	Transaminase increase Anemia
Ambrisentan	5 or 10	qd	LFTs quarterly, CBC quarterly	Transaminase increase Anemia Peripheral edema
Sildenafil	20	tid	—	—
Tadalafil	40	qd	—	Headache, myalgias, flushing

Abbreviations: bid, twice a day; CBC, complete blood count; LFT, liver function test; qd, every day; tid, 3 times a day.

Table 2
Efficacy of the 4 approved oral therapies for PAH

Drug	Dose	Placebo-corrected 6MWD (m)	mPAP (mm Hg)	PVR (dyn s.cm[5])	CI (L/min/m[2])	Change in WHO Functional Class	Reference
Bosentan	125 mg bid	76 44	−6.7 (−11.7 to −1.5)*	−415 (−608 to −221)	1.0 (0.6–1.4)	Yes	21,22
Ambrisentan	5 mg qd	51	NA	NA	NA	Yes in 1 of 2 trials	20
Sildenafil	20 mg tid	45	−2.1 (−4.3 to 0.0)	−122 (−217 to −27)	0.21 (0.04–0.8)	NS	63
Tadalafil	40 mg qd	33[a]	−4.3 (95% confidence interval, −8 to −1)	−209 (95% confidence interval, −406 to −13)	0.60 (95% confidence interval, 0.1–1.6)	NS	76

Abbreviations: NA, not available; NS, not significant.
* Hemodynamics obtained in Study 351, reference 21.
[a] Placebo-corrected increase in 6MWD for all patients treated with 40 mg tadalafil. For treatment-naive patients treated with 40 mg tadalafil, the difference was 44 m.
Data from Channick RN, Simonneau G, Sitbon O, et al. Effects of the dual endothelin-receptor antagonist bosentan in patients with pulmonary hypertension: a randomized placebo controlled study. Lancet 2001;358:1119–23.

and a PDE5 inhibitor, improvement in 6MWD was similar in 14 patients randomized to receive sildenafil (75 m) and 12 patients randomized to receive bosentan,[83] although the number of patients studied was too small to draw conclusions about differences in efficacy with any degree of confidence.

Compared with ERAs, the PDE5 inhibitors may be an easier class of medications to administer. Aside from nitrates, they have few interactions with other medications and can be obtained from most pharmacies without a third-party distributor. Adverse events are generally mild and self-limited and, unlike ERAs, monitoring of liver transaminases and/or pregnancy status is not required. In the United States, the commercial price for the approved dose of PDE5 inhibitors is less than half the cost of ERA therapy. Aside from sildenafil, which has recently become available in generic form, most third-party payers require preauthorization for both classes of medication and the cost to the patient may be no different depending on their insurance coverage.

Of the 2 PDE5 inhibitors currently approved for treatment of PAH, clinical efficacy of sildenafil and tadalafil seem to be comparable (see **Fig. 4**, **Table 2**). The overall clinical experience, particularly in treatment-naive patients, is greater with sildenafil, although a recent analysis reported the combined experience of 12 studies that included nearly 900 patients treated with tadalafil alone.[84] At this time, it is unclear whether or not the longer half-life of tadalafil has any clinical advantage compared with sildenafil, but the once-daily dosing of tadalafil may be more convenient to some patients.

The relative potency of sildenafil and tadalafil at their approved dosages is unclear The currently approved dosage of sildenafil for PAH is less than the lowest dosage of sildenafil used to treat ED, whereas the approved dosage of tadalafil for PAH is the highest dosage approved for ED. It is difficult to determine whether sildenafil and tadalafil at these dosages have similar pulmonary hemodynamic effects. In the study by Ghofrani and colleagues,[44] a single 50-mg dose of sildenafil had an acute pulmonary vasodilator effect that was similar to 40 mg of tadalafil. However, lower doses of sildenafil were not studied and hemodynamic measurements were recorded for only 2 hours. Change from baseline pulmonary hemodynamic measurements were assessed in all patients treated with sildenafil in the SUPER study and in subgroups of patients treated with each dose of tadalafil in the PHIRST study (see **Table 2**).[85] The mPAP and PVR decreased by 2.1 mm Hg and 122 dyn s.cm^5 after 12 weeks of sildenafil 20 mg 3 times a day, compared with a decrease of 4.3 mm Hg and 209 dyn s.cm^5 after 16 weeks of tadalafil 40 mg every day (see **Table 2**). CI increased by 0.21 L/min/m^2 (95% confidence interval, 0.04–0.8 L/min/m^2) with sildenafil 20 mg 3 times a day and 0.60 L/min/m^2 (95% confidence interval, 0.1–1.6 L/min/m^2) with tadalafil 40 mg every day (see **Table 2**). However, direct comparison between studies is difficult because of the smaller number of patients studied in the tadalafil study, the concomitant use of bosentan in some patients taking tadalafil, and the difference in time between baseline and repeat hemodynamic measurements between studies.

Some practitioners have also been concerned that the use of tadalafil at the highest approved dosage for ED and its longer half-life may increase the incidence of adverse events, particularly in the elderly or at the start of therapy. However, this does not seem to be the case. Post hoc analysis of data from the PHIRST study found no significant differences in adverse events between the 20-mg or 40-mg treatment groups.[85]

Another consideration is the lack of long-term data for patients taking the approved 20-mg dose of sildenafil. In the extension phase of the pivotal trial of sildenafil, patients were increased to the maximum dosage studied (80 mg 3 times a day) and improvement in 6MWD after 12 weeks, which was similar for all 3 dosages studied, was maintained for 12 months.[63] It is unclear whether this sustained improvement in walking distance would have occurred if patients were maintained on a lower dosage of sildenafil. As a result, many clinicians who are treating patients with PAH with sildenafil are compelled to increase the dosage gradually from 20 to 80 mg 3 times a day during the first year of therapy, which can be problematic because many third-party payers are unwilling to cover any dosage greater than the approved 20 mg 3 times a day. Additional studies are needed to determine whether it is necessary to increase the dosage of sildenafil during long-term treatment to maintain response to treatment.

SUMMARY

The development of oral therapies for PAH has been a breakthrough in management for this life-threatening condition. Diagnosis and institution of treatment at earlier stages of disease has likely improved outcomes. Although data are limited because of the rare nature of PAH and lack of head-to-head comparisons between the various oral therapies, long-term data and clinical experience unequivocally support their critical role and clinical benefits. Novel oral agents are being developed that may further advance the field.

REFERENCES

1. Yanagisawa M, Kurihara H, Kimura S, et al. A novel potent vasoconstrictor peptide produced by vascular endothelial cells. Nature 1988;332: 411–5.
2. Inoue A, Yanagisawa M, Kimura S, et al. The human endothelin family: three structurally and pharmacologically distinct isopeptides predicted by three separate genes. Proc Natl Acad Sci U S A 1989;86:2863–7.
3. Mattoli S, Mezzetti M, Riva G, et al. Specific binding of endothelin on human bronchial smooth muscle cells in culture and secretion of endothelin-like material from bronchial epithelial cells. Am J Respir Cell Mol Biol 1990;3:145–51.
4. Yu J, Davenport A. Secretion of endothelin-1 and endothelin-3 by human cultured vascular smooth muscle cells. Br J Pharmacol 1995;114:551–7.
5. Ehrenreich H, Anderson RW, Fox CH, et al. Endothelins, peptides with potent vasoactive properties, are produced by human macrophages. J Exp Med 1990;172:1741–8.
6. Miyauchi T, Masaki T. Pathophysiology of endothelin in the cardiovascular system. Annu Rev Physiol 1999;61:391–415.
7. Michael J, Markewitz B. Endothelins and the lung. Am J Respir Crit Care Med 1996;154:555–81.
8. Yoshimoto S, Ishizaki Y, Sasaki T, et al. Effect of carbon dioxide and oxygen on endothelin production by cultured porcine cerebral endothelial cells. Stroke 1991;22:378–83.
9. Takuwa Y, Kasuya Y, Takuwa N, et al. Endothelin receptor is coupled to phospholipase C via pertussis toxin insensitive guanine nucleotide binding regulatory protein in vascular smooth muscle cells. J Clin Invest 1990;85:653–8.
10. Chua BH, Krebs CJ, Chua CC, et al. Endothelin stimulates protein synthesis in smooth muscle cells. Am J Physiol 1992;262:E412–6.
11. Davie N, Haleen SJ, Upton PD, et al. ETA and ETB receptors modulate the proliferation of human pulmonary artery smooth muscle cells. Am J Respir Crit Care Med 2002;165:398–405.
12. Hirata Y, Emori T, Eguchi S. Endothelin receptor subtype B mediates synthesis of nitric oxide by cultured bovine endothelial cells. J Clin Invest 1993;91:1367–73.
13. Masaki T. Possible role of endothelin in endothelial regulation of vascular tone. Annu Rev Pharmacol Toxicol 1995;35:235–55.
14. Dupuis J, Jasmin JF, Prié S, et al. Importance of local production of endothelin-1 and of the ETB receptor in the regulation of pulmonary vascular tone. Pulm Pharmacol Ther 2000;13:135–40.
15. Giaid A, Yanagisawa M, Langleben D, et al. Expression of endothelin-1 in the lungs of patients with pulmonary hypertension. N Engl J Med 1993; 328:1732–9.
16. Bando K, Vijayaraghavan P, Turrentine MW, et al. Dynamic changes of endothelin-1, nitric oxide, and cyclic GMP in patients with congenital heart disease. Circulation 1997;96(Suppl 9):II-346–51.
17. Kim H, Yung GL, Marsh JJ, et al. Endothelin mediates pulmonary vascular remodelling in a canine model of chronic embolic pulmonary hypertension. Eur Respir J 2000;15:640–8.
18. Bauer M, Wilkens H, Langer F, et al. Selective upregulation of endothelin B receptor gene expression in severe pulmonary hyper- tension. Circulation 2002;105:1034–6.
19. Galié N, Badesch D, Oudiz R, et al. Ambrisentan therapy for pulmonary arterial hypertension. J Am Coll Cardiol 2005;46:529–35.
20. Galié N, Olschewski H, Oudiz RJ, et al. Ambrisentan for the treatment of pulmonary arterial hypertension: results of the ambrisentan in pulmonary arterial hypertension, randomized, double-blind, placebo-controlled, multicenter, efficacy (ARIES) study 1 and 2. Circulation 2008;117(23):3010–9.
21. Channick RN, Simonneau G, Sitbon O, et al. Effects of the dual endothelin-receptor antagonist bosentan in patients with pulmonary hypertension: a randomized placebo controlled study. Lancet 2001; 358:1119–23.
22. Rubin LJ, Badesch DB, Barst RJ, et al. Bosentan therapy for pulmonary arterial hypertension. N Engl J Med 2002;346(12):896–903.
23. Galié N, Rubin LJ, Hoeper M, et al. Treatment of patients with mildly symptomatic pulmonary arterial hypertension with bosentan (EARLY study): a double-blind, randomized controlled trial. Lancet 2008;37:2093–100.
24. Galié N, Beghetti M, Gatzoulis MA, et al. Bosentan therapy in patients with Eisenmenger syndrome: a multicenter, double-blind, randomized, placebo-controlled study. Circulation 2006;114(1):48–54.
25. McLaughlin VV, Sitbon O, Badesch DB, et al. Survival with first-line bosentan in patients with primary pulmonary hypertension. Eur Respir J 2005;25: 244–9.
26. Klinger JR. The nitric oxide/cGMP signaling pathway in pulmonary hypertension. Clin Chest Med 2007;28(1):143–67.
27. Frostell CG, Blomqvist H, Hedenstierna G, et al. Inhaled nitric oxide selectively reverses human hypoxic pulmonary vasoconstriction without causing systemic vasodilation. Anesthesiology 1993;78(3):427–35.
28. Wanstall JC, Hughes IE, O'Donnell SR. Evidence that nitric oxide from the endothelium attenuates inherent tone in isolated pulmonary arteries from rats with hypoxic pulmonary hypertension. Br J Pharmacol 1995;114(1):109–14.

29. Hill NS, Klinger JR, Warburton RR, et al. Brain natriuretic peptide: possible role in the modulation of hypoxic pulmonary hypertension. Am J Physiol 1994;266(3 Pt 1):L308–15.

30. Klinger JR, Warburton RR, Pietras L, et al. Targeted disruption of the gene for natriuretic peptide receptor-A worsens hypoxia-induced cardiac hypertrophy. Am J Physiol Heart Circ Physiol 2002; 282(1):H58–65.

31. Zhao L, Long L, Morrell NW, et al. NPR-A-deficient mice show increased susceptibility to hypoxia-induced pulmonary hypertension. Circulation 1999;99(5):605–7.

32. Charloux A, Chaouat A, Piquard F, et al. Renal hyporesponsiveness to brain natriuretic peptide: both generation and renal activity of cGMP are decreased in patients with pulmonary hypertension. Peptides 2006;27(11):2993–9.

33. Kharitonov SA, Cailes JB, Black CM, et al. Decreased nitric oxide in the exhaled air of patients with systemic sclerosis with pulmonary hypertension. Thorax 1997;52(12):1051–5.

34. Klinger JR, Abman SH, Gladwin MT. Nitric oxide deficiency and endothelial dysfunction in pulmonary arterial hypertension. Am J Respir Crit Care Med 2013. [Epub ahead of print].

35. Lincoln TM, Dey N, Sellak H. Invited review: cGMP-dependent protein kinase signaling mechanisms in smooth muscle: from the regulation of tone to gene expression. J Appl Physiol 2001; 91:1421–30.

36. Surks HK, Mochizuki N, Kasai Y, et al. Regulation of myosin phosphatase by a specific interaction with cGMP-dependent protein kinase I alpha. Science 1999;286(5444):1583–7.

37. Corbin JD, Turko IV, Beasley A, et al. Phosphorylation of phosphodiesterase-5 by cyclic nucleotide-dependent protein kinase alters its catalytic and allosteric cGMP-binding activities. Eur J Biochem 2000;267:2760–7.

38. Lugnier C. Cyclic nucleotide phosphodiesterase (PDE) superfamily: a new target for the development of specific therapeutic agents. Pharmacol Ther 2006;109(3):366–98.

39. Keravis T, Lugnier C. Cyclic nucleotide phosphodiesterases (PDE) and peptide motifs. Curr Pharm Des 2010;16(9):1114–25.

40. Kass DA, Champion HC, Beavo JA. Phosphodiesterase type 5: expanding roles in cardiovascular regulation. Circ Res 2007;101(11):1084–95.

41. Maclean MR, Johnston ED, Mcculloch KM, et al. Phosphodiesterase isoforms in the pulmonary arterial circulation of the rat: changes in pulmonary hypertension. J Pharmacol Exp Ther 1997;283(2): 619–24.

42. Hanson KA, Ziegler JW, Rybalkin SD, et al. Chronic pulmonary hypertension increases fetal lung cGMP phosphodiesterase activity. Am J Physiol 1998; 275:L931–41.

43. Mikhail GW, Prasad SK, Li W, et al. Clinical and haemodynamic effects of sildenafil in pulmonary hypertension: acute and mid-term effects. Eur Heart J 2004;25:431–6.

44. Ghofrani HA, Pepke-Zaba J, Barbera JA, et al. Nitric oxide pathway and phosphodiesterase inhibitors in pulmonary arterial hypertension. J Am Coll Cardiol 2004;43:68S–72S.

45. Michelakis E, Tymchak W, Lien D, et al. Oral sildenafil is an effective and specific pulmonary vasodilator in patients with pulmonary arterial hypertension: comparison with inhaled nitric oxide. Circulation 2002;105(20):2398–403.

46. Weimann J, Ullrich R, Hromi J, et al. Sildenafil is a pulmonary vasodilator in awake lambs with acute pulmonary hypertension. Anesthesiology 2000; 92(6):1702–12.

47. Zhao L, Mason NA, Morrell NW, et al. Sildenafil inhibits hypoxia-induced pulmonary hypertension. Circulation 2001;104(4):424–8.

48. Richalet JP, Gratadour P, Robach P, et al. Sildenafil inhibits altitude-induced hypoxemia and pulmonary hypertension. Am J Respir Crit Care Med 2005;171(3):275–81.

49. Angulo J, Gadau M, Fernandez A, et al. IC351 enhances nitric oxide-mediated relaxation of human arterial and trabecular penile smooth muscle. Diabetologia 2001;44(S1):A295.

50. Preston IR, Klinger JR, Landzberg MJ, et al. Vasoresponsiveness of sarcoidosis-associated pulmonary hypertension. Chest 2001;120:866–72.

51. Schermuly RT, Krupnik E, Tenor H, et al. Coaerosolization of phosphodiesterase inhibitors markedly enhances the pulmonary vasodilatory response to inhaled iloprost in experimental pulmonary hypertension. Maintenance of lung selectivity. Am J Respir Crit Care Med 2001;164:1694–700.

52. Schermuly RT, Roehl A, Weissmann N, et al. Combination of nonspecific PDE inhibitors with inhaled prostacyclin in experimental pulmonary hypertension. Am J Physiol Lung Cell Mol Physiol 2001; 281:L1361–8.

53. Ichinose F, Erana-Garcia J, Hromi J, et al. Nebulized sildenafil is a selective pulmonary vasodilator in lambs with acute pulmonary hypertension. Crit Care Med 2001;29:1000–5.

54. Preston IR, Hill NS, Gambardella LS, et al. Synergistic effects of ANP and sildenafil on cGMP levels and amelioration of acute hypoxic pulmonary hypertension. Exp Biol Med (Maywood) 2004;229: 920–5.

55. Sebkhi A, Strange J, Phillips S, et al. Phosphodiesterase type 5 as a target for the treatment of hypoxia-induced pulmonary hypertension. Circulation 2003;107:3230–5.

56. Schermuly R, Kreisselmeier K, Ghofrani H, et al. Chronic sildenafil treatment inhibits monocrotaline-induced pulmonary hypertension in rats. Am J Respir Crit Care Med 2004;169:39–45.

57. Zhao L, Mason N, Strange J, et al. Beneficial effects of phosphodiesterase 5 inhibition in pulmonary hypertension are influenced by natriuretic peptide activity. Circulation 2003;107:234–7.

58. Leuchte HH, Schwaiblmair M, Baumgartner RA, et al. Hemodynamic response to sildenafil, nitric oxide, and iloprost in primary pulmonary hypertension. Chest 2004;125:580–6.

59. Preston IR, Klinger JR, Houtches J, et al. Acute and chronic effects of sildenafil in patients with pulmonary arterial hypertension. Respir Med 2005;99:1501–10.

60. Wilkens H, Guth A, Konig J, et al. Effect of inhaled iloprost plus oral sildenafil in patients with primary pulmonary hypertension. Circulation 2001;104:1218–22.

61. Bharani A, Mathew V, Sahu A, et al. The efficacy and tolerability of sildenafil in patients with moderate-to-severe pulmonary hypertension. Indian Heart J 2003;55:55–9.

62. Sastry BK, Narasimhan C, Reddy NK, et al. Clinical efficacy of sildenafil in primary pulmonary hypertension: a randomized, placebo-controlled, double-blind, crossover study. J Am Coll Cardiol 2004;43:1149–53.

63. Galie N, Ghofrani HA, Torbicki A, et al. Sildenafil citrate therapy for pulmonary arterial hypertension. N Engl J Med 2005;353:2148–57.

64. Ricart A, Maristany J, Fort N, et al. Effects of sildenafil on the human response to acute hypoxia and exercise. High Alt Med Biol 2005;6:43–9.

65. Aldashev AA, Kojonazarov BK, Amatov TA, et al. Phosphodiesterase type 5 and high altitude pulmonary hypertension. Thorax 2005;60:683–7.

66. Ghofrani H, Schermuly R, Rose F, et al. Sildenafil for long-term treatment of nonoperable chronic thromboembolic pulmonary hypertension. Am J Respir Crit Care Med 2003;167:1139–41.

67. Ghofrani HA, Wiedemann R, Rose F, et al. Sildenafil for treatment of lung fibrosis and pulmonary hypertension: a randomised controlled trial. Lancet 2002;360:895–900.

68. Lepore JJ, Maroo A, Bigatello LM, et al. Hemodynamic effects of sildenafil in patients with congestive heart failure and pulmonary hypertension: combined administration with inhaled nitric oxide. Chest 2005;127:1647–53.

69. Skoumal R, Chen J, Kula K, et al. Efficacy and treatment satisfaction with on-demand tadalafil (Cialis) in men with erectile dysfunction. Eur Urol 2004;46(3):362–9.

70. Tolrà JR, Campaña JM, Ciutat LF, et al. Prospective, randomized, open-label, fixed-dose, crossover study to establish preference of patients with erectile dysfunction after taking the three PDE-5 inhibitors. J Sex Med 2006;3(5):901–9.

71. Ghofrani HA, Voswinckel R, Reichenberger F, et al. Differences in hemodynamic and oxygenation responses to three different phosphodiesterase-5 inhibitors in patients with pulmonary arterial hypertension: a randomized prospective study. J Am Coll Cardiol 2004;44(7):1488–96.

72. Palmieri EA, Affuso F, Fazio S, et al. Tadalafil in primary pulmonary arterial hypertension. Ann Intern Med 2004;141(9):743–4.

73. Mukhopadhyay S, Sharma M, Ramakrishnan S, et al. Phosphodiesterase-5 inhibitor in Eisenmenger syndrome: a preliminary observational study. Circulation 2006;114(17):1807–10.

74. Aggarwal P, Patial RK, Negi PC, et al. Oral tadalafil in pulmonary artery hypertension: a prospective study. Indian Heart J 2007;59(4):329–35.

75. Bharani A, Patel A, Saraf J, et al. Efficacy and safety of PDE-5 inhibitor tadalafil in pulmonary arterial hypertension. Indian Heart J 2007;59(4):323–8.

76. Galie N, Brundage BH, Ghofrani HA, et al. Tadalafil therapy for pulmonary arterial hypertension. Circulation 2009;11:2894–903.

77. Arneson C, McDevitt S, Klinger JR. Tadalafil in geriatric patients with pulmonary arterial hypertension. Chest 2010;138:367A.

78. Chen HC, Wang CS, Chuang SH, et al. Pulmonary embolism after tadalafil ingestion. Pharm World Sci 2008;30(5):610–2.

79. Tripathi A, O'Donnell NP. Branch retinal artery occlusion; another complication of sildenafil. Br J Ophthalmol 2000;84(8):934–5.

80. Akash R, Hrishikesh D, Amith P, et al. Case report: association of combined nonarteritic anterior ischemic optic neuropathy (NAION) and obstruction of cilioretinal artery with overdose of Viagra. J Ocul Pharmacol Ther 2005;21(4):315–7.

81. Peter NM, Singh MV, Fox PD. Tadalafil-associated anterior ischaemic optic neuropathy. Eye (Lond) 2005;19(6):715–7.

82. Bollinger K, Lee MS. Recurrent visual field defect and ischemic optic neuropathy associated with tadalafil rechallenge. Arch Ophthalmol 2005;123(3):400–1.

83. Wilkins MR, Paul GA, Strange JW, et al. Sildenafil versus Endothelin Receptor Antagonist for Pulmonary Hypertension (SERAPH) study. Am J Respir Crit Care Med 2005;171(11):1292–7.

84. Udeoji DU, Schwarz ER. Tadalafil as monotherapy and in combination regimens for the treatment of pulmonary arterial hypertension. Ther Adv Respir Dis 2013;7(1):39–49.

85. Oudiz RJ, Brundage BH, Galiè N, et al, PHIRST Study Group. Tadalafil for the treatment of pulmonary arterial hypertension: a double-blind 52-week uncontrolled extension study. J Am Coll Cardiol 2012;60(8):768–74.

Parenteral and Inhaled Prostanoid Therapy in the Treatment of Pulmonary Arterial Hypertension

Vallerie V. McLaughlin, MD[a], Harold I. Palevsky, MD[b],*

KEYWORDS

- Epoprostenol • Iloprost • Inhaled therapy • Intravenous therapy • Parenteral therapy
- Prostacyclins • Prostanoids • Treprostinil

KEY POINTS

- With the US Food and Drug Administration approval of continuous intravenous epoprostenol in 1995, prostanoids became the first class of drugs available for the treatment of pulmonary arterial hypertension (PAH).
- Although prostanoid therapies are constrained by a short half-lives, they are now available for intermittent inhalation and continuous subcutaneous and intravenous administration.
- Prostanoids are potent pulmonary vasodilators that inhibit platelet aggregation, and also seem to have antiproliferative effects.
- Continuous intravenous epoprostenol remains the only agent that has been shown to improve PAH survival in clinical trials.
- Although prostanoids are inconvenient, they remain the mainstay of therapy for patients with rapidly progressing or advanced (functional class IV) PAH.

INTRODUCTION

Prostacyclin therapy has transformed the care of patients with pulmonary arterial hypertension (PAH), an orphan disease for which there was no effective treatment option for most patients until 20 years ago.[1] More than 25 years ago, epoprostenol (prostaglandin I2 [PGI2]), a stable freeze-dried preparation of prostacyclin, was shown to reduce symptoms and improve hemodynamics in a woman with severe primary pulmonary hypertension (PPH) awaiting lung transplant.[2] Following small clinical trials and a pivotal trial that established the safety and efficacy in PPH, intravenous epoprostenol (Flolan) was approved for clinical use in PAH by the US Food and Drug Administration (FDA) in 1995.[3] The effectiveness of prostacyclin, a vasodilator and inhibitor of platelet aggregation, reflects the mechanisms thought to contribute substantially to the development of

Disclosures: V.V. McLaughlin, consulting for Actelion, Bayer, Gilead, Ikaria, Merck, United Therapeutics; speaking for Gilead, United Therapeutics; research funding for clinical trials to the University of Michigan from Actelion, Bayer, Ikaria, Novartis. H.I. Palevsky, consulting for Actelion, Aires, Bayer, United Therapeutics; research funding for clinical trials to the University of Pennsylvania from Actelion.
a Pulmonary Hypertension Program, Cardiovascular Center, University of Michigan Hospital and Health Systems, 1500 East Medical Center Drive, Room 2392, Ann Arbor, MI 48109-5853, USA; b Pulmonary Vascular Disease Program, Pulmonary, Allergy and Critical Care Medicine, Penn Presbyter Medical Center, 51 North 39th Street, Philadelphia, PA 19104-2699, USA
* Corresponding author.
E-mail address: harold.palevsky@uphs.upenn.edu

PAH. The evolution of prostanoid therapies with FDA approval has been rapid and now includes intravenous epoprostenol (Flolan, Veletri and generic forms), intravenous and subcutaneous (SC) treprostinil (Remodulin), inhaled iloprost (Ventavis), and inhaled treprostinil (Tyvaso).

PATHOPHYSIOLOGIC BASIS FOR PROSTACYCLIN USE

The complex pathobiology of PAH is thought to begin with endothelial dysfunction that results in chronically impaired production of vasodilators including nitric oxide (NO) and prostacyclin (PGI_2), and overexpression of the endogenous vasoconstrictor endothelin (ET)-1 and the pro-thrombotic thromboxane A_2.[4,5] Prostacyclin synthase expression is decreased in lungs from patients with severe PAH,[6] and smooth muscle proliferation and medial hypertrophy is associated with a decrease in smooth muscle cell (SMC) PGI_2 receptor activity.[7] Each of the pathways involved in the pathogenesis of PAH is a potential pharmacologic target.[8]

PGI_2 is a potent direct vasodilator of both the pulmonary and systemic vascular beds, as well as an inhibitor of platelet aggregation. There is also evidence that it has antiproliferative effects. Prostacyclin analogues have been shown in vitro to inhibit SMC growth.[9] The mechanism by which prostacyclins mediate vasodilation is ligand binding to a G-protein–coupled receptor with subsequent signal transduction inducing relaxation of vascular smooth muscle. Signal transduction via adenylate cyclase increases intracellular cyclic adenosine monophosphate (cAMP).

The benefit of PGI_2 in PAH was initially assumed to be related to the vasodilating effect produced by activating membrane-bound adenylate cyclase to increase cAMP, which results in SMC relaxation.[10] There is no relationship between the acute vasodilating response to epoprostenol and long-term benefit, so vasodilatation is not the sole, or even predominant, benefit.[11] Other putative benefits of prostacyclin include (1) reduction in the rate of remodeling by antiproliferative and antisecretive effects on SMCs,[9,12,13] (2) reduced endothelial cell dysfunction,[14] (3) reduced platelet aggregation,[14] (4) antithrombotic effects,[15] (5) decrease in extracellular matrix secretion by endothelial cells and SMC,[16] (6) reverse remodeling with reduction in smooth muscle mass,[7] and (7) increase in right heart inotropy.[17,18]

Intravenous Epoprostenol

Epoprostenol sodium (Flolan, GlaxoSmithKline, Research Triangle Park, NC; Veletri Actelion Pharmaceuticals Ltd, Allschwil, Switzerland), and generic epoprostenol sodium (Teva Pharmaceuticals, North Wales, PA), is the intravenous formulation of PGI_2. Intravenous epoprostenol was FDA approved in 1995 for idiopathic PAH (IPAH, then referred to as PPH) and the indication was subsequently expanded to include PAH related to the scleroderma spectrum of diseases. Intravenous epoprostenol is commonly used for many forms of World Health Organization (WHO) group I PAH. Intravenous epoprostenol is the PAH therapy for which the longest term and most robust data exist, and is considered the gold standard in patients with more advanced (functional class III and IV) disease.[8] Although originally thought to be simply a bridge to heart-lung or lung transplantation, long-term outcomes with intravenous epoprostenol have established it as a chronic therapy.

Pharmacokinetics

Epoprostenol is rapidly degraded in blood at a neutral pH into 2 primary metabolites (6-keto-$PGF_{1\alpha}$ and 6,15-diketo-13,14-dihydro-$PGF_{1\alpha}$), both of which are biologically inactive and excreted in the urine. The half-life of epoprostenol in humans is approximately 6 minutes. The 2 major pharmacologic actions of epoprostenol are inhibition of platelet aggregation and potent vasodilation of systemic and pulmonary vascular beds, both of which are mediated via stimulation of adenylate cyclase and increased production of cAMP.

Drug delivery

Epoprostenol sodium for injection (Flolan, generic) is supplied as a sterile freeze-dried powder in glass vials, available in 0.5 mg (500,000 ng) and 1.5 mg (1,500,000 ng) sizes, which must be stored at 15° to 25°C (59°F–77°F). More recently, a thermostable form of epoprostenol, formulated with L-arginine rather than glycine (Veletri) has been approved by the FDA. This formulation does not require ice packs, and cassettes may be mixed up to 7 days in advance of use.[19,20] Because of the need to maintain an uninterrupted infusion, long-term infusion is maintained via a tunneled, cuffed central venous catheter, although it may be given temporarily via a peripheral line (eg, in emergency situations). Intravenous epoprostenol is administered continuously via an ambulatory portable, battery-operated infusion pump, most commonly the CADD-Legacy pump (SIMS-Deltec [a division of Smiths Medical, St. Paul, MN]). The pump has low-battery, end-of-infusion, and occlusion alarms, and is positive pressure driven with intervals between pulses not exceeding 3 minutes to deliver the prescribed medication rate.

In most instances, insurance approval is obtained before the commencement of therapy. Most centers hospitalize patients for initiation of intravenous epoprostenol for monitoring as well as extensive teaching regarding sterile preparation of the medication, operation of the ambulatory infusion pump, and care of the central venous catheter.

Clinical trial data: randomized and observational

In 1982, Rubin and colleagues[21] investigated the hemodynamic effects of escalating doses of intravenous epoprostenol (2–12 ng/kg/min) in 7 patients with IPAH and severe hemodynamic compromise. At a mean dose of 5.7 ng/kg/min, epoprostenol reduced total pulmonary resistance (TPR) by approximately 43%, whereas cardiac output (CO) increased by 56%. Longer term infusions (1–25 months) led to hemodynamic improvement, clinical stabilization, and improved exercise capacity in patients with severe IPAH who were refractory to oral vasodilators, digoxin, and diuretic therapy.[2] These early observational studies led to the first randomized trial with epoprostenol in 1990.[22] Patients with IPAH (n = 23) were randomized to epoprostenol (mean dose, 7.1 ng/kg/min) or conventional therapy, and functional classification, 6-minute walk distance (6MWD), and cardiopulmonary hemodynamics were compared at baseline and 2 months after therapy. All 10 patients treated with epoprostenol improved by at least one functional class, and on average increased their 6MWD from 246 to 378 m. TPR decreased from 21.6 to 13.9 mm Hg/L/min and CO increased from 3.3 to 3.9 L/min. In contrast, most placebo-treated patients did not symptomatically improve, had a lesser increase in walk distance, with no significant changes in hemodynamics. Three patients in the placebo arm died over the 8-week study period versus 1 subject treated with epoprostenol. These findings also provided the impetus for the first prospective, multicenter, open-label trial, which randomized 81 patients with IPAH, functional class III or IV, to epoprostenol plus conventional therapy versus conventional therapy alone.[3] At 12 weeks, the epoprostenol-treated group (mean dose, 9.2 ng/kg/min) had improved quality-of-life scores, improved functional class, and increased median 6MWD (+31 m vs −29 m in conventional therapy group) versus conventional therapy alone. Pulmonary vascular resistance (PVR) decreased by approximately 25% (placebo increased 9%) and cardiac index (CI) increased by 15%, whereas mean systemic arterial pressure decreased by only 5%. Patients with the greatest hemodynamic

improvements over the study period tended to have the largest improvements in 6MWD. Eight patients died during the 12-week study period, all of whom had been randomized to the conventional therapy group. The hemodynamic and clinical improvements seen in the epoprostenol-treated patient were not predicted by short-term hemodynamic responsiveness to epoprostenol before randomization, confirming previous observations that the longer term effects of epoprostenol are not well predicted by short-term acute vasodilator responsiveness. The results of this study led to FDA approval of epoprostenol in 1995 for patients with IPAH.

Epoprostenol has also been studied specifically in a population with PAH related to the scleroderma spectrum of diseases. Badesch and colleagues[23] studied epoprostenol in 111 such patients in a randomized, open-label trial conducted over a 12-week period. The patients in the epoprostenol treatment group were ill at baseline, with a mean 6MWD of only 272 m, right atrial pressure of 13 mm Hg, and CI of 1.9 L/min/m². In response to epoprostenol (mean dose, 11.2 ng/kg/min), PVR declined by 32% and CI increased 0.5 L/min/m², whereas 6MWD increased (270–316 m). In patients treated with conventional therapy, the 6MWD declined (240–192 m), for a placebo-corrected 6MWD difference of +108 m. Unlike the results in IPAH, there were no survival differences detected (4 deaths in the epoprostenol group, 5 deaths in the conventional treatment group) over this short follow-up period, although neither study was powered to detect a survival benefit.

Longer term observational studies have shown improved outcomes in patients with IPAH treated with epoprostenol. Long-term survival on epoprostenol was assessed in a prospective cohort of 69 patients with IPAH in functional class III and IV who were followed for 330 to 770 days.[24] Survival at 1, 2, and 3 years was 80%, 76%, and 49% respectively. In a smaller observational study of patients treated with intravenous epoprostenol for more than a year, 26 of 27 patients had an improvement in functional class.[11] Improvements in exercise duration (142%), mean pulmonary artery pressure (mPAP; decreased by 22%), and CO (increased by 67%) were noted. Significant improvements in hemodynamics occurred in most patients despite the absence of an acute response to intravenous adenosine during acute vasodilator testing. In 2002, McLaughlin and colleagues[25] reported on the long-term clinical outcomes of 162 patients with IPAH treated with epoprostenol (median follow-up, 36 months). The observed survival at 1, 2, 3, and 5 years was 88%, 76%, 63%, and 47% and was significantly greater than the expected survival at 1, 2, and 3 years of 59%, 46%, and 35%, as predicted by the US National Institutes of Health registry.[1] Baseline predictors of survival included exercise capacity, right atrial pressure, and vasodilator responsiveness in response to adenosine. On follow-up, subjects who remained functional class I to II fared better (3-year and 5-year survival, 89% and 73%) than those who were class III (62%, 35%); patients who remained class IV did especially poorly (survival 42% at 2 years, 0% at 3 years). A total of 70 episodes of sepsis were reported, 4 of which were fatal; 1 patient died because of interruption of epoprostenol therapy. Sitbon and colleagues[26] similarly reported an overall survival rate at 1, 2, 3, and 5 years of 85%, 70%, 63%, and 55%, respectively, in 178 patients with IPAH treated with continuous intravenous epoprostenol. After 3 months on therapy, a history of right heart failure, persistence of class III or IV functional status, and a less than 30% decrease in TPR were associated with poor survival. These findings provide the basis for the recommendation for referral for lung transplantation in patients with PAH who remain class III or IV despite prostacyclin therapy. Observational series have also shown beneficial effects of epoprostenol in associated forms of PAH including congenital heart disease, human immunodeficiency virus, and portopulmonary hypertension, in addition to sarcoid-related and chronic thromboembolic pulmonary hypertension (CTEPH).[27–32]

Dosing/Dose titration

The optimal long-term dosing protocol for epoprostenol had not been established by randomized controlled trials. At the end of the 12-week randomized trials, patients were being treated with 9 to 11 ng/kg/min. In the series by Sitbon and colleagues,[26] mean dose at 12 weeks was 14 ng/kg/min, and at 1 year was 21 ng/kg/min. In the series by McLaughlin and colleagues[25] the dose was 34.5 and 51.7 ng/kg/min at 17 and 30 months respectively, although in patients who began treatment after 1998 these values were 21.9 and 27.2 ng/kg/min. Epoprostenol overdose can occur, typically manifesting clinically with stereotypical, but excessive, prostanoid side effects (diarrhea, flushing) and a high CO state by right heart catheterization.[33]

In general, intravenous epoprostenol is initiated in a monitored setting at 2 ng/kg/min. In a stable patient who is starting therapy electively, we typically titrate up by 2 ng/kg/min on a daily basis until side effects become intolerable or interfere with teaching sessions. Most of our patients are discharged on 4 to 8 ng/kg/min. If the patient is critically ill, dosing uptitration is more aggressive (**Box 1**).

Dosing is highly individualized and needs to be assessed for each patient based on the symptoms of pulmonary hypertension (PH) and side effects of intravenous epoprostenol. The nurse clinician plays a pivotal role in chronic outpatient management.

Adverse effects

The most common acute adverse effects noted during the clinical trials include flushing, headache, nausea/vomiting, and systemic hypotension. Jaw pain, often described as occurring with the first bite or two of food, is nearly universal and diarrhea is common also. These side effects associated with acute dosing can be present intermittently and tend to become less intense with the duration of therapy. Other side effects that may occur with longer term therapy include leg and foot pain, thrombocytopenia, weight loss, and (rarely) ascites.

Serious complications related to the delivery system include local catheter infections, bloodstream infections, catheter-related thrombosis, and paradoxic embolism. Symptoms of severe PH may recur after abrupt discontinuation of the infusion, and this can be fatal. This complication

---

Box 1
Hospital initiation and titration of intravenous epoprostenol

- Initiate at 2 ng/kg/min
- Titrate up by 2 ng/kg/min daily as tolerated
- Hospital stay generally 3 to 5 days, depending on patient ability to mix the epoprostenol and operate the pump
- Clinical nurse specialist calls weekly for first several months after discharge
- Intravenous epoprostenol is increased by 2 ng/kg/min once or twice weekly as tolerated
- First return visit at 4 to 12 weeks, depending on clinical status of the patient, and subsequently approximately every 3 months
- Dose increases continue based on symptoms of PAH and side effects of intravenous epoprostenol
- Dose at 1 year is generally 35 to 50 ng/kg/min
- Functional class and 6MWD with each clinic visit
- Right heart catheterization at 1 year

The dose varies depending on concentration and delivery rate options based on pump characteristics.

seems to be less common in the current era than it was previously, because many patients on intravenous therapy are on also on oral PAH-specific therapy.

SC Treprostinil

Treprostinil sodium (Remodulin, United Therapeutics Corporation, Research Triangle Park, NC) is a chemically stable, tricyclic benzindene analogue of prostacyclin.[16] SC treprostinil received a provisional FDA approval in 2002 for PAH in WHO class II to IV and full approval in 2006 after completion of a postapproval commitment study.[34] The potential advantages of SC treprostinil compared with intravenous prostanoids include there being no need for central venous access, small cassette pump, no risk of bacteremia, and no risk of catheter or venous thrombosis or thromboembolism. The potential disadvantages are related to the side effect of pain and erythema at the site of the SC infusion, and occasional abscess formation at infusion sites.

Pharmacokinetics

SC treprostinil is rapidly and completely absorbed with complete bioavailability.[35] A dose of 10 to 15 ng/kg/min results in rapid increase in plasma concentration and reaches maximum plasma concentration (C_{max}) within 2 to 3 hours of onset of infusion, and elimination half-life in healthy volunteers is 2.9 to 4.6 hours.[36] More recently, the clinical significance of the longer half-life of treprostinil has been called into question. In a case series of patients with PAH withdrawn from treprostinil in an intensive care unit setting, significant increases in mPAP and PVR were noted within 1 hour of treprostinil discontinuation.[37] SC treprostinil steady-state pharmacokinetics studies in patients with PAH show dose linearity within a range from 10 to 125 ng/kg/min.[38] In early studies designed to test the relative hemodynamic effects of prostanoids in patients with PPH, McLaughlin and colleagues[39] found that, at short-term maximal tolerated doses, intravenous epoprostenol and intravenous treprostinil resulted in a similar reduction in PVR acutely (22% and 20%, respectively). Intravenous treprostinil and SC treprostinil also showed comparable short-term decreases in PVR (23% and 28%, respectively).

Drug delivery

Treprostinil sodium is a sterile sodium salt with the same formulation for SC and intravenous administration, and is stable at room temperature with neutral pH. It is supplied in 20-mL multiuse vials in 4 strengths: 1 mg/mL, 2.5 mg/mL, 5 mg/mL, or 10 mg/mL of treprostinil. During use, a single reservoir (syringe) of undiluted treprostinil can be administered up to 72 hours at 37°C.

SC treprostinil is administered by continuous infusion via a self-inserted SC catheter using an infusion pump designed for SC drug delivery (eg, MiniMed, Sylmar, CA). The ambulatory infusion pump should be (1) small and lightweight; (2) adjustable to approximately 0.002 mL/h; (3) have occlusion/no-delivery, low-battery, programming error and motor malfunction alarms; (4) have delivery accuracy of ±6% or better; and (5) be positive pressure driven. The reservoir should be made of polyvinyl chloride, polypropylene, or glass.

As with other prostacyclins, once insurance approval has been secured, extensive patient education must be provided. In contrast with intravenous prostanoids, SC treprostinil can be started at home, although some patients are hospitalized for 2 or 3 days.

Clinical trial data: randomized and observational

The efficacy and safety of SC treprostinil was established in a pivotal 12-week, double-blind, placebo-controlled study, conducted in 24 PH centers throughout the United States, Europe, and Australia.[40] Four-hundred and seventy patients with PAH were randomized to receive SC treprostinil or placebo in addition to standard care. The primary efficacy end point of change in 6MWD was slightly greater with treprostinil than with placebo (between-group difference in median 6MWD, 16 m; $P = .006$). Compared with placebo, SC treprostinil treatment also improved the Borg dyspnea index score ($P<.0001$). The improvement in 6MWD was highly correlated with dose (36 m when dose at 12 weeks was >13.8 ng/kg/min).

The largest open-label, observational study of SC treprostinil was reported by Barst and colleagues[41] in 2006. The observational study was conducted in 860 patients with PAH who had participated in one of 3 placebo-controlled trials of SC treprostinil or were de novo patients with standard criteria for treprostinil. Patients continued in the study until (1) death; (2) transplantation; (3) initiation of intravenous, inhaled, or oral prostaglandins or their analogues; or (4) an intolerable adverse event. In the 860 patients who receive SC treprostinil for up to 4.5 years, Kaplan-Meier estimates for survival at 1, 2, 3, and 4 years were 87%, 78%, 71%, and 68%, respectively. The treatment was discontinued in 23% of patients because of adverse events, and 11% were switched to another prostanoid. A second PAH-specific treatment was added in 130 patients. More recently, a single-center observational registry evaluated long-term outcomes on 111 patients with PAH treated with SC treprostinil as their initial therapy.[42] Of these, 13 (12%) stopped therapy prematurely because of drug side effects, 11 (9.9%) went on to lung transplantation, and 49 (44.1%) died. The overall survival rates at 1 and 5 years were 84% and 33% respectively.

A subset of 90 of 470 patients (most WHO functional class III) participating in 2 placebo-controlled 12-week trials of SC treprostinil had PAH associated with a connective tissue disease (systemic lupus erythematosus, scleroderma, or mixed connective tissue disease/overlap). Treatment was associated with improved exercise capacity, reduced symptoms, and improved hemodynamics, including a decrease in PVR and an increase in CI.[43] Two open-label studies support a role for SC treprostinil in inoperable CTEPH.[44,45]

A multicenter withdrawal study was designed to assess the efficacy of SC treprostinil compared with intravenous epoprostenol. Patients with stable PAH receiving intravenous epoprostenol were hospitalized for 2 weeks to provide a safe environment for transition to SC treprostinil or placebo. Twenty-two patients were randomized in a 2:1 ratio (SC treprostinil and SC placebo). Patients were assessed on a daily basis regarding effort tolerance and examined by an experienced nurse and physician unaware of the treatment.[34] The mean epoprostenol dose at baseline was 22.3 ± 3.3 ng/kg/min in the treprostinil treatment group, and the mean maximum treprostinil dose over the 8-week study was 32.2 ± 4.9 ng/kg/min. Safety and tolerability results for patients transitioning to SC treprostinil were consistent with findings in de novo patients. The results of this trial led to the FDA amendment of this agent to include patients transitioning from epoprostenol treatment to treprostinil therapy. Vachiery and colleagues[46] showed that successful transitions can be done over short periods of time in the hospital setting. Transitions between prostacyclins should only be considered by physicians with extensive experience with both agents.

Dosing/Dose titration

Optimization of SC treprostinil dosing regimens has not been subjected to clinical trials. The FDA approved package insert recommends the rate be initiated at 1.25 ng/kg/min, which if necessary is reduced to 0.625 ng/kg/min. Infusion rate is increased in increments of 1.25 ng/kg/min per week for the first 4 weeks and then 2.5 ng/kg/min per week depending on clinical response. The goal of gradual chronic dosage adjustments is to establish a dose at which PAH symptoms are improved (optimally to WHO functional class I–II),

and excessive side effects (headache, nausea, emesis, restlessness, anxiety, and infusion site pain or reaction) are minimized. These recommendations are based on the pivotal trial in which SC treprostinil was initiated at 1.25 ng/kg/min and uptitrated slowly to a maximum dose of 22.5 ng/kg/min.[40]

The safety and efficacy of rate of titration was described in a randomized prospective study comparing a slow versus a rapid dose-escalation protocol in 23 patients with PAH.[47] The SC treprostinil slow-escalation group was initiated at 2 ng/kg/min, and increased weekly, if tolerated, by 1.25 to 2.0 ng/kg/min. The rapid-escalation group was initiated at 2.5 ng/kg/min, and increased by 2.5 ng/kg/min twice in the first week, with an additional increase of 2.5 ng/kg/min every 1 or 2 weeks. At week 12, the mean dose had reached 12.9 ± 2.7 ng/kg/min in the slow-escalation group (similar to the pivotal trial) and 20.3 ± 5.8 ng/kg/min in the rapid-escalation group. Improvements in exercise capacity at week 12 were significantly greater in the rapid-escalation group compared with the slow-escalation group ($P = .03$), and, contrary to expectation, infusion site pain was more common in the slow-escalation group (81.8%) compared with the rapid-escalation group (58.3%; $P = .04$).

Our protocol includes a rapid home or hospital titration and rapid subsequent titration (**Box 2**). Rapid titration facilitates the evaluation of clinical response to SC treprostinil within several months whether as monotherapy or as second-agent or third-agent combination therapy.

Although the half-life is about 4 hours, clinically significant changes in hemodynamics occur within an hour and patients and caregivers are told that abrupt cessation of SC treprostinil infusion should

---

Box 2
Home or hospital initiation and titration of SC treprostinil

- Initiate at 2 ng/kg/min
- Increase by 2 ng/kg/min twice weekly until first visit, provided patient tolerates dosage
- First visit at 6 to 8 weeks; if patient lives far away, first visit at 3 months
- Average dose after 6 months is about 60 ng/kg/min
- Clinic visits every 3 months
- Functional class and 6MWD at each visit
- Repeat right heart catheterization at 1 year

The dose varies depending on concentration and delivery rate options based on pump characteristics.

be avoided. The absorption of drug does not seem dependent on site or site duration. The historical recommendation was for a site change every 3 days. However, experienced patients use sites for up to 30 days without difficulty. Such sites are considered good sites and may be reused months later. Sites in which pain is intense within the first day and there is no relief by day 3 are considered bad sites and should be changed. Optimal sites vary between individuals. It is best to rotate to a distant site until site pain and inflammation are resolved. Examples of typical effective and ineffective sites are provided in **Table 1**.

Adverse effects

The most common adverse events reported for treprostinil and placebo in the 12-week study were infusion site pain (85%), infusion site reaction (83%), and infusion site bleeding/bruising (34%).[40] **Table 2** shows the methods of reducing pain and increasing site duration. Site-related pain is a common reason for therapy discontinuation. Other common adverse events were consistent with prostacyclin therapy and included diarrhea, jaw pain, flushing, and lower-limb edema. Safety and tolerability during long-term treatment were comparable with observations during the placebo-controlled studies.

Intravenous Treprostinil

Given the limitation of site pain/reaction from SC infusion, and that SC and intravenous treprostinil have virtually the same bioavailability and hemodynamic effects, long-term intravenous treprostinil has also been studied in PAH.[38] The pharmacology of intravenous treprostinil is identical to that described earlier for SC treprostinil. Based

Table 1
The best SC treprostinil infusion sites depend on SC fat

Preferred	Sites to Avoid
Abdomen (first site)	Stretch marks and scar tissue
Upper lateral buttocks	Edematous areas (pannus) and areas with erythema or induration
Lower flanks	Underneath waistbands or beltlines
Thigh and underside of upper arm if adequate fat	Sites with nodular or rubbery texture or previous abscess Boney prominences

Table 2
Local, topical, and systemic options to manage infusion site pain

Local/Topical	Systemic
Ice	Ibuprofen
Warm bath with Epsom salt	Gabapentin
PLO gel compounds[a] (current or old sites)	Pregabalin
Lidocaine 5% patches (current or old sites)	Loratadine
Diphenhydramine HCl, topical	Hydroxyzine pamoate (for severe itching)
Hemorrhoid ointment	Amitriptyline HCl and other antidepressants
Aloe vera gel	Tramadol HCl
Triamcinolone acetonide	Fexofenadine HCl
Fluticasone propionate nasal spray	Cetirizine HCl
Lidocaine/ prilocaine cream	Ranitidine HCl
Hydrocortisone cream	Famotidine
Pimecrolimus cream 1%	If fentanyl or other narcotics are required more than occasionally, consider intravenous prostacyclin therapy
Clobetasol propionate cream	—

Abbreviation: PLO, pluronic lecithin organogel.
[a] Contain ketoprofen, lidocaine, and gabapentin and may also contain ketamine, amitriptyline, and clonidine.
Courtesy of United Therapeutics; with permission.

on bioequivalence data, intravenous treprostinil is indicated in PAH for those unable to tolerate SC infusion.

Clinical trial data: randomized and observational

An investigator-initiated, open-label, uncontrolled trial with intravenous treprostinil in patients with PAH led to important observations in both naive and intravenous epoprostenol transition patients. Tapson and colleagues[48] reported on 16 patients with PAH treated with intravenous treprostinil as their initial therapy in an open-label, uncontrolled series. Over 12 weeks, the primary end point,

6MWD, improved from 319 to 400 m. There were also significant improvements in secondary end points, including Naughton-Blake protocol treadmill time, Borg dyspnea score, and hemodynamics. In an open-label uncontrolled trial, Gomberg-Maitland and colleagues[49] transitioned 31 patients with PAH on intravenous epoprostenol to intravenous treprostinil. Four patients were transitioned back to epoprostenol over the 12-week study. Among those 27 who remained on intravenous treprostinil, the 6MWD was unchanged, although the mPAP was higher and the CO was lower than baseline. At week 12, the mean dose of treprostinil was more than twice the dose of epoprostenol.

A placebo-controlled trial of intravenous treprostinil (2:1 randomization) was conducted in 44 patients with PAH at 14 sites in India.[50] However, this study was terminated early after the independent Rescue Therapy and Safety Committee reviewed all catheter-related complications, deaths, and other serious adverse events and recommended suspension of the trial pending implementation of a series of recommendations to increase patient safety. Only 45 of the planned 126 patients (36%) had been enrolled at the time of study termination.

Intravenous treprostinil may also be administered via low-flow pumps at rates as low as 0.1 mL/h. In a 12-week study, pump complications occurred in 5 of 12 patients receiving such therapy, although no catheter occlusions occurred.[51] Patients were anticoagulated to an International Normalized Ratio of at least 2.0 throughout that study. A recent case series of patients treated with intravenous treprostinil via an implantable pump was reported as a letter to the editor.[52] Further study of this concept is ongoing.

Dosing/Dose titration

Like intravenous epoprostenol, intravenous treprostinil is initiated in a monitored setting in the hospital. Like intravenous epoprostenol, it is generally started at a dose of 2 ng/kg/min and, in the stable patient, titrated up at a dose of 2 ng/kg/min on a daily basis. Chronic outpatient care is similar to that described for epoprostenol, although generally doses are at least twice as high as those for intravenous epoprostenol.

Adverse effects

With the exception of the local site reactions, the adverse effects for intravenous treprostinil include those listed earlier for SC treprostinil. In addition, the adverse effects of the continuous intravenous delivery system described earlier for intravenous epoprostenol may occur with intravenous treprostinil. Although bloodstream infection is a concern with intravenous agents, a concern for an increased risk of gram-negative infections has been raised with intravenous treprostinil.[53] This risk was further evaluated in the large REVEAL registry (Registry to Evaluate Early and Long Term PAH Disease Management).[54] Of the 3518 patients enrolled in REVEAL, 1146 received intravenous prostanoid therapy. Bloodstream infection rates were significantly increased in patients receiving intravenous treprostinil versus intravenous epoprostenol (0.36 vs 0.12 per 1000 treatment days; $P<.001$). This finding was primarily attributed to gram-negative organisms (0.20 vs 0.03 per 1000 treatment days; $P<.001$). Multivariate analysis adjusting for age, causes of PAH, and year of bloodstream infection found that treatment with intravenous treprostinil was associated with a 3.08-fold increase (95% confidence interval, 2.05 to 4.62; $P<.001$) in bloodstream infections of any type and a 6.86-fold increase (95% confidence interval, 3.60–13.07; $P<.001$) in gram-negative infections compared with treatment with intravenous epoprostenol.

The Clinical Perspective

Using the parenteral prostanoids in PAH requires a thorough understanding of the diagnosis and natural history of the disease, the pharmacology, experience in monitoring response, and other treatment options including transplant. Despite the advances in oral and parenteral treatment options for PAH, the 5-year mortality remains high, and most participants in placebo-controlled trials of oral PAH-specific therapies were WHO functional class II and III.

Treatment options for PAH have been formulated into guidelines by consensus of US and European expert panels.[55–58] There is general agreement within the cardiology, pulmonology, and rheumatology communities that, before treatment decisions, the diagnosis and prognosis need to be assessed and or confirmed by physicians experienced in PH. PH centers have multidisciplinary groups of physicians and unique support by nurses in both the outpatient and inpatient settings.

Patients who have advanced symptoms (WHO functional class IV), who fail an oral PAH-specific drug after a trial and remain WHO functional class III, or those who progress on oral therapy should be referred to an experienced center for consideration of parenteral prostanoid therapy. Other poor prognostic indicators, including high right atrial pressure, low CI, and low 6MWD, influence the decision to proceed to parenteral prostacyclin therapy.[8,55] Much of the clinical trial results and metrics for risk stratification in PAH are based on IPAH and scleroderma, but apply to other associated diseases with the exception of congenital heart disease, which generally has a better prognosis. Monitoring of the response to a strategy and decision for advancing therapies requires a considerable amount of clinical experience and the ability to interpret testing including the 6-min hall walk, echo-Doppler, chest computed tomography, pulmonary function tests, cardiopulmonary exercise testing, biomarkers such as brain natriuretic peptide (BNP) and N-terminal BNP (NT-BNP), renal and hepatic function, and baseline and on-treatment hemodynamic indices.

Criteria for Initiating the Parenteral Prostanoids

Before considering parenteral prostanoids, the patient, family members, and participating physician(s) need to consider the patient's physical and emotional status, support system, and provider issues, which are listed in **Box 3**.

The most essential are an understanding of prognosis, treatment options, and availability of insurance. It is essential that patients and family

---

Box 3
Considerations before initiating parenteral prostanoids

- Patient related
  - Understanding prognosis
  - Understanding treatment options and expectations
  - Understanding complexity and potential complications of treatment
  - Adequate physical ability (eg, scleroderma)
  - Emotional stability
  - Bleeding risk
  - End-of-life decisions
  - Insurance coverage
- Support system
  - Significant other or available close friend
  - Experienced home health care agency
  - Local PH support group
- Treating physician
  - Experience in prostanoid therapy
  - Experienced nursing team
  - Reliable testing facilities

---

members understand that there is no cure for PAH, and that they are not given undue expectations. They are told that prostacyclin therapy may improve symptoms within days to months, and, if so, will likely prolong life expectancy. In those without a lung transplant option (eg, age and associated diseases), the patient and family members need to have an understanding that end-of-life decisions in PAH are complex and the hospice option may not be possible on parenteral prostacyclins. The choice between parenteral prostanoids depends on patient preference, physician experience, and hemodynamic instability. Because of the short half-life (4–6 minutes) and experience with rapid dose titration in critically ill patients, intravenous epoprostenol is preferred rather than intravenous treprostinil in hemodynamically unstable patients and those rapidly deteriorating to WHO class IV requiring emergent hospitalization. There are fewer clinical trial data and a higher rate of catheter infection with treprostinil than epoprostenol. The alternative of SC treprostinil may have advantages in WHO class III patients who may want to avoid the central venous catheter.

The education requirements for patients and family members are summarized in **Box 4**.

Intravenous prostacyclin can be initiated via a midline or peripherally inserted central catheter (PICC), but long-term treatment requires a central catheter. The infusion catheter should have a single lumen, be tunneled, and be placed no farther than the superior vena cava right atrial junction under fluoroscopic guidance. The exit site should be in the subclavicular-pectoral region on the nondominant side to allow for patient use of the dominant arm/hand. When patients are not certain about long-term use or a trial is necessary to determine safety, a PICC line is preferable and can be used for up to a few months.

Prostacyclin, the pump, and the catheter are generally well tolerated. The monitoring team must have a high index of suspicion for catheter-associated bacteremia, the only sign of which can be loss of energy and mild increase in dyspnea. Practice guidelines for prevention of catheter-related infection associated with the prostanoids have been developed.[59] In addition, practice guidelines may help reduce prostacyclin administration errors in the inpatient setting.[60]

Dosing and cost-related issues
The ideal dose of parenteral prostacyclin is highly individualized, and many experts titrate the dose to achieve an improvement in symptoms (to functional class 1 or 2) and a normal CO. In general, after more than 1 year of treatment with epoprostenol,

---

Box 4
Educational requirements for patient and significant other before discharge

- Response to emergencies
  - Catheter dislodgement or pump alarm
  - Worsening of symptoms
  - Use of local hospital and emergency services
  - Home health care agency
  - Contact and access with PH office staff 24 hours a day, 7 days a week
- Use of the pump
  - Rate adjustments
  - Need for backup pump
- Central access site
  - Sterile techniques
  - Signs of infections
  - Securing sutures
- Prostacyclin
  - Reconstitution of epoprostenol
  - Handling of vials with treprostinil
  - Handling tubing/connect/disconnect
  - Site care for subcutaneous treprostinil
  - Plans for dose titration
- Expected side effects
  - Minor
  - Major

---

doses typically decrease into the range of 30 to 55 ng/kg/min. Few long-term data are available for treprostinil, but doses are generally approximately twice as high as for epoprostenol. Oudiz and Farber[61] conducted a survey of treating physicians and found that the most common dose range for epoprostenol was 30 to 39 ng/kg/min, whereas the most common dose range for treprostinil was 60 to 69 ng/kg/min. They also compared the annual cost (for the drug and diluent only) of epoprostenol and treprostinil for a 70-kg individual and found treprostinil to be more expensive, particularly when dosing differences were considered. For example, the annual cost of epoprostenol at 30 ng/kg/min was $48,027, whereas the annual cost of the same dose of treprostinil was $71,175. However, the treprostinil dose of 60 ng/kg/min, which is more comparable with the 30 ng/kg/min does of epoprostenol was $142,350.

Inhaled Iloprost

Inhaled iloprost, a synthetic analogue of prostacyclin, was approved for use as an inhalation agent, Ventavis (Actelion Pharmaceuticals, Ltd, Allschwil, Switzerland), in the European Union and Australia (in 2003) and in the United States (2004). Its approval in the United States is for adult patients with PAH and functional class III or IV symptoms.

Pharmacokinetics

Inhaled iloprost, as with other prostanoids, dilates both the pulmonary arterial and systemic arterial vascular beds. It has a serum half-life of 20 to 25 minutes. Because of the proximity of the alveoli to the intra-acinar pulmonary arteries, iloprost can be administered by inhalation as well as intravenously.[62,63] With the inhalational route of administration, inhaled iloprost eliminates the need for SC or central venous access and the pump delivery systems required for parenteral prostanoid use. In addition, by potentially increasing pulmonary arterial flow to well-ventilated lung units, inhalational therapy may improve pulmonary ventilation-perfusion matching. Similar to other prostacyclin analogues, iloprost seems to inhibit platelet aggregation and cell proliferation.[9,64] Its short elimination half-life requires that, as an inhalation agent, doses be administered 6 to 9 times daily.[62]

The initial trial of inhaled iloprost, in 6 patients (4 IPAH, 2 scleroderma Associated Pulmonary Arterial Hypertension [APAH]) showed a reduction in PVR, with improved CO. Arterial oxygen saturations were increased with inhaled prostanoids, but remained unchanged after intravenous prostanoids. The effects of inhaled iloprost lasted longer than those seen with inhaled prostacyclin.[65]

Drug delivery

Inhaled iloprost is presently inhaled through a unique nebulizer device, the I-neb AAD (adaptive aerosol delivery) system (Philips Respironics, Tangmere, Chichester, United Kingdom). This device is portable, battery powered, and rechargeable, and contains a chip that maintains data on treatment frequency, duration, and completeness.

Inhaled iloprost is administered 6 to 9 times a day in doses of either 2.5 μg or 5.0 μg per treatment. It is manufactured in single-dose ampules at a concentration of either 10 μg/mL (for either the 2.5 μg or 5.0 μg doses) or 20 μg/mL (for only 5.0 μg doses). The 20 μg/mL concentration was introduced to decrease inhalation treatment time, to increase patient adherence to the prescribed treatment regimen, and to improve patient satisfaction.

Most patients are up-titrated to the 5.0 μg/treatment dose, with a goal of 6 or more treatments per day. A recent study of low-dose (2.5 μg/treatment;

6 treatments per day) from China suggested that inhaled low-dose iloprost could be effective in early PAH (functional class II).[66]

Clinical trial data

FDA approval of inhaled iloprost was based on a single multicenter trial conducted in Europe and enrolling 203 patients with either CTEPH (57 patients) or PAH (146 patients)[67]; the review and approval in the United States was based solely on the patients with PAH.

Patients received iloprost inhalations at 2.5 or 5.0 μg (median inhaled dose, 30 μg per day) or placebo between 6 and 9 times daily for 12 weeks. The mean frequency of inhalation was 7.5 times a day. The primary end point was a combined measure of improvement of at least 1 functional class and at least 10% improvement in a 6MWD from baseline to week 12 in the absence of deterioration in the clinical condition or death during the 12 weeks of the study. Secondary end points included the 6MWD, the New York Heart Association (NYHA) functional class, Mahler Dyspnea Index, hemodynamic variables, and quality of life. The combined clinical end point was met by 17% of subjects receiving inhaled iloprost and 5% of subjects receiving placebo (P<.05). Inhaled iloprost significantly increased mean 6MWD compared with placebo (36 m, P = .004). Inhaled iloprost treatment also resulted in a significant improvement in cardiopulmonary hemodynamics, functional class, dyspnea, and quality of life (Euro-Qol scale).

Longer term data regarding inhaled iloprost are conflicting. They suggest that although inhaled iloprost is clearly beneficial to patients, only a minority of patients remain stable on inhaled iloprost, particularly if used as monotherapy.[68] In a 1-year, open, uncontrolled study of 24 patients with IPAH, aerosolized iloprost at a daily dose of 100 to 150 μg, 6 to 8 inhalations per day, improved exercise capacity (mean increase in 6MWD, 75 m) and pulmonary hemodynamics.[69] A prospective study followed 76 patients with NYHA class II or III IPAH treated with inhaled iloprost for up to 5 years. During the follow-up period of 535 ± 61 days, 11 patients (14%) died, 6 patients (9%) underwent transplantation, 25 patients (33%) were switched to intravenous prostanoids, 16 patients (23%) received additional oral PAH therapies, and 12 patients (17%) discontinued inhaled iloprost for other reasons. Event-free survival rates at 1, 2, and 5 years were 53%, 29%, and 13% respectively.[70]

Inhaled iloprost has been studied in patients who remained symptomatic (NYHA functional class III or IV) while receiving oral bosentan for at least 3 months.[71] In this multicenter trial, 67 patients with PAH (94% NYHA functional class III; mean baseline 6MWD, 355 m) were randomized to receive inhaled iloprost (5 μg; 6–9 times per day), or placebo. After 12 weeks, the primary efficacy measure, postinhalation 6MWD, improved by 30 m in the inhaled iloprost group and 4 m in the placebo group, for a placebo-adjusted difference of +26 m (P = .051). There were also improvements in NYHA functional class (P = .002), and postinhalation mPAP (P<.001) and PVR (P<.001). This combination therapy seemed to be safe and well tolerated.

Inhaled iloprost has also been studied (acutely) in combination with the oral phosphodiesterase type 5 inhibitor sildenafil. Five patients with IPAH, 4 of whom had been on inhaled iloprost for more than 2 years, were studied after an iloprost inhalation to determine their hemodynamic response to the inhaled iloprost, and the effects of administration of sildenafil (doses of 25 mg and 50 mg). The combination of iloprost plus sildenafil lowered the mPAP significantly more than iloprost alone (13.8 ± 1.4 vs 9.4 ± 1.3 mm Hg; P<.009). There was a no difference in PVR. The investigators concluded that small doses of phosphodiesterase type 5 inhibitor may be a useful adjunct to inhaled iloprost in the management of pulmonary hypertension.[72]

Inhaled iloprost has, on occasion, provided a means to transition patients off intravenous or SC prostanoid therapy. This transition may be because of clinical improvement allowing transition from a parenteral prostanoid, because of patient request, or because of adverse events related to parenteral prostanoid or the delivery system. A recent retrospective study of 37 patients, all on background oral PAH therapy, who had been transitioned from parenteral prostanoid therapy to inhaled iloprost (only 7 [18.9%] transitioned for clinical improvement), found that, at 1 year, 78.4% of the patients continued on inhaled iloprost, and 81.1% were free of clinical worsening.[73]

Adverse effects

Inhaled iloprost is generally well tolerated. Side effects relate to the inhalational route of administration (ie, cough) and to prostanoid side effects related to systemic absorption of the inhaled medications (ie, headache, flushing [systemic vasodilatation], jaw pain and syncope).

Cost

The annual cost (in the United States) for inhaled iloprost therapy depends on the number of medication vials (treatments) a patient is doing each day. Data from the Massachusetts Executive

Office of Health and Human Services (2011) showed that the average annual cost per claim for inhaled iloprost as of early 2011 was approximately \$120,000 to \$135,000.

A recent analysis of the cost-effectiveness of prostacyclin therapy (intravenous epoprostenol, SC treprostinil, and inhaled iloprost) in PAH, found that, in Spain, in most clinical simulations, initiating prostanoid treatment with inhaled iloprost was the least costly option.[74] In particular, inhaled iloprost was assessed to be a more effective and less costly alternative compared with SC treprostinil.

Inhaled Treprostinil

In 2009, an inhaled form of treprostinil, Tyvaso (United Therapeutics Corporation, Research Triangle Park, NC), was approved in the United States for use in patients with PAH in functional class III.

Pharmacokinetics
The pharmacokinetics of inhaled treprostinil are similar to those of SC and intravenous treprostinil, as discussed earlier.[75]

Drug delivery
Treprostinil by inhalation is delivered through a unique device, the OptiNeb portable nebulizer, which is portable, battered powered, and rechargeable.

Inhaled treprostinil is administered 4 times per day with 3 to 9 breaths (each delivering approximately 6 μg of treprostinil) per treatment. A day's supply of inhaled treprostinil is contained in a single ampoule, which is emptied into the OptiNeb once a day. The device is cleaned and recharged at the end of each day.

Studies of the possibility of administering inhaled treprostinil via a metered-dose inhaler are ongoing.[76]

Clinical trial data
Inhaled treprostinil was initially studied as an add-on therapy in 12 patients with PAH who remained symptomatic despite oral bosentan therapy. Four times daily of either 30 μg or 45 μg of inhaled treprostinil was safe and well tolerated. Therapy was associated with an improvement in 6MWD, functional class, and pulmonary hemodynamics (measured at peak postinhalation times).[77] Inhaled treprostinil was also studied for use in combination with oral sildenafil in 28 patients with PAH and 17 patients with CTEPH.[78] This study concluded that the combination of inhaled treprostinil and sildenafil was well tolerated and induced synergistic improvement in pulmonary hemodynamics.

Inhaled treprostinil was approved for use in the United States from a single clinical trial; the

TRIUMPH-1 (Treprostinil Sodium Inhalation Used in the Management of Pulmonary Arterial Hypertension 1) study.[79] This 12-week study randomized 235 adults with PAH who remained in NYHA functional class III (98%) or IV despite background oral therapy with bosentan (67%) or sildenafil (33%) to receive 4 daily inhalations of treprostinil sodium or placebo. Inhaled treprostinil improved the placebo-corrected median improvement in peak 6MWD at week 12 by 10 m ($P = .0004$). This treatment effect was more pronounced in the patients receiving background bosentan therapy, although the study was not powered for this subgroup analysis. Quality of life significantly improved on 2 subscales, but there were no improvements in time to clinical worsening, Borg dyspnea score, functional class, or PAH signs and symptoms.

An open-label extension trial that followed patients who had participated in the TRIUMPH-1 trial reported that, in the 118 patients who continued use of inhaled treprostinil for 24 months, the median improvement in 6MWD was 18 m.[80]

Inhaled treprostinil, on occasion, has provided a means to transition patients off intravenous or SC prostanoid therapy. A recent retrospective review of 18 patients with PAH transitioned from intravenous epoprostenol (n = 3) or intravenous or SC treprostinil (n = 15) because of issues with these therapies found that, at a mean follow-up of 7 ± 2 months, there was no difference in 6MWD or BNP; however, there was a trend toward worsening of NYHA function class, and of NT-BNP. Two patients required reinitiation of parenteral prostanoid therapy during the follow-up period.[81]

Patients have also been transitioned from inhaled iloprost to inhaled treprostinil.[82] A study of 73 patients with PAH on inhaled iloprost (56% functional class II; 42% function class III symptoms) found that 38% of patients reported treatment frequency of less than the labeled rate of 6 to 9 times daily. On inhaled treprostinil, daily treatment time was reduced compared with when on inhaled iloprost and clinical status was maintained.[82]

Adverse effects
Inhaled treprostinil is generally well tolerated. Side effects relate to the inhalation route of administration (ie, cough and throat irritation or pharyngolaryngeal pain) and to prostanoid side effects related to systemic absorption of the inhaled medications (ie, headache, nausea, dizziness, and flushing).[79]

Cost
Data from the Massachusetts Executive Office of Health and Human Services (2011) showed that the average annual cost per claim for inhaled

treprostinil as of early 2011 was approximately $142,000.

SUMMARY

Over the past 3 decades, the development of prostanoids has changed the prognosis for patients with PAH. Prostanoids were the first medications to alter disease progression and the outlook for patients with PAH, and they remain the mainstay of therapy for patients with advanced (ie, functional class IV) disease. The availability of different routes of administration for the various prostanoids has expanded the role of these agents into a broader group of patients with PAH. Although expensive, prostanoid therapy (intravenous epoprostenol) is unique among PAH treatments in having shown improvement in short-term survival. The varied routes of prostanoid administration allow for a stepwise and incremental use of this class of agents if PAH progresses. They will remain a major component of PAH therapy for the foreseeable future.

REFERENCES

1. D'Alonzo GE, Barst RJ, Ayres SM, et al. Survival in patients with primary pulmonary hypertension. Results from a national prospective registry. Ann Intern Med 1991;115(5):343–9.
2. Higenbottam T, Wheeldon D, Wells F, et al. Long-term treatment of primary pulmonary hypertension with continuous intravenous epoprostenol (prostacyclin). Lancet 1984;1(8385):1046–7.
3. Barst RJ, Rubin LJ, Long WA, et al. A comparison of continuous intravenous epoprostenol (prostacyclin) with conventional therapy for primary pulmonary hypertension. N Engl J Med 1996;334:296–301.
4. Christman BW, McPherson CD, Newman JH, et al. An imbalance between the excretion of thromboxane and prostacyclin metabolites in pulmonary hypertension. N Engl J Med 1992;327:70–5.
5. Humbert M, Morrell NW, Archer SL, et al. Cellular and molecular pathobiology of pulmonary arterial hypertension. J Am Coll Cardiol 2004;43(12 Suppl S):13S–24S.
6. Tuder RM, Cool CD, Geraci MW, et al. Prostacyclin synthase expression is decreased in lungs from patients with severe pulmonary hypertension. Am J Respir Crit Care Med 1999;159(6):1925–32.
7. Hoshikawa Y, Voelkel NF, Gesell TL, et al. Prostacyclin receptor-dependent modulation of pulmonary vascular remodeling. Am J Respir Crit Care Med 2001;164(2):314–8.
8. McLaughlin VV, McGoon MD. Pulmonary arterial hypertension. Circulation 2006;114(13):1417–31.
9. Clapp LH, Finney P, Turcato S, et al. Differential effects of stable prostacyclin analogs on smooth muscle proliferation and cyclic AMP generation in human pulmonary artery. Am J Respir Cell Mol Biol 2002;26(2):194–201.
10. Best LC, Martin TJ, Russell RG, et al. Prostacyclin increases cyclic AMP levels and adenylate cyclase activity in platelets. Nature 1977;267(5614):850–2.
11. McLaughlin VV, Genthner DE, Panella MM, et al. Reduction in pulmonary vascular resistance with long-term epoprostenol (prostacyclin) therapy in primary pulmonary hypertension. N Engl J Med 1998;338:273–7.
12. Jeffery TK, Morrell N. Molecular and cellular basis of pulmonary vascular remodeling in pulmonary hypertension. Prog Cardiovasc Dis 2002;45(3):173–202.
13. Fetalvero KM, Martin KA, Hwa J. Cardioprotective prostacyclin signaling in vascular smooth muscle. Prostaglandins Other Lipid Mediat 2007;82(1–4):109–18.
14. Friedman R, Mears JG, Barst RJ. Continuous infusion of prostacyclin normalizes plasma markers of endothelial cell injury and platelet aggregation in primary pulmonary hypertension. Circulation 1997;96:2782–4.
15. Boyer-Neumann C, Brenot F, Wolf M, et al. Continuous infusion of prostacyclin decreases plasma levels of t-PA and PAI-1 in primary pulmonary hypertension. Thromb Haemost 1995;73(4):735–6.
16. Olschewski H, Rose F, Schermuly R, et al. Prostacyclin and its analogues in the treatment of pulmonary hypertension. Pharmacol Ther 2004;102(2):139–53.
17. Fassina G, Tessari F, Dorigo P. Positive inotropic effect of a stable analogue of PGI2 and of PGI2 on isolated guinea pig atria. Mechanism of action. Pharmacol Res Commun 1983;15(8):735–49.
18. Fontana M, Olschewski H, Olschewski A, et al. Treprostinil potentiates the positive inotropic effect of catecholamines in adult rat ventricular cardiomyocytes. Br J Pharmacol 2007;151(6):779–86.
19. Lambert O, Bandilla D. Stability and preservation of a new formulation of epoprostenol sodium for treatment of pulmonary arterial hypertension. Drug Des Devel Ther 2012;6:235–44.
20. Fuentes A, Coralic A, Dawson KL. A new epoprostenol formulation for the treatment of pulmonary arterial hypertension. Am J Health Syst Pharm 2012;69(16):1389–93.
21. Rubin LJ, Groves BM, Reeves JT, et al. Prostacyclin-induced acute pulmonary vasodilation in primary pulmonary hypertension. Circulation 1982;66(2):334–8.
22. Rubin LJ, Mendoza J, Hood M, et al. Treatment of primary pulmonary hypertension with continuous intravenous prostacyclin (epoprostenol). Results

of a randomized trial. Ann Intern Med 1990;112(7): 485–91.

23. Badesch DB, Tapson VF, McGoon MD, et al. Continuous intravenous epoprostenol for pulmonary hypertension due to the scleroderma spectrum of disease. Ann Intern Med 2000;132:425–34.

24. Shapiro SM, Oudiz RJ, Cao T, et al. Primary pulmonary hypertension: improved long-term effects and survival with continuous intravenous epoprostenol infusion. J Am Coll Cardiol 1997;30:343–9.

25. McLaughlin VV, Shillington A, Rich S. Survival in primary pulmonary hypertension: the impact of epoprostenol therapy. Circulation 2002;106:1477–82.

26. Sitbon O, Humbert M, Nunes H, et al. Long-term intravenous epoprostenol infusion in primary pulmonary hypertension: prognostic factors and survival. J Am Coll Cardiol 2002;40:780–8.

27. Robbins IM, Gaine SP, Schilz RJ, et al. Epoprostenol for treatment of pulmonary hypertension in patients with systemic lupus erythematosus. Chest 2000;117:14–8.

28. McLaughlin VV, Genthner DE, Panella MM, et al. Compassionate use of continuous prostacyclin in the management of secondary pulmonary hypertension: a case series. Ann Intern Med 1999;130: 740–3.

29. Petitpretz P, Brenot F, Azarian R, et al. Pulmonary hypertension in patients with human immunodeficiency virus infection: comparison with primary pulmonary hypertension. Circulation 1994;89:2722–7.

30. Aguilar RV, Farber HW. Epoprostenol (prostacyclin) therapy in HIV-associated pulmonary hypertension. Am J Respir Crit Care Med 2000;162(5):1846–50.

31. Rosenzweig EB, Kerstein D, Barst RJ. Long-term prostacyclin for pulmonary hypertension with associated congenital heart defects. Circulation 1999; 99:1858–65.

32. Kuo PC, Johnson LB, Plotkin JS, et al. Continuous intravenous infusion of epoprostenol for the treatment of portopulmonary hypertension. Transplantation 1997;63:604–16.

33. Rich S, McLaughlin VV. The effects of chronic prostacyclin therapy on cardiac output and symptoms in primary pulmonary hypertension. J Am Coll Cardiol 1999;34:1184–7.

34. Rubenfire M, McLaughlin VV, Allen RP, et al. Transition from IV epoprostenol to subcutaneous treprostinil in pulmonary arterial hypertension: a controlled trial. Chest 2007;132(3):757–63.

35. Wade M, Baker FJ, Roscigno R, et al. Absolute bioavailability and pharmacokinetics of treprostinil sodium administered by acute subcutaneous infusion. J Clin Pharmacol 2004;44(1):83–8.

36. Wade M, Baker FJ, Roscigno R, et al. Pharmacokinetics of treprostinil sodium administered by 28-day chronic continuous subcutaneous infusion. J Clin Pharmacol 2004;44(5):503–9.

37. Walkey AJ, Fein D, Horbowicz KJ, et al. Differential response to intravenous prostacyclin analog therapy in patients with pulmonary arterial hypertension. Pulm Pharmacol Ther 2011;24(4):421–5.

38. McSwain CS, Benza R, Shapiro S, et al. Dose proportionality of treprostinil sodium administered by continuous subcutaneous and intravenous infusion. J Clin Pharmacol 2008;48(1):19–25.

39. McLaughlin VV, Gaine SP, Barst RJ, et al. Efficacy and safety of treprostinil: an epoprostenol analogue for primary pulmonary hypertension. J Cardiovasc Pharmacol 2003;41(2):293–9.

40. Simonneau G, Barst RJ, Galie N, et al. Continuous subcutaneous infusion of treprostinil, a prostacyclin analogue, in patients with pulmonary arterial hypertension. Am J Respir Crit Care Med 2002;165:800–4.

41. Barst RJ, Galie N, Naeije R, et al. Long-term outcome in pulmonary arterial hypertension patients treated with subcutaneous treprostinil. Eur Respir J 2006;28(6):1195–203.

42. Sadushi-Kolici R, Skoro-Sajer N, Zimmer D, et al. Long-term treatment, tolerability, and survival with sub-cutaneous treprostinil for severe pulmonary hypertension. J Heart Lung Transplant 2012; 31(7):735–43.

43. Oudiz R, Schilz RJ, Barst RJ, et al. Treprostinil, a prostacyclin analogue, in pulmonary arterial hypertension associated with connective tissue disease. Chest 2004;126:420–7.

44. Skoro-Sajer N, Bonderman D, Wiesbauer F, et al. Treprostinil for severe inoperable chronic thromboembolic pulmonary hypertension. J Thromb Haemost 2007;5(3):483–9.

45. Lang I, Gomez-Sanchez M, Kneussl M, et al. Efficacy of long-term subcutaneous treprostinil sodium therapy in pulmonary hypertension. Chest 2006;129(6):1636–43.

46. Vachiery JL, Hill N, Zwicke D, et al. Transitioning from IV epoprostenol to subcutaneous treprostinil in pulmonary arterial hypertension. Chest 2002; 121:1561–5.

47. Skoro-Sajer N, Lang IM, Harja E, et al. A clinical comparison of slow- and rapid-escalation treprostinil dosing regimens in patients with pulmonary hypertension. Clin Pharm 2008;47(9):611–8.

48. Tapson VF, Gomberg-Maitland M, McLaughlin VV, et al. Safety and efficacy of IV treprostinil for pulmonary arterial hypertension: a prospective, multicenter, open-label, 12-week trial. Chest 2006; 129(3):683–8.

49. Gomberg-Maitland M, Tapson VF, Benza RL, et al. Transition from intravenous epoprostenol to intravenous treprostinil in pulmonary hypertension. Am J Respir Crit Care Med 2005;172(12):1586–9.

50. Hiremath J, Thanikachalam S, Parikh K, et al. Exercise improvement and plasma biomarker changes

with intravenous treprostinil therapy for pulmonary arterial hypertension: a placebo-controlled trial. J Heart Lung Transplant 2010;29(2):137–49.

51. Tapson VF, McLaughlin VV, Gomberg-Maitland M, et al. Delivery of intravenous treprostinil at low infusion rates using a miniaturized infusion pump in patients with pulmonary arterial hypertension. J Vasc Access 2006;7(3):112–7.

52. Ewert R, Halank M, Bruch L, et al. A case series of patients with severe pulmonary hypertension receiving an implantable pump for intravenous prostanoid therapy. Am J Respir Crit Care Med 2012;186(11):1196–8.

53. Kallen AJ, Lederman E, Balaji A, et al. Bloodstream infections in patients given treatment with intravenous prostanoids. Infect Control Hosp Epidemiol 2008;29(4):342–9.

54. Kitterman N, Poms A, Miller DP, et al. Bloodstream infections in patients with pulmonary arterial hypertension treated with intravenous prostanoids: insights from the REVEAL REGISTRY(R). Mayo Clin Proc 2012;87(9):825–34.

55. McLaughlin VV, Archer SL, Badesch DB, et al. ACCF/AHA 2009 expert consensus document on pulmonary hypertension a report of the American College of Cardiology Foundation Task Force on Expert Consensus Documents and the American Heart Association developed in collaboration with the American College of Chest Physicians; American Thoracic Society, Inc.; and the Pulmonary Hypertension Association. J Am Coll Cardiol 2009;53(17):1573–619.

56. Badesch DB, Abman SH, Simonneau G, et al. Medical therapy for pulmonary arterial hypertension: updated ACCP evidence-based clinical practice guidelines. Chest 2007;131(6):1917–28.

57. Galie N, Hoeper MM, Humbert M, et al. Guidelines for the diagnosis and treatment of pulmonary hypertension: the Task Force for the Diagnosis and Treatment of Pulmonary Hypertension of the European Society of Cardiology (ESC) and the European Respiratory Society (ERS), endorsed by the International Society of Heart and Lung Transplantation (ISHLT). Eur Heart J 2009;30(20):2493–537.

58. Barst RJ, Gibbs JS, Ghofrani HA, et al. Updated evidence-based treatment algorithm in pulmonary arterial hypertension. J Am Coll Cardiol 2009; 54(Suppl 1):S78–84.

59. Doran AK, Ivy DD, Barst RJ, et al. Guidelines for the prevention of central venous catheter-related blood stream infections with prostanoid therapy for pulmonary arterial hypertension. Int J Clin Pract 2008;(160):5–9.

60. Kingman MS, Tankersley MA, Lombardi S, et al. Prostacyclin administration errors in pulmonary arterial hypertension patients admitted to hospitals

in the United States: a national survey. J Heart Lung Transplant 2010;29(8):841–6.

61. Oudiz RJ, Farber HW. Dosing considerations in the use of intravenous prostanoids in pulmonary arterial hypertension: an experience-based review. Am Heart J 2009;157(4):625–35.

62. Krause W, Krais T. Pharmacokinetics and pharmacodynamics of the prostacyclin analogue iloprost in man. Eur J Clin Pharmacol 1986;30(1):61–8.

63. John J, Palevsky H. Clinical pharmacology and efficacy of inhaled iloprost for the treatment of pulmonary arterial hypertension. Expert Rev Clin Pharmacol 2011;4(2):197–205.

64. Beghetti M, Reber G, de MP, et al. Aerosolized iloprost induces a mild but sustained inhibition of platelet aggregation. Eur Respir J 2002;19(3): 518–24.

65. Olschewski H, Walmrath D, Schermuly R, et al. Aerosolized prostacyclin and iloprost in severe pulmonary hypertension. Ann Intern Med 1996;124(9): 820–4.

66. Sun YJ, Xiong CM, Shan GL, et al. Inhaled low-dose iloprost for pulmonary hypertension: a prospective, multicenter, open-label study. Clin Cardiol 2011; 35(6):365–70.

67. Olschewski H, Simonneau G, Galie N, et al. Inhaled iloprost for severe pulmonary hypertension. N Engl J Med 2002;347(5):322–9.

68. Olschewski H. Inhaled iloprost for the treatment of pulmonary hypertension. Eur Respir Rev 2009; 18(111):29–34.

69. Hoeper MM, Schwarze M, Ehlerding S, et al. Long-term treatment of primary pulmonary hypertension with aerosolized iloprost, a prostacyclin analogue. N Engl J Med 2000;342(25):1866–70.

70. Opitz CF, Wensel R, Winkler J, et al. Clinical efficacy and survival with first-line inhaled iloprost therapy in patients with idiopathic pulmonary arterial hypertension. Eur Heart J 2005;26(18): 1895–902.

71. McLaughlin VV, Oudiz RJ, Frost A, et al. Randomized study of adding inhaled iloprost to existing bosentan in pulmonary arterial hypertension. Am J Respir Crit Care Med 2006;174(11):1257–63.

72. Wilkens H, Guth A, Konig J, et al. Effect of inhaled iloprost plus oral sildenafil in patients with primary pulmonary hypertension. Circulation 2001;104(11): 1218–22.

73. Channick R, Frantz R, Kawut S, et al. A multicenter, retrospective study of patients with pulmonary arterial hypertension transitioned from parenteral prostacyclin therapy to inhaled iloprost. Pulm Circ 2013; 3:381–8.

74. Roman A, Barbera JA, Escribano P, et al. Cost effectiveness of prostacyclins in pulmonary arterial hypertension. Appl Health Econ Health Policy 2012;10(3):175–88.

75. Channick RN, Voswinckel R, Rubin LJ. Inhaled tre-prostinil: a therapeutic review. Drug Des Devel Ther 2012;6:19–28.

76. Voswinckel R, Reichenberger F, Gall H, et al. Me-tered dose inhaler delivery of treprostinil for the treatment of pulmonary hypertension. Pulm Phar-macol Ther 2009;22(1):50–6.

77. Channick RN, Olschewski H, Seeger W, et al. Safety and efficacy of inhaled treprostinil as add-on therapy to bosentan in pulmonary arterial hyper-tension. J Am Coll Cardiol 2006;48(7):1433–7.

78. Voswinckel R, Reichenberger F, Enke B, et al. Acute effects of the combination of sildenafil and inhaled treprostinil on haemodynamics and gas ex-change in pulmonary hypertension. Pulm Pharma-col Ther 2008;21(5):824–32.

79. McLaughlin VV, Benza RL, Rubin LJ, et al. Addition of inhaled treprostinil to oral therapy for pulmonary arterial hypertension: a randomized controlled clin-ical trial. J Am Coll Cardiol 2010;55(18):1915–22.

80. Benza RL, Seeger W, McLaughlin VV, et al. Long-term effects of inhaled treprostinil in patients with pulmonary arterial hypertension: the Treprostinil Sodium Inhalation Used in the Management of Pul-monary Arterial Hypertension (TRIUMPH) study open-label extension. J Heart Lung Transplant 2011;30(12):1327–33.

81. de Jesus Perez VA, Rosenzweig E, Rubin LJ, et al. Safety and efficacy of transition from systemic prostanoids to inhaled treprostinil in pulmonary arterial hypertension. Am J Cardiol 2012;110(10):1546–50.

82. Bourge RC, Tapson VF, Safdar Z, et al. Rapid tran-sition from inhaled iloprost to inhaled treprostinil in patients with pulmonary arterial hypertension. Car-diovasc Ther 2013;31(1):38–44.

Combination Therapy in Pulmonary Arterial Hypertension

Meredith E. Pugh, MD, MSCI, Anna R. Hemnes, MD,
Ivan M. Robbins, MD*

KEYWORDS

- Pulmonary arterial hypertension • Combination therapy • Endothelin receptor antagonists
- Prostacyclin • Phosphodiesterase-5 inhibitors • Treatment

KEY POINTS

- Multiple open-label, small, and often single-center studies describing results with combination therapy in pulmonary arterial hypertension (PAH) have been published. The results of these studies are mixed, although most suggest a benefit without significant toxicity.
- Several multicenter, randomized, placebo-controlled studies have also been performed, also with mixed results, although the largest of these studies, TRIUMPH-1 and PACES, showed significant improvement in exercise capacity, and the latter in hemodynamics and survival, although with the caveat that the dose of sildenafil used was higher than that approved for use.
- Regardless of the mixed results of published studies, combination therapy is used in a sizable proportion of patients with PAH and will likely be used in even greater numbers of patients as more drugs for PAH are approved.
- Other than the BREATHE-2 study, randomized trials have not raised issues of safety with combination therapy. The IMPRES study reported a large number of subdural hematomas in patients receiving imatinib, but this appears more likely to be related to the drug itself rather than combination therapy. Both of these studies enrolled very sick patients with more severe hemodynamic impairment, suggesting that this may be an important factor with regard to the severe adverse events seen.
- Several large, long-term studies with a variety of medications should provide more robust data in the near future, especially with regard to oral therapy combinations and upfront versus add-on combination therapy.

Despite the availability of multiple agents for the treatment of pulmonary arterial hypertension (PAH), PAH remains a progressive disease with unacceptably high morbidity and mortality. Although the complete pathobiology of PAH is not known, therapies targeting 3 pathways (endothelin, nitric oxide, and prostacyclin pathways) have been evaluated, and have shown benefit in the treatment of PAH. Currently approved therapies for the treatment of PAH in the United States include endothelin receptor antagonists (ambrisentan [Letairis], bosentan [Tracleer]), phosphodiesterase-5 (PDE5)

Conflicts of Interest: M.E. Pugh has received consulting fees from Gilead and funding from the NIH; A.R. Hemnes has served as a consultant for United Therapeutics, Actelion, and Pfizer, and has received grants from the NIH, United Therapeutics, and Pfizer; I.M. Robbins has received consulting fees from United Therapeutics, Gilead, and Actelion for attending advisory board meetings, and has received grants from the NIH.
Division of Allergy, Pulmonary and Critical Care Medicine, Department of Medicine, Vanderbilt University, T1218 Medical Center North, 1161 21st Avenue South, Nashville, TN 37232, USA
* Corresponding author.
E-mail address: ivan.robbins@vanderbilt.edu

Clin Chest Med 34 (2013) 841–855
http://dx.doi.org/10.1016/j.ccm.2013.08.007
0272-5231/13/$ – see front matter © 2013 Elsevier Inc. All rights reserved.

inhibitors (sildenafil [Revatio], tadalafil [Adcirca]), and prostacyclin derivatives (epoprostenol [Flolan, Veletri], iloprost [Ventavis], treprostinil [Remodulin, Tyvaso]).[1,2] These agents improve PAH symptoms, exercise capacity, and hemodynamic outcomes over the short term,[3–9] and are available as oral agents (ambrisentan, bosentan, tadalafil, sildenafil), inhaled therapies (iloprost, treprostinil), subcutaneous infusions (treprostinil), and intravenous infusions (epoprostenol, treprostinil).

Even with use of these diverse agents, many patients on PAH monotherapy continue to worsen, develop right heart failure, and, too often, die of the disease. Targeting more than 1 pathway with combination therapy to improve outcome, similar to the way in which other chronic disorders such as congestive heart failure and cancer are treated, is a natural extension of the treatment algorithm of PAH.[2,10] There are data to support a synergistic interaction with PAH-approved medications; this has been demonstrated with the combination of a PDE5 inhibitor and a prostaglandin in animals, and in acute studies in humans with pulmonary hypertension (PH).[11–14] Although not providing a basis for all combinations, the synergistic effect that was demonstrated acutely provided support and impetus for combining agents in the treatment of PAH. Combinations include concomitant use of endothelin receptor antagonists (ERAs) and PDE5 inhibitors (PDE5-Is), prostanoids and ERAs or PDE5-Is, and all 3 classes of agents (prostanoids + ERA + PDE5-I). In addition, 2 recent studies have evaluated the addition of the tyrosine kinase inhibitor, imatinib (Gleevec) to the regimen of patients treated with approved PAH therapy.

Use of combination therapy in clinical practice is widespread, but although it is a logical next step in the treatment of PAH, there are presently few data to support the benefit of this approach. Numerous small, open-label studies or case series have been published with varying results, and even the results of randomized clinical trials of combination therapy in PAH have not consistently supported this approach. In addition, the results of randomized studies of certain combinations, in particular combination oral therapy, are not yet available. Most studies have evaluated the benefit of sequential add-on therapy, and only a few published studies have evaluated initial treatment with combination therapy. Data from the REVEAL registry show a high prevalence of the use of combination therapy for PAH, with the majority of patients on PAH treatment receiving multiple agents at registry enrollment.[15] Combination therapy is recommended in consensus guidelines for patients who are not responding to initial monotherapy.[10] Which combination of agents is most beneficial is not known, and

whether combination therapy is best initiated as sequential (or add-on) therapy or as first-line combination therapy is also uncertain at present. Although combination therapy seems to be well tolerated in many patients in clinical practice, the question of when to consider this strategy remains largely unanswered. Several ongoing multicenter studies should provide more robust results in the near future that will help guide treatment decisions. This review examines the current evidence regarding combination therapy in PAH, and discusses which patients may benefit from this strategy.

PROSTACYCLIN ANALOGUES + ENDOTHELIN RECEPTOR ANTAGONISTS
Small or Nonrandomized Trials and Case Series

Several uncontrolled studies report a beneficial effect of additive therapy with ERAs and prostacyclin analogues. In a study of 20 idiopathic PAH (IPAH) patients who had evidence for declining clinical status on nonparenteral prostanoid therapy, either inhaled iloprost or oral beraprost (the latter not approved in the United States), Hoeper and colleagues[16] showed that the addition of bosentan lead to significant improvement in 6-minute walk distance (6MWD) after 3 months of follow-up (346 ± 106 m baseline vs 404 ± 101 m, $P<.0001$). In addition, treatment with bosentan resulted in improvements in several end points, including maximal oxygen consumption (Vo_2) and anaerobic threshold, during cardiopulmonary exercise testing. Combination therapy was well tolerated in all patients, including a subset followed for up to 6 months.

The beneficial effect of the addition of bosentan to prostanoid therapy was also seen in a smaller study of 16 patients with PH, which included 9 with IPAH and 5 with chronic thromboembolic PH (CTEPH).[17] In this study, patients with clinical deterioration on stable doses of prostanoids (beraprost, inhaled iloprost, or intravenous iloprost) were given bosentan for a median follow-up of 13.5 months (range 9–22 months). Significant improvement in 6MWD (increase in 42.5 ± 66 m at 6 months and 44.6 ± 66 m at maximal follow-up, $P<.05$) was observed. Improvement in right ventricular function on echocardiogram was also seen. No significant side effects were reported in this group of patients.

A pilot study of 11 PAH patients, stable on monotherapy with bosentan, evaluated the effect of add-on therapy with inhaled treprostinil 4 times daily on 6MWD, hemodynamics, and heart failure symptoms at 12 weeks.[18] Both the preinhalation and postinhalation 6MWD after 12 weeks of inhaled treprostinil therapy were significantly improved (increase in 49 m, $P = .009$ and 67 m, $P = .01$, respectively). Significant reduction in postinhalation mean pulmonary artery pressure (-10% change) and improvement in functional class (FC) in 9 of 11 patients was also seen. Combination therapy was well tolerated in this small cohort of patients.

In a retrospective review of IPAH patients treated with first-line bosentan, Provencher and colleagues[19] report outcomes of 36 patients in whom prostanoid therapy (intravenous epoprostenol in 30 patients, inhaled iloprost in 6 patients) was added to bosentan because of a deteriorating clinical course. After 3 months of combination therapy, improvement in 6MWD (from 310 ± 108 to 347 ± 117 m, $P = .031$), cardiac index (2.22 ± 0.45 to 2.64 ± 0.63 L/min/m^2, $P = .002$), and, less impressively, mean pulmonary artery pressure (mPAP) (60 ± 12 to 56 ± 11 mm Hg, $P = .014$) was noted. In addition, 39% of patients on combination therapy improved by 1 or more FC. This same group also reported their experience with upfront combination therapy of epoprostenol and bosentan in 23 patients of FC III or IV with IPAH or anorexigen-associated PAH.[20] After 4 months, the investigators found significant improvement in 6MWD and pulmonary vascular resistance (PVR), which was maintained out to 30 ± 19 months. The 1-, 2-, and 3-year transplant-free survival estimates were 96%, 85%, and 77%, respectively, which are higher than those previously reported for epoprostenol therapy alone. Compared with 43 matched controls started on epoprostenol monotherapy, there was a significantly greater decrease in PVR in the combination group at initial follow-up ($P = .0001$) and, with long-term follow-up, a trend toward improvement in survival ($P = .07$). Combination therapy was well tolerated with similar epoprostenol doses in both groups, without increased epoprostenol side effects. Two of 23 patients receiving bosentan had an increase in transaminases to greater than 8 times the upper limit of normal.

Several studies adding ERAs to therapy for adults as well as children receiving subcutaneous or intravenous prostanoids have been published. Improved hemodynamics were reported in a small case series of 8 FC II adult IPAH patients receiving high-dose epoprostenol after the addition of bosentan 62.5 mg twice daily, half of the recommended dose.[21] There was no significant change in 6MWD or brain natriuretic peptide (BNP) levels. The dose of epoprostenol was decreased in the majority of patients because of side effects (mainly flushing and nausea). One patient discontinued bosentan because of an increase in liver enzymes.

Two larger studies, one in adults and one in children, have reported benefit with the addition of bosentan to either continuous treprostinil or epoprostenol therapy. Benza and colleagues[22] reported the results of a single-center retrospective review of 19 PAH patients (IPAH, associated PAH, or chronic thromboembolic PH, 76% World Health Organization [WHO] FC III), receiving long-term subcutaneous treprostinil. Bosentan was added either because patients remained in FC III or had intolerable prostaglandin side effects that limited dose increases. In the patients in whom bosentan was added, there was improvement in both mPAP (from 56 ± 16 to 47 ± 11 mm Hg) and right atrial pressure (from 10 ± 7 to 5 ± 4 mm Hg) ($P<.001$ for both). 6MWD also improved, from 333 ± 80 to 374 ± 110 m, but did not reach statistical significance ($P = .071$). Twelve patients were FC III before the addition of bosentan, and 7 improved to FC II. Combination therapy in this cohort was safe and well tolerated without an increase in transaminases.

In the only study exclusively looking at children, Ivy and colleagues[23] reported the outcome of 86 patients (36 with IPAH, 48 with congenital heart disease–associated PAH, and 2 with connective tissue disease [CTD]-associated PAH) treated with bosentan, either as monotherapy (n = 42) or added on to continuous prostaglandin therapy, intravenous epoprostenol, or subcutaneous treprostinil. There was no standardized protocol for adding bosentan to prostaglandin therapy; this was done according the treating physician's clinical judgment. The median exposure time to bosentan was 24 months, and the study design allowed for a decrease in the dose of epoprostenol or treprostinil. Excluding the 2 CTD patients, 53% of patients receiving bosentan and prostanoid therapy discontinued bosentan during the study period, most commonly because of lack of efficacy (28%). Bosentan was well tolerated, and was discontinued in only 2 patients because of side effects and in 3 because of an asymptomatic elevation in transaminases. Though with significant limitations, these small case series and single-center reviews confirm that combination therapy with bosentan and prostanoids is generally well tolerated, and suggest a beneficial effect in patients with inadequate response to either agent alone.

Randomized Trials

The first trial to evaluate the efficacy of combination therapy was the BREATHE-2 study (Bosentan Randomized trial of Endothelin Antagonist Therapy for PAH), a double-blind, placebo-controlled study in which 33 patients from 7 centers were studied over 16 weeks (**Table 1**).[24] This trial

Table 1
Summary of randomized trials that included combination therapy for pulmonary arterial hypertension

Authors,[Ref.] Year	Combination	Number Enrolled	PAH Etiology	Study Duration (wk)	Primary End Point	End Point Met?	Other Key Results
Humbert et al,[24] 2004 (BREATHE-2)	Eoprostenol and bosentan initiated together	33	IPAH, CTD	16	Decrease in TPR	No	Two deaths in active treatment arm
McLaughlin et al,[25] 2006 (STEP)	Inhaled Iloprost added to bosentan	67	IPAH, CTD, HIV, CHD, anorexigen use, HIV infection	12	Change in 6MWD	No	More improvement in FC and less clinical deterioration in iloprost group
Hoeper et al,[26] 2006 (COMBI)	Inhaled Iloprost added to bosentan	40	IPAH	12	Change in 6MWD	No	Study stopped early owing to futility Greater improvement in median 6MWD in iloprost group, 25 m vs 5 m
McLaughlin et al,[27] 2010 (TRIUMPH-1)	Inhaled treprostinil added to either sildenafil or bosentan	235	IPAH, CTD, "other" in 27 patients	12	Change in 6MWD	Yes	Greater decreased in NT proBNP in iloprost group
Simonneau et al,[33] 2008 (PACES)	Sildenafil added to eoprostenol	267	IPAH, CTD, "other" in 10 patients	16	Change in 6MWD	Yes	Mortality benefit and less clinical worsening in the sildenafil group
Iversen et al,[48] 2010	Sildenafil added to bosentan	21	CHD	12	Change in 6MWD	No	Improvement in sildenafil group in peripheral saturation, 2.9 vs −1.8% in placebo, $P > .01$. Crossover study design

Study	Intervention	N	Population	Weeks	Primary Endpoint	Met	Comments
Galie et al,[9] 2009 (PHIRST)	Tadalafil added to bosentan	216	IPAH, CTD, HIV, CHD, anorexigen use	16	Change in 6MWD	No	—
Ghofrani et al,[50] 2010	Imatinib added to an ERA and/or sildenafil and/or prostaglandin	29	IPAH/HPAH, CTD, "other" in 5 patients	24	Change in 6MWD	No	Post hoc subgroup analysis suggested patients with PVR $\geq$12.5 had a greater hemodynamic response and significant improvement in 6MWD
Hoeper et al,[51] 2013 (IMPRES)	Imatinib added to ERA and/or PDE5I and/or prostaglandin in patients with a PVR >10 U	202	IPAH, CTD, HIV, CHD, anorexigen use	24	Change in 6MWD	Yes	Subdural hematoma in 8 patients in imatinib group (6 in open-label extension, all on warfarin) Greater discontinuation of imatinib because of AEs, 27% vs 9% for placebo
Simonneau et al,[52] 2012	Selexipag added to ERA and/or PDE5-I	43	IPAH/HPAH, CTD, CHD, anorexigen use	17	Change in PVR	Yes	—
Tapson et al,[53] 2013 (FREEDOM-C2)	Oral treprostinil added to ERA and/or PDE5-I	310	IPAH/HPAH, CTD, HIV, CHD	16	Change in 6MWD	No	Greater discontinuation of treprostinil because of AEs, 11% vs 5% for placebo

Abbreviations: 6MWD, 6-minute walk distance; AEs, adverse events; CHD, congenital heart disease; CTD, connective tissue disease; ERA, endothelin receptor antagonist; FC, functional class; HIV, human immunodeficiency virus; HPAH, heritable PAH; IPAH, idiopathic PAH; NT proBNP, N-terminal prohormone of brain natriuretic peptide; PAH, pulmonary arterial hypertension; PDE5-I, phosphodiesterase-5 inhibitor; PVR, pulmonary vascular resistance; TPR, total pulmonary resistance.

represents the only combination study involving prostanoids in which all patients were treatment naïve. All patients were started on epoprostenol at a dose of 2 ng/kg/min, and 2 days later were randomized in a 2:1 ratio to receive bosentan or placebo. Epoprostenol was titrated over the study period to a goal of 12 to 16 ng/kg/min. Hemodynamics, 6MWD, and FC were assessed at baseline and at the conclusions of the study, and the primary end point of the study was change in total pulmonary resistance (TPR).

The study population consisted of WHO FC III (76%) and IV (24%) patients with PAH, 27 of whom had IPAH and the rest CTD-associated PAH. Eighteen of 22 patients in the bosentan arm and 10 of 11 patients in the placebo group completed the hemodynamic evaluation at week 16. TPR decreased in both groups, and although the decrease was greater in the bosentan group ($-36.3\% \pm 4.3\%$) than in the placebo group ($22.6\% \pm 6.2\%$), the difference was not statistically significant ($P = .08$). 6MWD increased similarly in each arm with a median increase in the bosentan arm of 68 m, compared with 74 m in the placebo group. There was also a similar percentage of patients with improvement in FC in both arms.

Side effects were most frequently those known to occur with epoprostenol and were similar in both groups except for diarrhea, which was reported more frequently in those receiving bosentan (55% vs 27%). Lower extremity edema also occurred more frequently in the active treatment group (27% vs 9%). Of note, a higher percentage of patients in the placebo arm developed asymptomatic increases in hepatic transaminases (18% vs 9%), and 2 patients from each group were withdrawn from the study because of this. Serious adverse events (AEs) were also similar in the two groups; however, 2 patients receiving bosentan died during the study and an additional patient died following withdrawal from the study for worsening PAH, whereas none treated with epoprostenol alone died. These deaths were not considered to be related to the study treatment.

The BREATHE-2 study showed some trends for greater hemodynamic improvement with the combination of bosentan and epoprostenol; however, the study appeared to be underpowered to show a significant difference. The combination of an ERA and intravenous epoprostenol was well tolerated for the most part. Three deaths in bosentan group, although not thought to be related to the study drug, does raise some concern, but this was a small study and the group of patients enrolled was appreciably ill with no lower limit of 6MWD as an exclusion criteria. Unfortunately, it is unlikely that an additional combination study with an ERA and intravenous or subcutaneous prostaglandins will be undertaken.

Subsequent to the BREATHE-2 study, 2 randomized trials were undertaken to evaluate the addition of inhaled iloprost in patients already on background therapy with bosentan. The 12-week, multicenter STEP study (Safety and pilot efficacy Trial in combination with bosentan for Evaluation in Pulmonary arterial hypertension) randomized 67 stable patients to treatment with iloprost (6 to 9 inhalations daily) or placebo on top of background bosentan therapy.[25] Nearly all patients (94%) in this study were FC III; 55% had IPAH and 45% had associated PAH. The addition of iloprost to bosentan was associated with a placebo-adjusted difference in 6MWD of 26 m ($P = .051$). Improvements in FC, time to clinical worsening, and hemodynamics (postinhalation mPAP and PVR) were also seen in the combination therapy group. Combination therapy was well tolerated and appeared safe in this study. Specifically, syncope was reported in only 1 patient on iloprost, less commonly than in the Aerosolized Iloprost Randomized (AIR) study.[8]

The benefits of the addition of iloprost to bosentan seen in the STEP trial were not seen in a multicenter, open-label trial restricted to IPAH patients. In the COMBI trial (Combination therapy for bosentan and aerosolized iloprost in idiopathic PAH), patients with IPAH (FC III), on stable background therapy with bosentan, were randomized to the addition of inhaled iloprost (6 inhalations daily) or continuation of background monotherapy.[26] This trial was stopped after enrollment of 40 patients, after a futility analysis predicted a low likelihood of meeting the primary end point (change in 6MWD by 45 m). In this trial, the placebo-adjusted 6MWD at 12 weeks was -10 m in favor of the bosentan monotherapy group ($P = .49$). No significant differences were seen in WHO FC, time to clinical worsening, and cardiopulmonary exercise test assessments. This trial was limited by an open-label design and the small sample size, which was inadequately powered to detect a treatment benefit.

A more recent 12-week randomized, controlled trial evaluated the safety and efficacy of inhaled treprostinil in IPAH, heritable PAH (HPAH), or associated PAH patients on background therapy with sildenafil or bosentan.[27] In the TRIUMPH-1 study (TReprostinil sodium Inhalation Used in the Management of Pulmonary arterial Hypertension), 235 patients were randomized to inhaled treprostinil 4 times daily or placebo inhalation in addition to stable background ERA or PDE5-I therapy. Most participants (56%) had IPAH or HPAH, and nearly all were WHO FC III. A minority of patients were on background sildenafil therapy: 33% of patients in the inhaled treprostinil group, and 27% in the placebo group. The addition of inhaled treprostinil improved exercise capacity (between-treatment median difference in change from baseline to peak 6MWD of 20 m at week 12, P = .0004). Of interest, patients with the lowest quartile for baseline 6MWD had the greatest treatment effect with inhaled treprostinil (between-treatment median difference of 49 m, P = .0003). Although the improvement in 6MWD appeared greater in the bosentan + treprostinil group, the study was not powered to detect differences in response to inhaled treprostinil between ERA and PDE5-I background therapy. No significant differences in FC, time to clinical worsening, or Borg dyspnea scores were seen between patients treated with inhaled treprostinil or placebo. In addition to improved exercise capacity, the inhaled-treprostinil group did have improved quality-of-life measures and N-terminal pro-BNP measurements. Similar to the trials of inhaled iloprost, the addition of inhaled treprostinil was associated with a greater number of side effects, including cough and prostanoid class effects (eg, headache, flushing).

Although the aforementioned studies are not completely consistent in their conclusions, at least the 2 larger of these randomized trials of inhaled prostanoids added to stable oral therapy with bosentan (STEP, TRIUMPH-1) or sildenafil (TRIUMPH-1) suggest that the sequential addition of an inhaled prostacyclin analogue to ERA or PDE5-I therapy may have some benefit in exercise capacity in IPAH and associated PAH. Although the COMBI trial did not show this same benefit, this study was limited by a small sample size and lack of a placebo-controlled group. It is not clear whether this combination strategy improves WHO FC or time to clinical worsening. Despite these limitations and somewhat contradictory data, all 3 studies seem to demonstrate that combining inhaled prostanoid therapy with an ERA or PDE5-I is safe and generally well tolerated. In clinical practice, combination therapy with addition of inhaled prostacyclin to oral therapy is frequently used, as demonstrated by the very low rate of inhaled prostanoid monotherapy in registry studies.[15]

PROSTACYCLIN ANALOGUES + PDE5-IS
Small or Nonrandomized Trials and Case Series

The potential benefit of combining the PDE5-I, sildenafil, to inhaled iloprost therapy was seen in several small, proof-of-concept, acute hemodynamic studies.[12,13] A small study of 11 patients (8 with IPAH and 3 with PAH associated with toxic oil syndrome) with deterioration despite treatment with prostaglandin therapy (either epoprostenol, treprostinil, or inhaled iloprost) reported improvement in 6MWD of 36 ± 11 m (P = .02) following the addition of sildenafil at 12 months.[28] In another study of combination therapy with a PDE5-I and prostanoids, Ruiz and colleagues[29] reported significant improvement in exercise capacity and FC when sildenafil was added for 20 patients on a variety of prostanoid regimens (8 subcutaneous treprostinil, 7 intravenous epoprostenol, 5 inhaled iloprost) who had evidence of clinical deterioration despite prostanoid therapy. Patients were followed for 2 years, and a significant improvement in 6MWD of 79 m at 1 year and 105 m at 2 years after the addition of sildenafil was reported. Mean FC also significantly improved at both the 1- and 2-year time points. In addition to the significant limitations of small sample size and uncontrolled design, the dosing of background prostanoid was able to be adjusted during the follow-up interval, which makes it difficult to determine whether the beneficial effects seen were related to higher prostanoid dosing or to sildenafil add-on therapy.

Ghofrani and colleagues[30] evaluated the effect of sildenafil (25–50 mg 3 times daily) in 14 patients with PAH (9 IPAH, 4 CTD-associated PAH) with clinical deterioration on inhaled iloprost therapy. In each patient, 6MWD improved and remained improved up to 12 months after the initiation of sildenafil (346 ± 26 m at 3 months vs 256 ± 30 m at baseline, P = .002; 349 ± 32 m at 9–12 months, P = .002). In addition, PVR was significantly reduced compared with pre-sildenafil values. Combination therapy was well tolerated without any serious AEs reported.

Two additional small, open-label studies have reported improvement with the addition of sildenafil administration to patients treated chronically with either subcutaneous treprostinil or intravenous epoprostenol. Nine PAH patients (WHO FC II or III) receiving long-term subcutaneous treprostinil had sildenafil added, starting at a dose of 25 mg 3 times daily and increasing to 50 mg 3 times daily after 2 weeks.[31] Patients were followed for 12 weeks; 1 patient withdrew early from the study because of side effects from sildenafil. In the remaining 8 patients, there was a 42% improvement in the primary end point of treadmill walking time, and all patients demonstrated an increase. Combination therapy was well tolerated with minimal side effects in the 8 patients who completed the study. In another open-label study, sildenafil, increased to a dose of 25 mg 3 times daily over several weeks, was added in 5 patients receiving epoprostenol for longer than 12 months.[32] These patients were considered nonresponders to epoprostenol (defined by failure to improve FC and mean right atrial pressure increases to ≥8 mm Hg). Improvement in FC and hemodynamics was noted in the 3 patients undergoing repeat evaluation 3 months after adding sildenafil. No increase in transaminases or other side effects were reported.

Randomized Trials

The largest combination study of prostanoids and oral therapy is the PACES study (Pulmonary Arterial Hypertension Combination Study of Epoprostenol and Sildenafil) (see **Table 1**).[33] Two-hundred sixty-seven PAH patients with PAH (79%, IPAH and 17% CTD-associated PAH), were enrolled in this multicenter, double-blind, placebo-controlled 16-week study. Study subjects had to be on a stable dose of epoprostenol for 3 months before entry into the study, and were randomized to receive either sildenafil, starting at a dose of 20 mg 3 times daily and increasing to 80 mg 3 times daily by week 8, or placebo with dummy dose escalations. The primary end point of the study was change in 6MWD, although hemodynamics and time to clinical worsening were also evaluated. Patients were also stratified by baseline 6MWD (<325 or ≥325 m). Ten of 133 patients randomized to the placebo group did not complete the study (2 were not treated and 8 were lost to follow-up), whereas only 1 of 134 patients in the sildenafil group did not complete the study. The median dose of epoprostenol at randomization was similar in both groups, and the mean duration of treatment was close to 3 years for both groups.

The patients treated with sildenafil demonstrated a significantly greater improvement in 6MWD at 16 weeks compared with the control group, 29.8 m versus 1.0 m (P<.001). Most of the improvement occurred in patients with a baseline walk of 325 m or further, with a placebo-adjusted increase of 39.9 m (95% CI 24.4–55.5 m) compared with only 3.0 m (95% CI 32.3–38.4 m) in those patients with a baseline walk of less than 325 m. Hemodynamic improvement, while modest in both arms, was significantly greater in the sildenafil group. Eight patients receiving sildenafil, compared with 24 in the placebo group, had clinical worsening during the study (P = .002). Of note, 7 deaths occurred in the placebo group in comparison with none in the sildenafil group. All 7 patients had severe disease with a mean walk of 182 m (range 108–238 m), considerably less than the entire group. Several side effects observed

previously with sildenafil occurred more frequently in the active treatment group, including headache, dyspepsia and nausea; however, more patients in the placebo group than in the sildenafil group (14 vs 7 patients) discontinued the study because of side effects.

The PACES study demonstrated improvement in exercise capacity, hemodynamics, and survival with the addition of sildenafil in patients treated chronically with epoprostenol therapy. Although the increase in 6MWD is greater than in most combination studies, the results are mitigated somewhat by the fact that patients were treated with 80 mg sildenafil 3 times daily, whereas the approved dose is only 20 mg 3 times daily; therefore, it is unknown how effective adjunctive sildenafil at the approved dose would be in patients treated with chronic epoprostenol. The PACES study is only the second study in PAH patients to show a survival benefit; however, survival was not a prespecified end point.

The TRIUMPH-1 study was a randomized, placebo-controlled clinical trial in 235 PAH patients, which evaluated the safety and efficacy of inhaled treprostinil added to either chronic therapy with bosentan or sildenafil.[27] This trial is discussed in more detail in the section on prostacyclin analogues + ERAs. Only about 30% of patients in the study were receiving sildenafil. Although this study demonstrated improved exercise capacity with the addition of inhaled treprostinil for the entire study group, patients on background sildenafil therapy did not show significant improvement in peak 6MWD at weeks 6 or 12 of the study (between-treatment median difference of 11 and 9 m, P not significant). As it was not designed to assess for differences in response between background sildenafil and bosentan therapy, definitive conclusions cannot be made from this study regarding the combination of inhaled treprostinil and sildenafil therapy.

ORAL COMBINATION THERAPY

Oral combination therapy is an attractive option for practitioners treating PAH. PDE5-Is (sildenafil and tadalafil) and ERAs (ambrisentan and bosentan) have been used in combination extensively in PAH management. Oral combination therapy is generally well tolerated and offers patient convenience with relatively infrequent dosing. It is frequently used in large PH centers, as demonstrated by the REVEAL registry,[15] and also in the community, where recent work has shown that dual oral therapy is used in as much as 28% of patients.[34,35] Although commonly used in the treatment of PAH, there are few published randomized trials, and those that do exist involve small numbers of patients. For this reason, there remain many unanswered questions about oral combination therapy in PAH. This section summarizes prior clinical experience with, and clinical trial data supporting, oral combination therapy, mainly with PDE5-Is and ERAs, although there are several recent studies presenting data on newer oral agents.

Although there is potential benefit to targeting different pathways in PAH, it is possible that there may be a drug-drug interaction that limits plasma levels or efficacy of one or another drug class. Initial oral-therapy combination studies focused on sildenafil and bosentan, as these were initially the only options in their respective drug classes. Paul and colleagues[36] demonstrated in PAH patients that treatment with bosentan was associated with an increase in sildenafil clearance, thereby decreasing sildenafil plasma levels. These findings were recapitulated with tadalafil and bosentan in healthy volunteers, in whom tadalafil plasma levels decreased with bosentan coadministration.[37] Sildenafil is known to be eliminated by the cytochrome P450 enzyme CYP3A4, whose expression is induced by bosentan in the liver.[35] Thus the putative mechanism for the drug-drug interaction is through increased CYP3A4 expression driving higher clearance of PDE5-Is. Ambrisentan, by contrast, does not induce CYP3A4, and when administered in combination with tadalafil in healthy volunteers has not been shown to decrease PDE5-I concentrations.[38] Despite these theoretical concerns, in clinical use there does not appear to be a meaningful drug-drug interaction between any of the PDE5-Is and ERAs. This finding was corroborated by a study of invasive hemodynamics in PAH patients on chronic therapy with bosentan in whom acute sildenafil and inhaled nitric oxide pulmonary vascular responses were compared.[39] Both inhaled nitric oxide and oral sildenafil decreased PVR similarly, suggesting no important acute attenuation of sildenafil's efficacy in the pulmonary vasoconstriction.

Small or Nonrandomized Trials and Case Series

There are several published case series of sequential addition of PDE5-Is and ERAs in PAH patients, usually sildenafil added to bosentan.[40–44] Initial reports demonstrated that the addition of sildenafil to bosentan increased 6MWD in general, but the effect may be greater in IPAH patients than in those with scleroderma-associated PAH.[40,41] Keogh and colleagues[42] recently published the effect of sequential combination therapy (primarily the addition of sildenafil

to bosentan) in an Australian PAH cohort of 112 patients, predominantly FC III and IV, deteriorating on oral monotherapy. About half of the patients had IPAH and about a quarter had scleroderma. Twelve months after the addition of a second agent (2 oral agents in 83% of patients), there was marked improvement in 6MWD, with similar improvement in IPAH or heritable PAH (HPAH, increase from 315 ± 122 to 407 ± 138 m) and scleroderma (from 285 ± 103 to 374 ± 119 m). However, 12- and 24-month survival was better in IPAH/HPAH (93% and 79%, respectively), than in scleroderma-related PAH (72% and 48%, respectively). This cohort study design or others like it[45] cannot demonstrate definitively that combination therapy is less effective in scleroderma-associated PAH, but, along with data from Mathai and colleagues,[40] does suggest potentially less efficacy of the combination of bosentan and sildenafil in scleroderma-associated PAH, at least in terms of survival.

Two case series on the combination of bosentan and sildenafil have been published.[46,47] Lunze and colleagues[46] treated 11 PAH patients (6 with congenital heart disease [CHD], 4 with IPAH, 1 with CTEPH) with bosentan and sildenafil, either as combination therapy to start or with sildenafil added on to bosentan therapy, although it is not stated which patients started on combination therapy. Eight of the 11 patients were younger than 18 years. There was improvement in FC, peripheral saturation, Vo_2 uptake, and hemodynamics. More recently, the results of a single-center study of sildenafil added to bosentan were reported in 32 patients with CHD-associated PH.[47] After 6 months of combination therapy, there was mild but significant hemodynamic improvement, most pronounced in the PVR index, which decreased from 24 ± 16 U/m^2 to 19 ± 9 U/m^2 ($P = .003$). There was also an impressive increase in 6MWD from 293 ± 68 m to 360 ± 51 m ($P = .005$). No serious AEs were reported in either of these studies. Although not randomized, the results of these open-label studies and case series suggest that combination therapy with a PDE5-I and ERA is safe and may be beneficial, particularly in IPAH but also in other conditions associated with the development of PAH.

Randomized Trials

There has been one small randomized, placebo-controlled trial of the addition of sildenafil or placebo for patients treated initially with bosentan, which included only CHD-associated PAH.[48] Twenty-one patients were enrolled in the study, all of whom were initially treated with bosentan for

3 months. Following this, sildenafil or placebo was added for 3 months, and patients were then crossed over to the other treatment for the last 3 months. There were no differences between sildenafil and placebo in 6MWD, the primary end point. Oxygen saturation at rest did improve in the sildenafil group (2.9% vs −18% in the placebo group, $P<.01$), potentially suggesting improved pulmonary hemodynamics. There are no publications on the use of combination therapy in other types of associated PAH such as portopulmonary, human immunodeficiency virus, or schistosomiasis.

Although the initial trials of sildenafil and bosentan were placebo controlled and did not allow additional specific PAH therapy,[4,7] more recent studies have frequently included patients on other oral PAH therapy. This trend has allowed additional observations on the efficacy of addition of PDE5-I to ERA in the PHIRST trial (Pulmonary Arterial Hypertension and Response to Tadalafil).[9] In this 16-week, double-blind, placebo-controlled study, 405 patients with PAH (IPAH or associated PAH), either treatment-naïve or on background therapy with the ERA bosentan, were randomized to receive either placebo or tadalafil at 1 of 4 doses. About 60% of patients had IPAH and 20% CTD-associated PAH, and 53% of the patients enrolled in the study were treated with background bosentan. The primary end point of the study was change in 6MWD, and separate analyses of treatment-naïve patients and tadalafil as add-on to bosentan were prespecified. The placebo-adjusted change in treatment-naïve patients receiving tadalafil was 44 m (95% CI 20–69, $P<.01$), substantially greater than the 23 m (95% CI −2 to 48, $P = .09$) for patients on background bosentan, and showed no significant increase in 6MWD after the addition of tadalafil in patients already on background therapy with bosentan.[49] Of importance, this subgroup analysis did not find increased rates of treatment-related AEs in patients in whom tadalafil was added on to bosentan when compared with treatment-naïve patients treated with tadalafil alone. Comparing IPAH and CTD-associated PAH patients on background bosentan therapy, the investigators did find that there was a significant increase in 6MWD with addition of tadalafil in the IPAH patients but not in the CTD-associated PAH patients. This finding echoes the earlier case-series results, and may represent either differences in underlying pathobiology in CTD-associated PAH or other differences in patient phenotype that make this subgroup more difficult to successfully treat, either with monotherapy or combination therapy.

Several recent phase III clinical trials have recently been completed in PAH patients, allowing double or triple combination therapy with oral PDE5-Is, ERAs, or both. These agents include the tissue-selective ERA macitentan, the soluble guanylate cyclase stimulator riociguat, the tyrosine kinase inhibitor imatinib, selexipag (an oral prostaglandin I_2 receptor agonist), and oral treprostinil. Multicenter studies with all of these compounds are well under way, and published results from two studies with imatinib, one with treprostinil and one with selexipag, are presently available. The first study with imatinib was a phase II, 24-week randomized, double-blind, placebo-controlled study of 59 patients with PAH, only 42 of whom completed the trial. Just over 80% of patients had IPAH/HPAH, and one-third of enrollees were treated with the combination of a PDE5-I and ERA.[50] The primary end point of the study was improvement in 6MWD, and there was no difference between those receiving imatinib and those on placebo. There was improvement in hemodynamics in the imatinib cohort, with a greater response in patients starting out with worse hemodynamics. The study did not include a specific subgroup analysis of this cohort, but no increased AEs were reported in this subgroup.

Based on the findings of the initial imatinib study, the IMPRES study (Imatinib in Pulmonary Arterial Hypertension, a Randomized, Efficacy Study) was undertaken.[51] This randomized, double-blind, placebo-controlled trial enrolled 202 patients with severe PAH defined by treatment with 2 or more PAH therapies and a PVR of at least 800 dyn/s/cm^{-5} at screening. Approximately 75% of patients had IPAH/HPAH. Patients received imatinib or placebo for 24 weeks, and 29% of patients were on the combination of ERA and PDE5-I. Overall, there was a statistically significant improvement in the primary end point of change in 6MWD; however, in patients receiving dual oral therapy, the change in 6MWD was not statistically significant. There were also significant hemodynamic improvements in patients receiving imatinib, but no subgroup analysis was reported. Of importance, there was a high rate of subdural hematomas in patients in the imatinib group, who were also receiving warfarin, a finding that has tempered enthusiasm for this drug in the treatment of PAH.

Selexipag was evaluated in a phase II study of 43 PAH patients (IPAH or associated PAH) receiving a PDE5-I and/or an ERA.[52] Patients were randomized 3:1 to receive selexipag or placebo in addition to background therapy and were followed for 17 weeks. The primary end point of the study was percentage change in PVR. Compared with placebo, there was a 30.3% decrease in PVR ($P = .005$). Selexipag was well tolerated, with side effects expected from its pharmacologic effect. A larger phase III study (the GRIPHON trial) is currently under way. Recently, the results of the FREEDOM-C2 study (Efficacy and Safety of Oral UT-15C Tablets to Treat Pulmonary Arterial Hypertension) were published.[53] Oral treprostinil or placebo was added on to background therapy with PDE5-Is and/or ERAs (40% of patients were receiving both), and the primary end point was change in 6MWD after 16 weeks of treatment. Two-thirds of the patients had IPAH/HPAH, and the remainder had associated PAH. The primary end point of the study was not met, with a placebo-corrected median difference in 6MWD of 10 m ($P = .089$). Side effects of prostaglandin medications were common, but tolerated by most patients.

In summary, although there are limited data to support the use of dual oral combination therapy in PAH, this combination is widely used in the community and at academic centers. There are no clinical data to suggest AEs related to dual oral combination therapy or that the combination is poorly tolerated. In the upcoming years, results of larger and longer-lasting (years as opposed to months) placebo-controlled studies will help to clarify whether (1) combination therapy is more effective than single-agent therapy in PAH, (2) combination should be first line or sequentially added, and (3) certain subgroups (eg, CTD-associated PAH) are less likely to achieve benefit from dual oral combination therapy.

COMBINATION THERAPY TO FACILITATE TRANSITION FROM INTRAVENOUS/SUBCUTANEOUS INFUSED THERAPY TO ORAL THERAPY

Whereas combination therapy is most frequently used to prevent disease decline or to improve exercise capacity in deteriorating patients already on PAH therapy, an alternative strategy is to use combinations of oral and infused therapies to facilitate transition to oral therapy alone. Several small studies have shown that a minority of carefully selected, stable patients on intravenous epoprostenol or subcutaneous treprostinil can successfully be transitioned to bosentan monotherapy after a period of dual-agent therapy.[54–57] Other case series have reported the use of sildenafil in combination with infused therapy to successfully wean to oral therapy alone.[58–60] Although the specific infused prostanoid–oral therapy combination used in these studies differed, these case series provide additional support for the safety and feasibility of treatment approaches involving combinations of agents.

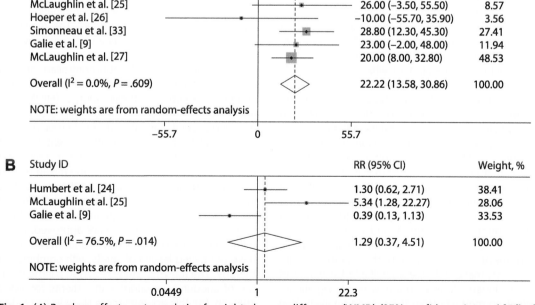

Fig. 1. (*A*) Random-effects meta-analysis of weighted mean difference (WMD) (95% confidence interval [CI]) of 6-minute walking distance: combination therapy versus controls. Sizes of data markers indicate the weight of each study in the analysis. (*B*) Random-effects meta-analysis of relative risk (RR) (95% CI) of functional class improvement: combination therapy versus controls.

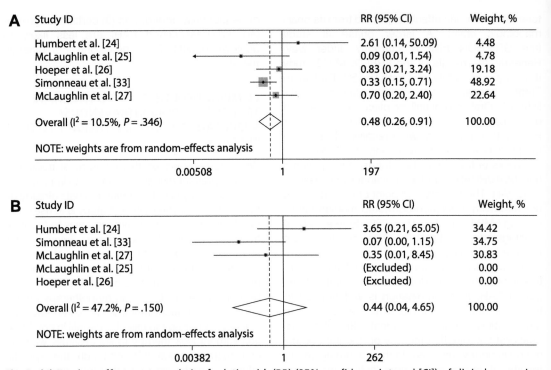

Fig. 2. (*A*) Random-effects meta-analysis of relative risk (RR) (95% confidence interval [CI]) of clinical worsening: combination therapy versus controls. (*B*) Random-effects meta-analysis of RR (95% CI) of mortality: combination therapy versus controls.

COMBINATION THERAPY META-ANALYSIS

There has been one published meta-analysis of randomized controlled trials evaluating combination therapy for PAH.[61] In this study, published before several of the more recent trials reviewed herein, the investigators identified 7 trials meeting their inclusion criteria, 1 of which included only subjects with congenital heart disease that was excluded from the final analysis. The remaining 6 studies,[9,24–27,33] already discussed in detail in this article, included 495 patients in the combination treatment group and 363 patients in the control group. 6MWD was the primary end point in 5 of the 6 studies. Using random-effects modeling, the investigators concluded that combination therapy significantly improved 6MWD and incidence of clinical worsening in comparison with the control group (**Figs. 1** and **2**). Combination therapy did reduce right atrial pressure, PVR, and mPAP compared with the control group; however, these data were available for only 3 of the included studies. There was no significant effect on mortality from the pooled analysis (see **Fig. 2**). Similar to each of the smaller, individual studies, no significant increase in AEs was seen with combination therapy in this meta-analysis.

SUMMARY

Multiple open-label, small, and often single-center studies describing results with combination therapy in PAH have been published. The results of these studies are mixed, although most suggest a benefit without significant toxicity. Several multicenter, randomized, placebo-controlled studies have also been performed, also with mixed results, although the largest of these studies, TRIUMPH-1 and PACES, showed significant improvement in exercise capacity, and the latter in hemodynamics and survival, although with the caveat that the dose of sildenafil used was higher than that approved for use. Regardless of the mixed results of published studies, combination therapy is used in a sizable proportion of patients with PAH and will likely be used in even greater numbers of patients as more drugs for PAH are approved. Other than the BREATHE-2 study, randomized trials have not raised issues of safety with combination therapy. The IMPRES study reported a large number of subdural hematomas in patients receiving imatinib, but this appears more likely to be related to the drug itself rather than combination therapy. Both of these studies enrolled appreciably sick patients with more severe hemodynamic impairment, so this may be an important factor with regard to the severe AEs noted. Several large, long-term studies with a variety of medications should provide more robust data in the near future, especially with regard to oral therapy combinations and up-front versus add-on combination therapy.

REFERENCES

1. Humbert M, Sitbon O, Simonneau G. Treatment of pulmonary arterial hypertension. N Engl J Med 2004;351:1425–36.
2. Barst RJ, Gibbs JS, Ghofrani HA, et al. Updated evidence-based treatment algorithm in pulmonary arterial hypertension. J Am Coll Cardiol 2009;54: S78–84.
3. Barst RJ, Rubin LJ, Long WA, et al. A comparison of continuous intravenous epoprostenol (prosta-cyclin) with conventional therapy for primary pulmonary hypertension. N Engl J Med 1996;334: 296–301.
4. Rubin LJ, Badesch DB, Barst RJ, et al. Bosentan therapy for pulmonary arterial hypertension. N Engl J Med 2002;346:896–903.
5. Simonneau G, Barst RJ, Galie N, et al. Continuous subcutaneous infusion of treprostinil, a prostacyclin analogue, in patients with pulmonary arterial hypertension: a double-blind, randomized, placebo-controlled trial. Am J Respir Crit Care Med 2002; 165:800–4.
6. Galie N, Olschewski H, Oudiz RJ, et al. Ambrisen-tan for the treatment of pulmonary arterial hypertension: results of the ambrisentan in pulmonary arterial hypertension, randomized, double-blind, placebo-controlled, multicenter, efficacy (ARIES) study 1 and 2. Circulation 2008;117:3010–9.
7. Galie N, Ghofrani HA, Torbicki A, et al. Sildenafil citrate therapy for pulmonary arterial hypertension. N Engl J Med 2005;353:2148–57.
8. Olschewski H, Simonneau G, Galie N, et al. Inhaled iloprost for severe pulmonary hypertension. N Engl J Med 2002;347:322–9.
9. Galie N, Brundage BH, Ghofrani HA, et al. Tadalafil therapy for pulmonary arterial hypertension. Circulation 2009;119:2894–903.
10. McLaughlin VV, Archer SL, Badesch DB, et al. ACCF/AHA 2009 expert consensus document on pulmonary hypertension: a report of the American College of Cardiology foundation task force on expert consensus documents and the American Heart Association developed in collaboration with the American College of Chest Physicians; American Thoracic Society, Inc; and the Pulmonary Hypertension Association. J Am Coll Cardiol 2009; 53:1573–619.
11. Schermuly RT, Roehl A, Weissmann N, et al. Combination of nonspecific PDE inhibitors with inhaled prostacyclin in experimental pulmonary hypertension. Am J Physiol Lung Cell Mol Physiol 2001; 281(6):L1361–8.
12. Wilkens H, Guth A, Konig J, et al. Effect of inhaled iloprost plus oral sildenafil in patients with primary pulmonary hypertension. Circulation 2001;104: 1218–22.
13. Ghofrani HA, Wiedemann R, Rose F, et al. Combination therapy with oral sildenafil and inhaled ilo-prost for severe pulmonary hypertension. Ann Intern Med 2002;136:515–22.
14. Kuhn KP, Wickersham NE, Robbins IM, et al. Acute effects of sildenafil in patients with primary pulmonary hypertension receiving epoprostenol. Exp Lung Res 2004;30:135–45.
15. Badesch DB, Raskob GE, Elliott CG, et al. Pulmonary arterial hypertension: baseline characteristics from the reveal registry. Chest 2010;137:376–87.
16. Hoeper MM, Taha N, Bekjarova A, et al. Bosentan treatment in patients with primary pulmonary hypertension receiving nonparenteral prostanoids. Eur Respir J 2003;22:330–4.
17. Seyfarth HJ, Pankau H, Hammerschmidt S, et al. Bosentan improves exercise tolerance and Tei index in patients with pulmonary hypertension and prostanoid therapy. Chest 2005;128:709–13.
18. Channick RN, Olschewski H, Seeger W, et al. Safety and efficacy of inhaled treprostinil as add-on therapy to bosentan in pulmonary arterial hypertension. J Am Coll Cardiol 2006;48:1433–7.
19. Provencher S, Sitbon O, Humbert M, et al. Long-term outcome with first-line bosentan therapy in idiopathic pulmonary arterial hypertension. Eur Heart J 2006;27:589–95.
20. Kemp K, Savale L, O'Callaghan DS, et al. Usefulness of first-line combination therapy with epoprostenol and bosentan in pulmonary arterial hypertension: an observational study. J Heart Lung Transplant 2012;31(2):150–8.
21. Akagi S, Matsubara H, Miyaji K, et al. Additional effects of bosentan in patients with idiopathic pulmonary arterial hypertension already treated with high-dose epoprostenol. Circ J 2008;72:1142–6.
22. Benza RL, Rayburn BK, Tallaj JA, et al. Treprostinil-based therapy in the treatment of moderate-to-severe pulmonary arterial hypertension: long-term efficacy and combination with bosentan. Chest 2008;134:139–45.
23. Ivy DD, Rosenzweig EB, Lemarie JC, et al. Long-term outcomes in children with pulmonary arterial hypertension treated with bosentan in real-world clinical settings. Am J Cardiol 2010; 106:1332–8.
24. Humbert M, Barst RJ, Robbins IM, et al. Combination of bosentan with epoprostenol in pulmonary arterial hypertension: BREATHE-2. Eur Respir J 2004;24:353–9.

25. McLaughlin VV, Oudiz RJ, Frost A, et al. Randomized study of adding inhaled iloprost to existing bosentan in pulmonary arterial hypertension. Am J Respir Crit Care Med 2006;174:1257–63.

26. Hoeper MM, Leuchte H, Halank M, et al. Combining inhaled iloprost with bosentan in patients with idiopathic pulmonary arterial hypertension. Eur Respir J 2006;28:691–4.

27. McLaughlin VV, Benza RL, Rubin LJ, et al. Addition of inhaled treprostinil to oral therapy for pulmonary arterial hypertension: a randomized controlled clinical trial. J Am Coll Cardiol 2010;55:1915–22.

28. Jimenez Lopez-Guarch C, Escribano Subias P, Tello de Meneses R, et al. Efficacy of oral sildenafil as rescue therapy in patients with severe pulmonary arterial hypertension chronically treated with prostacyclin. Long-term results. Rev Esp Cardiol 2004;57:946–51 [in Spanish].

29. Ruiz MJ, Escribano P, Delgado JF, et al. Efficacy of sildenafil as a rescue therapy for patients with severe pulmonary arterial hypertension and given long-term treatment with prostanoids: 2-year experience. J Heart Lung Transplant 2006;25:1353–7.

30. Ghofrani HA, Rose F, Schermuly RT, et al. Oral sildenafil as long-term adjunct therapy to inhaled iloprost in severe pulmonary arterial hypertension. J Am Coll Cardiol 2003;42:158–64.

31. Gomberg-Maitland M, McLaughlin V, Gulati M, et al. Efficacy and safety of sildenafil added to treprostinil in pulmonary hypertension. Am J Cardiol 2005;96:1334–6.

32. Kataoka M, Satoh T, Manabe T, et al. Oral sildenafil improves primary pulmonary hypertension refractory to epoprostenol. Circ J 2005;69:461–5.

33. Simonneau G, Rubin LJ, Galie N, et al. Addition of sildenafil to long-term intravenous epoprostenol therapy in patients with pulmonary arterial hypertension: a randomized trial. Ann Intern Med 2008;149:521–30.

34. Copher R, Cerulli A, Watkins A, et al. Treatment patterns and healthcare system burden of managed care patients with suspected pulmonary arterial hypertension in the United States. J Med Econ 2012;15:947–55.

35. Angalakuditi M, Edgell E, Beardsworth A, et al. Treatment patterns and resource utilization and costs among patients with pulmonary arterial hypertension in the United States. J Med Econ 2010;13:393–402.

36. Paul GA, Gibbs JS, Boobis AR, et al. Bosentan decreases the plasma concentration of sildenafil when coprescribed in pulmonary hypertension. Br J Clin Pharmacol 2005;60:107–12.

37. Wrishko RE, Dingemanse J, Yu A, et al. Pharmacokinetic interaction between tadalafil and bosentan in healthy male subjects. J Clin Pharmacol 2008;48:610–8.

38. Spence R, Mandagere A, Harrison B, et al. No clinically relevant pharmacokinetic and safety interactions of ambrisentan in combination with tadalafil in healthy volunteers. J Pharm Sci 2009;98:4962–74.

39. Gruenig E, Michelakis E, Vachiery JL, et al. Acute hemodynamic effects of single-dose sildenafil when added to established bosentan therapy in patients with pulmonary arterial hypertension: results of the COMPASS-1 study. J Clin Pharmacol 2009;49:1343–52.

40. Mathai SC, Girgis RE, Fisher MR, et al. Addition of sildenafil to bosentan monotherapy in pulmonary arterial hypertension. Eur Respir J 2007;29:469–75.

41. Porhownik NR, Al-Sharif H, Bshouty Z. Addition of sildenafil in patients with pulmonary arterial hypertension with inadequate response to bosentan monotherapy. Can Respir J 2008;15:427–30.

42. Keogh A, Strange G, Kotlyar E, et al. Survival after the initiation of combination therapy in patients with pulmonary arterial hypertension: an Australian collaborative report. Intern Med J 2011;41:235–44.

43. Hoeper MM, Faulenbach C, Golpon H, et al. Combination therapy with bosentan and sildenafil in idiopathic pulmonary arterial hypertension. Eur Respir J 2004;24:1007–10.

44. Minai OA, Arroliga AC. Long-term results after addition of sildenafil in idiopathic PAH patients on bosentan. South Med J 2006;99:880–3.

45. Launay D, Sitbon O, Le Pavec J, et al. Long-term outcome of systemic sclerosis-associated pulmonary arterial hypertension treated with bosentan as first-line monotherapy followed or not by the addition of prostanoids or sildenafil. Rheumatology (Oxford) 2010;49:490–500.

46. Lunze K, Gilbert N, Mebus S, et al. First experience with an oral combination therapy using bosentan and sildenafil for pulmonary arterial hypertension. Eur J Clin Invest 2006;36(Suppl 3):32–8.

47. D'Alto M, Romeo E, Argiento P, et al. Bosentan-sildenafil association in patients with congenital heart disease-related pulmonary arterial hypertension and Eisenmenger physiology. Int J Cardiol 2012;155:378–82.

48. Iversen K, Jensen AS, Jensen TV, et al. Combination therapy with bosentan and sildenafil in Eisenmenger syndrome: a randomized, placebo-controlled, double-blinded trial. Eur Heart J 2010;31:1124–31.

49. Barst RJ, Oudiz RJ, Beardsworth A, et al. Tadalafil monotherapy and as add-on to background bosentan in patients with pulmonary arterial hypertension. J Heart Lung Transplant 2011;30:632–43.

50. Ghofrani HA, Morrell NW, Hoeper MM, et al. Imatinib in pulmonary arterial hypertension patients with inadequate response to established therapy. Am J Respir Crit Care Med 2010;182(9):1171–7.

51. Hoeper MM, Barst RJ, Bourge RC, et al. Imatinib mesylate as add-on therapy for pulmonary arterial hypertension: results of the randomized IMPRES study. Circulation 2013;127:1128–38.

52. Simonneau G, Torbicki A, Hoeper MM, et al. Selexipag: an oral, selective prostacyclin receptor agonist for the treatment of pulmonary arterial hypertension. Eur Respir J 2012;40(4):874–80.

53. Tapson VF, Jing ZC, Xu KF, Rubin On Behalf of the FREEDOM-C2 Study Team. Oral treprostinil for the treatment of pulmonary arterial hypertension in patients on background endothelin receptor antagonist and/or phosphodiesterase type 5 inhibitor therapy (The FREEDOM-C2 study): a randomized controlled trial. Chest 2013;144:952–8.

54. Suleman N, Frost AE. Transition from epoprostenol and treprostinil to the oral endothelin receptor antagonist bosentan in patients with pulmonary hypertension. Chest 2004;126:808–15.

55. Steiner MK, Preston IR, Klinger JR, et al. Conversion to bosentan from prostacyclin infusion therapy in pulmonary arterial hypertension: a pilot study. Chest 2006;130:1471–80.

56. Safdar Z. Outcome of pulmonary hypertension subjects transitioned from intravenous prostacyclin to oral bosentan. Respir Med 2009;103:1688–92.

57. Ivy DD, Doran A, Claussen L, et al. Weaning and discontinuation of epoprostenol in children with idiopathic pulmonary arterial hypertension receiving concomitant bosentan. Am J Cardiol 2004;93:943–6.

58. Johnson RF, Loyd JE, Mullican AL, et al. Long-term follow-up after conversion from intravenous epoprostenol to oral therapy with bosentan or sildenafil in 13 patients with pulmonary arterial hypertension. J Heart Lung Transplant 2007;26:363–9.

59. Keogh AM, Jabbour A, Weintraub R, et al. Safety and efficacy of transition from subcutaneous treprostinil to oral sildenafil in patients with pulmonary arterial hypertension. J Heart Lung Transplant 2007;26:1079–83.

60. Diaz-Guzman E, Heresi GA, Dweik RA, et al. Long-term experience after transition from parenteral prostanoids to oral agents in patients with pulmonary hypertension. Respir Med 2008;102:681–9.

61. Bai Y, Sun L, Hu S, et al. Combination therapy in pulmonary arterial hypertension: a meta-analysis. Cardiology 2011;120:157–65.

Lung Transplantation and Atrial Septostomy in Pulmonary Arterial Hypertension

Stephanie G. Norfolk, MD[a], David J. Lederer, MD, MS[b,c],
Victor F. Tapson, MD[d],*

KEYWORDS

- Pulmonary hypertension • Pulmonary arterial hypertension • Atrial septostomy • Lung transplant
- Heart-lung transplant

KEY POINTS

- Surgical options should be considered for patients with pulmonary hypertension with severe disease or those who are failing medical management.
- Atrial septostomy can be considered at experienced centers for patients with right ventricular failure secondary to pulmonary hypertension who meet criteria.
- Referral for lung transplantation should be considered in all patients receiving maximal medical therapy, or for those with New York Heart Association functional class III or IV or rapidly progressive disease.
- Bilateral lung transplantation and combined heart-lung transplantation are the preferred procedures for pulmonary hypertension, with individualized decisions influenced by patient hemodynamics and individual center practice.

INTRODUCTION

Pulmonary hypertension (PH) is defined as a mean pulmonary artery pressure of greater than or equal to 25 mm Hg during right heart catheterization.[1] The revised World Health Organization (WHO) classification further divides PH into 5 subclasses, groups 1 through 5 (**Box 1**).[1] Group I is pulmonary arterial hypertension (PAH), and this develops as the sequela of vascular remodeling and proliferation leading to increased resistance and right ventricular (RV) compromise and includes a pulmonary capillary wedge pressure (PCWP) less than 15 mm Hg to exclude left heart disease as the underlying cause. Idiopathic PAH (IPAH) is a rare disease with recent registry data in the United Kingdom/Ireland listing an incidence of 1.1 cases per million per year with a prevalence of 6.6 cases

Funding Sources: None.
Conflicts of Interest: Dr S.G. Norfolk, none; Dr D.J. Lederer, consulting for ImmuneWorks related to lung transplantation; Dr V.F. Tapson, (previous 3 years) consulting with companies involved in medical therapy for pulmonary arterial hypertension (Actelion, Bayer, Gilead, Lung LLC, Novartis, United Therapeutics).
a Division of Pulmonary and Critical Care, Duke University Medical Center, DUMC 102342, Durham, NC 27710, USA; b Department of Medicine, Columbia University Medical Center, PH Room 14-104, 622 West 168th Street, New York, NY 10032, USA; c Department of Epidemiology, Columbia University Medical Center, PH Room 14-104, 622 West 168th Street, New York, NY 10032, USA; d Division of Pulmonary and Critical Care, Duke University Medical Center, 330 Trent Drive, Room 128 Hanes House, DUMC 102351, Durham, NC 27710, USA
* Corresponding author.
E-mail address: victor.tapson@dm.duke.edu

Clin Chest Med 34 (2013) 857–865
http://dx.doi.org/10.1016/j.ccm.2013.09.002
0272-5231/13/$ – see front matter © 2013 Elsevier Inc. All rights reserved.

Box 1	
Revised WHO classification of PH	
Group	**Associated Diagnoses**
1	Pulmonary arterial hypertension Examples: idiopathic, familial, related to connective tissue disease, HIV or anorexigens, congenital shunts, portal hypertension (includes PVOD, PCH)
2	Left-sided (systolic or diastolic dysfunction) heart or valvular disease
3	Parenchymal lung disease and/or hypoxemia Examples: COPD, ILD, OSA
4	Chronic thromboembolic or embolic disease
5	Miscellaneous Examples: sarcoidosis, vascular compression from adenopathy or mass, histiocytosis X, lymphangioleiomyomatosis

Abbreviations: COPD, chronic obstructive pulmonary disease; HIV, human immunodeficiency virus; ILD, interstitial lung disease; OSA, obstructive sleep apnea; PCH, pulmonary capillary hemangiomatosis; PVOD, pulmonary veno-occlusive disease.

Box 2
Risk factors for mortality in PAH

- NYHA functional class III or IV
- Poor 6MWT or cardiopulmonary exercise testing
- High right atrial pressure/low cardiac index
- Clinical evidence of RV failure
- Increased N-terminal pro-BNP/BNP
- Scleroderma

Abbreviation: BNP, brain natriuretic peptide.

per million,[2] and France giving an incidence of 2.4 cases per million per year and 15 cases per million.[3] The Registry to Evaluate Early and Long-term PAH Disease Management (REVEAL), the United States registry, which began enrollment in 2006, identified more than 2500 adult patients in its first year, more than 50% of whom had New York Heart Association (NYHA) functional class III or IV symptoms.[4] The development of novel pharmacologic treatment options over the past 2 decades has significantly improved mortality in group 1 patients.[5] Current estimated survival at 1, 3, and 5 years is 88%, 73%, and 64% respectively, with median survival of 7 years based on recent REVEAL data,[6] compared with 68%, 48%, and 34% with median survival 2.8 years from patients followed in the National Institutes of Health (NIH) registry between 1981 and 1985.[7] However, even with current drug therapy, mortality is estimated at 15% within 1 year of diagnosis[1] in the presence of certain risk factors (**Box 2**). Surgical therapy for PH can include thromboendarterectomy, atrial septostomy, and both heart and lung transplantation and should be considered for patients in the appropriate clinical circumstance. Thromboendarterectomy for group 4 PH is not covered in this article because it is discussed by Marshall and colleagues elsewhere in this issue.

Although patients with underlying parenchymal lung disease in group 3 of the PH classification often have some degree of PH, this article focuses on those patients with group 1 PH (PAH).

ATRIAL SEPTOSTOMY

Atrial septostomy was first described by Rich and Lam[8] in 1983 in a 22-year-old woman with refractory PAH[8] based on the suggestion that patients with PH and a patent foramen ovale had better clinical function based on their right-to-left shunt off-loading a failing right heart. The procedure is performed percutaneously either by using a blade-tipped or a balloon-tipped catheter to create a hole in the right atrium.[9–11] Increased systemic oxygen transport from improved cardiac output can result in improved hemodynamics and functional status. If the left ventricular end-diastolic pressure increases to 18 mm Hg or more or if the saturation of atrial oxygen (Sao_2) decreases more than 10% from baseline or less than 80% on room air the procedure is stopped.[9] Early reports listed associated mortality as high as 16%.[10] However, more recent data show significant improvement in mortality (5.4%) with documented improvement in cardiac index (CI), NYHA function, and decreased right atrial pressure (RAP).[9,12] Law and colleagues,[12] presented data on a series of 43 younger patients (aged 3 months to 30 years, with median age of 12.5 years) in whom they performed 46 procedures and recommended caution in proceeding with patients with a mean RAP of more than 18 mm Hg. In 2011, Sandoval and colleagues[13] published an adult cohort of 34 patients in whom 50 procedures were performed with only 1 periprocedural death and a median survival of 60 months, with 88% of survivors showing clinical improvement and the remaining 12% showing no change. A variety of techniques, including transesophageal and intracardiac ultrasound,[14,15] have been used for a variety of cardiac procedures requiring controlled intra-atrial perforation in an attempt to limit complications such as inadvertent tearing of the septum or perforation of the free wall or other structures. Newer technologies, including radiofrequency ablation, which has come into use at some centers for left atrial catheterization for percutaneous valvuloplasty and ablation procedures,[16–18] are also being used, with a recent Italian cohort of 11 patients with PAH undergoing successful atrial septostomy, albeit with 2 expiring within an 8-month follow-up period.[19] The procedure, which can be considered in patients with group I disease as a palliative measure in refractory disease or as a bridge to transplant, has clear contraindications (**Box 3**). In addition, given the risk of complications, it is recommended that the procedure be done at a facility with a high degree of experience.[20–22]

LUNG AND HEART-LUNG TRANSPLANTATION

The first successful heart-lung transplantation (HLT) was performed in 1981 in a patient with PAH.[23] Lung transplantation and combined HLT remain important surgical options for these patients. Of all HLT procedures performed since 1982, 877 (27.6%) have been performed in patients with PAH, whereas 1064 lung transplant procedures worldwide (3.1% of the total) have been performed for PAH.[24] In the United States, patients with PAH made up 6.9% of the waiting list and accounted for 4.4% of lung transplantations performed in 2011.[25] Transplantation is a controversial therapy for PAH for the following reasons:

Box 3
Contraindications to atrial septostomy[a]

1. Impending death with severe RV failure

2. Mean RAP greater than 20 mm Hg

3. Pulmonary vascular resistance greater than 15 Wood units

4. One-year survival estimated at less than 40%

5. Baseline arterial oxygen saturation less than 90% on room air

[a] Experience with this technique is essential; it is performed for patients with severe pulmonary hypertension with RV compromise, but as RV failure worsens the risk of the procedure increases.

Data from Sandoval J, Rothman A, Pulido T. Atrial septostomy for pulmonary hypertension. Clin Chest Med 2001;22(3):547–60; and Law MA, Grifka RG, Mullins CE, et al. Atrial septostomy improves survival in select patients with pulmonary hypertension. Am Heart J 2007;153(5):779–84.

- Lung transplantation for PAH is associated with high risks of early complications and mortality compared with outcomes after lung transplantation for other indications, such as interstitial lung disease (ILD) and chronic obstructive pulmonary disease (COPD).
- Patients with PAH may not be appropriately prioritized on the lung transplant waiting list in the United States.
- Because of variation in referral practices around the United States, some patients with PAH are referred for lung transplantation with end-stage disease, when they may be too sick to safely undergo lung transplantation.

Data on waiting lists and posttransplant outcomes of adults with PAH are discussed later, followed by recommendations for the timing of referral for lung transplantation.

WAITING LIST OUTCOMES IN PAH

In the past, waiting list times among different transplant centers have been variable.[25] Until May 2005, priority for lung transplantation in the United States was based on the number of days of waiting time accrued since the patient's placement on the lung transplant waiting list; a candidate who had been on the list for 30 days would have had higher priority than a candidate on the list for 2 days, regardless of clinical acuity.[26] In May 2005, the Organ Procurement and Transplantation Network (OPTN)/United Network of Organ Sharing UNOS) implemented a lung allocation scoring system (LAS) that prioritized candidates based on both medical urgency (predicted waiting list mortality) and transplant benefit (predicted improvement in survival time with lung transplantation).[26] Although waiting times decreased for all groups in the LAS system era, it became clear early on that transplantation rates for patients with PAH (the so-called group B patients in the LAS system) did not improve as much as those with other indications for lung transplantation, such as COPD (group A), cystic fibrosis (CF; group C), and ILD (group D).[25,27] It was not until 2010 that transplantation rates for patients with PAH began to approach those of patients with COPD (**Fig. 1**).[25] Nevertheless, patients with CF and ILD undergo transplantation at rates 2 to 3 times those of patients with PAH (see **Fig. 1**).[25] As a result, in 2011, only 48.4% of patients with PAH received a lung transplant within 1 year of listing, compared with 71.2% for ILD and 63.3% for CF.[25]

The low transplantation rate for patients with PAH has been attributed to shortcomings of the

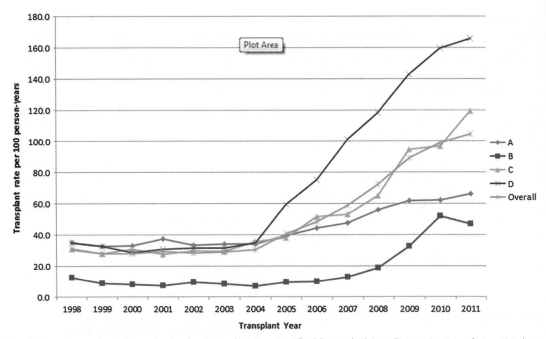

Fig. 1. Lung transplantation rates in the United States stratified by underlying diagnosis. A = obstructive lung diseases; B = pulmonary vascular diseases; C = cystic fibrosis; D = interstitial lung diseases.

LAS, which may not accurately predict mortality in PAH, because measures of RV function are not included.[26] Based on analyses of the REVEAL registry showing increased mortality in patients with idiopathic PAH with a mean RAP greater than or equal to 14 mm Hg or 6-minute walk test (6MWT) distance of 300 m or less,[28] modifications to the LAS, such as inclusion of RAP, CI, brain natriuretic peptide (BNP), and a continuous (rather than binary) 6MWT distance, have been proposed in order to more accurately represent disease-specific risk for this group.[25,27] A soon-to-be-released update to the LAS calculation will include serum bilirubin (reflecting hepatic congestion), interval change in serum bilirubin, central venous pressure, and CI.[29] If inclusion of these measures leads to a more accurate estimation of medical urgency for patients with PAH, transplantation rates for these patients may increase in the coming years.

In line with what is perceived to be an unacceptably long waiting time for transplantation, registry data suggest that the waiting list mortality in PAH may have increased in the LAS era, reversing a downward trend observed before 2006 (**Fig. 2**).[25] Two factors have likely contributed to this finding: removal of healthier patients from the waiting list who were too well for transplantation (thereby diminishing the denominator in the waiting list mortality calculation) and the continued listing of more severely affected individuals at high risk of death without transplantation. Although

unfortunate, particularly for patients with PAH who seem to have had the steepest increase in mortality rates over time, Schaffer and colleagues[30] recently suggested that the risk of death for patients with PAH on the waiting list has decreased in the LAS era. Differences between the Scientific Registry of Transplant Recipients analysis[25] and the latter analysis may be related to the use of a competing risk model in the model by Schaffer and colleagues,[30] an analysis method that may provide more meaningful event rates.

OUTCOMES AFTER LUNG TRANSPLANTATION

Most single-center and registry studies show higher early mortality for patients with PAH undergoing lung transplantation compared with other transplant indications.[26,27] In Franke's single-center study, survival at 30 days as well as at 1 year was significantly lower for patients with idiopathic PAH compared with patients with other subgroups of PH (ie, Eisenmenger and chronic thromboembolic pulmonary hypertension [CTEPH]).[31] More recent data from one center's experience with lung transplant for PH more than 14 years showed significantly decreased 30-day mortality after transplantation for patients transplanted after 2005 compared with earlier years but noted worse 10-year survival for patients with IPAH compared with other transplant recipients (42% compared with 70%; P = .01).[32] The most

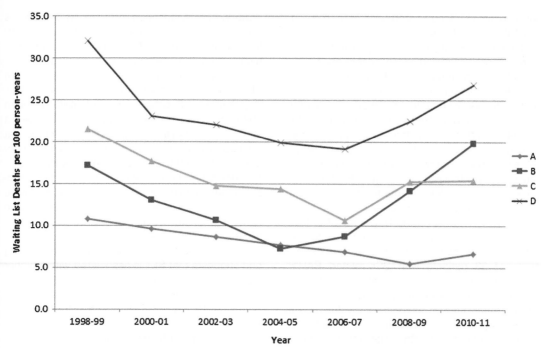

Fig. 2. Mortality rates for adults listed for lung transplantation in the United States. A = obstructive lung diseases; B = pulmonary vascular diseases; C = cystic fibrosis; D = interstitial lung diseases.

recent International Society of Heart Lung Transplantation (ISHLT) registry report, which includes survival data for worldwide transplant recipients since 1990, shows that patients with IPAH have the lowest 1-year (70%) and 3-year (59%) survival rates among all disease groups.[24] US data from the 2005 to 2006 cohort suggests better survival for patients with IPAH: 1-year survival of 78% and 3-year survival of 66%.[25] Much of the earlier mortality among patients with PAH is attributable to a high rate of primary graft dysfunction (a form of ischemia-reperfusion pulmonary edema that occurs within the first 72 hours of lung transplantation and shares key clinical and pathologic features with the acute respiratory distress syndrome).[33] In a recent multicenter prospective cohort study of more than 1300 lung transplant recipients, PAH was independently associated with an odds ratio of 3.5 for primary graft dysfunction.[33] Furthermore, several additional independent risk factors for primary graft dysfunction, such as bilateral (vs single) lung transplantation, use of intraoperative cardiopulmonary bypass, and blood product transfusion, are almost universally present in patients with PAH undergoing lung transplantation.[33] Additional risk factors for primary graft dysfunction include longer cold ischemic time,[34] pretransplantation obesity,[35] and use of lungs from a donor with a history of cigarette smoking.[33] Transplant surgery for patients with PAH is often complicated by bleeding, the

need for cardiopulmonary bypass, and hemodynamic instability. Despite poorer early outcomes, medium-term and long-term survival rates for patients with PAH after lung transplantation are similar to survival rates for patients undergoing transplantation for other indications,[21] including risks of acute and chronic rejection.[36–38] Increasing evidence supports the use of azithromycin to slow the development and/or progression of chronic rejection.[39,40]

Patients with connective tissue disease (CTD)–related PAH have additional potential risk factors that must be taken into consideration, specifically the incidence of esophageal dysmotility. Pre-LAS revision data showed increased waiting list mortality but no statistically significant mortality increase in patients with CTD-related PAH after transplant[26]; more recent data from the REVEAL registry show that although patients with CTD-related PAH have improved 1-year survival overall compared with those with idiopathic disease, patients with systemic sclerosis (SSc)-PAH had the lowest 1-year survival compared with other CTD-PAH subgroups.[41] Although the incidence of PAH in patients with rheumatoid arthritis, dermatomyositis and polymyositis, and lupus is ill defined,[42,43] the incidence in some registries of PAH associated with SSc is as high as 73% with 3-year survival in these patients significantly less than in those with lupus and dermatomyositis or polymyositis (47% compared with 74%, $P = .01$, and 100%, $P = .03$, respectively).[43]

Studies have suggested progression of pulmonary parenchymal disease secondary to uncontrolled gastroesophageal reflux disease (GERD) and microaspiration, and evaluation of patients with SSc with concomitant severe esophageal dysfunction indicates progression of ILD compared with their counterparts with only mild to moderate dysmotility.[44] Data suggesting recurrence of acute rejection and worsening lung function after transplant in patients with GERD have led some centers to refer patients for early Nissen in the preoperative or perioperative period.[45–47] Some centers, including the University of California at San Francisco, have published data that indicate similar survival statistics at 3 years in a group of 23 patients with SSc-related PAH[48]; they also noted no significant difference in rates of acute rejection or bronchiolitis obliterans score (BOS). Equal rates of esophageal dysfunction in the SSc group in this retrospective cohort were noted compared with other patients with CTD-related PAH at the same center (52% vs 41%, $P = .47$). Data on early fundoplication in 11 patients with CTD who underwent transplantation from the same center did not yield increased complications at the end of their 24-month follow-up period in terms of acute rejection episodes or BOS, although sample size was limited; however, 10 of the 11 patients were still alive at the end of the follow-up period.[48] Given the degree of esophageal involvement in the SSc group, estimated at between 6% and 60%,[41] evaluation of esophageal function in these patients is considered to be of prime importance.[47–49]

TYPE OF TRANSPLANT PROCEDURE

Discussion regarding optimal surgical treatment (single lung transplantation [SLT] vs bilateral lung transplantation [BLT] vs HLT) is ongoing and center dependent. In a 2001 review of transplant centers in the United States, Canada, Europe, and Israel, bilateral lung transplantation was preferred in the United States whereas HLT was preferred in Europe and Israel.[25] Franke and colleagues,[31] compared outcomes in 63 patients with IPAH, secondary PH, CTEPH, and Eisenmenger who underwent transplantation between 1988 and 1998 at their center in Germany. Of the patients with IPAH, there was lower survival with BLT versus HLT, but this finding did not reach statistical significance.[31] There is evidence that patients undergoing SLT for PH show signs of RV functional recovery,[50] which supports the possibility of SLT as well as the need for HLT only in cases of profound RV dysfunction. A review of 58 patients with IPAH and secondary PH who underwent transplantation at the University of Pittsburgh between 1989 and 1996 showed no statistically significant survival benefit of BLT compared with SLT.[51] However, subsequent data from Johns Hopkins on 57 patients transplanted between 1995 and 2000, 15 of whom had IPAH, showed a statistically significant survival advantage at 4 years in those who had received bilateral lung transplants (100% compared with 50%, $P<.001$).[52] Ninety five percent of lung transplants performed in 2010 for PH were bilateral and there was a statistically significant survival advantage compared with patients undergoing SLT ($P<.0003$) based on recent ISHLT data.[24] A subsequent analysis of UNOS data confirms this finding and suggests that SLT is associated with a higher mortality than BLT for PAH.[53] Given the limited number of organs available for transplantation, combined HLT is generally reserved for those patients in the United States with congenital heart disease or left ventricular failure.

RECOMMENDATIONS FOR TIMING OF REFERRAL AND LISTING FOR LUNG TRANSPLANTATION

Box 4 presents criteria for referral for lung transplant evaluation and listing in patients with PH as established by the ISHLT in 2006.[54,55] Based on the authors' clinical experience, we recommend referring patients with PAH for lung transplant

---

Box 4
ISHLT lung transplantation selection guidelines in PAH

Referral Criteria	Transplant Criteria
NYHA functional class III or IV	Persistent NYHA functional class III or IV despite maximal medical therapy
Rapidly progressive disease	Low (less than 350 m) or declining 6MWT
	Failure of intravenous epoprostenol or equivalent
	CI less than 2 L/min/meter²
	Mean RA pressure greater than 15 mm Hg

Abbreviation: RA, right atrial.
Data from Orens JB, Estenne M, Arcasoy S, et al. International guidelines for the selection of lung transplant candidates: 2006 update–a consensus report from the Pulmonary Scientific Council of the International Society for Heart and Lung Transplantation. J Heart Lung Transplant 2006;25(7):745–55.

evaluation once they meet one or more of the following criteria:

- Patients receiving parenteral prostanoids regardless of symptoms or NYHA functional class
- Patients with NYHA functional class III or IV symptoms despite escalating therapy
- Patients with rapidly progressive disease
- Patients with known or suspected pulmonary veno-occlusive disease or pulmonary capillary hemangiomatosis, given the lack of viable medical therapies and poor prognosis

Although newer therapies for PAH have improved survival, when these drugs are failing, patients should be transplanted.

SUMMARY

Surgical options for PH to other than CTEPH include atrial septostomy and lung transplantation as well as combined HLT. Atrial septostomy should be considered for suitable patients with significant RV compromise as a palliative measure or bridge to transplantation. Transplant referral should be considered for any patient with high NYHA functional impairment or rapidly progressive disease. Given the high mortality that can be associated with the disease, referral for transplantation should be considered early. If the patient is able to be stabilized on medical therapy, the need for transplantation may be delayed if not obviated. Type of transplant (single vs bilateral vs heart-lung) depends on patient characteristics and center preference.

REFERENCES

1. McLaughlin VV, Archer SL, Badesch DB, et al. ACCF/AHA 2009 expert consensus document on pulmonary hypertension: a report of the American College of Cardiology Foundation Task Force on Expert Consensus Documents and the American Heart Association developed in collaboration with the American College of Chest Physicians; American Thoracic Society, Inc.; and the Pulmonary Hypertension Association. J Am Coll Cardiol 2009; 53(17):1573–619.

2. Ling Y, Johnson MK, Kiely DG, et al. Changing demographics, epidemiology, and survival of incident pulmonary arterial hypertension: results from the pulmonary hypertension registry of the United Kingdom and Ireland. Am J Respir Crit Care Med 2012;186(8):790–6.

3. Humbert M, Sitbon O, Chaouat A, et al. Pulmonary arterial hypertension in France: results from a national registry. Am J Respir Crit Care Med 2006;173(9):1023–30.

4. Badesch DB, Raskob GE, Elliott CG, et al. Pulmonary arterial hypertension: baseline characteristics from the REVEAL Registry. Chest 2010;137(2): 376–87.

5. Shapiro SM, Oudiz RJ, Cao T, et al. Primary pulmonary hypertension: improved long-term effects and survival with continuous intravenous epoprostenol infusion. J Am Coll Cardiol 1997;30(2):343–9.

6. Benza RL, Miller DP, Barst RJ, et al. An evaluation of long-term survival from time of diagnosis in pulmonary arterial hypertension from the REVEAL Registry. Chest 2012;142(2):448–56.

7. D'Alonzo GE, Barst RJ, Ayres SM, et al. Survival in patients with primary pulmonary hypertension. Results from a national prospective registry. Ann Intern Med 1991;115(5):343–9.

8. Rich S, Lam W. Atrial septostomy as palliative therapy for refractory primary pulmonary hypertension. Am J Cardiol 1983;51(9):1560–1.

9. Sandoval J, Gaspar J, Pulido T, et al. Graded balloon dilation atrial septostomy in severe primary pulmonary hypertension. A therapeutic alternative for patients nonresponsive to vasodilator treatment. J Am Coll Cardiol 1998;32(2):297–304.

10. Rothman A, Beltran D, Kriett JM, et al. Graded balloon dilation atrial septostomy as a bridge to lung transplantation in pulmonary hypertension. Am Heart J 1993;125(6):1763–6.

11. Kerstein D, Levy PS, Hsu DT, et al. Blade balloon atrial septostomy in patients with severe primary pulmonary hypertension. Circulation 1995;91(7): 2028–35.

12. Law MA, Grifka RG, Mullins CE, et al. Atrial septostomy improves survival in select patients with pulmonary hypertension. Am Heart J 2007;153(5): 779–84.

13. Sandoval J, Gaspar J, Pena H, et al. Effect of atrial septostomy on the survival of patients with severe pulmonary arterial hypertension. Eur Respir J 2011;38(6):1343–8.

14. Unger P, Stoupel E, Vachiery JL, et al. Atrial septostomy under transesophageal guidance in a patient with primary pulmonary hypertension and absent right superior vena cava. Intensive Care Med 1996;22(12):1410–1.

15. Bidoggia H, Maciel JP, Alvarez JA. Transseptal left heart catheterization: usefulness of the intracavitary electrocardiogram in the localization of the fossa ovalis. Cathet Cardiovasc Diagn 1991; 24(3):221–5.

16. Esch JJ, Triedman JK, Cecchin F, et al. Radiofrequency-assisted transseptal perforation for electrophysiology procedures in children and adults with repaired congenital heart disease. Pacing Clin Electrophysiol 2013;36(5):607–11.

17. Sakata Y, Feldman T. Transcatheter creation of atrial septal perforation using a radiofrequency transseptal system: novel approach as an alternative to transseptal needle puncture. Catheter Cardiovasc Interv 2005;64(3):327–32.

18. Sherman W, Lee P, Hartley A, et al. Transatrial septal catheterization using a new radiofrequency probe. Catheter Cardiovasc Interv 2005;66(1):14–7.

19. Baglini R. Atrial septostomy in patients with end-stage pulmonary hypertension. No more needles but wires, energy and close anatomical definition. J Interv Cardiol 2013;26(1):62–8.

20. Sandoval J, Rothman A, Pulido T. Atrial septostomy for pulmonary hypertension. Clin Chest Med 2001; 22(3):547–60.

21. Klepetko W, Mayer E, Sandoval J, et al. Interventional and surgical modalities of treatment for pulmonary arterial hypertension. J Am Coll Cardiol 2004;43(12 Suppl S):73S–80S.

22. Barst RJ, Gibbs JS, Ghofrani HA, et al. Updated evidence-based treatment algorithm in pulmonary arterial hypertension. J Am Coll Cardiol 2009; 54(Suppl 1):S78–84.

23. Reitz BA. The first successful combined heart-lung transplantation. J Thorac Cardiovasc Surg 2011; 141(4):867–9.

24. Christie JD, Edwards LB, Kucheryavaya AY, et al. The Registry of the International Society for Heart and Lung Transplantation: 29th adult lung and heart-lung transplant report-2012. J Heart Lung Transplant 2012;31(10):1073–86.

25. Valapour M, Paulson K, Smith JM, et al. OPTN/SRTR 2011 Annual Data Report: lung. Am J Transplant 2013;13(Suppl 1):149–77.

26. Egan TM, Murray S, Bustami RT, et al. Development of the new lung allocation system in the United States. Am J Transplant 2006;6(5 Pt 2): 1212–27.

27. Chen H, Shiboski SC, Golden JA, et al. Impact of the lung allocation score on lung transplantation for pulmonary arterial hypertension. Am J Respir Crit Care Med 2009;180(5):468–74.

28. Benza RL, Miller DP, Frost A, et al. Analysis of the lung allocation score estimation of risk of death in patients with pulmonary arterial hypertension using data from the REVEAL Registry. Transplantation 2010;90(3):298–305.

29. Chan KM. Idiopathic pulmonary arterial hypertension and equity of donor lung allocation in the era of the lung allocation score. Am Journal Respir Crit Care Med 2009;180:385–7.

30. Schaffer JM, Singh SK, Joyce DL, et al. Transplantation for idiopathic pulmonary arterial hypertension: improvement in the lung allocation score era. Circulation 2013;127:2503–13.

31. Franke U, Wiebe K, Harringer W, et al. Ten years experience with lung and heart-lung transplantation

32. de Perrot M, Granton JT, McRae K, et al. Outcome of patients with pulmonary arterial hypertension referred for lung transplantation: a 14-year single-center experience. J Thorac Cardiovasc Surg 2012;143(4):910–8.

33. Diamond JM, Lee JC, Kawut SM, et al. Clinical risk factors for primary graft dysfunction after lung transplantation. Am J Respir Crit Care Med 2013; 187:527–84.

34. Thabut G, Mal H, Cerrina J, et al. Graft ischemic time and outcome of lung transplantation: a multicenter analysis. Am J Respir Crit Care Med 2005; 171(7):786–91.

35. Lederer DJ, Kawut SM, Wickersham N, et al. Obesity and primary graft dysfunction after lung transplantation: the Lung Transplant Outcomes Group Obesity Study. Am J Respir Crit Care Med 2011;184(9): 1055–61.

36. Bando K, Paradis IL, Komatsu K, et al. Analysis of time-dependent risks for infection, rejection, and death after pulmonary transplantation. J Thorac Cardiovasc Surg 1995;109(1):49–57 [discussion: 57–9].

37. Boehler A, Estenne M. Obliterative bronchiolitis after lung transplantation. Curr Opin Pulm Med 2000; 6(2):133–9.

38. Kroshus TJ, Kshettry VR, Savik K, et al. Risk factors for the development of bronchiolitis obliterans syndrome after lung transplantation. J Thorac Cardiovasc Surg 1997;114(2):195–202.

39. Yates B, Murphy DM, Forrest IA, et al. Azithromycin reverses airflow obstruction in established bronchiolitis obliterans syndrome. Am J Respir Crit Care Med 2005;172(6):772–5.

40. Gerhardt SG, McDyer JF, Girgis RE, et al. Maintenance azithromycin therapy for bronchiolitis obliterans syndrome: results of a pilot study. Am J Respir Crit Care Med 2003;168(1):121–5.

41. Chung L, Liu J, Parsons L, et al. Characterization of connective tissue disease-associated pulmonary arterial hypertension from REVEAL: identifying systemic sclerosis as a unique phenotype. Chest 2010;138(6):1383–94.

42. Fagan KA, Badesch DB. Pulmonary hypertension associated with connective tissue disease. Prog Cardiovasc Dis 2002;45(3):225–34.

43. Condliffe R, Kiely DG, Peacock AJ, et al. Connective tissue disease-associated pulmonary arterial hypertension in the modern treatment era. Am J Respir Crit Care Med 2009;179(2): 151–7.

44. Marie I, Dominique S, Levesque H, et al. Esophageal involvement and pulmonary manifestations in systemic sclerosis. Arthritis Rheum 2001;45(4): 346–54.

in primary and secondary pulmonary hypertension. Eur J Cardiothorac Surg 2000;18(4):447–52.

45. Hadjiliadis D, Duane Davis R, Steele MP, et al. Gastroesophageal reflux disease in lung transplant recipients. Clin Transplant 2003;17(4):363–8.

46. Gasper WJ, Sweet MP, Golden JA, et al. Lung transplantation in patients with connective tissue disorders and esophageal dysmotility. Dis Esophagus 2008;21(7):650–5.

47. Hoppo T, Jarido V, Pennathur A, et al. Antireflux surgery preserves lung function in patients with gastroesophageal reflux disease and end-stage lung disease before and after lung transplantation. Arch Surg 2011;146(9):1041–7.

48. Sottile PD, Iturbe D, Katsumoto TR, et al. Outcomes in systemic sclerosis-related lung disease after lung transplantation. Transplantation 2013; 95(7):975–80.

49. Hassoun PM. Pulmonary arterial hypertension complicating connective tissue diseases. Semin Respir Crit Care Med 2009;30(4):429–39.

50. Kramer MR, Valantine HA, Marshall SE, et al. Recovery of the right ventricle after single-lung transplantation in pulmonary hypertension. Am J Cardiol 1994;73(7):494–500.

51. Gammie JS, Keenan RJ, Pham SM, et al. Single-versus double-lung transplantation for pulmonary hypertension. J Thorac Cardiovasc Surg 1998; 115(2):397–402 [discussion: 402–3].

52. Conte JV, Borja MJ, Patel CB, et al. Lung transplantation for primary and secondary pulmonary hypertension. Ann Thorac Surg 2001;72(5):1673–9 [discussion: 1679–80].

53. Force SD, Kilgo P, Neujahr DC, et al. Bilateral lung transplantation offers better long-term survival, compared with single-lung transplantation, for younger patients with idiopathic pulmonary fibrosis. Ann Thorac Surg 2011;91:244–9.

54. Orens JB, Estenne M, Arcasoy S, et al. International guidelines for the selection of lung transplant candidates: 2006 update-A consensus report from The Pulmonary Scientific Council of the International Society for Heart and Lung Transplantation. J Heart Lung Transplant 2006;25(7):745–55.

55. Pielsticker EJ, Martinez FJ, Rubenfire M. Lung and heart-lung transplant practice patterns in pulmonary hypertension centers. J Heart Lung Transplant 2001;20(12):1297–304.

Novel Medical Therapies for Pulmonary Arterial Hypertension

Caroline O'Connell, MB[a],*,
Dermot S. O'Callaghan, MB, MD[a],
Marc Humbert, MD, PhD[b,c,d]

KEYWORDS

- Endothelial progenitor cells • Endothelin receptor antagonists • Guanylate cyclase stimulators
- Prostacyclin receptor agonists • Rho-kinase inhibitors • Tyrosine kinase inhibitors

KEY POINTS

- Macitentan (Opsumit) is a new dual endothelin receptor antagonist with reduced risk of hepatotoxicity and drug interactions, that only requires once-daily dosing. The phase III SERAPHIN trial showed this drug reduced a combined morbidity and mortality end point in pulmonary arterial hypertension by 50% compared with controls.
- Previously developed oral prostacyclin analogues have limited efficacy. However, prostacyclin I receptor agonists, of which selexipag (ACT-293987) is the first in class, may be more effective. A phase II study of this orally active agent showed a 30% reduction in pulmonary vascular resistance, and a phase III study is underway.
- Riociguat (BAY63-2521) is a guanylate cyclase stimulator that has demonstrated positive effects on exercise capacity in phase III studies evaluating patients with pulmonary arterial hypertension and chronic thromboembolic pulmonary hypertension.
- Other new potential treatments that require further investigation include rho-kinase inhibitors, dichloroacetate, angiotensin-converting enzyme 2 inhibitors, receptors for advanced glycation end products (RAGE) inhibitors, chemical chaperones for mutations associated with pulmonary arterial hypertension, and endothelial progenitor cells.

INTRODUCTION

Pulmonary arterial hypertension (PAH) is a disease of the pulmonary microvasculature characterized by a pathologic increase in pulmonary vascular resistance (PVR) that eventually causes the right side of the heart to fail.[1] The French pulmonary hypertension registry reported a 3-year survival of 58% for incident cases of idiopathic, familial, or anorexigen-associated PAH diagnosed in early 2002 to 2003.[2] This figure is significantly higher than that reported by the US National Institutes of Health registry in 1991, which found a median survival of 2.8 years in a similar patient group that was studied in the late 1980s before the general availability of targeted therapies for PAH.[3] Although currently licensed agents have been shown to improve patient symptoms, exercise capacity, and pulmonary hemodynamics, a cure for PAH remains elusive and there is an acute need for even more effective treatments.

[a] Department of Respiratory Medicine, Mater Misericordiae University Hospital, 56 Eccles Street, Dublin 7, Ireland; [b] Faculty of Medicine, Paris-South University, 63 rue Gabriel Peri, 94276 Le Kremlin-Bicêtre cedex, France; [c] AP-HP, DHU Thorax Innovation, Department of Respiratory Medicine, Bicêtre Hospital, 78 rue du General Leclerc, 94275 Le Kremlin-Bicêtre cedex, France; [d] INSERM U999, LabEx LERMIT, 133 Avenue de la Resistance, 92350 Le Plessis-Robinson, France
* Corresponding author.
E-mail address: caroline1597@hotmail.com

Clin Chest Med 34 (2013) 867–880
http://dx.doi.org/10.1016/j.ccm.2013.08.002
0272-5231/13/$ – see front matter © 2013 Elsevier Inc. All rights reserved.

Much of the historical PAH research focus was on the detrimental role of endothelial dysfunction and in particular the importance of the imbalance between endothelial-derived vasodilators and vasoconstrictors. These endeavors led to the clinical development and eventual approval of currently available PAH therapies, which variously aim to restore this imbalance by targeting the prostacyclin, nitric oxide (NO), and endothelin pathways, respectively. In general, novel drug development strategies for PAH fall into two broad categories: identification of agents that act on one or more of these three pathways yet have greater efficacy and tolerability than treatments currently in use; and novel drugs that are characterized by enhanced antiproliferative activity that target the intimal fibrosis, smooth muscle hypertrophy and proliferation associated with PAH.

Several candidate drugs are currently being tested and there is hope that over the next decade treatments with greater clinical efficacy will enter the clinical arena (**Table 1**). Encouragingly, most agents under investigation are delivered either orally or by the inhaled route, suggesting that the next era of PAH management will be well-represented by therapies that are more acceptable to patients with respect to modes of administration.

NEW DRUGS IN THE FINAL STAGES OF DRUG DEVELOPMENT
The Endothelin Pathway

Endothelin-1 is a protein that promotes vasoconstriction and smooth muscle proliferation overexpressed in the pulmonary arteries of patients with PAH.[4] Bosentan (Tracleer) and ambrisentan (Volibris; Letairis) are endothelin receptor antagonists (ERA) that act by blocking the deleterious effects of endothelin-1 in the pulmonary microvasculature. Bosentan blocks endothelin receptors A

and B (dual antagonism), whereas ambrisentan preferentially targets the A receptor. Both treatments confer improvements in functional class, exercise capacity, and hemodynamics, and delay time to clinical worsening in patients with PAH. These agents are orally active and generally well tolerated, although both are teratogenic and have the potential to cause elevation in liver transaminases (up to 10% of cases with bosentan).[5]

Macitentan (Opsumit; in review at the Federal Drug Administration; not yet approved) is a new dual ERA that is also taken orally but has higher tissue penetration than bosentan (**Fig. 1**). Prolonged local tissue activity permits single daily dosing. Because macitentan does not interfere with normal bile acid secretion, the risk of hepatotoxicity is reduced.[6] A phase II trial that examined macitentan as a potential therapy for idiopathic pulmonary fibrosis demonstrated that the incidence of liver enzyme abnormalities was similar to that in patients receiving placebo (5.1% and 3.4%, respectively).[7] Moreover, because there is reduced hepatic drug accumulation, potential for drug-drug interaction is lower. In a monocrotaline-induced pulmonary hypertension rat model, macitentan reduced pulmonary artery pressures and right ventricular hypertrophy, and conferred improved survival in comparison with bosentan-treated animals.[8] Macitentan demonstrates dose-dependent pharmacokinetics and in phase I and II trials the most common adverse effect was headache.[9–11] The phase III SERAPHIN trial was a multicenter, double-blind, event-driven study of macitentan that used a combined morbidity and mortality end point and is to date the largest trial carried out in patients with PAH.[12] A total of 742 patients were randomized to either 3 or 10 mg of macitentan or placebo, in addition to usual PAH treatments (other than ERAs). Treatment was continued for up to 3.5 years. The primary end

Table 1
Summary of important clinical trials

Trial	Drug Name	No. of Patients	Length of Study	End Points
SERAPHIN (phase III)	Macitentan	742	3.5 y	45% reduction in morbidity/mortality
FREEDOM-M (phase III)	Treprostinil diethanolamine	349	12 wk	23-m improvement in 6MWD, no change functional class/time to clinical worsening
Phase II	Selexipag	43	17 wk	30% reduction in PVR
PATENT-1 (phase III)	Riociguat	443	12 wk	36-m improvement in 6MWD
IMPRES (phase III)	Imatinib	202	24 wk	6MWD improved 32-m, cardiac output improved 0.88 L/min

Abbreviations: 6MWD, 6-minute walk distance; PVR, pulmonary vascular resistance.

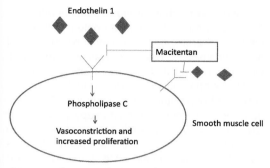

Fig. 1. Mechanism of action of macitentan.

point was reached with a reduction in morbidity/mortality of 30% (P = .0108) and 50% (P<.0001) for the 3- and 10-mg doses of macitentan, respectively, compared with placebo. Both of these doses showed similar adverse event rates. The most common adverse effects were headache, nasopharyngitis, and anemia. Approval of macitentan by regulatory authorities is expected in the near future.

The Prostacyclin Pathway

Prostaglandin I_2 (prostacyclin) is a potent pulmonary vasodilator that also exerts antithrombotic, antiproliferative, antimitogenic, and immunomodulatory activity. The normal production of prostacyclin by endothelial cells from arachidonic acid in the cell membranes is impaired in patients with PAH.[13] Epoprostenol (Flolan) is a synthetic prostacyclin analogue and was the first targeted therapy to be used in PAH after demonstrating a survival advantage compared with placebo. Epoprostenol has a very short half-life (4–5 minutes) that necessitates continuous infusion by an indwelling central venous catheter with the attendant potentially fatal complications of catheter-related bloodstream infections, thrombosis, and catheter dislodgement.[14] Administration of epoprostenol also necessitates a storage cassette that must be changed daily or twice daily. Recently, a thermostable formulation of epoprostenol (Veletri) has been developed, which has the advantage of remaining stable at room temperature for at least 24 hours and only requires cassettes to be changed every second day. This novel preparation is being studied in an open-label, single-arm, safety, efficacy, and quality-of-life study of 20 patients with PAH.[15] Preliminary results of a study testing the effects of switching from the original to the new epoprostenol formulation indicate that transition has no negative effect on hemodynamics or functional class after 3 months.[16]

Although considered the gold standard of PAH treatments, introduction of intravenous or subcutaneous prostanoids in patients with advanced or worsening disease despite oral therapy remains an underused strategy, as demonstrated by data from the US REVEAL registry.[17] An effective orally active prostanoid remains a clear unmet need. Treprostinil diethanolamine (UT-15C) is an oral sustained-release form of treprostinil that is under investigation, although clinical trial experience to date has been disappointing. The safety and efficacy of adding oral treprostinil to a type 5 phosphodiesterase inhibitor (PDE5I) or an ERA was examined in 354 patients with PAH in the phase III placebo-controlled FREEDOM-C trial.[18] The primary end point of change in 6-minute walk distance (6MWD) was not reached, although there was a large dropout rate caused by adverse events that may have impacted results. Even though the subsequent FREEDOM-C2 study used smaller incremental doses,[19] the primary end point was not met with a placebo-adjusted change in median 6MWD of only 10 m (P = .089).[20] A third phase III trial (FREEDOM-M) looked at the efficacy of oral treprostinil monotherapy in 349 patients with PAH. This showed a placebo-adjusted improvement in 6MWD of 23 m (P = .0125) at 12 weeks when performed at peak serum drug levels, but no change in functional class or time to clinical worsening.[21] FREEDOM-EV, a phase III, double-blind, placebo-controlled, event-driven study, will compare the time to clinical worsening in patients with PAH receiving oral treprostinil in combination with a PDE5-I or ERA with a PDE5-I or ERA alone.[22] The study is planned to enroll 858 newly diagnosed patients with PAH. The Food and Drug Administration declined approval of this drug in 2012 because of the lack of evidence of clinical efficacy.

Beraprost is another oral prostacyclin analogue, which was has been approved for use in Japan and Korea. Clinical studies have shown only modest efficacy with this agent,[23] although a sustained-release preparation is being investigated.[24]

A metered dose inhaler formulation of inhaled treprostinil has been tested in a placebo-controlled study of 39 patients with PAH and chronic thromboembolic PH (CTEPH). Acute administration of 30, 45, or 60 µg led to significant reductions in mean pulmonary arterial pressure (mPAP) and PVR, which mirrored the effect of 20 ppm of inhaled NO. Unlike inhaled iloprost, pulmonary selectivity was also confirmed, with patients experiencing no systemic adverse effects, even at higher doses.[25] The efficacy and safety of treprostinil delivered by metered dose inhaler awaits evaluation in a long-term randomized trial.

Selexipag (ACT-293987)

Given the generally disappointing results of trials evaluating oral prostacyclin analogues, investigators have sought to evaluate alternative pharmacologic strategies targeting the prostacyclin pathway. Selexipag is a first in class orally active prostacyclin I receptor agonist that has low affinity for the vasoconstrictor prostaglandin E receptor 3.[26] Selexipag is a prodrug that is activated in the liver resulting in lower tendency to gastrointestinal side effects. A long half-life allows for only twice-daily dosing. In a phase I study of five healthy volunteers, headache was the most common adverse event.[27] A proof of concept phase II multicenter study of 43 patients with PAH showed that 17 weeks of selexipag treatment led to a 30.3% reduction in PVR ($P<.0045$) and an increase in cardiac index (2.4 ± 0.6 L/min/m^2 at baseline; 2.7 ± 0.6 L/min/m^2 at week 17).[28,29] Modest improvements in 6MWD were also observed with treatment, although the study was not designed to analyze this end point. A phase III, multicenter, double-blind, placebo-controlled trial (GRIPHON) looking at time to clinical worsening with selexipag in 1150 patients with PAH is ongoing.[30]

The NO Pathway

NO upregulates cyclic guanosine 5'-monophosphate (cGMP) activity by soluble guanylate cyclase (sGC) resulting in smooth muscle relaxation, inhibition of smooth muscle cell proliferation and platelet aggregation, and activation of proapoptotic pathways.[31] Inhaled NO has demonstrated favorable effects on pulmonary hemodynamics in the acute setting in PAH. Small observational studies have found beneficial effects on hemodynamics, functional class, and brain natriuretic peptide (BNP) levels with continuous pulsed NO delivered by nasal cannula in ambulatory patients with few side effects.[32,33] However, the requirement for continuous administration by means of cumbersome delivery systems limits its potential for use in the outpatient setting.

Phosphodiesterase inhibitors (PDE5I), widely used in the treatment of erectile dysfunction, have also been extensively studied in PAH. This class of agent confers its beneficial effects by acting on the NO signaling pathway, by inhibiting cGMP breakdown to GMP. The PDE5Is sildenafil (Revatio) and tadalafil (Adcirca) have been approved for use in PAH based on positive results from phase III clinical trials.[34,35] Vardenafil (Levitra) is another PDE5I that has demonstrated more potent inhibition of PDE5 than either of the existing licensed agents in pharmacodynamic studies.[36] In

an open-label study involving 45 patients with PAH, 1 year of vardenafil treatment conferred improvements in exercise capacity, functional class, and hemodynamics.[37] The drug was well tolerated, with no withdrawals because of adverse events. A Chinese phase III randomized, double-blind, placebo-controlled study of patients with PAH randomized to vardenafil monotherapy (N = 44) or placebo (N = 22) showed that the treatment group had improved hemodynamics (mean placebo-corrected cardiac index +0.39 L/min/m^2; mPAP −5.3 mm Hg; PVR −4.7 Wood units) and 6MWD (+69 m; $P<.001$) after 12 weeks.[36] Interestingly, those receiving vardenafil were also less likely to develop clinical worsening, although the study was not designed to address this issue. A 12-week open-label continuation phase of the study demonstrated that improvement in exercise capacity was maintained through 24 weeks.[38]

Riociguat (BAY63-2521)

A potential drawback of PDE5I therapy is that activity is mediated downstream of NO, thereby limiting efficacy.[39] Riociguat is a first in class orally active stimulator of sGC that overcomes this issue by increasing sensitivity of sGC to NO.[40] Furthermore, this activity is mediated independent of NO levels (**Fig. 2**). Administration of riociguat to a Sugen5416 and hypoxia rat model of pulmonary hypertension resulted in greater improvements in hemodynamics and reduction of pulmonary vascular remodeling compared with sildenafil.[41]

A preliminary acute hemodynamic study showed that riociguat conferred greater improvements in PVR, mPAP, and cardiac output compared with inhaled NO in 19 patients with moderate to severe pulmonary hypertension of different etiologies (PAH, distal CTEPH, and patients with pulmonary hypertension caused by interstitial lung disease).[40] A phase II, multicenter, open-label study of 74 patients with functional class II to III PAH or CTEPH showed reduced PVR (−215 dyn.s.cm^{-5} from baseline; $P<.0001$); improved 6MWD (+55 m; $P<.0001$); and NT-proBNP levels (−212.83 pg/ml; $P<.0001$).[42] An extension study showed that these improvements persisted for 15 months.[43]

An important side effect of riociguat is a tendency for reduction in systolic blood pressure. Although patients generally develop tolerance to this over time, dose titration must nevertheless be undertaken with caution. However, at doses of 2.5 mg thrice daily or less, treatment is generally well tolerated, with dyspepsia, headache, and nasal congestion the most common adverse effects. A phase III, randomized, multicenter,

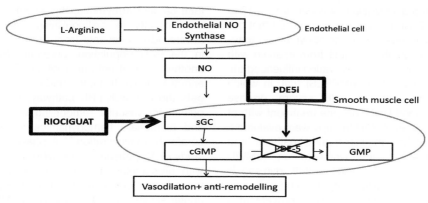

Fig. 2. Mechanism of action of riociguat.

placebo-controlled study of riociguat (PATENT-1) enrolled 443 patients who were either treatment naive or on background ERA or nonintravenous prostanoid therapy.[44] The primary efficacy end point was reached, with treated patients showing a placebo-adjusted improvement in 6MWD of 36 m (P<.0001) after 12 weeks. There were also statistically significant improvements in PVR, functional class, NT-proBNP levels, and time to clinical worsening, with no unexpected adverse drug effects observed. Results from the extension phase of this study, PATENT-2, are expected in late 2013.

CHEST-1 was a phase III multicenter study involving 261 patients with either inoperable or persistent CTEPH post–pulmonary endarterectomy randomized to receive riociguat or placebo. After 16 weeks, the primary end point of a significant improvement in exercise capacity was reached in the treatment group (6MWD improved by 46 m; P<.0001).[45] A 5-year extension study is also planned. Although it is reasonable to imagine that riociguat and PDE5Is might act synergistically, use of such a combination may be limited by systemic hypotension.[46] The PATENT-PLUS phase II trial should help clarify if this risk is excessive or not.[47] Regulatory approval in the United States and Europe for riociguat is expected to be granted shortly.

β-Blockers

It is currently generally recommended that β-adrenergic receptor blockers be avoided in pulmonary hypertension because of known negative inotropic effects. However, as has been clearly demonstrated in left heart failure, there are emerging data suggesting potential merit in such a treatment approach for pulmonary hypertensive patients. In a monocrotaline rat model, bisoprolol (Cardicor) administration helped delay development of right heart failure and was associated

with preservation of right ventricular function.[48] Data from a recent prospective study of 94 patients with PAH also found no difference in mortality rates, presence of heart failure, 6MWD, or hemodynamics whether or not this class of drug was part of background therapy.[49] Until more definitive data emerge, however, beta-blockers remain contraindicated in PAH.

NEW DRUGS LESS LIKELY TO REACH CLINICAL USE
Imatinib (Gleevec)

Platelet-derived growth factor (PDGF) is a potent endothelial and smooth muscle mitogen that plays a key role in angiogenesis. Because PDGF receptor expression is increased in the lungs of patients with PAH, blockade of this target has been tested as a potential strategy to reverse vascular remodeling.[50] Imatinib, an oral tyrosine kinase inhibitor (TKI) that binds to the tyrosine kinase domain on PDGF-R, Bcr-Abl kinase, and c-kit, has been evaluated as a potential PAH treatment. Administration of imatinib to monocrotaline rats and mice with hypoxic pulmonary hypertension is associated with reductions in mPAP, right ventricular hypertrophy, and pulmonary vascular remodeling.[51]

In a phase II double-blind, placebo-controlled, 24-week study of 59 patients with idiopathic or heritable PAH and persistent functional class II to IV symptoms despite standard therapy, imatinib failed to significantly improve exercise capacity but did significantly improve hemodynamics.[52] Seventeen patients did not complete the study, although adverse drug effects were not considered contributory. Nausea, headache, and peripheral edema were the most commonly reported problems. Patients receiving imatinib were more likely to develop anemia, which was compensated for by increased mixed venous oxygen levels. A long-term extension phase of the study showed continued improvement in functional class at 12 to 24 months. Post hoc analyses suggested that patients with the most severe hemodynamic impairment derived greatest benefit from imatinib with respect to 6MWD. This observation influenced the design of the phase III (IMPRES) trial, in which 202 high-risk patients with severe disease (PVR>12.5 Wood Units) despite treatment with at least two classes of PAH therapy were evaluated. After 24 weeks, imatinib-treated patients had placebo-corrected improvements in 6MWD (+32 m; P = .002); PVR (−379 dyn.sec^{-5}; $P<.001$); and cardiac output (+0.88 L/min; $P<.001$).[53] However, there was no improvement in time to clinical worsening or quality of life. Furthermore, there was a high number of dropouts from the study, raising concerns regarding the tolerability of the drug. The main adverse effects reported were edema (peripheral, periorbital, and facial); diarrhea; vomiting; hypokalemia; and anemia.

In addition to questions regarding the clinical efficacy of TKIs, there are significant concerns regarding the potential toxicity with this therapeutic class. An increased incidence of subdural hematomas reported in the IMPRES trial has fueled speculation that there may be excessive risk associated with imatinib in PAH. Cardiotoxicity has also been reported in some patients treated by imatinib for chronic myeloid leukemia, although this phenomenon was not observed in the phase II and III PAH trials. Inhibition of bcr-abl has been suggested as a potential mechanism that accounts for the cardiac effects of TKIs, and a redesigned PDGF inhibitor that lacks activity against bcr-abl demonstrated no cardiotoxic effects.[54] Lastly, imatinib is a CYP450 3A4 inhibitor and treatment may result in important potential drug-drug interactions when warfarin, sildenafil, and/or bosentan are coadministered. All of these concerns may ultimately prevent imatinib from becoming approved for clinical use.

Other TKIs

Despite the disappointing clinical experience to date with imatinib, there is ongoing interest in the potential of the TKI class in PAH. Nilotinib (Tasigna) has a different safety profile overall than imatinib, although cases of QT prolongation and sudden cardiac death have been reported.[55] A 24-week multicenter phase II study of nilotinib, with change in PVR as the primary end point, was terminated early because of the death of a study participant after an episode of ventricular tachycardia.[56] Although the Data Monitoring Committee review concluded that it was unlikely that nilotinib caused the development of the ultimately

fatal cardiac arrhythmia, this event underscores the difficulty in distinguishing disease-related severe adverse events from drug-related events in the PAH population. Sorafenib (Nexavar) is another TKI that not only inhibits PDGF, vascular endothelial growth factor, and c-Kit, but also targets the Raf/MEK/ERK pathway. In rat models, pulmonary vascular remodeling was attenuated and pulmonary hemodynamics improved after sorafenib administration.[57] A phase I open-label study of 12 patients with PAH previously treated with prostanoids and/or sildenafil showed that the addition of sorafenib for 16 weeks did not confer significant improvements in 6MWD.[58] The most frequent side effects were diarrhea, hand-foot syndrome, rash, and alopecia. A reduction in cardiac index was also reported. A further caution against the off-label use of this class of drugs is the reports of cases of PAH in patients with chronic myelogenous leukemia receiving the TKI dasatanib.[59,60]

Serotonin

For many years, serotonin has been suspected of playing a pathophysiologic role in PAH. However, serotonin metabolism is complex, with a transporter and several distinct receptors that orchestrate multiple functions in different organ systems. Serotonin causes vasoconstriction, smooth muscle and endothelial cell proliferation, and platelet aggregation; serotonin and its associated 5-hydroxytryptamine-2B receptor are also increased in idiopathic PAH.[61,62] Accordingly, targeting this pathway might be beneficial as a treatment strategy.[63] Several 5-hydroxytryptamine-2B receptor agonists, such as the appetite suppressant fenfluramine, have been withdrawn from the market because of an association with the development of PAH.[64] Another potential therapeutic target is the serotonin transporter, because certain alleles of the transporter have been linked to an increased risk of developing pulmonary hypertension.[65,66] The selective serotonin receptor inhibitor fluoxetine (Prozac) is a serotonin transporter inhibitor that protects against smooth muscle proliferation in animal models.[67] Registry data from the United States indicate that patients treated by selective serotonin receptor inhibitors are overall at reduced risk of development of pulmonary hypertension and have better survival if the disease develops, although compelling evidence of a definite treatment effect is lacking.[68]

Terguride is a type 2 serotonin receptor antagonist and partial dopamine agonist used for treatment of hyperprolactinemia. Preclinical studies have shown terguride has anti-inflammatory, anti-proliferative, and antifibrotic effects and inhibits the development and progression of pulmonary hypertension in animal models.[69] However, a multicenter randomized placebo-controlled phase II trial evaluating the safety and efficacy of terguride at 12 weeks in 84 patients with PAH with functional class II to IV showed no improvement in hemodynamics, time to clinical worsening, or exercise capacity, but an increased incidence of adverse events.[70] It remains to be determined whether targeting serotonin can provide a viable therapeutic option in the future.

Vasoactive intestinal peptide

Vasoactive intestinal peptide (VIP) is a neurotransmitter hormone with vasodilatory, antiproliferative, and anti-inflammatory activity. It binds to VIP receptors 1 and 2 (VPAC1 and VPAC2) and increases intracellular cyclic adenosine monophosphate and cGMP, leading to vasodilation. VIP also downregulates endothelin expression and regulates several genes involved in vascular remodeling, including the bone morphogenetic protein receptor (BMPR) type 2.[71] The wide range of pathways targeted by VIP has led to considerable interest as to its therapeutic potential in PAH. VIP-depleted mice develop pulmonary vascular remodeling and pulmonary hypertension, and these changes are attenuated when VIP is replaced.[72] When compared with oral bosentan, intraperitoneal VIP was more effective at reversing monocrotaline-induced pulmonary hypertension in rats; there is also evidence of a synergistic effect between these two treatments.[73] In patients with PAH, VIP levels are reduced and VIP receptor expression is upregulated.[74]

Aviptadil (Senatek) is a synthetic analogue of VIP that is administered either parenterally or by inhalation. In a 24-week pilot study of eight treatment-naive patients, treatment with inhaled VIP improved hemodynamics (increase in cardiac index by 0.8 L/min/m^2 [$P<.05$] and reduction in mPAP by 10 mm Hg [$P<.01$]); 6MWD (from 296 m to 409 m at 3 months); and dyspnea levels.[74] However, a subsequent phase II study examining the effect of addition of inhaled aviptadil to ERA and PDE5I in 56 patients with pulmonary hypertension failed to meet its primary end point of reduction in PVR after 12 weeks.[75] Furthermore, there was no change observed in 6MWD, BNP levels, or functional class.

Statins

Statins are 3-hydroxy-3-methylglutaryl-coenzyme A reductase inhibitors with pleiotropic effects that are potentially of benefit to patients with PAH. This pharmacologic class is known to promote anti-inflammatory, antioxidant, and antithrombotic effects and is capable of reducing vascular cell proliferation. An additional effect is the blockade of mevalonate and isoprenoid synthesis, which are required for Rho-kinase pathway activation.[76] The relatively low cost, wide availability, and established safety profile of statins make them an especially attractive therapeutic option. Encouraging results using simvastatin in animal models[77,78] prompted investigators to test the potential of this agent as an adjunct to standard PAH therapy in 16 patients. Three months of open-label therapy led to improvements in right ventricular systolic pressures and 6MWD overall.[76] However, subsequent larger trials have shown no consistent benefit with the use of simavastatin in PAH.[79,80] Moreover, in a randomized, placebo-controlled study of 220 patients with PAH and CTEPH, treatment with a low dose (10 mg) of atorvastatin (Lipitor) had no effect on pulmonary hemodynamics or functional class and was associated with a worsening of 6MWD after 6 months.[81]

Cicletanine

Cicletanine is a systemic antihypertensive with vasodilator and diuretic properties that increases vascular NO production, stimulates endothelial NO synthase, increases prostacyclin synthesis, inhibits PDE-1 and -5, blocks calcium channels, and promotes scavenging of endothelial-derived superoxide. Improved hemodynamics was previously found in a small number of patients with chronic obstructive pulmonary disease associated pulmonary hypertension treated with cicletanine.[82] This led to a phase II, randomized, double-blind, placebo-controlled dose-ranging trial of 162 functional class II and III patients with PAH already taking PAH-targeted therapies. However, the primary end point of change in 6MWD did not reach clinical significance, nor did the secondary analyses of functional class, NT-proBNP or hemodynamics.[83] As a result, development of this drug has been terminated.

NEW DRUGS IN THE EARLY STAGES OF DEVELOPMENT
Rho-Kinase Pathway

Rho-kinase is an enzyme that increases calcium ion sensitivity by an activity on myosin-phosphatase, resulting in smooth muscle contraction. Increased levels of Rho-kinase have been found in patients with PAH.[84] The use of Rho-kinase inhibitors in animal models of pulmonary hypertension reduces smooth muscle contraction and proliferation, modulates endothelial dysfunction, impedes migration of inflammatory cells, and improves survival.[85,86] Fasudil (HA-1077), administered by either the intravenous or inhaled route, selectively inhibits Rho-kinase. To date, however, data supporting its potential use in humans with PAH are limited. In a study of eight patients with severe PAH, administration of intravenous fasudil led to acute reduction of PVR by 20%.[86] Inhaled fasudil also has favorable acute effects on the pulmonary vasculature in PAH and seems to show greater pulmonary selectivity than when given parenterally.[87,88] Further evidence of the efficacy of this drug in longer-term trials is required however. Azaindole-1 is another highly selective Rho-kinase inhibitor with therapeutic promise that is orally active, although to date evidence of its potential efficacy has been confined to animal models.[88,89]

Dichloroacetate

Dichloroacetate is a small-molecule inhibitor of mitochondrial pyruvate dehydrogenase kinase that is capable of inducing a switch from antiapoptotic glycolytic metabolism toward a proapoptotic oxidative phosphorylation and potential reversal of pathologic pulmonary vascular remodeling. In animal models of pulmonary hypertension, dichloroacetate treatment reduced PVR and right ventricular hypertrophy and improved survival.[90,91] The first human dose-ranging phase 1 study is ongoing, designed to assess the safety and tolerability of the addition of dichloroacetate to standard therapy in advanced PAH.[92]

Angiotension-Converting Enzyme 2

Angiotensin II is a vasoconstrictor and smooth muscle mitogen produced by the action of angiotensin-converting enzyme (ACE) on angiotensin I in the lungs. The activity of angiotensin II is controlled by ACE2, which protects against cardiac remodeling, exerts antiproliferative effects on vascular smooth muscle cells, attenuates endothelial dysfunction, and reduces inflammatory cytokines.[93] Experimental models show ACE2 may have a protective effect against the disease and the presence of ACE2 antibodies may increase the risk of developing PAH in patients with connective tissue diseases.[94] Recently, a study in patients with PAH caused by congenital heart disease found that ACE2 levels decreased as pulmonary artery pressures increased.[95]

The administration of ACE2 in monocrotaline and BMPR2 R899X-induced pulmonary hypertension attenuated right ventricular hypertrophy and reduced right ventricular pressure[96–98] suggesting a therapeutic possibility with agents acting on this pathway.

Rituximab (Rituxan)

Rituximab is a monoclonal antibody directed at the CD20 cell receptor that results in B lymphocyte depletion. Currently licensed for use in non-Hodgkin lymphoma, chronic lymphocytic leukemia, and rheumatoid arthritis, there are also preclinical data and case reports of the benefit of rituximab in connective tissue disease–associated PAH.[99] A phase II, randomized, double-blind, placebo-controlled clinical trial is underway to test the effect of 24 weeks of rituximab in 80 scleroderma-associated patients with PAH, with change in PVR established as the primary study end point.[100]

Other Potential Targets

There are several new pathways recently identified in pulmonary hypertension that may translate into effective therapeutic targets. Molecules that improve the trafficking of mutated receptors to cell surfaces have been successfully developed as therapies in other lung diseases, such as cystic fibrosis. Such a therapeutic concept might also theoretically be applied in PAH. Heritable and idiopathic PAH can be caused by mutations of the gene coding for the BMPR type II (BMPR-II), which leads to cell-specific alterations in growth responses to bone morphogenetic proteins. Chemical chaperones that enhance trafficking of the receptors to the cell surface, such as sodium 4-phenylbutyrate and thapsigargin, are under investigation in this regard.[101] Ataluren (PTC124) promotes ribosomal read-through in the presence of premature stop codons, allowing full production of the protein.[102] Although such drugs are in the early stages of development, they have the potential to restore normal bone morphogenetic protein signaling. Even if normalization of BMPR function is achievable by this means, however, restoration of normal pulmonary vascular function may not be achievable, because BMPR-II mutations in isolation are not sufficient to trigger PAH (the so-called "two-hit" or "multiple-hit" hypotheses). As a result, the efficacy of such drugs may be limited. Nevertheless, this therapeutic approach seems worthy of pursuit.

Receptors for advanced glycation end-products (RAGE) have recently been shown to be elevated in patients with PAH and to attenuate BMPR-II signaling.[103] These molecules form part of a family of immunoglobulin cell surface proteins and are involved in inflammation, proliferation, and migration of cells. RAGE inhibition in experimental models of pulmonary hypertension is associated with reductions in pulmonary vascular remodeling, PAP, and right ventricular hypertrophy. RAGE inhibitors are already in clinical use, such as for the treatment of Alzheimer's disease. Studying this class of agent in PAH may eventually prove fruitful.

There are also several other agents already licensed for other indications that may have additional potential as PAH treatments. Sirolimus (Rapamycin) has been shown to reduce pulmonary artery smooth muscle proliferation in animal studies.[104] Histone deacetylation inhibitors (eg, valproic acid) effectively reduce mPAP and attenuate pulmonary artery smooth muscle cell growth in hypoxic rats and human pulmonary smooth muscle cells, although they may negatively affect right ventricular function.[105,106] Sapropterin dihydrochloride, the active form of NO synthase cofactor tetrahydrobiopterin, has also been evaluated as a potential treatment option. An open-label study of 18 patients with PAH and CTEPH who were given oral sapropterin in addition to an ERA or PDE5I showed a significant improvement in 6MWD and the drug was well tolerated.[107]

Endothelial progenitor cells

Research into gene therapy has been hindered in the past by the absence of an effective vector to deliver the gene to the target cells. Cell-based gene therapy, in which healthy bone marrow–derived endothelial cells are introduced into the pulmonary vasculature to promote healing and restoration of vascular homeostasis is an intriguing potential treatment option for PAH. This strategy is also based on evidence that bone marrow–derived endothelial cells are part of normal healing, whereby these populations are attracted to areas of vascular injury by growth factors and cytokines secreted by injured endothelial cells.[108] Pulmonary vascular endothelial cell dysfunction and dysregulated hematopoiesis are key components of PAH pathobiology, highlighting the potential therapeutic value of targeting this cellular population.[109,110]

Reversal of vascular remodeling and improved survival was shown when endothelial progenitor cells transfected with the endothelial NO synthase gene were engrafted to distal pulmonary arterioles of rodents with monocrotaline-induced PAH.[111] A Chinese study found a 48-m improvement in 6MWD and 17% reduction in PVR in patients with idiopathic PAH at 12 weeks using this stem cell–based therapy.[112] The PHACeT trial has recently been completed in Canada looking at the safety of endothelial progenitor cells gene transfer of endothelial NO synthase in 18 PAH patients with advanced disease.[113] The results of this study are awaited.

SUMMARY

The therapeutic options for patients with PAH have been transformed over the last two decades (**Fig. 3**). Approval for two novel oral agents, macitentan and riociguat, is expected in the near future after positive results from placebo-controlled multicenter trials.[12,44,45] Some treatments that showed initial promise as treatments for the disease, however, have either failed to demonstrate clinical efficacy or proved to be

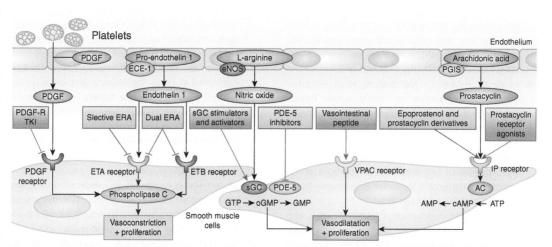

Fig. 3. Summary of current and emerging therapies for PAH. AC, adenylate cyclase; cAMP, cyclic AMP; cGMP, cyclic GMP; ECE-1, endothelin converting enzyme 1; eNOS, endothelial nitric oxide synthase; ETA, endothelin receptor type A; ETB, endothelin receptor type B; ERA, endothelin receptor antagonists; IP, prostaglandin I2; PDE-5, phosphodiesterase type 5; PDGF, platelet-derived growth factor; PDGF-R TKI, PDGF receptor tyrosine kinase inhibitors; PGIS, prostaglandin I synthase; sGC, soluble guanylate cyclase; VPAC, vasointestinal peptide receptor. (*From* O'Callaghan D, Savale L, Montani D, et al. Treatment of pulmonary arterial hypertension with targeted therapies. Nat Rev Cardiol 2011;8:526–38.)

potentially harmful when formally evaluated in randomized trials, underscoring the importance of rigorous testing of potential agents. A host of others agents are undergoing preclinical and clinical evaluation in clinical studies and there is optimism that some of these will become part of the future drug arsenal.

REFERENCES

1. O'Callaghan D, Savale L, Montani D, et al. Treatment of pulmonary arterial hypertension with targeted therapies. Nat Rev Cardiol 2011;8: 526–38.
2. Humbert M, Sitbon O, Chaouat A, et al. Survival in patients with idiopathic, familial, and anorexigen-associated pulmonary arterial hypertension in the modern management era. Circulation 2010; 122(2):156–63.
3. D'Alonzo G, Barst R, Ayres S, et al. Survival in patients with primary pulmonary hypertension. Results from a national prospective registry. Ann Intern Med 1991;115(5):343–9.
4. Giaid A, Yanagisawa M, Langleben D, et al. Expression of endothelin-1 in the lungs of patients with pulmonary hypertension. N Engl J Med 1993; 328(24):1732–9.
5. Humbert M, Segal E, Kiely D, et al. Results of European post-marketing surveillance of bosentan in pulmonary hypertension. Eur Respir J 2007;30(2): 338–44.
6. O'Connell C, O'Callaghan D, Gaine S. New drugs for pulmonary hypertension. Eur Respir Monogr 2012;57(19):233–46.
7. Raghu G, Million-Rousseau R, Morganti A, et al. Macitentan for the treatment of idiopathic pulmonary fibrosis: the randomised controlled MUSIC trial. Eur Respir J 2013. http://dx.doi.org/10.1183/09031936.00104612. [Epub ahead of print].
8. Iglarz M, Binkert C, Morrison K, et al. Pharmacology of macitentan, an orally active tissue-targeting dual endothelin receptor antagonist. J Pharmacol Exp Ther 2008;327(3):736–45.
9. Kummer O, Haschke M, Hammann F, et al. Comparison of the dissolution and pharmacokinetic profiles of two galenical formulations of the endothelin receptor antagonist macitentan. Eur J Pharm Sci 2009;38(4):384–8.
10. Sidharta P, van Giersbergen P, Halabi A, et al. Macitentan: entry-into-humans study with a new endothelin receptor antagonist. Eur J Clin Pharmacol 2011;67(10):977–84.
11. Raja S. Macitentan, a tissue-targeting endothelin receptor antagonist for the potential oral treatment of pulmonary arterial hypertension and idiopathic pulmonary fibrosis. Curr Opin Investig Drugs 2010;11(9):1066–73.
12. Pulido T, Adzerikho I, Channick R, et al. Macitentan and morbidity and mortality in pulmonary arterial hypertension. N Engl J Med 2013;369(9):809–18.
13. Christman B, McPherson C, Newman J, et al. An imbalance between the excretion of thromboxane and prostacyclin metabolites in pulmonary hypertension. N Engl J Med 1992;327(2):70–5.
14. Barst R, Rubin L, McGoon M, et al. Survival in primary pulmonary hypertension with long-term continuous intravenous prostacyclin. Ann Intern Med 1994;121(6):409–15.
15. US NIH ClinicalTrials.gov. Study of a new thermo stable formulation of epoprostenol sodium to treat pulmonary arterial hypertension (PAH). Available at: http://www.clinicaltrials.gov/ct2/show/NCT01462565?term=veletri&rank=12011. Last updated October 18, 2012. Last Accessed September 29, 2013.
16. Sitbon O, Delcroix M, Bergot E, et al. EPITOME-2, An open-label study evaluating a new formulation of epoprostenol sodium in pulmonary arterial hypertension patients switched from Flolan. Am J Resp Crit Care Med 2012. http://dx.doi.org/10.1164/ajrccm-conference.2012.185.1_MeetingAbstracts. A2500.
17. Farber H, Miller D, Meltzer L, et al. Treatment of patients with pulmonary arterial hypertension at the time of death or deterioration to functional class IV: Insights from the REVEAL registry. J Heart Lung Transplant 2013. pii: S1053-2498(13)01392-2. [Epub ahead of print].
18. Tapson V, Torres F, Kermeen F, et al. Oral treprostinil for the treatment of pulmonary arterial hypertension in patients on background endothelin receptor antagonist and/or phosphodiesterase type 5 inhibitor therapy (the FREEDOM-C study): a randomized controlled trial. Chest 2012;142(6):1383–90.
19. US NIH ClinicalTrials.gov. A 16-week, international, multicenter, double-blind, randomized, placebo-controlled study of the efficacy and safety of oral UT-15C sustained release tablets in subjects with pulmonary arterial hypertension (FREEDOM-C2). Available at: http://www.clinicaltrials.gov/ct2/show/NCT00887978?term=FREEDOM-C2&rank=12011. Last updated December 7, 2012. Last Accessed September 29, 2013.
20. United Therapeutics. UT-15C treprostinil diethanolamine sustained release tablets (oral treprostinil). Available at: http://www.unither.com/oral-treprostinil-for-pah. Last Accessed September 29, 2013.
21. US NIH ClinicalTrials.gov. FREEDOM - M: oral treprostinil as monotherapy for the treatment of pulmonary arterial hypertension (PAH). Available at: http://www.clinicaltrials.gov/ct2/show/NCT00325403?term=FREEDOM-M&rank=12012. Last updated February 12, 2013. Last Accessed September 29, 2013.

22. US NIH ClinicalTrials.gov. Trial of the early combination of oral treprostinil with a PDE-5 inhibitor or ERA in subjects with pulmonary arterial hypertension (FREEDOM-Ev) [Internet]. Available at: www.clinicaltrials.gov/ct2/show/NCT01560624?term=FREEDOM-Ev&;rank=1. Last updated September 20, 2013. Last Accessed September 29, 2013.

23. Barst R, McGoon M, McLaughlin V, et al. Beraprost therapy for pulmonary arterial hypertension. J Am Coll Cardiol 2003;41(12):2119–25.

24. US NIH Clinicaltrials.gov. A multinational, multicenter study to assess the efficacy and safety of BPS-314d-MR in subjects with pulmonary arterial hypertension currently receiving treatment with an endothelin receptor antagonist and or a phosphodiesterase-5 inhibitor. Available at: clinicaltrialsfeeds.org/clinical-trials/show/NCT01458236. Last updated September 26, 2013. Last Accessed September 29, 2013.

25. Voswinckel R, Reichenberger F, Gall H, et al. Metered dose inhaler delivery of treprostinil for the treatment of pulmonary hypertension. Pulm Pharmacol Ther 2009;22(1):50–6.

26. Gomberg-Maitland M, Olschewski H. Prostacyclin therapies for the treatment of pulmonary arterial hypertension. Eur Respir J 2008;31(4):891–901.

27. Kuwano K, Hashino A, Asaki T, et al. 2-[4-[(5,6-diphenylpyrazin-2-yl)(isopropyl)amino]butoxy]-N-(methylsulfonyl)acetamide (NS-304), an orally available and long-acting prostacyclin receptor agonist prodrug. J Pharmacol Exp Ther 2007;322(3):1181–8.

28. Simonneau G, Torbicki A, Hoeper M, et al. Selexipag, an oral, selective IP receptor agonist for the treatment of pulmonary arterial hypertension. Eur Respir J 2012;40(4):874–80.

29. McLaughlin V. Looking to the future: a new decade of pulmonary arterial hypertension therapy. Eur Respir Rev 2011;20(122):262–9.

30. US NIH ClinicalTrials.gov. ACT-293987 in pulmonary arterial hypertension. Available at: http://www.clinicaltrials.gov/ct2/show/NCT01106014?term=GRIPHON&rank=1. Last updated September 3, 2013. Last Accessed September 29, 2013.

31. Archer S, Michelakis E. Phosphodiesterase type 5 inhibitors for pulmonary arterial hypertension. N Engl J Med 2009;361(19):1864–71.

32. Ivy D, Parker D, Doran A, et al. Acute hemodynamic effects and home therapy using a novel pulsed nasal nitric oxide delivery system in children and young adults with pulmonary hypertension. Am J Cardiol 2003;92(7):886–90.

33. Channick R, Newhart J, Johnson F, et al. Pulsed delivery of inhaled nitric oxide to patients with primary pulmonary hypertension: an ambulatory delivery system and initial clinical tests. Chest 1996;109(6):1545–9.

34. Galie N, Ghofrani H, Torbicki A, et al. Sildenafil citrate therapy for pulmonary arterial hypertension. N Engl J Med 2005;353(20):2148–57.

35. Galie N, Brundage B, Ghofrani H, et al. Tadalafil therapy for pulmonary arterial hypertension. Circulation 2009;119(22):2894–903.

36. Corbin J, Beasley A, Blount M, et al. Vardenafil: structural basis for higher potency over sildenafil in inhibiting cGMP-specific phosphodiesterase-5 (PDE5). Neurochem Int 2004;45(6):859–63.

37. Jing Z, Jiang X, Wu B, et al. Vardenafil treatment for patients with pulmonary arterial hypertension: a multicentre, open-label study. Heart 2009;95(18):1531–6.

38. Jing Z, Yu Z, Shen J, et al. Vardenafil in pulmonary arterial hypertension: a randomized, double-blind, placebo-controlled study. Am J Respir Crit Care Med 2011;183(12):1723–9.

39. Evgenov O, Pacher P, Schmidt P, et al. NO-independent stimulators and activators of soluble guanylate cyclase: discovery and therapeutic potential. Nat Rev Drug Discov 2006;5(9):755–68.

40. Grimminger F, Weimann G, Frey R, et al. First acute haemodynamic study of soluble guanylate cyclase stimulator riociguat in pulmonary hypertension. Eur Respir J 2009;33(4):785–92.

41. Lang M, Kojonazarov B, Tian X, et al. The soluble guanylate cyclase stimulator riociguat ameliorates pulmonary hypertension induced by hypoxia and SU5416 in rats. PLoS One 2012;7(8):e43433.

42. Ghofrani H, Hoeper M, Halank M, et al. Riociguat for chronic thromboembolic pulmonary hypertension and pulmonary arterial hypertension: a phase II study. Eur Respir J 2010;36(4):792–9.

43. Rubin L, Galie N, Grimminger F, et al. Riociguat for the treatment of pulmonary arterial hypertension (PAH): a phase III long-term extension study (PATENT-2). Am J Respir Crit Care Med 2013. Available at: www.atsjournals.org/doi/abs/10.1164/ajrccm-conference.2013.187.1_MeetingAbstracts.A3531.

44. Ghofrani H, Galie N, Grimminger F, et al. Riociguat for the treatment of pulmonary arterial hypertension. N Engl J Med 2013;369:330–40.

45. Ghofrani H, D'Armini A, Grimminger F, et al. Riociguat for the treatment of chronic thromboembolic pulmonary hypertension. N Engl J Med 2013;369:319–29.

46. Ghofrani H, Osterloh I, Grimminger F. Sildenafil: from angina to erectile dysfunction to pulmonary hypertension and beyond. Nat Rev Drug Discov 2006;5(8):689–702.

47. US NIH ClinicalTrials.gov. Evaluation of the pharmacodynamic effect of the combination of

sildenafil and riociguat on blood pressure and other safety parameters (PATENT PLUS). Available at: http://clinicaltrials.gov/ct2/show/NCT01179334. Last updated May 21, 2013. Last Accessed September 29, 2013.

48. de Man F, Handoko M, van Ballegoij J, et al. Bisoprolol delays progression towards right heart failure in experimental pulmonary hypertension. Circ Heart Fail 2012;5(1):97–105.

49. So P, Davies R, Chandy G, et al. Usefulness of beta-blocker therapy and outcomes in patients with pulmonary arterial hypertension. Am J Cardiol 2012;109(10):1504–9.

50. Perros F, Montani D, Dorfmuller P, et al. Platelet-derived growth factor expression and function in idiopathic pulmonary arterial hypertension. Am J Respir Crit Care Med 2008;178(1):81–8.

51. Schermuly R, Dony E, Ghofrani H, et al. Reversal of experimental pulmonary hypertension by PDGF inhibition. J Clin Invest 2005;115(10):2811–21.

52. Ghofrani H, Morrell N, Hoeper M, et al. Imatinib in pulmonary arterial hypertension patients with inadequate response to established therapy. Am J Respir Crit Care Med 2010;182(9):1171–7.

53. Hoeper M, Barst R, Bourge R, et al. Imatinib mesylate as add-on therapy for pulmonary arterial hypertension: results of the randomized IMPRES study. Circulation 2013;127(10):1128–38.

54. Fernández A, Sanguino A, Peng Z, et al. An anticancer C-Kit kinase inhibitor is reengineered to make it more active and less cardiotoxic. J Clin Invest 2007;117(12):4044–54.

55. Kim T, le Coutre P, Schwarz M, et al. Clinical cardiac safety profile of nilotinib. Haematologica 2012;97(6):883–9.

56. US NIH ClinicalTrials.gov. Efficacy, safety, tolerability and pharmacokinetics (PK) of nilotinib (AMN107) in pulmonary arterial hypertension. Available at: http://clinicaltrials.gov/ct2/show/NCT01179737?term=Nilotinib+pulmonary&rank=12010. Last updated March 25, 2013. Last Accessed September 29, 2013.

57. Moreno-Vinasco L, Gomberg-Maitland M, Maitland M, et al. Genomic assessment of a multikinase inhibitor, sorafenib, in a rodent model of pulmonary hypertension. Physiol Genomics 2008; 33(2):278–91.

58. Gomberg-Maitland M, Maitland M, Barst R, et al. A dosing/cross-development study of the multikinase inhibitor sorafenib in patients with pulmonary arterial hypertension. Clin Pharmacol Ther 2010; 87(3):303–10.

59. Humbert M, Simonneau G, Dinh-Xuan A. Whistleblowers. Eur Respir J 2011;38(3):510–1.

60. Montani D, Bergot E, Gunther S, et al. Pulmonary arterial hypertension in patients treated by Dasatinib. Circulation 2012;125(17):2128–37.

61. Herve P, Launay J, Scrobohaci M, et al. Increased plasma serotonin in primary pulmonary hypertension. Am J Med 1995;99(3):249–54.

62. Launay J, Herve P, Peoc'h K, et al. Function of the serotonin 5-hydroxytryptamine 2B receptor in pulmonary hypertension. Nat Med 2002;8(10): 1129–35.

63. Dempsie Y, MacLean M. Pulmonary hypertension: therapeutic targets within the serotonin system. Br J Pharmacol 2008;155(4):455–62.

64. Roth BL. Drugs and valvular heart disease. N Engl J Med 2007;356(1):6–9.

65. Eddahibi S, Humbert M, Fadel E, et al. Serotonin transporter overexpression is responsible for pulmonary artery smooth muscle hyperplasia in primary pulmonary hypertension. J Clin Invest 2001; 108(8):1141–50.

66. Eddahibi S, Chaouat A, Morrell N, et al. Polymorphism of the serotonin transporter gene and pulmonary hypertension in chronic obstructive pulmonary disease. Circulation 2003;108(15):1839–44.

67. Zhai F, Zhang X, Wang H. Fluoxetine protects against monocrotaline-induced pulmonary arterial hypertension: potential roles of induction of apoptosis and upregulation of Kv1.5 channels in rats. Clin Exp Pharmacol Physiol 2009;36(8):850–6.

68. Shah S, Gomberg-Maitland M, Thenappan T. Selective serotonin reuptake inhibitors and the incidence and outcome of pulmonary hypertension. Chest 2009;136(3):694–700.

69. Dumitrascu R, Kulcke C, Konigshoff M, et al. Terguride ameliorates monocrotaline-induced pulmonary hypertension in rats. Eur Respir J 2011; 37(5):1104–18.

70. Ghofrani H, Al-Hitit H, Vonk-Noordegraaf H, et al. Proof-of-concept study to investigate the efficacy, haemodynamics and tolerability of teguride vs placebo in subjects with pulmonary arterial hypertension: results of a double-blind randomised, prospective IIa study. Am J Respir Crit Care Med 2012;185:A2496.

71. Hamidi S, Prabhakar S, Said S. Enhancement of pulmonary vascular remodelling and inflammatory genes with VIP gene deletion. Eur Respir J 2008; 31(1):135–9.

72. Said S, Hamidi S, Dickman K, et al. Moderate pulmonary arterial hypertension in male mice lacking the vasoactive intestinal peptide gene. Circulation 2007;115(10):1260–8.

73. Hamidi S, Lin R, Szema A, et al. VIP and endothelin receptor antagonist: an effective combination against experimental pulmonary arterial hypertension. Respir Res 2011;12:141.

74. Petkov V, Mosgoeller W, Ziesche R, et al. Vasoactive intestinal peptide as a new drug for treatment of primary pulmonary hypertension. J Clin Invest 2003;111(9):1339–46.

75. Galie N, Badesch D, Fleming T, et al. Effects of inhaled aviptadil (vasoactive intestinal peptide) in patients with pulmonary arterial hypertension (PAH): results from a phase II study. http://dx.doi.org/10.1164/ajrccm-conference.2010.181.1_Meeting Abstracts.A2516.

76. Kao PN. Simvastatin treatment of pulmonary hypertension: an observational case series. Chest 2005; 127(4):1446–52.

77. Laufs U, Marra D, Node K. 3-Hydroxy-3-methylglutaryl-CoA reductase inhibitors attenuate vascular smooth muscle proliferation by preventing rho GTPase-induced down-regulation of p27(Kip1). J Biol Chem 1999;274(31):21926–31.

78. Zhao L, Sebkhi A, Ali O, et al. Simvastatin and sildenafil combine to attenuate pulmonary hypertension. Eur Respir J 2009;34(4):948–57.

79. Wilkins MR, Ali O, Bradlow W, et al. Simvastatin as a treatment for pulmonary hypertension trial (SiPHT). Am J Respir Crit Care Med 2010;181(10):1106–13.

80. Kawut SM, Bagiella E, Lederer DJ, et al. Randomized clinical trial of aspirin and simvastatin for pulmonary arterial hypertension: ASA-STAT. Circulation 2011;123(25):2985–93.

81. Zeng W, Xiong C, Zhao L, et al. Atorvastatin in pulmonary arterial hypertension (APATH) study. Eur Respir J 2012;40(1):67–74.

82. Saadjian A, Philip-Joet F, Paganelli F. Long-term effects of cicletanine on secondary pulmonary hypertension. J Cardiovasc Pharmacol 1998;31(3): 364–71.

83. US NIH ClinicalTrials.gov. Study of cicletanine for pulmonary arterial hypertension (PAH). Available at: www.clinicaltrials.gov/show/NCT/00832507. Last updated August 22, 2012. Last Accessed September 29, 2013.

84. Guilluy C, Eddahibi S, Agard C, et al. RhoA and Rho kinase activation in human pulmonary hypertension: role of 5-HT signaling. Am J Respir Crit Care Med 2009;179(12):1151–8.

85. Oka M, Fagan K, Jones P. Therapeutic potential of RhoA/Rho kinase inhibitors in pulmonary hypertension. Br J Pharmacol 2008;155(4):444–54.

86. Abe K, Shimokawa H, Morikawa K, et al. Long-term treatment with a Rho-kinase inhibitor improves monocrotaline-induced fatal pulmonary hypertension in rats. Circ Res 2004;94(3):385–93.

87. Fukumoto Y, Matoba T, Ito A, et al. Acute vasodilator effects of a Rho-kinase inhibitor, fasudil, in patients with severe pulmonary hypertension. Heart 2005;91(3):391–2.

88. Hardavella G, Dionellis G, Kantza C. Latest therapeutic novelties and patents in pulmonary hypertension. Recent Pat Cardiovasc Drug Discov 2011;6(1):55–60.

89. Dahal B, Kosanovic D, Pamarthi P, et al. Therapeutic efficacy of azaindole-1 in experimental pulmonary hypertension. Eur Respir J 2010; 36(4):808–18.

90. McMurtry M, Bonnet S, Wu X, et al. Dichloroacetate prevents and reverses pulmonary hypertension by inducing pulmonary artery smooth muscle cell apoptosis. Circ Res 2004;95(8):830–40.

91. Dewachter L, Dewachter C, Naeije R. New therapies for pulmonary arterial hypertension: an update on current bench to bedside translation. Expert Opin Investig Drugs 2010;19(4):469–88.

92. US NIH ClinicalTrials.gov. Dichloroacetate (DCA) for the treatment of pulmonary arterial hypertension. Available at: http://clinicaltrials.gov/ct2/show/NCT01083524?term=Dichloroacetate&rank=1. 2010. Last updated November 3, 2011. Last Accessed September 29, 2013.

93. Shenoy V, Qi Y, Katovich M, et al. ACE2, a promising therapeutic target for pulmonary hypertension. Curr Opin Pharmacol 2011;11(2):150–5.

94. Takahashi Y, Haga S, Ishizaka Y, et al. Autoantibodies to angiotensin-converting enzyme 2 in patients with connective tissue diseases. Arthritis Res Ther 2010;12(3):R85.

95. Dai H, Guo Y, Guang X, et al. The changes of serum angiotensin-converting enzyme 2 in patients with pulmonary arterial hypertension due to congenital heart disease. Cardiology 2013;124(4):208–12.

96. Yamazato Y, Ferreira A, Hong K, et al. Prevention of pulmonary hypertension by angiotensin-converting enzyme 2 gene transfer. Hypertension 2009;54(2): 365–71.

97. Johnson J, Perrien A, Schuster M, et al. Cytoskeletal defects in BMPR2-associated pulmonary arterial hypertension. Am J Physiol Lung Cell Mol Physiol 2012;302(5):L474–84.

98. Ferreira A, Shenoy V, Yamazato Y, et al. Evidence for angiotensin-converting enzyme 2 as a therapeutic target for the prevention of pulmonary hypertension. Am J Respir Crit Care Med 2009; 179(11):1048–54.

99. Hennigan S, Channick R, Silverman G. Rituximab treatment of pulmonary arterial hypertension associated with systemic lupus erythematosus: a case report. Lupus 2008;17(8):754–6.

100. US NIH ClinicalTrials.gov. Rituximab for treatment of systemic sclerosis-associated pulmonary arterial hypertension (SSc-PAH). Available at: clinicaltrials.gov/ct2/show/NCT01086540. 2013. Last updated August 17, 2013. Last Accessed September 29, 2013.

101. Sobolewski A, Rudarakanchana N, Upton P, et al. Failure of bone morphogenetic protein receptor trafficking in pulmonary arterial hypertension: potential for rescue. Hum Mol Genet 2008;17(20): 3180–90.

102. Drake K, Dunmore B, McNelly L, et al. Correction of nonsense BMPR2 and SMAD9 mutations by

ataluren in pulmonary arterial hypertension. Am J Respir Cell Mol Biol 2013;49(3):403–9.

103. Meloche J, Courchesne A, Barrier M, et al. Critical role for the advanced glycation end-products receptor in pulmonary arterial hypertension etiology. J Am Heart Assoc 2013;2(1):e005157.

104. Houssaini A, Abid S, Mouraret N, et al. Rapamycin reverses pulmonary-artery smooth-muscle-cell proliferation in pulmonary hypertension. Am J Respir Cell Mol Biol 2013;48(5):568–77.

105. Zhao L, Chen C, Hajji N, et al. Histone deacetylation inhibition in pulmonary hypertension: therapeutic potential of valproic acid and suberoylanilide hydroxamic acid. Circulation 2012;126(4):455–67.

106. Bogaard H, Mizuno S, Hussaini A, et al. Suppression of histone deacetylases worsens right ventricular dysfunction after pulmonary artery banding in rats. Am J Respir Crit Care Med 2011;183(10): 1402–10.

107. Robbins I, Hemnes A, Gibbs J, et al. Safety of sapropterin dihydrochloride (6r-bh4) in patients with pulmonary hypertension. Exp Lung Res 2011; 37(1):26–34.

108. Schatteman G, Dunnwald M, Jiao C. Biology of bone marrow-derived endothelial cell precursors.

Am J Physiol Heart Circ Physiol 2007;292(1): H1–18.

109. Launay J, Herve P, Callebert J, et al. Serotonin 5-HT2B receptors are required for bone-marrow contribution to pulmonary arterial hypertension. Blood 2011;119(7):1772–80.

110. Gambaryan N, Perros F, Montani D, et al. Targeting of c-kit+ haematopoietic progenitor cells prevents hypoxic pulmonary hypertension. Eur Respir J 2011;37(6):1392–9.

111. Zhao Y, Courtman D, Deng Y, et al. Rescue of monocrotaline-induced pulmonary arterial hypertension using bone marrow-derived endothelial-like progenitor cells: efficacy of combined cell and eNOS gene therapy in established disease. Circ Res 2005;96(4):442–50.

112. Wang X, Zhang F, Shang Y, et al. Transplantation of autologous endothelial progenitor cells may be beneficial in patients with idiopathic pulmonary arterial hypertension: a pilot randomized controlled trial. J Am Coll Cardiol 2007;49(14):1566–71.

113. US NIH ClinicalTrials.gov. Pulmonary hypertension: assessment of cell therapy (PHACeT). Available at: http://clinicaltrials.gov/ct2/show/NCT00469027? term=PHACeT&rank=12010. Last updated March 7, 2013. Last Accessed September 29, 2013.

Index

Note: Page numbers of article titles are in **boldface** type

Clin Chest Med 34 (2013) 881–886
http://dx.doi.org/10.1016/S0272-5231(13)00160-3
0272-5231/13/$ – see front matter © 2013 Elsevier Inc. All rights reserved.

chestmed.theclinics.com

United States Postal Service
Statement of Ownership, Management, and Circulation
(All Periodicals Publications Except Requestor Publications)

1. Publication Title	2. Publication Number	3. Filing Date
Clinics in Chest Medicine	0 0 0 - 7 0 0 6	9/14/13

4. Issue Frequency	5. Number of Issues Published Annually	6. Annual Subscription Price
Mar, Jun, Sep, Dec	4	$329.00

7. Complete Mailing Address of Known Office of Publication (*Not printer*) (*Street, city, county, state, and ZIP+4®*)

Elsevier Inc.
360 Park Avenue South
New York, NY 10010-1710

Contact Person
Stephen R. Bushing

Telephone (Include area code)
215-239-3688

8. Complete Mailing Address of Headquarters or General Business Office of Publisher (*Not printer*)

Elsevier Inc., 360 Park Avenue South, New York, NY 10010-1710

9. Full Names and Complete Mailing Addresses of Publisher, Editor, and Managing Editor (*Do not leave blank*)

Publisher (*Name and complete mailing address*)

Linda Belfus, Elsevier, Inc., 1600 John F. Kennedy Blvd. Suite 1800, Philadelphia, PA 19103-2899

Editor (*Name and complete mailing address*)

Katie Saunders, Elsevier, Inc., 1600 John F. Kennedy Blvd. Suite 1800, Philadelphia, PA 19103-2899

Managing Editor (*Name and complete mailing address*)

Adrianne Brigido, Elsevier, Inc., 1600 John F. Kennedy Blvd. Suite 1800, Philadelphia, PA 19103-2899

10. Owner (*Do not leave blank. If the publication is owned by a corporation, give the name and address of the corporation immediately followed by the names and addresses of all stockholders owning or holding 1 percent or more of the total amount of stock. If not owned by a corporation, give the names and addresses of the individual owners. If owned by a partnership or other unincorporated firm, give its name and address as well as those of each individual owner. If the publication is published by a nonprofit organization, give its name and address.*)

Full Name	Complete Mailing Address
Wholly owned subsidiary of	1600 John F. Kennedy Blvd, Ste. 1800
Reed/Elsevier, US holdings	Philadelphia, PA 19103-2899

11. Known Bondholders, Mortgagees, and Other Security Holders Owning or Holding 1 Percent or More of Total Amount of Bonds, Mortgages, or Other Securities. If none, check box ☐ None

Full Name	Complete Mailing Address
N/A	

12. Tax Status (*For completion by nonprofit organizations authorized to mail at nonprofit rates*) (*Check one*)
The purpose, function, and nonprofit status of this organization and the exempt status for federal income tax purposes:
☐ Has Not Changed During Preceding 12 Months
☐ Has Changed During Preceding 12 Months (*Publisher must submit explanation of change with this statement*)

PS Form 3526, September 2007 (Page 1 of 3 (Instructions Page 3)) PSN 7530-01-000-9931 PRIVACY NOTICE: See our Privacy policy in www.usps.com

---

13. Publication Title	14. Issue Date for Circulation Data Below
Clinics in Chest Medicine	September 2013

15. Extent and Nature of Circulation		Average No. Copies Each Issue During Preceding 12 Months	No. Copies of Single Issue Published Nearest to Filing Date
a. Total Number of Copies (*Net press run*)		1,279	1,289
b. Paid Circulation (By Mail and Outside the Mail)	(1) Mailed Outside-County Paid Subscriptions Stated on PS Form 3541. (*Include paid distribution above nominal rate, advertiser's proof copies, and exchange copies*)	757	846
	(2) Mailed In-County Paid Subscriptions Stated on PS Form 3541 (*Include paid distribution above nominal rate, advertiser's proof copies, and exchange copies*)		
	(3) Paid Distribution Outside the Mails Including Sales Through Dealers and Carriers, Street Vendors, Counter Sales, and Other Paid Distribution Outside USPS®	238	242
	(4) Paid Distribution by Other Classes Mailed Through the USPS (e.g. First-Class Mail®)		
c. Total Paid Distribution (*Sum of 15b (1), (2), (3), and (4)*)		995	1,088
d. Free or Nominal Rate Distribution (By Mail and Outside the Mail)	(1) Free or Nominal Rate Outside-County Copies Included on PS Form 3541	56	66
	(2) Free or Nominal Rate In-County Copies Included on PS Form 3541		
	(3) Free or Nominal Rate Copies Mailed at Other Classes Through the USPS (e.g. First-Class Mail)		
	(4) Free or Nominal Rate Distribution Outside the Mail (Carriers or other means)		
e. Total Free or Nominal Rate Distribution (*Sum of 15d (1), (2), (3) and (4)*)		56	66
f. Total Distribution (*Sum of 15c and 15e*)		1,051	1,154
g. Copies not Distributed (*See instructions to publishers #4 (page #3)*)		228	135
h. Total (*Sum of 15f and g*)		1,279	1,289
i. Percent Paid (*15c divided by 15f times 100*)		94.67%	94.28%

16. Publication of Statement of Ownership

☐ If the publication is a general publication, publication of this statement is required. Will be printed in the December 2013 issue of this publication.   ☐ Publication not required

17. Signature and Title of Editor, Publisher, Business Manager, or Owner

Stephen R. Bushing

Stephen R. Bushing – Inventory Distribution Coordinator

Date
September 14, 2013

I certify that all information furnished on this form is true and complete. I understand that anyone who furnishes false or misleading information on this form or who omits material or information requested on the form may be subject to criminal sanctions (including fines and imprisonment) and/or civil sanctions (including civil penalties).

PS Form 3526, September 2007 (Page 2 of 3)

Moving?

Make sure your subscription moves with you!

To notify us of your new address, find your **Clinics Account Number** (located on your mailing label above your name), and contact customer service at:

Email: journalscustomerservice-usa@elsevier.com

800-654-2452 (subscribers in the U.S. & Canada)
314-447-8871 (subscribers outside of the U.S. & Canada)

Fax number: 314-447-8029

**Elsevier Health Sciences Division
Subscription Customer Service
3251 Riverport Lane
Maryland Heights, MO 63043**

*To ensure uninterrupted delivery of your subscription, please notify us at least 4 weeks in advance of move.

Printed and bound by CPI Group (UK) Ltd, Croydon, CR0 4YY

03/10/2024

01040375-0004